# MASTERING THE NURSING PROCESS:
# A CASE METHOD APPROACH

# MASTERING THE NURSING PROCESS: A CASE METHOD APPROACH

**Jean D'Meza Leuner M.S., R.N.**
Assistant Professor
MGH Institute of Health Professions
Boston, Massachusetts

**Anne Keiran Manton M.S., R.N., CEN**
Assistant Professor
MGH Institute of Health Professions
Boston, Massachusetts

**Dorothy Bagnell Kelliher M.S., R.N.**
Lecturer
MGH Institute of Health Professions
Boston, Massachusetts

**Sharon P. Sullivan M.S., R.N.**
Former Lecturer, MGH Institute of Health Professions
Staff, Massachusetts General Hospital
Boston, Massachusetts

**Meg Doherty M.S., R.N.**
Former Lecturer, MGH Institute of Health Professions
Administrative Supervisor
Norwell Visiting Nurse Association Inc.
Norwell, Massachusetts

 F.A. DAVIS COMPANY • PHILADELPHIA

Printed in the United States of America

Last digit indicates print number: 10 9 8 7 6 5 4 3 2 1

NOTE: As new scientific information becomes available through basic and clinical research, recommended treatments and drug therapies undergo changes. The author(s) and publisher have done everything possible to make this book accurate, up-to-date, and in accord with accepted standards at the time of publication. However, the reader is advised always to check product information (package inserts) for changes and new information regarding dose and contraindications before administering any drug. Caution is especially urged when using new or infrequently ordered drugs.

Illustrations for Case Study 23
© Beth Anne Willert, M.S.

Library of Congress Cataloging-in-Publication Data


Mastering the nursing process : a case method approach / Jean D'Meza
    Leuner ... [et al.].
        p.    cm.
    Includes bibliographical references.
    ISBN 0-8036-5588-6
    1. Nursing.  2. Nursing care plans.    I. Leuner, Jean D'Meza.
    [DNLM: 1. Nursing Process.    WY 100 M423]
    RT41.M42  1990
    610.73--dc20
    DNLM/DLC
    for Library of Congress                                    89-71523
                                                                    CIP

*To my husband Rick and children Kirstyn and Kyle for their unfailing love and support.*
**JDL**

*To Judee, Suzanne, Sean and mostly to Jack for their unconditional love and for giving meaning to my life.*
**AKM**

*To my loving family John, Erin, Kara and Caitlin, thank you for your encouragement and interest in this endeavor.*
**DBK**

*To my husband Steven for his love and patience.*
**SPS**

*To Danny, Meaghan, Griffin, and Elo for your support, understanding, and love.*
**MD**

# FOREWORD

This book is a major contribution that will assist in the teaching of clinical reasoning and judgment in nursing. The authors have selected materials that are vivid representations of clinical situations encountered in nursing practice. They present materials that can be used in a case method approach to learning and provide guidelines for case analyses.

Clinical reasoning and judgment have become the hallmark of professional nursing practice. The importance of these abilities is highly emphasized in the American Association of Colleges of Nursing publication on Essentials of College and University Education for Nursing, is supported by the American Nurses Association definition of professional nursing as involving diagnostic-therapeutic judgment, and is inherent in professional standards of practice published in the last two decades. Thus, it behooves us as educators and clinicians to find ways of helping students and current practitioners to increase their clinical judgment abilities.

The authors organize the clinical simulations in this book in a way that will facilitate the use of the case method approach. This method uses a practice-feedback loop for teaching the critical thinking skills needed in professional nursing practice. It requires active participation of the learner. Case data can provide faculty with rich clinical materials to use at various levels of education and with various teaching methodologies.

Clinical reasoning and judgment require the collection, organization, and analysis of health-related information. The functional health pattern assessment format for information collection is used to organize assessment data in this book; these patterns represent an integrative level of human functioning that is beyond the purely biological and the purely psychosocial. Health patterns provide an organizing framework for the collection and analysis of clinical information. This framework is used in a variety of clinical settings both nationally and internationally. In addition, a number of curricula and textbooks organize nursing content within the functional health pattern framework. The authors have indexed cases on the basis of frequently occurring medical problems. They provide the learner with clinical case information organized within a set of categories that facilitate data analysis. The case materials are comprehensive and present health pattern information in the context of the client's age-developmental level, sex, and biomedical condition, thus integrating biomedical and functional data. A strength of the book is that nursing diagnoses are used as a basis for planning nursing interventions and that the rationale for interventions is based on nursing research.

With the American Nurses Association adoption of the NANDA Taxonomy as the diagnostic classification system for the profession, students and clinicians will find the nursing diagnosis-based treatment and outcomes in the case materials useful. The case method approach should facilitate students' participation in the learning process and their development of clinical judgment skills.

Marjory Gordon, Ph.D., R.N., F.A.A.N.
Professor, Boston College School of Nursing

# ACKNOWLEDGEMENTS

The writing of this book has been a collegial effort involving the five of us who are its authors as well as those who have written contributions to it and those who, as consultants, have helped us to refine the presentation. This effort has required, in full measure, the time and talents of us all. Although the authors' duties may have differed from one to another, we have shared the same goal of producing a book that would help students breathe life into the nursing process. With the publication of this book, we can each take pride in the knowledge that our efforts have been successful.

The authors wish to acknowledge with gratitude the following people who have contributed in so many ways to the creation of this book:

- Marjory Gordon, for her work in nursing assessment and diagnosis and for communicating it so well.

- Our nursing colleagues, especially those at the MGH Institute of Health Professions and the Massachusetts General Hospital. To our contributors, we owe a particular debt of gratitude for their enthusiasm and participation in this project.

- Our nursing students, past and present, whose creative work in using case studies well assures us continually of the benefits of this approach in nursing education.

- Cindy Murphy who served as typist extraordinaire for so much of this project, not only with skill but with humor.

- And last to the F.A. Davis family for their belief in this project and their ongoing support.

# CONTRIBUTORS

**Gloria F. Antall, M.S., R.N.**
Assistant Professor
Simmons College School of Nursing
Boston, Massachusetts

**Julia Hodsdon Basque, M.S., R.N.**
Unit-Based Clinical Nurse Specialist
Massachusetts General Hospital
Boston, Massachusetts

**Maria N. Bueche, Ph.D., R.N.C.**
Associate Professor
Graduate Program in Primary Health Care Nursing
Graduate School of Health Studies
Simmons College
Boston, Massachusetts

**Susan Caloggero, B.S.N., M.S.N., R.N.**
Staff Nurse/AIDS Liason Nurse
Massachusetts General Hospital
Boston, Massachusetts

**Marie Femino Esposito, M.S., R.N., CPNP**
Maternal Child Coordinator
Cambridge Visiting Nurses Association
Cambridge, Massachusetts

**Alice Lucille Rose, M.S.N., R.N.**
Assistant Director of Nursing for Professional Development
The Dana Farber Cancer Institute
Boston, Massachusetts

**J. Elaine Souder, Ph.D., R.N., C.S.**
Research Associate in Gerontological Nursing
University of Pennsylvania
Philadelphia, Pennsylvania

# CONSULTANTS

**Jane Bliss-Holtz, D.N.Sc., R.N.**
Assistant Professor
Rutgers—The State University of New Jersey
College of Nursing
Newark, New Jersey

**Irene L. Bond, R.N., M.S.N.**
Nursing Coordinator
Manatee Community College
Bradenton, Florida

**Sharon A. Brown, Ph.D., R.N.**
Associate Dean of Research
University of Texas Health Sciences Center
Houston, Texas

**Patricia Broadway Caldwell, B.S.N., M.Ed.**
Outreach Coordinator
Presbyterian Hospital School of Nursing
Charlotte, North Carolina

**Katherine Camaco Carr, R.N., C.N.M., Ph.D.**
Consultant-Midwifery and Perinatal Nursing
Seattle, Washington

**Mardell Davis, R.N., M.S.N., C.E.T.N.**
Assistant Professor
University of Alabama—Birmingham
School of Nursing
Birmingham, Alabama

**M. Tita De La Cruz, R.N., M.S.N.**
Assistant Professor
Gwynedd-Mercy College
Gwynedd Valley, Pennsylvania

**Pamela R. Jeffries, R.N., M.S.N.**
Assistant Professor
Indiana University School of Nursing
Indianapolis, Indiana

**Toni J. Galvan, R.N., M.S.N., CCRN**
Assistant Professor
Texas Tech Health Sciences Center
School of Nursing
Lubbock, Texas

**Nicola S. Gilboy, R.N., M.S., C.E.N.**
Nurse Educator
Emerson Hospital
Concord, Massachusetts

**Shirley J. Jones, R.N., M.S.**
Doctoral Candidate
University of Michigan
Ann Arbor, Michigan

**Gail B. Lewis, R.N., M.S.N.**
Faculty
Barnes School of Nursing
St. Louis, Missouri

**Barbara C. Long, M.S.N., R.N.**
Associate Professor Emerita
Case Western Reserve University
Cleveland, Ohio

**Leslie Mancuso, R.N., M.S.N.**
Associate Director of Nursing
Project Hope
Millwood, Virginia

**Patricia R. Raynor, R.N., M.S.**
Curriculum Coordinator
Presbyterian Hospital School of Nursing
Charlotte, North Carolina

**Ellen M. Strauman, R.N., M.S.N.**
Staff Development Instructor
St. Agnes Medical Center
Philadelphia, Pennsylvania

**Daryl L.N. Sutton, R.N., M.S.N.**
Chairperson
Department of Nursing and Allied Health
Los Angeles Pierce College
Woodland Hills, California

**Jean Tillman, R.N., B.S.N., M.S.N.**
Professor of Nursing
Holyoke Community College
Holyoke, Massachusetts

# TABLE OF CONTENTS

# INTRODUCTION

## THE CASE METHOD APPROACH TO TEACHING/LEARNING

The case method approach on which this book is based has been used by educators in many disciplines. Perhaps law schools and schools of business and management have become most noted for their successful use of this teaching strategy; however, it has also been used successfully in teaching health care professionals, for example at the Harvard Medical School. Some of the reasons for using the case method approach have been described in the literature by its proponents and deserve consideration here.

The case method approach engages the students in the learning process; it is active rather than passive learning. We believe that much information needs to be communicated to students through lecture and readings. We also agree, however, with the point of view that states that no amount of information by itself can improve insight and clinical judgment, or increase one's ability to act wisely under various conditions. The knowledge and insight told by others cannot be used effectively, it must be one's own insight and knowledge that is used and which has become one's own through the process of active thought and consideration. It is a questionable assumption that knowledge can be passed on in a useful form by the process of telling. If the learning process is to be effective, something dynamic must take place in the learner (Andrews, 1953). The case study approach provides the student the opportunity to make the knowledge and insight related in the classroom her/his own; it enables something dynamic to take place in that individual.

As a result of the student's active participation in the learning process through use of the case method approach, there are many achievements that may be expected. These include:

- the development of sound thinking, reasoning, and creative ability, i.e. the case study method is not so much intended to impart knowledge as to teach student's how to think critically
- learning at the application level, the ability to apply previously introduced knowledge
- an increased awareness of the importance of data collection
- the ability to classify information, to recognize its degree of relevance, and also to recognize the relevance of missing information
- the enhancement of problem identification skills and improvement in the problem-solving process
- the development of synthesis and evaluation skills (Masoner, 1988)

In addition, several student achievements may be realized due to the seminar method, used for case study discussion. These seminar-related accomplishments include:

- the development of oral communication skills and the ability to articulate the rationale for one's conclusions

- improved listening, observing, and data gathering skills
- increased ability to learn from peers, to learn to work together, and to appreciate the value of working together
- increased confidence in expressing ideas

# THE CASE METHOD APPROACH IN NURSING EDUCATION

In view of the anticipated accomplishments that derive from use of the case method approach, its usefulness in nursing education can be readily appreciated. As nurses, the students will be expected to be able to carry out the nursing process with each of the patients in their care. By the use of case studies and seminar discussions, students can learn, in a safe environment, to recognize signs and symptoms of problems, identify those problems, determine priorities, decide on a plan of care, and evaluate the effectiveness of various interventions. The case method approach allows students to apply in a non-clinical setting, knowledge which has been previously presented, so that once faced with the ambiguities and stresses of the clinical setting, the student will be better prepared to act on that knowledge and the patient will thus be advantaged.

In their work with expert nurses' clinical judgments, Benner and Tanner (1987) describe intuitive judgment as that which distinguishes expert human judgment from decisions that might be made by a beginner or a machine. They cite Dreyfus's six key aspects of intuitive judgment as pattern recognition, similarity recognition, commonsense understanding, skilled know-how, sense of salience, and deliberative rationality. The question is asked, "Can we teach intuition?", and the answer is provided: "The kinds of pattern recognition described in this article cannot be taught in lectures nor broken down into procedural rules. However, such pattern recognition *can* be developed through case studies . . ." (Benner & Tanner, 1987, p. 31). The authors of this text suggest that all six of the aspects of intuitive judgment as described can be enhanced by the use of the case method approach.

Through the use of the case studies, students learn to synthesize the data presented, to consider what other information might be helpful, and to arrive at nursing diagnoses based on the information at hand. This use of the case studies augments the developing skills of students in the assessment and diagnostic phases of the nursing process.

Given the case study as a "real" patient situation, students are able to plan the nursing care of the patient, to determine priorities, to identify appropriate interventions and possible driving and restraining forces associated with selected interventions, and to establish criteria by which the effectiveness of the interventions would be evaluated. Because the case discussion takes place in a seminar format, students are able to discuss with each other and with faculty the rationale for their decisions in all phases of the nursing process. Students are able to think critically about each patient situation, to weigh the relative advantages and disadvantages of care giving decisions, and to hear how others might approach the same patient in a different manner.

## Educator's Role

The importance of the educator's role in the successful use of the case method approach is worth considering. The role of the educator is not limited to the preparation and selection of cases. It is essential for the educator to create an environment that is favorable for analyzing and discussing cases and applying the nursing process. The seminar must be perceived by the students to be a place in which they can put forth ideas and questions, and offer opinions freely. In order for the appropriate climate to prevail, students must feel secure that they and the ideas they put forth will be treated with respect and tolerance by the educator and each other. This is not to suggest that opinions should not be challenged or debated, but rather, that the exchange of ideas should be conducted in a respectful and thoughtful way. It is by articulating one's opinions, ideas, and the rationale to support them, that one learns to think critically and by listening to and questioning others that one learns from others.

More specific aspects of the educator's role in the case method approach include:

- preparing and/or selecting cases
- selecting reading assignments in keeping with major conceptual issues to be stressed in the case discussion, including relevant research
- establishing rapport with the class
- clarifying expectations and ground rules for the class
- asking frequent questions related to the case data

- summarizing discussion at intervals in order to verify understanding and help to maintain discussion focus, without directing the discussion
- assuring that all students are included in the discussion
- being alert for "errors" and making corrections tactfully
- helping students to develop points
- assisting the students to develop a research awareness as a result of the case discussion, either as potential areas for research or for research utilization

Christensen (1981) summarizes perhaps the most important aspects of the educator's role, "Teaching is not only the art of thinking and speaking. It is also the art of listening and understanding. Nor by listening is meant just the act of keeping still. Keeping still is a technique; listening is an art." (p. 48).

## Student's Role

The student's role is also important to the success of the case method approach. While lecture presentations allow the student to come to class unprepared, the case method approach does not. Thoughtful preparation is essential for this teaching/learning approach, which means that careful consideration must be given to the issues identified in the case. In addition to reading the case in preparation for seminar, students are expected to read from the literature related to the case topic. Whether the readings are assigned or unassigned may depend on the proficiency level of the students in the seminar. Active participation by each student in the seminar group is essential. Participation includes not only recognizing facts, but also determining their meaning in the context of the case study. Students must also engage in active problem solving, questioning and responding to the questions and ideas of others. Although discussion and debate are encouraged, students must listen to and respect the ideas and opinions of others.

We view the case method approach as suitable for all levels of nursing education. Of necessity, the focus and depth of discussion will vary with different educational and experiential levels. The achievements, previously discussed, which can be anticipated as a result of the case method approach, are important at all levels of nursing education and nursing practice.

# USING THIS BOOK IN A CASE METHOD APPROACH

The cases selected for inclusion in this book represent a broad sampling of patients and illness which the practicing nurse may encounter. Although the cases are predominantly associated with medical-surgical issues, the settings have been varied. Also included are cases related to pediatric, obstetrical, community health, and psychiatric nursing practice. These are not meant to be all inclusive, but rather, to be representative of patients in those specialty areas.

The selection of the nursing diagnoses developed in the nursing care plans was not based on perceived priority for that particular patient; rather, the nursing diagnoses were varied throughout the book in an attempt to include a broader range of nursing concerns and appropriate nursing care plans. Faculty using this text may wish to have students develop care plans for the other diagnoses that may be present, or to discuss prioritization of the nursing diagnoses as they would address them if they were actually caring for the patient.

Each unit in this book contains two case studies. Each case study is accompanied by information that will enhance the reader's ability to critically examine the case presentation. It should be noted that all of the case study patients are fictitious. The names and places of residence have been created by the authors. Similarity with actual patients is coincidental.

The supplemental information that precedes each case study begins with an overview of anatomy, physiology, and pertinent pathophysiology. Risk factors and common clinical findings as well as treatment modalities are incorporated in the preliminary information in each chapter to present a broad view of relevant clinical information. The inclusion of this information at the beginning of each chapter emphasizes the importance of a knowledge base for nursing practice. Clinical information should be considered using a systematic, organized approach. In order to accomplish this goal, chapters have been organized using a consistent format. The reader is able to consider this information as it relates to the specific case study patient, as well as other patients one might encounter in a clinical situation.

## Patient Assessment Data Base

The patient assessment data base section of this book provides the information to be evaluated in order to describe the status of the case study patient's health and plan individualized patient care. The data base consists of three components; the health history, organized by functional health patterns; the physical examination; and laboratory data with diagnostic studies.

## FUNCTIONAL HEALTH PATTERNS (HEALTH HISTORY)

The functional health pattern assessment format is used throughout this book. Proposed by Marjory Gordon, 11 pattern areas constitute the functional health pattern assessment system that facilitates the organization of assessment data regarding common health pattern areas regardless of the patient's age or medical problem. This systematic health pattern assessment system is considered to have the following advantages:

1. It does not have to be continually relearned (application is expanded as clinical knowledge accumulates).
2. It leads directly to nursing diagnoses.
3. It encompasses a holistic approach to human functional assessment in any setting with any age group at any point in the health-illness continuum (Gordon, 1987, p. 91).

The functional health assessment format considers sequences of behavior across time which in turn creates a pattern. A pattern is created using the subjective data from the patient and observations from the nurse. Using a focused approach for the patient interview, data is gathered for each pattern area. Pattern development has particular significance in that it prevents the collection of superficial data that can often lead to an error in defining a diagnosis. Patterns are always subject to change as new information is identified. The development of a pattern is not an isolated event with a finite set of elements. (Gordon, 1987, p. 92). The functional health pattern assessments included in this book often contain more information than one would obtain in practice. This was done to provide the reader with a comprehensive data base.

The following is a brief overview of the functional health pattern format.

- Health Perception–Health Management Pattern
  Describes the patient's perceived health status and practices he/she uses to manage health.
- Nutrition–Metabolic Pattern
  Describes the patient's dietary habits and indicators of nutrition and/or metabolic alterations.
- Elimination Pattern
  Describes the patient's regularity and control of bladder and bowel function and an assessment of routines and practices.
- Activity–Exercise Pattern
  Describes patterns of exercise and activity. Leisure and recreational activities are assessed as well as activities of daily living that require energy consumption. Cardiac risk factors are assessed.
- Sleep–Rest Pattern
- Describes the patient's patterns of sleep and rest and level of satisfaction with both. Routines and methods to promote sleep and rest are assessed.
- Cognitive–Perceptual Pattern
  Describes the status of the senses: hearing, vision, smell, taste, and touch. The patient's cognitive state is assessed, as is learning style and ability to manage pain.
- Self-Perception–Self-Concept Pattern
  Describes the patient's perception of self worth, personal identity, and self-concept.
- Role–Relationship Pattern
  Describes the patient's role in the family, at work, and in the community.
- Sexuality–Reproductive Pattern
  Describes the patient's level of satisfaction with sexual and reproductive patterns and associated problems or concerns.
- Coping–Stress Tolerance Pattern
  Describes the patient's coping patterns and perception of stressful life events.
- Value–Belief Pattern
  Describes the patient's values and beliefs. This includes an assessment of religious and philosophical beliefs (Gordon, 1987, p. 93).

## PHYSICAL EXAMINATION AND LABORATORY STUDIES

The information that is obtained from the patient or significant other, the patient history or functional health pattern assessment, serves to direct the physical examination that the nurse will conduct. Information gleaned from a physical examination provides additional assessment data for the nurse thus strengthening the data base. A patient history should always be considered in conjunction with the physical examination. The development of a plan of care should come directly from the assessment data base, and a complete assessment data base is necessary to develop a plan with the patient that is appropriate and individualized.

Laboratory tests and diagnostic studies are performed to supplement the data base that is developed for each patient. The findings from pertinent tests are presented in each chapter without differentiating normal from abnormal findings. The presentation of this data in a non-descriptive format suggests the importance of being able to readily understand and interpret the tests that are performed on patients as well as test results.

## Collaborative Plan of Care

A collaborative plan of care includes patient interventions that are both multidisciplinary and interdisciplinary. Health care professionals work with patients for health promotion, maintenance, and restoration. As professionals work with patients, a collaborative relationship emerges. A plan of care is defined for a specific individual, which may require a variety of actions. For consistency within this book, the collaborative plan of care has been written in a specific format. This will enable the reader to quickly identify the components of the collaborative plan for each case study patient.

## Nursing Diagnoses in this Book

Three nursing diagnoses are defined for each case study in this book. The nursing diagnoses that have been developed emerge from dysfunctional health pattern assessment data. The nursing diagnoses that have been developed in the nursing care plans are not necessarily the priority nursing diagnoses for the particular patient in the case study. The authors of this book specifically chose a range of diagnoses to be developed. Some diagnoses have been repeated in the book to demonstrate how each care plan is specific for the patient in the case study.

## Additional Nursing Diagnoses

Each chapter includes a list of additional nursing diagnoses to be considered by the reader. These diagnoses are suggested by the assessment data that is presented in the case study. These diagnoses may be developed by the reader using the information contained in the case study. The reader should consider what additional information or assessment data is needed to fully develop the additional nursing diagnoses for the specific patient. Providing a list of nursing diagnoses for consideration reminds the reader that the three diagnoses prepared for each case study are not the only pertinent diagnoses to be considered when planning patient care.

## Nursing Care Plans for Identified Nursing Diagnoses

In each case study, nursing care plans have been developed for the three nursing diagnoses selected by the author. Diagnostic statements are presented with each diagnosis to more clearly define the problem that is of concern. The etiological ("related to") factors are presented and defining characteristics are evidenced by the cluster of subjective and objective patient signs and symptoms that support the identification of a specific nursing diagnosis. The defining characteristics can be identified as the "evidenced by" portion of the diagnostic statement.

Desired patient outcomes are defined for each nursing care plan. Outcomes may be appropriate for the family as well as the patient and therefore they may be defined for the patient/family unit. The outcome statement is presented as a realistic and appropriate objective or goal for the patient and is projected prior to implementing a plan of care. Outcome statements are presented at the beginning of the care plan in order to guide the actions or nursing interventions that follow.

Evaluation criteria are defined at the beginning of the nursing care plan. These criteria are derived from the desired patient outcomes and provide a measurement for the effectiveness of the nursing interventions. By referring to the evaluation criteria, it is possible to determine whether the desired outcome was achieved.

Each nursing diagnosis developed in this book has a plan for nursing care with specific nursing interventions. The interventions have been written specifically for the patient in the case study to present an individualized approach to patient care. The interventions are accompanied by rationale statements from the literature in order to support the selected interventions. The rationale statements provide the reader with an understanding as to why a particular intervention has been selected. Thus, the documentation of a rationale statement in parallel with an intervention statement demonstrates the fact that the nursing interventions are grounded from a theoretical perspective. The ability to articulate a rationale for one's actions will serve to assist the nurse to communicate clearly with patients, family, and other health care professionals concerning the plan for patient care.

# Questions for Discussion

A list of questions is presented at the end of each case study. These questions refer specifically to the case study patient and are provided to stimulate discussion. The answers to these questions should be focused on the patient information provided in each case study.

Additional generic questions for the reader to consider follow. These questions apply to all of the case studies provided in this book.

- What are the defining characteristics and signs and symptoms for the additional diagnoses to be considered?
- Are there additional nursing diagnoses present for the case study patient?
- Discuss nursing care implications that are not specifically addressed in the collaborative plan of care and not associated with the nursing diagnoses (e.g., the side effects and nursing implications for the prescribed medications).
- What is the significance of the abnormal physical exam findings with the case study patient?
- What is the significance of the diagnostic/laboratory data presented for the case study patient?
- Are there additional health care professionals or support groups with whom you would consult in caring for the patient?
- What research findings would assist you in caring for the case study patient?

Neither the list of specific questions nor the list of generic questions is meant to be all-inclusive of the questions that could be posed concerning the case presentations. Readers are encouraged to identify additional questions that would enhance the understanding of the case presentations and stimulate discussion.

## REFERENCES

Andrews, KR: The Case Method of Teaching Human Relations and Administration. Harvard University Press, Cambridge, MA, 1953.

Benner, P and Tanner, C: Clinical judgment: How expert nurses use intuition. Am J Nurs 87:23–31, 1987.

Christensen, CR: Teaching by the Case Method. Division of Research, Harvard Business School. Cambridge, MA, 1981.

Gordon, M: Nursing Diagnosis: Process and Application, ed 2. McGraw Hill Inc., St. Louis, 1987.

Masoner, M: An Audit of the Case Study Method. Praeger Publishers, New York, 1988.

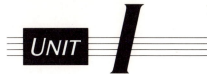

# THE PATIENT WITH COGNITIVE PERCEPTUAL ALTERATIONS

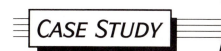
*1*

# A PATIENT WITH ALZHEIMER'S DISEASE

Meg Doherty, M.S., R.N.

Alzheimer's disease is a progressive, degenerative disorder of cognition and widespread brain atrophy, resulting in irreversible dementia and associated with high mortality. There are over 50 diseases causing dementia and more than half of all patients with dementia have Alzheimer's disease. Afflicting 1.5 to 2 million persons annually, it is the fourth or fifth leading cause of total disability in the United States (Fig. 1–1).

## PATHOPHYSIOLOGY

Pathological changes involve widespread death of neurons (responsible for nerve conduction) in the

• Basal ganglia, which are areas of gray matter located at the base of each hemisphere that are responsible for regulating and integrating motor tone and gross intentional movements.

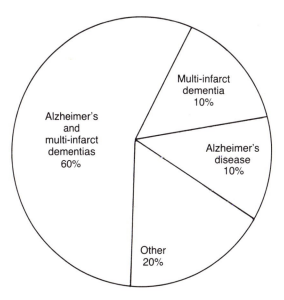

**FIGURE 1–1.** Causes of dementia. (Adapted from Nursing 88, 18(5):10, May, 1988.)

- Substantia nigra, 1 of 3 nuclear masses located in the upper midbrain and considered part of the basal ganglia system since it is connected to the basal ganglia by important neuronal pathways.
- Cortex, the gray matter of the brain made up of nerve cell bodies, responsible for higher cerebral functions such as memory, cognition, and thought.

Other notable anatomical changes include enlarged ventricles and loss of brain weight. Microscopically, neurofibrillary tangles and senile plaque formation are present throughout the cerebral cortex and hippocampus.

Physiologically, neurotransmission in the hippocampus and cortex becomes impaired by a profound reduction in the neurotransmitters somatostatin and acetyltransferase.

Recent research findings indicate that Alzheimer's disease may be genetically based. The isolation and characterization of a gene on chromosome 21 as a coding for part of a protein that may be a precursor for amyloid, which is unusually abundant in the brains of Alzheimer's patients, support this theory. Neither the action of amyloid in cells nor its abundance in the Alzheimer-stricken brain is understood. Chromosome 21, when present in triplicate, causes Down's syndrome. Most Down's syndrome patients who live past the age of 30 develop neurological signs of what appears to be Alzheimer's disease. Alzheimer's disease may also be hereditary, but it is a difficult theory to prove partly because the affliction so often strikes late in life and carriers of the gene simply may not live long enough to develop the symptoms.

Other popular causal theories include the brain's generalized reaction to a toxin, slow virus, or metal deposit, or an immunological dysfunction. Another research focus has been on the role of neurotransmitters since a deficiency of acetylcholine has been identified in the brains of affected patients. Research endeavors also include methods of early detection.

# RISK FACTORS

The risk for developing dementia increases with age. Risk factors specifically and seemingly related to Alzheimer's disease are advancing age and perhaps heredity.

# COMMON CLINICAL FINDINGS

In the early stages of Alzheimer's disease, patients experience difficulty concentrating and have subtle short-term memory problems. They may be somewhat depressed, withdrawn, and a little forgetful. Abstract thinking and decision making gradually become more difficult. Irritability, mood swings, flattened affect, and agitation are common. A person's ability to function independently may not be seriously impaired at this point. Patchy loss of cortical neurons results in memory loss. The neuronal damage is symmetrical, preventing opposite hemisphere compensation.

As loss of frontal and temporal lobe function increases, problems in memory, reasoning, judgment, and social interaction become more overt. This second stage of Alzheimer's disease, usually developing 2 to 4 years later, demonstrates itself when the patient becomes lost, loses coordination and the ability to speak and write, and develops poor hygiene, eating habits, and elimination patterns. The ability to see, hear, and feel pain may become impaired. Hyperorality (ie, excessive use of the mouth, putting things in the mouth), difficulty swallowing, and seizures may occur.

During the third and terminal stage, the patient becomes mute and unresponsive, anorectic, and unable to carry out a learned, voluntary act. Aspiration pneumonia is the usual cause of death.

Clinical diagnosis remains presumptive, confirmed only by microscopic postmortem examination. Since over 100 reversible conditions may mimic irreversible dementia, it is imperative that a thorough dementia assessment be performed, including complete physical, neurological, and psychiatric evaluation. A brain scan is useful in ruling out a curable disorder as well as demonstrating signs of normal age-related changes such as brain shrinkage due to reduction or death of brain cells as a natural course of events, which is not necessarily a sign of disease.

Research methods of diagnosis, specifically the use of brain biopsy, pose legal and ethical dilemmas. The therapeutic benefit of current treatment modalities and obtaining informed consent from a demented patient for invasive procedures are at issue.

# TREATMENT MODALITIES

Currently there is no cure for Alzheimer's disease; however, there is still much that can be done to help the patient and family cope. Careful use of drugs can lessen agitation, anxiety, and depression and improve sleeping patterns if this is needed. The person should be encouraged to maintain daily routines, physical activities, and social contacts, and should not be discouraged from trying new things. Often, stimulating the patient by supplying information on the time of day, place of residence, and what is going on in the immediate environment and in world events, encourages the use of the skill and information that remain. This in turn may keep brain activity from failing at a more rapid pace. Providing memory aids helps people to help themselves in day-to-day living. The loneliness, the frustrations, the lack of information and resources for good medical care for patients and their families, have led to the development of family groups around the country. The Alzheimer's Disease and Related Disorders Association (7 East Lake Street, Chicago, IL 60601), which has more than 100 chapters across the country, encourages research, education, and family services.

# PATIENT ASSESSMENT DATA BASE

## Health History

*Client:*
Mr. Norman Streeter

*Address:* 61 Libbey Street, Seattle, WA 98195
*Telephone:* 206-555-6695
*Contact:* Regina Streeter (wife)
*Address of contact:* 61 Libbey Street, Seattle, WA 98195
*Telephone of contact:* 206-555-6695
*Age:* 75    *Sex:* Male    *Race:* White
*Educational background:* MBA from University of Washington
*Religion:* Methodist    *Marital status:* Married
*Usual occupation:* First Vice President, Seattle Credit Union
*Present occupation:* Retired
*Source of income:* Pension plus salary
*Insurance:* Aetna
*Source of referral:* Grandson, John Deering (medical student)
*Source of history:* Wife and medical record
*Reliability of historian:* Reliable
*Date of interview:* 2/7/90
Reason for visit/Chief complaint: Routine follow-up (Alzheimer's disease); further discussion re: nursing home placement; local or last medical doctor, office visit

## HEALTH PERCEPTION/HEALTH MANAGEMENT PATTERN

*Present Health Status*

Since last visit, 1/31/90, the patient's condition continues to deteriorate. He no longer recognizes his wife. His speech is incoherent and he speaks jibberish. Urinary incontinence continues and he is increasingly more agitated.

*Progression of Disease*
*8/87.* Mr. Streeter first sought help for a 6-month history of recent memory loss. "I don't remember where I put things." The patient denies any other physical complaints.

*12/87.* The patient continues to experience problems with memory loss. Although he has been politically active, he cannot re-

## Present Health Status—Continued

member who is the president of the United States, the governor, or the current mayor. "I had a question to ask you, Doctor, but now I can't remember it." His memory is slightly worse. Computed tomography (CT) scan is negative.

4/88. Recent memory loss continues. Mrs. Streeter voices concern about these changes in her husband, stating that "he can remember things that I can't from years ago."

8/88. Patient is still working every day but is increasingly relying on his wife for appropriate dressing and other activities of daily living (ADLs). He has great difficulty with serial 7's but is able to do simple subtractions. He cannot recite the days of the week or months of the year.

1/89. The patient is becoming more forgetful and more difficult to deal with. He is no longer able to work. He and his wife argue about his ability to drive and he becomes very upset about his inability to remember. He recalls a single number 10 minutes later but cannot recall sequence. He appears physically well but his wife states that "he is becoming very unsteady on his feet."

4/89. The patient has deteriorated remarkably over the past 4–5 days. According to the family, he is hallucinating, confabulating, and speaking jibberish. He is frequently agitated, and is unable to decide whether to sit or stand, or get dressed or undressed. His recent memory is completely gone; he is unable to answer questions because he can't remember the question. Today he does know his wife.

5/89. The patient is now incontinent of urine and exhibits agitated outbursts. His wife states that he falls frequently. The evening dose of haloperidol (Haldol) is increased to 2 mg.

8/89. The patient continues to deteriorate. He is noticeably weaker, requiring assistance with feeding and dressing. Alice Leavitt, MSW, discussed the possibilities of home health care, the availability of a family support group, and eventual long-term care alternatives. Mrs. Streeter is reluctant to discuss or pursue any of these suggestions. Gross neurological examination demonstrates poor recent memory, and progressive motor weakness in the upper extremities.

9/89. The patient does not recognize his wife and other family members, nor does he realize where he is. Wife continues with total care at home; he is still continent of feces at this time.

1/90. Mr. Streeter is intermittently belligerent and confused. His wife performs most of the patient's ADLs with family member assistance at times. Patient is incontinent of urine and requires diapers. Sleep patterns are erratic. Haldol increased to 3 mg tid.

## Past Health Status

**General Health.** No major health problems. The family states "he has always been healthy until this."
**Prophylactic Medical/Dental Care.** Annual physical examination and dental examination every 6 months.
**Childhood Illnesses.** "Routine": measles, mumps, chickenpox.
**Immunizations.** All childhood. Last tetanus shot, "At least 20 years ago."

### Major Illnesses/Hospitalizations
*1975:* Transurethral resection of the prostate (TURP)
*1960:* Bilateral cataract removal
*1955:* Hemorrhoidectomy

### Current Medications
*Prescription:* Haloperidol decanoate (Haldol) 3 mg tid.
*Nonprescription:* Milk of magnesia (MOM) (occasionally).
**Allergies.** None known to food or medications.

### Habits
*Alcohol:* Occasional highball.
*Caffeine:* None.
*Drugs:* See Current Medications.
*Tobacco:* Denies past or present use.

### Family Health History

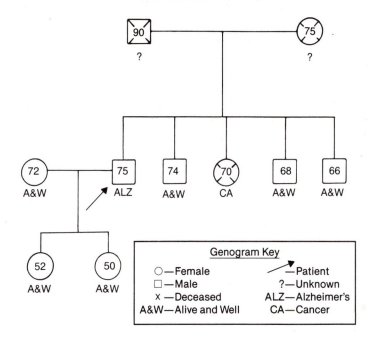

Genogram Key
○ —Female          —Patient
□ —Male           ? —Unknown
x —Deceased       ALZ—Alzheimer's
A&W—Alive and Well  CA—Cancer

## NUTRITIONAL/METABOLIC PATTERN

*Nutritional*

Mr. Streeter used to eat 3 "well balanced" meals a day. For the past several months he has been eating sporadically: refusing, picking, or eating ravenously.

### Usual Daily Menu
*Breakfast:* Cup of coffee, toast, eggs or cereal, orange juice.
*Lunch:* Sandwich (cheese, meat, or fish); fruit, pudding, or cookies; milk.
*Snack:* Cookies, cake, or graham crackers; juice or milk.
*Dinner:* Salad, meat (now usually hamburger or chicken) or fish, green vegetable, potato, dessert, milk or a soft drink.

**Dentition:** Excellent.

*Metabolic*

The patient has lost 10 lb (4.5 kg) in the past 2 months. *Height:* 5 ft 10 in (178 cm). *Weight:* usually 178 lb (84 kg), now 175 lb (77.5 kg).

## Elimination Pattern

*Bowel*

Slightly constipated at times; requires the use of laxatives approximately once/week.*

*Bladder*

Urinary incontinence; intermittent since 5/88. At present wears diapers constantly.

## Activity/Exercise Pattern

*Activity/Exercise*

Recent full retirement due to deterioration in mental/physical condition. Patient is extremely restless and agitated interspersed with weakness and confusion. He can perform no ADL by himself; is totally cared for by his wife and daughter.

### Self-Care Ability

Feeding—II          Grooming—II
Bathing—II          General mobility—II
Toileting—II        Cooking—IV
Bed mobility—0       Home maintenance—IV
Dressing—II         Shopping—IV

Self-care abilities are not expected to improve.

> ### Functional Levels Code
> 0—Full self-care
> I—Requires use of equipment or device
> II—Requires assistance or support from another person
> III—Requires assistance or support from another person and equipment or device
> IV—Is dependent and does not participate

*Oxygenation/Perfusion*

**Last chest x-ray:** 12/87—negative; no history of pulmonary problems.
**PPD:** read 1/3/87—negative.
**ECG:** 12/87—within normal limits.
**Normal sinus rhythm:** rate 68.
**ECG:** 8/88—slightly irregular; transient sinus arrythmia.
**BP:** consistent at 130–140/76–84 left arm.

### Cardiac Risk Factors

|                              | Positive | Negative |
|------------------------------|----------|----------|
| Sedentary life-style         |          | X        |
| Hyperlipidemia               |          | X        |
| Cigarette smoking            |          | X        |
| Diabetes                     |          | X        |
| Obesity                      |          | X        |
| Hypertension                 |          | X        |
| Hypervigilant personality    | X        |          |
| Family history of heart disease |       | X        |

---

*Bowel incontinence occurs if patient is unable to locate the bathroom.

## SLEEP/REST PATTERN

### Sleep/Rest

Wife reports sporadic sleeping patterns even with the use of Haldol. At times Mr. Streeter sleeps 6–8 hours during the day with increased agitation and activity at night; he may sleep 3–4 hours at night. Usually 1 family member or another is awake during the night. Wife states, "He was such a creature of habit. This is the hard part to deal with."

## COGNITIVE/PERCEPTUAL PATTERN

### Hearing

No history of hearing problems.

### Vision

Wears glasses; bilateral cataract removal 27 years ago; last eye examination 10/87.

### Sensory Perception

Mr. Streeter is right hand dominant. Extensive cognitive deterioration as described above. He is seemingly unaware of his surroundings; is unable to remember from moment to moment; has intermittent, incoherent speech and a progressively unsteady gait.

### Learning Style

Unable to assess.

## SELF-PERCEPTION/SELF-CONCEPT PATTERN

### Self-Perception/Self-Concept

Wife describes her husband as being very independent and hard-working. "It was very difficult for him to understand why he was forgetting everything. He would get so frustrated. He always took care of every detail. He was an excellent husband and provider for the girls and me. If he realized what he looked like and what he was doing, he would be so upset."

## ROLE/RELATIONSHIP PATTERN

### Role/Relationship

Daughters and grandson are constantly at their parents' home, frequently spending the night. "If it weren't for my daughters I'd have to hire someone." The family has encouraged Mrs. Streeter to seek help and consider the possibility of health-facility placement, since caring for the patient at home has become increasingly more difficult. Mrs. Streeter states, "He always took care of us . . . we can't turn our backs on him now." The daughters describe the home environment as "chaotic." Close friends and business associates have dwindled over the past 2 years. Wife has devoted her every minute to caring for Mr. Streeter, without social outlet. "She is overwrought and exhausted."

## SEXUALITY/REPRODUCTIVE PATTERN

### Sexuality/Reproductive

Mrs. Streeter states that she and her husband "have a close relationship and are extremely compatible. Our married life has been a very happy one." Sexual relations have been sporadic over the past 10 years, without any in the past 3 years. Mr. and Mrs. Streeter have 2 grown, married daughters.

## COPING/STRESS TOLERANCE PATTERN

### Coping/Stress Tolerance

"My husband was the strong one in the family; we always looked to him for help and support and he never failed us," states his

*Coping/Stress Tolerance—*
*Continued*

wife. "This illness has been difficult for him because he forgets things. Later when we remind him he becomes very upset." Wife and daughters describe the patient as very intelligent and as someone who "always knew the right thing to do. I have learned what it means to cope now! I hope to continue to have the strength to carry on. I've really never done well with change and this is a drastic change in our lives."

## VALUE/BELIEF PATTERN

*Value/Belief*

"We are a very close and religious family; without God I don't know how we would get through all this. We have taken good care of ourselves; I still can't believe that this has happened to us. I thought when we reached this age we would be enjoying ourselves puttering around our yard and maybe traveling . . . How could God let us end up this way?"

# Physical Examination

*General Survey*

Seventy-five-year-old male, appearing stated age in no acute distress but obviously confused, unsteady, and unaware of his surroundings.

*Vital Signs*

*Temperature:* 98.2°F (36.7°C) (oral)
*Pulse:* 64 regular (apical)
*Respirations:* 16 regular
*BP:* 140/76 (R) arm; 140/78 (L) arm, sitting.

*Integument*

*Skin.* Skin on head, arms, and torso is dry, warm, and supple and without lesions or scarring. Skin on the lower extremities is dry, warm, slightly scaling, and with small bruised areas on the shins bilaterally.
*Mucous Membranes.* Pink and moist.
*Nails.* Nails on hands and feet are well groomed and healthy in appearance.

*HEENT*

*Head.* Scalp has no palpable masses; symmetrical in shape. Hair is thinning and gray, neatly groomed. Face is symmetrical without drooping or swelling. No tenderness or crepitus on palpation. Temporomandibular joint (TMJ) is freely movable.
*Eyes.* Extraocular movements (EOMs) intact; pupils equal, round, reactive to light and accommodation (PERRLA). Visual acuity 20/30 (R), 20/30 (L) with glasses in place (Rosenbaum chart).
*Ears.* Able to hear whisper at 2 ft (61 cm) in both ears; ears are symmetrical in size and shape. Weber-Rinne test: air conduction > bone conduction. Canals are clear; tympanic membranes are intact and without scarring.
*Nose.* Nostrils are patent, without septal deviation.
*Mouth/Throat.* Mucosa is pink and moist; uvula midline; excellent dentition with multiple gold crowns; tonsils nonvisual.

*Neck*

Trachea is midline; thyroid nonpalpable. No palpable nodes.

**Pulmonary**

Symmetrical, normal chest expansion; no abnormalities in the rate or rhythm of breathing. Lungs are clear to auscultation and percussion.

**Breast**

Normal male breasts, without masses or tenderness.

**Cardiovascular**

Regular, slow rhythm, with a grade II systolic murmur, best heard at the apex. No rub; point of maximal impulse (PMI) at the 5th intercostal space, midclavicular line.

**Peripheral Vascular**

Pulses in upper extremities are within normal limits; no cyanosis or pallor noted. Pulses in lower extremities are bilaterally equal and within normal limits. No edema noted.

*Peripheral Pulses*
Temporal—4 bilaterally
Carotid—4 bilaterally
Brachial—4 bilaterally
Radial—4 bilaterally
Femoral—4 bilaterally
Popliteal—4 bilaterally
Posterior tibial—4 bilaterally
Dorsalis pedis—4 bilaterally

*Peripheral Pulse Scale*

| |
|---|
| 0—Absent |
| 1—Markedly diminished |
| 2—Moderately diminished |
| 3—Slightly diminished |
| 4—Normal |

**Abdomen**

Hyperactive bowel sounds; nonpalpable liver, kidneys, and spleen. No masses, bruits, or tenderness noted.

**Musculoskeletal**

Normal muscle mass in both upper and lower extremities. Upper and lower extremities are somewhat rigid with distal weakness.

**Neurological**

*Mental Status.* Total loss of recall, complete confusion, not oriented to time, place, or person. Does not recognize wife; intermittent belligerence, more agitated in the late afternoon and early evening.
*Cranial Nerves.* Intact.
*Motor.* Gait unsteady; upper and lower extremity rigidity.
*Sensory.* Difficult to assess. Patient not able to provide accurate responses.

*Deep Tendon Reflexes*

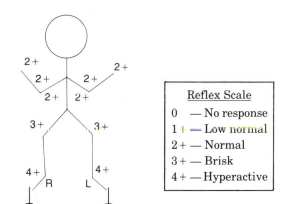

Reflex Scale
0 — No response
1+ — Low normal
2+ — Normal
3+ — Brisk
4+ — Hyperactive

**Rectal**          Prostate is slightly enlarged, smooth, nontender, non-nodular. Guaiac test: stool negative.

**Genitalia**          Normal male genitalia.

## Laboratory Data/Diagnostic Studies

**Laboratory Data**

*Glucose:* 98 mg/dl          *Urinalysis:* negative
*BUN:* 12 mg/dl          *Vitamin $B_{12}$:* 820 pg/ml
*Creatinine:* 1.0 mg/dl          *Na:* 142 mEq/L
*Acid Phos:* 2 Bodansky          *K:* 4.6 mEq/L
  units/ml
*Alk Phos:* 4 Bodansky          *Cl:* 108 mEq/L
  units/ml
*SGOT:* 16 U/L          *$T_4$:* 6.8 μg/dl
*SGPT:* 10 U/L          *Thyroxine:* negative
*LDH:* 148 IU/L

**Diagnostic Studies**          12/87. Computed cranial tomography negative for mass, hemorrhage; mild cortical atrophy.

9/89. Computed cranial tomography with contrast — negative for mass, lesions, midline shift, or extra- or intracerebral hemorrhage; evidence of loss of tissue visualized by increase in size of the ventricles and increase of the sulci. Contrast — findings consistent with above.

## COLLABORATIVE PLAN OF CARE

*1/90:* Referral to the Seattle Visiting Nurse Association.

**Home Visit**          To assess and evaluate efficacy of increased dose of Haldol.
To assess and evaluate the need for Home Health Aide assistance.
To assess nutritional intake.
To assess and evaluate environmental safety.
To assess the need for Social Service intervention.

## NURSING DIAGNOSES DEVELOPED IN CARE PLAN

Ineffective Coping, Wife, p. 13
Potential for Injury, p. 14
Alteration in Elimination Patterns (Bowel and Urine), p. 15

## ADDITIONAL NURSING DIAGNOSES TO BE CONSIDERED

Altered Family Processes
Altered Nutrition: Less Than Body Requirements
Anticipatory Grieving (Family)
Bathing/Hygiene Self-Care Deficit
Dressing/Grooming Self-Care Deficit
Impaired Physical Mobility
Impaired Verbal Communication

# NURSING CARE PLAN BASED ON IDENTIFIED NURSING DIAGNOSES

| | |
|---|---|
| **Ineffective Coping, Wife** | ***Related to:*** Inaccurate appraisal of the situation; inability to deal with the tangible consequences of the illness; lack of objective responsiveness to the situation. <br> ***Evidenced by:*** Wife's refusal to accept social supports; overdependence on family members: "we cannot turn our backs on him now"; "chaotic" home situation as described by other family members. |
| **Desired Patient/Family Outcomes** | **The Wife Will:** <br> • Develop an objective understanding of husband's illness and its impact on their relationship, lifestyle, and other family members. <br> • Develop an increased ability to problem-solve as husband's disease progresses. <br> • Develop realistic plans for comprehensive care during the final stage of husband's illness. |
| **Evaluation Criteria** | ***By the Third Home Visit, the Wife Will:*** <br> • Verbalize an accurate understanding of husband's disease process. <br> • Verbalize stressors associated with husband's disease that affect husband, herself, and other family members. <br> • Identify and begin to utilize appropriate assistive resources. <br> • Identify all available health care options for husband. <br><br> ***By the Fifth Home Visit, the Wife Will:*** <br> • Initiate investigation of health care options for the terminal care of her husband. <br> • Utilize support systems (family members, identified resources) to assist with the development of realistic plans. |

## Interventions

Assess wife's perception of her husband's illness by encouraging description, questions, and verbalization.

Provide accurate information, utilizing consultation with medical, social services, legal, financial, and local support groups to assist with interpretations.

Assist wife with identification of feelings and fears associated with emotional responses to stresses of husband's illness.

## Rationale

Knowledge deficits may be influenced by stressors. Perception may be altered by psychological stress. Significant other "may not be physically, emotionally, or mentally capable" of learning (Doenges and Moorhouse, 1988, p. 228).

Experiences increase the person's knowledge and ability to cope. "Both patients and families benefit from being provided with information on self-help groups, as well as being given lists of other available community support groups and resources. Self-help and support groups can also assist patients and families in coping with the stigmatizing that occurs with certain health problems." (Thompson, et al, 1989, p. 1812) Just being with other people who are going through the same ordeal can help family members feel less isolated (Gray-Vickrey, 1988, p. 39).

Problem-solving behavior becomes less effective in coping . . . when the person focuses less on acquiring and processing information and more on emotional responses (Thompson, et al, 1986, p. 1896).

## Interventions

Provide support and feedback.

## Rationale

Appropriate feedback facilitates understanding and agreement between communicators (Thompson, et al, 1986, p. 1862). Significant others need a lot of support and understanding. Information about support facilities is helpful. Various books written for the lay public help significant others understand and cope with a person who has Alzheimer's disease (Luckmann and Sorensen, 1987, p. 491).

Provide wife and family with a realistic needs assessment, their options, and resources, emphasizing consistent, safe, comprehensive supervision.

"Full-time assistance at home is ideal; part-time assistance is essential. At this stage, the health professional should be prepared to discuss the option of institutionalizing the patient. Institutions can sometimes provide a higher level of care than the most devoted family" (Reisberg, 1984, p. 228).

Assist decision making by providing support.

If a person needs placement in a long-term care facility, significant others need considerable support and understanding with this decision. Help them examine all options and provide information (Luckmann and Sorensen, 1987, p. 491).

---

**Potential for Injury**

*Related to:* Stage 2, Alzheimer's disease.
*Evidenced by:* Unsteady gait, bruised shins; distal extremity weakness; cognitive and perceptual deficits as stated in health history.

**Desired Patient/Family Outcomes**

• Patient injury will be prevented by minimization and/or elimination of risk factors.

**Evaluation Criteria**

*Family Members Will:*
• Identify and recognize the physiological, cognitive/perceptual, and environmental factors that increase the risk of injury.
• Identify and develop protective strategies to reduce the risk of injury.
• Monitor for and report any untoward physiological responses to increased dose of Haldol.
• Modify environment to reduce the risk of injury.
• Provide return demonstration of appropriate body mechanics.

---

## Interventions

Identify with family actual/potential:

• Physiologic risk factors:
  (increasing loss of motor control, decreasing muscle strength, agitation)

## Rationale

Maintaining a safe environment is a major priority (Kneisl and Ames, 1986, p. 1173). The patient is at risk for falls since coordination is lost and balance is unsteady. Swallowing may become more difficult. The person has a slowed metabolic rate and is more susceptible to cold. Avoid negative experiences (e.g., arguments, criticism) to decrease aggressive behaviors. Dressing is less complicated with slip-on clothing; foods should be cut into small pieces and finger foods will require less coordination. Assistance with eating may be necessary (Luckmann and Sorensen, 1987, pp. 490–491). Significant others need a lot of support to safely manage the person at home for as long as possible. Physically and mentally disabled individuals with Alzheimer's disease are at risk for accidents and infection (Kneisl and Ames, 1986, p. 491).

## Interventions

- Cognitive/perceptual risk factors: (increasing confusion, impaired judgment, auditory, visual, sensation deficits, inability to verbalize needs)

- Environmental risk factors: (lighting, stairways, cluttered areas, loose objects, dangerous materials, chemicals, firearms, matches, hot water, medications)

Instruct family about the use of identification methods, for example, ID bracelet, name and address sewn to clothing, name tag.

Teach family about the potential side effects of an increased dose of Haldol and associated risk factors.

Identify assistive devices and instruct family in appropriate body mechanics.

Identify and refer family to local resources for adjunct equipment and structural alterations.

## Rationale

A confused individual is prone to accidental injury because of the inability to take responsibility for basic safety needs or to evaluate the unforeseen consequences (Doenges, Moorhouse, and Geissler, 1989, p. 315). Since the person may not be able to verbalize needs, physiologic signs (e.g., pain, cold) must be observed for. Sometimes the person may ask a question that is really a personal statement, for example, "Are you hungry?", meaning, I am hungry. Severe memory loss causes the person to forget to eat, drink, toilet, recognize surroundings (Luckmann and Sorensen, 1987, pp. 489–491). Patients may lose portions of their ability to see, to hear, and to feel pain. The client will have marked communication and perceptual deficits as well as behavioral problems. The nurse can best assist families by helping them to identify effective coping strategies, to assess support systems, and to seek legal and financial counseling (Kneisl and Ames, 1986, p. 1173).

Precautions to prevent injuries include using night lights; communication devices such as a bell to alert family when person wanders into unsafe area; safety locks; keeping gates or doors to stairways closed; keeping dangerous materials locked up; avoiding scatter rugs and cluttered areas (Kneisl and Ames, 1986, p. 1174; Luckmann and Sorensen, 1987, p. 491).

Confused patients may wander off and not be able to identify themselves (Kneisl and Ames, 1986, p. 1174).

Mental confusion may increase and muscle coordination may decrease until drug response is known. Haldol may cause orthostatic hypotension. Close observation is imperative when doses are changed (Govoni and Hayes, 1988, p. 586).

Minimize potential for injury to patient and caregivers as the physical demands of care increase.

Most family members become exhausted and distressed by the overwhelming demands of day-to-day care. Simply knowing about available resources is helpful (Gray-Vickrey, 1988, p. 39).

---

| *Alteration in Elimination Patterns (Bowel and Urine)* | *Related to:* Forgetfulness, loss of neurological function. *Evidenced by:* Urinary incontinence: wears diapers; bowel incontinence if unable to locate bathroom, and is sometimes constipated. |
| --- | --- |
| *Desired Patient/Family Outcomes* | • The patient will become less constipated and be able to locate the bathroom. <br> • The family will be able to manage problems associated with elimination. |
| *Evaluation Criteria* | *The Patient Will:* <br> • Be less frequently constipated. <br> • Be able to locate the bathroom with or without direction. |

***The Family Will:***
- Expect elimination problems as part of the disease process.
- Identify methods of preventing constipation.
- Identify and implement methods of assisting the patient with finding the bathroom.
- Identify patient's nonverbal cues for need for elimination.

## Interventions

Teach family that elimination problems are to be expected.

Assist family with clearly identifying bathroom and orienting patient to it.

Teach family methods of preventing constipation.

Assist family with recognizing nonverbal cues for the need to eliminate.

Assess family's desires regarding patient's bladder control management.

## Rationale

A person with Alzheimer's disease may become incontinent or constipated. This may be due to an inability to locate the bathroom or forgetfulness about elimination habits (Luckmann and Sorensen, 1987, p. 491). Expect confused people to use any convenient container or the floor for elimination purposes (Luckmann and Sorensen, 1987, p. 490).

Location, adequate lighting signs, and/or color coding enhance orientation. Make bright signs showing the person where the bathroom is and regularly take the person there. Provide adequate lighting, especially at night (Doenges, Moorhouse, and Geissler, 1989, p. 325; Luckmann and Sorensen, 1987, p. 490). Adherence to a daily and regular schedule may prevent accidents (Doenges, Jeffries, and Moorhouse, 1984, p. 215).

Encourage adequate fluid intake, increased dietary fiber, stool softeners, and exercise to avoid constipation (Doenges, Moorhouse, and Geissler, 1989, p. 325; Luckmann, 1987, p. 490).

Restlessness, holding self, and picking at clothes may indicate elimination need (Luckmann and Sorensen, 1987, p. 490).

If bladder control is involved, limit fluid intake during the late evening and at bedtime (Luckmann and Sorensen, 1987, p. 490). Avoid caffeinated beverages especially and limit fluids after 8 PM to minimize nocturnal incontinence (Gray-Vickrey, 1988, p. 39).

# QUESTIONS FOR DISCUSSION

1. Identify the symptoms that would determine the transition from stage 1 to stage 2 Alzheimer's disease.
2. Identify the most likely nursing diagnoses, both actual and potential, for stage-2 Alzheimer's disease.
3. Outline a plan of care for the hospitalized patient with stage-2 Alzheimer's disease.
4. What is the major risk for the patient in terminal, stage-3 Alzheimer's disease? Identify preventative nursing measures.
5. Identify the physical parameters used in assessing the nutritional status of the patient. How would you advise the family with regard to meeting the patient's nutritional needs?
6. Identify ways in which you would reorient a patient with stage 1–2 Alzheimer's disease.
7. How would you provide care for the caregivers in this case study?
8. Since Mr. Streeter is insured by Medicare, how would you financially advise this family in order to obtain supportive help in their home?

# REFERENCES

Doenges, M, Moorhouse, MF, Geissler, A: Nursing Care Plans: Nursing Diagnosis in Planning Patient Care. FA Davis, Philadelphia, 1989.

Govoni, L and Hayes, J: Drugs and Nursing Implications. Appleton-Century-Crofts, Norwalk, Conn, 1988.

Gray-Vickrey, P: Evaluating Alzheimer's patients. Nursing '88 18:12, 1988.

Kneisl, C and Ames, S: Adult health nursing. Addison-Wesley, Reading, Mass, 1986.

Luckmann, J and Sorensen, K: Medical-Surgical Nursing: A Psychophysiologic Approach. WB Saunders, Philadelphia, 1987.

Reisberg, B: Stages of cognitive decline. AJN 84:2, 1984.

Thompson J, et al: Clinical Nursing. CV Mosby, St. Louis, 1989.

# BIBLIOGRAPHY

Amato, I: Alzheimer's disease: Scientists report research advances. Science News, Nov 22, 1986.

Beam, I: Helping families survive. Am J Nurs 84:2, 1984.

Beck, C and Heacock, P: Nursing interventions for patients with Alzheimer's disease. Nurs Clin N Am 23:1, 1988.

Brunner, L and Suddarth, D: Textbook of Medical-Surgical Nursing, ed 6. JB Lippincott, Philadelphia, 1988.

Carpenito, L: Nursing Diagnosis: Application to Practice, ed 2. JB Lippincott, Philadelphia, 1987.

Dietsch, L: Alzheimer's disease: Advances in clinical nursing. J Gerontol Nurs 8:2, 1982.

Dodson, J: The slow death: Alzheimer's disease. J Neurosurg Nurs 16:5, 1984.

Fischbach, F: Manual of Laboratory Diagnostic Tests, ed 3. JB Lippincott, Philadelphia, 1988.

Gordon, M: Nursing Diagnosis: Process and Application, ed 2. McGraw-Hill, New York, 1987.

Guyton, A: Textbook of Medical Physiology. WB Saunders, Philadelphia, 1983.

Hall, G: Care of the patient with Alzheimer's disease living at home. Nurs Clin N Am 23:1, 1988.

Hickey, J: The Clinical Practice of Neurological and Neurosurgical Nursing, ed 2. JB Lippincott, Philadelphia, 1986.

Ninos, M and Makohon, R: Functional assessment of the patient. Geriatr Nurs 6:3, 1985.

Pajk, M: Alzheimer's disease: Inpatient care. Am J Nurs 84:2, 1984.

Pluckhaw, M: Alzheimer's disease: Helping the patient's family. Nursing '86 11, 1986.

Price, S and Wilson, L: Pathophysiology: Clinical Concepts of Disease Processes. McGraw-Hill, New York, 1986.

Redder, M: Nursing update on Alzheimer's disease. J Neurosurg Nurs 7:3, 1985.

Schafer, S: Modifying the environment. Geriatr Nurs 6:3, 1985.

Schneider, E and Emr, M: Alzheimer's disease: Research highlights. Geriatr Nurs 6:3, 1985.

Tinkham C: Community Health Nursing: Evolution and Process in the Family and Community, ed 3. Appleton-Century-Crofts, Norwalk, Conn, 1984.

Weiner, H and Levitt, L: Neurology for the House Officer. Williams & Wilkins, Baltimore, 1983.

Williams, L: Alzheimer's: The need for caring. J Gerontol Nurs 12:2, 1986.

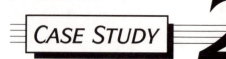

# 2

# A PATIENT WITH CHRONIC OTITIS MEDIA

Dorothy Bagnell Kelliher, M.S., R.N.

## ANATOMY AND PHYSIOLOGY OF THE EAR

The *external ear* has two parts, the auricle, also called the pinna, and the external auditory canal. The ear is located on each side of the head. The height alignment of the pinna is measured by drawing an imaginary line from the outer orbit of the eye to the occiput of the skull. The top of the pinna should meet or cross this line. Low-set ears are commonly associated with renal anomalies or mental retardation. Normally the pinna extends slightly outward from the skull.

Other landmarks of the pinna are the helix, the prominent outer rim of the pinna; the antihelix, a second curved rim that is adjacent and almost parallel to the helix; the concha, the deep cavity that leads into the external auditory canal; the tragus, which lies anterior to the concha; the antitragus, which lies just opposite the tragus; and the lobule (earlobe), which is just below the antitragus and is the fleshy part of the ear.

The external auditory canal is about 2.5 cm (1 in) long and terminates at the tympanic membrane (eardrum). The walls of the external auditory canal are pink. They are more pigmented in dark-skinned persons. Glands in the canal secrete cerumen (earwax). Cerumen helps to capture foreign material and protects the canal epithelium.

The tympanic membrane is a translucent, light, pearly pink, or gray color and is the gateway to the middle ear. Attached to the eardrum are the three auditory ossicles (bones) called the malleus, incus, and stapes. The stapes inserts into the oval window, which is the first part of the inner ear.

The other very important part of the middle ear is the eustachian tube. The eustachian tube connects the middle ear to the nasopharynx and serves to equalize air pressure between the middle ear and the external ear. The eustachian tubes of the infant and young child are shorter, wider, and more horizontally placed than that of the adult (Fig. 2–1). This anatomical difference is felt to be the reason for the increased susceptibility of infants and very young children to ear infections. As the child develops, the facial structure changes, causing the inner ear to be located more deeply and the eustachian tube to develop a more vertical direction.

The *inner ear* is a series of fluid-containing channels located in the temporal bones. The most important structures of the inner ear are the semicircular canals, cochlea, and auditory nerves. The semicircular canals maintain equilibrium and balance. The cochlea and the auditory nerves are responsible for hearing.

The basic *physiology of hearing* involves sound waves, collected by the auricle and directed by the external auditory canal to the tympanic membrane, which in turn stimulates this membrane to vibrate. The vibration sets the ossicles in motion. The stapes, at its position at the oval window, causes a fluid wave that is transmitted into the cochlea, a spiral chamber where the sound waves are coded by the neural tissue. It is in the cochlea that most of the reception and processing of sound occurs. The cochlea, the hardest bone in the body, contains the sensory cells of sound perception along with the vestibular apparatus concerned with orientation and posture of the body. The vestibulo-cochlear nerves, when stimulated, send messages by way of the medulla, pons, and midbrain to the temporal lobes of the cortex, where the impulses are interpreted as sound.

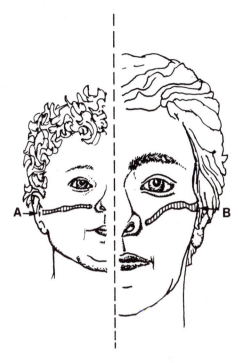

**FIGURE 2–1.** Anatomic developmental difference of the eustachian tube in the child versus the adult. (***A***) child's tube lies horizontally (***B***) adult's tube lies at a more vertical angle. (Adapted from Servonsky, J, and Opas S: Nursing Management of Children. Jones and Bartlett Publishers, Boston, 1987.)

Sound waves may be conducted through air or bone. Both stimulate the organ of Corti (spiral organ). Air conduction is the normal event of sound waves in air striking the tympanic membrane, setting in motion the ossicles and initiating the events of sound processing in the inner ear. In bone conduction, sound waves move through the skull to the inner ear, bypassing the middle ear.

## PATHOPHYSIOLOGY OF OTITIS MEDIA

Otitis media is primarily a result of dysfunction of the eustachian tubes. The eustachian tubes have 3 important functions related to the middle ear. They protect the middle ear from nasopharyngeal secretions, promote drainage of secretions produced in the middle ear into the nasopharynx, and ventilate the middle ear to equalize pressure between the middle ear and the outer ear. If the eustachian tube develops an obstruction or opens inappropriately, it may cause an accumulation of secretions in the middle ear or allow a reflux of bacteria from the nasopharynx into the middle ear. Eustachian tube obstruction results in negative middle ear pressure and if prolonged it causes a transudative middle ear effusion. Drainage is inhibited by sustained negative pressure and impaired ciliary transport within the eustachian tube. If the tube is partially obstructed contamination of the middle ear can take place by reflux of secretions, aspiration, sneezing, nose blowing, and swallowing when the nose is obstructed. If bacteria invade the middle ear and the tube remains blocked, the accumulated fluid will result in increased middle ear pressure. The tympanic membrane bulges outward and may perforate and drain fluid into the external auditory canal.

Chronic otitis media results from middle ear effusion lasting longer than 3 months. It usually involves a chronic infection of the middle ear and mastoid cells. The condition is frequently painless. If the posterior margin of the tympanic membrane is ruptured, epithelial tissue from the external canal can grow into the middle ear forming a cholesteatoma. This in turn can cause erosion of adjacent bones and tissues resulting in ossicular or neurological damage.

## RISK FACTORS

Factors that predispose infants and young children (those under 7 years of age) to the occurrence of otitis media include anatomical features of the eustachian tubes, that is, they are short, wide, relatively straight tubes that lie in a horizontal position; undeveloped cartilage leading to inappropriate opening of the eustachian tubes; enlarged lymphoid tissue in the nasopharynx that may obstruct the tubes; immature humoral defense response that may increase risk of infection; and the lying-down position of infants, when bottle-fed, which favors pooling of formula in the pharyngeal cavity.

Adults may also develop otitis media. Usually this is due to blockage of the eustachian tube during an upper respiratory tract infection. Chronic otitis media is most often seen in adults with a previous history of acute otitis media.

Otitis media is one of the most prevalent of early childhood diseases. Statistics indicate that 70% of children have at least 1 episode and 33% have 3 or more episodes by age 3. The incidence is highest between the ages of 6 months and 2 years. Then the incidence seems to decrease with age, except that a small increase is seen at age 5-6 when children enter school. After age 7, otitis media becomes less common or may become chronic otitis media. Preschool boys seem more affected than girls. The incidence of otitis media is highest in the winter; crowded household conditions also seem to increase its incidence. Some researchers have found a higher incidence of otitis media in children whose parents or siblings have a history of chronic otitis media.

## COMMON CLINICAL FINDINGS

Clinical findings are a result of an increase of fluid in the middle ear. Pain is usually present as pressure increases on surrounding structures. Infants frequently indicate an ear problem by rolling their heads or tugging on their ears. Young children verbally complain of discomfort. A temperature elevation is usually present and may go as high as 104°F (40°C). Glands in the neck may be enlarged. Other signs of an upper respiratory tract infection may also be present. Appetite is decreased due to the discomfort caused by chewing and sucking. If the tympanic membrane ruptures, a sharp decrease in pain is noted, the fever abates, and a purulent discharge is seen in the external auditory canal.

Occasionally a person will complain of a feeling of fullness in the ear, or a popping sensation when swallowing. If air is also present, a sensation of motion within the ear may be noted. These symptoms are not usually accompanied by pain or fever when the underlying cause is otitis media with effusion.

On otoscopic examination, significant changes in the tympanic membrane may give an indication of the developing disease. Marked erythema of the eardrum may indicate suppurative otitis media. A dull, non-transparent, grayish color may indicate serious otitis media, or ashen gray areas may indicate areas of scarring from previous perforations of the eardrum. A black area is suggestive of a perforation of the tympanic membrane that has not healed. Slight redness in the newborn is normal and is due to increased vascularity. Slight redness may also be evident in older infants and young children as a result of crying and should not be interpreted as inflammation.

Mobility of the tympanic membrane is markedly reduced when there is presence of fluid or high negative pressure within the middle ear. This decrease in mobility is a reliable and significant indication of middle ear effusion.

Conductive hearing loss may accompany prolonged ear disorders. The causes of this type of hearing loss are attributed to negative middle ear pressure, presence of middle ear effusion, and rupture of the tympanic membrane.

## TREATMENT MODALITIES

When otitis media is diagnosed, the treatment of choice is antibiotic therapy. The drug of choice is a 10-14-day course of penicillin or amoxicillin. Other antibiotics may also be used in conjunction with the aforementioned drugs. Most children respond in 2-3 days. If no response is noted the child should be reevaluated for a change in medication or change in diagnosis. Analgesic/antipyretic drugs are prescribed for fever and discomfort. Decongestants are recommended for relief of nasal allergic responses. Ear drops are seldom used.

If acute episodes of otitis media with effusion are frequent and/or close together, not only should antibiotic therapy be used but other additional treatment should be instituted. This includes myringotomy with insertion of tympanotomy tubes to improve middle ear ventilation and drainage. The goal is to allow the eustachian tubes time to recover while the tubes provide pressure equalization.

The use of tympanotomy tubes, while a common practice in the United States, is not without its foes. Some physicians are reluctant to use them because the tubes tend to plug easily, often require reinsertion, need to be inserted under anesthesia thus introducing surgical risks, increase the risk of secondary infection, and no hard data exist to support the long-range benefits of the procedure.

If cholesteatoma has developed as a result of prolonged and repeated ear infections, the treatment is surgical excision of the entire cholesteatoma and a tympanoplasty to repair the ruptured tympanic membrane.

# PATIENT ASSESSMENT DATA BASE

## Health History

*Client:*
Caitlin Lisieux

*Address:* 63 Maple Street, Hingham, MA 01103
*Telephone:* 617-555-3468
*Contact:* Darcy (mother)
*Address of contact:* Same
*Telephone of contact:* Same
*Age:* 6   *Sex:* Female   *Race:* White
*Educational background:* 1st Grade
*Religion:* Roman Catholic   *Marital status:* Single
*Usual occupation:* Student
*Present occupation:* Does not apply
*Source of income:* Parents
*Insurance:* Blue Cross/Blue Shield Health Plus
*Source of referral:* Pediatrician
*Source of history:* Mother of patient
*Reliability of historian:* Reliable
*Date of interview:* 1/30/90
*Reason for visit/Chief complaint:* "Caitlin's ear started draining profusely a month ago. The discharge was a thick yellow material. We took her to her pediatrician who recommended that she see Dr. P., the ear specialist. We saw him last week and we are here today to discuss the results of his findings. I think he is going to tell us that some type of surgery is necessary."

### HEALTH PERCEPTION/HEALTH MANAGEMENT PATTERN

**Present Health Status**

Caitlin's mother said that she is essentially a very healthy child with the exception of these recurring ear infections. During this past year, she reports that Caitlin had 2 very "bad" episodes in the spring and they were treated with ampicillin. In August, Caitlin had an episode of ear drainage but strangely, it was not associated with pain. The drainage was grayish yellow and foul smelling. Again, she was treated with ampicillin. The pediatrician also suggested that she not go swimming for the remainder of the summer.

*Progression of Disease*
*10/89.* In October, Caitlin developed more painless ear drainage; this time she was treated with amoxicillin. These episodes were localized to her right ear and were not always accompanied by an elevated temperature.

*12/26/89.* On the morning of December 26, Caitlin again experienced thick, grayish yellow drainage from her right ear. She was seen first by her pediatrician, who has referred her to Dr. P. for further evaluation.

**Past Health Status**

*General Health.* Essentially Caitlin is a healthy child. She has experienced the usual upper respiratory infections (URI). When she was very young (infant to 3 years) her mother noted that her colds often turned into bronchitis. They were treated with penicillin and then she was "just fine." After 3 years of age, Caitlin's respiratory infections were more often followed by acute otitis

**Past Health Status—Continued**

media. One or both ears might be involved. These attacks were usually treated with ampicillin and sometimes with amoxicillin.

*Prophylactic Medical/Dental Care.* Caitlin sees her own pediatrician for a yearly checkup and as necessary. First visit to the dentist was at age 5—no caries noted. She is due to see the dentist next month.

*Childhood Illnesses. Bronchitis:* Age 13 months and then 3 to 4 times per year, usually following a URI. Since age 3 the bronchitis has occurred less often. *Acute otitis media:* Usually associated with a URI; these occurred more from age 2 and up to the present. At least 3 to 4 episodes a year. *Chickenpox:* Age 5—mild case.

*Immunizations.* Diphtheria-pertussis-tetanus (DPT)—age 6 months. Measles, mumps, and rubella—Can't remember exactly, but were given on schedule by pediatrician.

*Major Illnesses.* See Childhood Illnesses.

### Current Medications

*Prescription:* Amoxicillin—250 mg q8h PO (has been taking since 12/26).

*Nonprescription:* Pseudoephedrine HCl (Sudafed)—30 mg PO q4–6h.

Multivitamin † tab per day during winter months.

Baby aspirin—2 tabs q4h PO prn for temperature or pain.

*Allergies.* None.

### Habits

Is not a "thumb sucker" and did not use a pacifier.

*Alcohol:* No.
*Caffeine:* No.
*Drugs:* No.
*Tobacco:* No.

### *Family Health History*

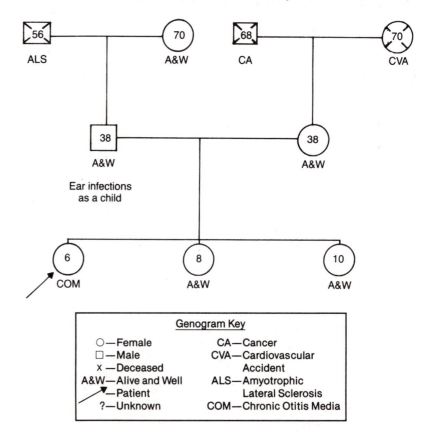

| Genogram Key | |
|---|---|
| ○—Female | CA—Cancer |
| □—Male | CVA—Cardiovascular |
| X—Deceased |     Accident |
| A&W—Alive and Well | ALS—Amyotrophic |
| ↖—Patient |     Lateral Sclerosis |
| ?—Unknown | COM—Chronic Otitis Media |

## NUTRITIONAL/METABOLIC PATTERN

*Nutritional*

Caitlin is a good eater. She enjoys most foods and will try new foods. Favorite foods are pizza, hamburger, and chicken. She is not a "sweets eater."

***Usual Daily Menu***
*Breakfast:* Cornflakes (½ cup) with milk, 1 English muffin with margarine, 1 large glass of orange juice.
*Lunch:* Peanut butter and marshmallow sandwich, ½ orange, 2 Oreo cookies, milk.
*Dinner:* Spaghetti and meatballs (medium helping), 2 slices bread, small tossed salad with Italian dressing, 1 large glass of milk, no dessert.

*Metabolic*

At present: *Height:* 47 inches (119.4 cm). *Weight:* 48 lb (21.8 kg).

## ELIMINATION PATTERN

*Bowel*

One to two brown formed stools a day. No constipation; diarrhea only when associated with gastrointestinal upset. Kaopectate has been taken on occasion for this.

*Bladder*

Clear, light yellow in color; no odor; seldom wakes at night to go to the bathroom.

## ACTIVITY/EXERCISE PATTERN

*Activity/Exercise*

Very active child. She participates in all gym and school sports activities; her energy level is excellent; enjoys being outdoors playing with friends, bike riding, jump rope, swimming, etc.

***Self-Care Ability***

| | |
|---|---|
| Feeding—0 | Grooming—0 |
| Bathing—0 | General mobility—0 |
| Toileting—0 | Cooking—IV |
| Bed mobility—0 | Home maintenance—IV |
| Dressing—0 | Shopping—IV |

> ***Functional Levels Code***
> 0—Full self-care
> I—Requires use of equipment or device
> II—Requires assistance or support from another person
> III—Requires assistance or support from another person and equipment or device
> IV—Is dependent and does not participate

*Oxygenation/Perfusion*

***Last chest x-ray:*** 1/85—no exertional dyspnea.
No rheumatic fever; no family history of diabetes.

***Cardiac Risk Factors***

| | Positive | Negative |
|---|---|---|
| Sedentary life-style | | X |
| Hyperlipidemia | | X |
| Cigarette smoking | | X |
| Diabetes | | X |
| Obesity | | X |
| Hypertension | | X |
| Hypervigilant personality | | X |
| Family history of heart disease | X | |

## SLEEP/REST PATTERN

*Sleep/Rest*

Sleeps 10–11 hours per night; goes to bed at approximately 7:30 PM and sleeps until 6:30 AM. She awakes easily and is "cheerful and ready to go." Seldom has nightmares; sleeps soundly.

## COGNITIVE/PERCEPTUAL PATTERN

*Hearing*

Caitlin has had frequent earaches over the past 3 years. She complains of a "blocked" ear frequently, and also complains that her ear clicks and pops when she swallows. Her mother has noticed that when she has had ear infections her hearing is decreased from 1–6 weeks after the episode. This last year she has had some difficulty in school when trying to learn her vowel sounds. Kindergarten and first grade teachers noted that she seemed to be "daydreaming or not listening and sometimes did not respond or follow directions appropriately." Caitlin had no difficulty passing the school hearing test in October, 1988 (kindergarten); but she did not pass the hearing test in October of 1989 (1st grade). The school nurse notified Mrs. Lisieux that there was a significant drop in hearing in the right ear. Her pediatrician was notified and he felt this was the result of some fluid and it would clear up in another few weeks. He suggested Caitlin be seated in front of the teacher until this problem resolved. At no time did he consider putting in ear tubes. He felt they just got plugged up or fell out. He felt the risks outweighed the benefits of the tubes.

*Vision*

No problem.

*Sensory Perception*

Caitlin notices a "blocked ear" sensation in her right ear; describes the sensation feels like "water in the ear." No pain felt during the last couple of episodes of otitis media.

*Learning Style*

Learns best by audiovisual and repetition; she seems to be losing some of the audio benefits. Struggles with sounds and spelling. Reading is on grade level.

## SELF-PERCEPTION/SELF-CONCEPT PATTERN

*Self-Perception/Self-Concept*

Caitlin is a happy, outgoing child according to her mother. She has many school friends, and is included in birthday parties and weekend sleep-overs. She enjoys inviting friends over to play at her house, etc.

She is a warm affectionate child with family and friends. Will spontaneously hug her parents. Tends to be shy and reserved around strangers.

## ROLE/RELATIONSHIP PATTERN

*Role/Relationship*

Caitlin lives with her mother and father and 2 sisters in a single family home in a coastal suburb of Boston. She is the youngest of the 3 girls. Her sisters are 8 and 10 years of age. She gets along quite well with them. They do have the usual "fights and tears" but they pass quickly. She and her family enjoy beaching and sailing. This has been a bit of a problem since Caitlin has been restricted from swimming since the beginning of August. Mrs. Lisieux admits she is torn between going to the beach and not allowing Caitlin to swim or just making everyone "skip the beach." She said she was really happy to have school start this year for more than one reason!

## SEXUALITY/REPRODUCTIVE PATTERN

### Sexuality/Reproductive

Normal female development for child of 6 years. No signs of precocious puberty.

## COPING/STRESS TOLERANCE PATTERN

### Coping/Stress Tolerance

Caitlin is a fairly easygoing child. She has handled most childhood frustrations by speaking out, crying, and sometimes by fighting with her sisters. She does not "hold grudges," and pouting or sulking is of brief duration.

She did have a hard time accepting the fact that she could not go swimming at the end of last summer with her family and friends. Her mother said she did tend to be "out of sorts" when she was "left behind." Her parents tried to plan non-water-related fun to ease her disappointment.

Washing Caitlin's hair has tended to present some aggravation for both mother and daughter. Caitlin finally realizes that she just can't "stick her head under the faucet" because water might get into her ear.

Parents and her teacher have noticed that Caitlin seems to be inattentive at times and sometimes does not answer questions appropriately. This had been a source of concern to them. The children have occasionally laughed at her responses and this has left Caitlin bewildered and unsure of what was going on.

## VALUE/BELIEF PATTERN

### Value/Belief

Education is highly valued in Caitlin's family. Caitlin also wants to do well and to bring home good grades and a good report card. She did not receive the type of report that she expected this last marking period. This is an area of concern to parents, teacher, and Caitlin herself. Good health is also highly valued by this family as evidenced by appropriate visits by all to doctor and dentist and by good health practices in general.

# Physical Examination

### General Survey

Six-year-old white female. Cheerful expression although somewhat anxious about the examination. Posture is good; walks with a well-coordinated stride. Follows directions well; occasionally responds inappropriately or asks to have questions repeated. Her weight is 48 lb (21.8 kg) and her height is 47 in (119.4 cm).

### Vital Signs

*Temperature:* 98°F (36.5°C) (oral)
*Pulse:* 86 regular (apical)
*Respirations:* 22 regular
*BP:* 85/48 (left arm, sitting).

### Integument

*Skin.* Warm, dry; no birthmarks or blemishes, no bruises or scars.
*Mucous Membranes.* Smooth, moist, pink.
*Nails.* Well trimmed, no evidence of nail biting; color—pink.

### HEENT

*Head.* Well-shaped head; size appropriate for age. Scalp clean and smooth; no evidence of pediculi, no areas of tenderness. Very shiny, thick, curly blond hair, shoulder length. Facial features are well aligned; expression is appropriate to situation.
*Eyes.* Acuity (Snellen chart)—20/30 both eyes; pupils equal, round, reactive to light and accommodation (PERRLA)—

### *HEENT — Continued*

extraocular movements (EOMs)—normal; color vision—normal; sclera clear, conjunctiva pink.

***Ears.*** External canals are pink. Ⓡ external ear shows some scaling of skin; slight otorrhea (sour odor). Tympanic membrane —dull, gray; perforation noted in central area; decreased mobility; landmarks obliterated.

*Weber test:* Sound localized to Ⓡ ear; Ⓛ ear within normal limits (WNL).

*Rinne test:* Ⓡ ear AC* < BC; Ⓛ ear AC > BC.

*Whisper test:* Ⓡ ear—unable to hear at 1 ft (30 cm); Ⓛ ear—can hear at 2 ft (60 cm).

*Watch tick test:* Ⓡ ear—unable to hear at 1 inch (2.5 cm); Ⓛ ear—can hear at 3 inches (7.5 cm).

***Nose.*** Mucous membrane is somewhat indurated and inflamed; draining yellow mucous; sniffs frequently.

***Mouth/Throat.*** Mucous membrane is moist and pink; missing Ⓛ and Ⓡ central incisor in lower jaw; no caries. Parotid gland is intact; tongue pink and moist. Uvula is midline; tonsils and adenoids are present and are slightly indurated and inflamed; mucous drainage observed at back of oropharynx.

### *Neck*

Trachea is midline; supple, full range of motion; thyroid not palpable; no nodes felt.

### *Pulmonary*

Anteroposterior (AP) and lateral diameter 1:2; respiratory rate —22–24; rhythm—regular; lungs clear on auscultation; slight hyperresonance on posterior and anterior chest percussion.

### *Breast*

Normal female child.

### *Cardiovascular*

Good capillary return; skin color pink. Relaxed posture; able to lie down; no change in respirations. $S_1$ and $S_2$ heard; no murmurs or extra sounds. Apical rate—86 regular.

### *Peripheral Vascular*

All pulses strong and regular; no bruits. Extremities warm; no mottling, good capillary return.

***Peripheral Pulses***
Temporal—4 bilaterally
Carotid—4 bilaterally
Brachial—4 bilaterally
Radial—4 bilaterally
Femoral—4 bilaterally
Poplitial—4 bilaterally
Posterior tibialis—4 bilaterally
Dorsalis pedis—4 bilaterally

***Peripheral Pulse Scale***

0—Absent
1—Markedly diminished
2—Moderately diminished
3—Slightly diminished
4—Normal

### *Abdomen*

Slightly rounded and symmetrical, umbilicus centrally placed; no skin rashes or scars. Bowel sounds in all 4 quadrants; tympanic on percussion; no bruits.

### *Musculoskeletal*

Muscular development and skeletal structure are bilaterally equal and normal for age. No joint deformity or tenderness; full active range of motion. Normal spinal curve; no deviation noted; Good muscle tone and strength bilaterally.

*AC = air conduction; BC = bone conduction.

**Neurological**

*Mental Status.* Very alert, cooperative 6-year-old; is quite a good historian regarding her ear condition.
*Cranial Nerves.* I–XII (with exception of VIII cranial) intact; no problems elicited. See ear evaluation for VIII cranial nerve.
*Sensory.* Able to distinguish between pain and light touch in all body areas.

*Deep Tendon Reflexes*

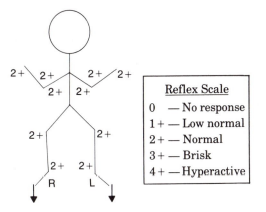

**Rectal**

Deferred.

**Genitalia**

Deferred.

# Laboratory Data/ Diagnostic Studies

**Laboratory Data**

*Hematocrit:* 38%   *Hemoglobin:* 14 g/dl
*RBC Count:* 4.3 million/mm³   *WBC Count:* 10,800/mm³
*Platelet Count:* 400,000/mm³   *Clotting Time:* 4 minutes
*PPT:* 24 seconds   *PT:* 13 seconds
*Ear Culture: Streptococcus pneumoniae*

**Diagnostic Studies**

*Auditory.* Ⓡ ear responds at 35 dB; Ⓛ ear at 15 dB — indicates mild hearing loss in Ⓡ ear.
*Pneumatic Otoscopy.* Decreased mobility of tympanic membrane Ⓡ ear; Ⓛ ear WNL.
*Chest X-Ray.* Lungs clear.

**Additional Data**

Caitlin is diagnosed as having chronic otitis media complicated by the development of a cholesteatoma. She is scheduled for surgical removal of the cholesteatoma and a tympanoplasty on 2/12/90.

# COLLABORATIVE PLAN OF CARE

**Diet**

Diet as tolerated.

**Medications**

Amoxicillin — 250 mg PO q8h to continue to date of surgery.
Acetaminophen — 320 mg PO q4–6h prn for fever/pain.

| | |
|---|---|
| *Intravenous Therapy* | Does not apply. |
| *Therapeutic Measures* | Cleanse external auditory canal with hydrogen peroxide prn for otorrhea. <br> Prevent water from entering ear. <br> Preoperative teaching for patient and parents on 2/11/90. |
| *Consults* | Does not apply. |
| *Preoperative Plan* | NPO after midnight. <br> Promethazine 25 mg PO on call with sip of water. <br> Meperidine 25 mg PO on call with sip of water. |

## NURSING DIAGNOSES DEVELOPED IN CARE PLAN

Potential for Infection, p. 28
Fear, p. 29
Sensory-Perceptual Alteration: Auditory, p. 30

## ADDITIONAL NURSING DIAGNOSES TO BE CONSIDERED

Altered Growth and Development
Knowledge Deficit—Surgery
Noncompliance
Pain
Potential Impaired Skin Integrity
Powerlessness: Child and Parents
Self-Esteem Disturbance

## NURSING CARE PLAN BASED ON IDENTIFIED NURSING DIAGNOSES

| | |
|---|---|
| *Potential for Infection* | *Related to:* A ruptured right tympanic membrane. <br> *Evidenced by:* Otorrhea. |
| *Desired Patient Outcome* | The patient will remain free from bacterial invasion. |
| *Evaluation Criteria* | Prior to entering the hospital for surgery and during hospital admission, the patient will remain free of bacterial infection by use of the following methods: |

- Parent and child will verbalize correct techniques to avoid water from entering ears.
- Child demonstrates gentle nose blowing.
- Parent continues to administer antibiotic as prescribed and verbalizes knowledge of reason to complete prescription.
- Ear packs are changed as necessary and skin of the right ear canal remains intact.
- Nurses and parents are observed washing their hands before and after patient care.
- Parents and child verbalize ways to prevent infection while at home, at school, and in the hospital.

## Interventions

Prevent water from entering affected ear during shampoos, bathing, or showering. Place two pieces of cotton in the ear; the first piece is dry, and the second piece is saturated with petroleum jelly (Vaseline).

Teach patient to blow nose gently and keep *both* nostrils open.

Administer antibiotics as ordered.

Teach parents that antibiotic therapy must be carried out until **all** the prescribed medicine is taken.

If the ear is draining, place cotton loosely in the outer ear to collect drainage; replace when moist. Cleanse external canal with sterile swabs soaked in hydrogen peroxide; protect auricle with Vaseline or zinc oxide.

Wash hands before and after changing cotton packs.

Instruct and involve the family and child in infection control strategies.

## Rationale

Parents are instructed to plug the child's ears lightly with sterile cotton coated with petroleum jelly during baths or shampooing to keep water from entering the ear canal. Also, diving or swimming deeply under water is not permitted because it leads to contamination of the middle ear (Foster, et al, 1989, p. 1206). Bath and shampoo water should not enter the ear because soap reduces surface tension of the water, thus facilitating its entry through the tympanic opening (Whaley and Wong, 1987, p. 1353).

Infected material from the nasopharynx will not be forced into the middle ear if children are taught to blow their noses properly during respiratory infections, e.g., not to hold one nostril closed while blowing their nose (Foster, et al, 1989, p. 1206).

Antibiotics are the drugs of choice for otitis media (Fischer, 1985, p. 474).

Although the child looks well in 2–3 days, the infection is not completely eradicated until all the prescribed medication is taken (Whaley and Wong, 1987, p. 1353).

Ear packs should be loose enough to allow accumulated drainage to flow out of the ear to prevent infection being transferred to the mastoid process (Whaley and Wong, 1987, p. 1352; Phipps et al, 1983, p. 905). Skin surrounding the ear and the auricle may become excoriated from exudate (Whaley and Wong, 1987, p. 1352).

Handwashing is the single most important means of preventing the spread of infection (Atkinson and Murray, 1985, p. 342).

Learning occurs quickly when the learner perceives both a need and a way to meet that need (Atkinson and Murray, 1985, p. 163). Understanding increases compliance (Gettrust, 1985, p. 113).

---

**Fear**

**Related to:** Impending separation from family, and hospitalization and surgery.
**Evidenced by:** Increased apprehension, nervousness and reluctance to let her mother out of her sight.

**Desired Patient/Family Outcome**

• The child and family will be prepared to understand the hospital and surgical experience.

**Evaluation Criteria**

• The child and parents will verbalize a decrease in fear produced by hospitalization and surgery beginning with the first day of admission.

---

## Interventions

Provide orientation to the hospital unit and surgical routine on day of admission.

## Rationale

Based on the principle that fear of the unknown (fantasy) exceeds fear of the known. Thus if fear is decreased, children are able to direct energies toward dealing with other unavoidable stresses of hospitalization and to benefit optimally from the growth potential of the experience (Whaley and Wong, 1987, p. 1085).

## Interventions

Provide opportunity for child and parents to ask questions and verbalize fears that remain after orientation.

Provide information regarding "rooming in" opportunity for parents.

Explain the operative experience — right ear will be operated on; emphasize that left ear and other parts of the body *will not* be touched.

Explain postoperative events for this type of surgery, that is:

• Teach child to lie on affected side as much as possible.
• Encourage child to change position slowly.

Explain discharge care plan to parents. Include specifics of care of ear dressing, available community resources, and follow-up plan.

## Rationale

Allows parents and child to relax and further clarify areas of uncertainty (Whaley and Wong, 1987, p. 1086).

A child's anxiety may be allayed by the presence of supportive parents. If parents can "room-in" with their child, many of the fears are dispelled (Foster, et al, 1989, p. 944).

School-age children fear disability, loss of body parts, possibility of negative surprises, and physical discomfort (Servonsky and Opas, 1987, p. 380).

Knowledge reduces or alleviates fear of the unknown (Whaley and Wong, 1987, p. 1077).

Lying on affected side will facilitate drainage into bulky head dressing (Whaley and Wong, 1987, p. 1353).
Avoidance of sudden movements will possibly eliminate nausea, dizziness, and vomiting (Mott, 1985, p. 1613).

Information reduces parental anxiety when their child returns home, provides them with resources, and enables them to reorganize family functioning, which was disrupted by child's illness and hospitalization (Waechter, 1985, p. 91).

---

| *Sensory-Perceptual Alteration: Auditory* | *Related to:* Decreased hearing and repeated ear infections.<br>*Evidenced by:* Daydreaming; not always responding to voice stimuli; difficulty with some classroom learning. |
|---|---|
| *Desired Patient/Family Outcomes* | *The Child and Parents Will:*<br>• Identify practices that enhance hearing.<br>• Know how to avoid contamination of the ear. |
| *Evaluation Criteria* | *The Child and Parents Will:*<br>• Demonstrate and verbalize measures to assess and enhance hearing.<br>• Verbalize knowledge of methods to avoid contamination of the ear and prevent further hearing loss. |

---

## Interventions

Avoid practices that can cause ear infections, that is, instruct about shampoo, shower, and swimming restrictions; eliminate tobacco smoke from environment; prevent injury to ear or eardrum.

Teach parents and child to report signs of middle ear problems to their doctor: feeling of fullness, pain, fever, or drainage.

## Rationale

The primary nursing role is prevention of infections such as chronic otitis media, which is the most common cause of hearing loss in children (Whaley and Wong, 1987, p. 1017).

At the risk of alarming parents, it is important to stress the potential complications of otitis media, especially hearing loss, which can be prevented with adequate treatment and follow-up care (Whaley and Wong, 1987, p. 1353).

## Interventions

Teach parents to evaluate child's hearing and assess the need for intervention by communicating problem with school and teacher, or the doctor.

## Rationale

Even mild hearing loss significantly reduces vocabulary growth, articulation skills, the use of grammar and syntax, and auditory memory skill (Foster, et al, 1989, p. 2019). Asking to have statements repeated or answering them incorrectly are signs suggestive of hearing impairment in young children (Whaley and Wong, 1987, p. 1918). Assess parents' reports of suspected hearing loss, past history of ear infections, and behavior patterns (Whaley and Wong, 1987, p. 1017).

Administer hearing test and refer the patient for audiometry.

The school nurse should supervise the hearing screening program, recognizing its limitations to discover hearing loss and pathology in its early stages. Pure-tone audiometry should be supplemented with the observations and concerns of parents and teachers (Foster, et al, 1989, p. 2025).

Practice good communication techniques to facilitate hearing for the hearing impaired child:

- Talk directly to the child, and attract his or her attention before speaking.
- Speak in a normal tone.
- Repeat statements when in a group situation.
- Speak toward the better ear.
- When in a classroom or group situation have the child sit close to and facing the teacher/speaker. Be sure the speaker's face is well lit.

A child's ability to speech read is improved if adequate lighting falls on the speaker's face and if natural speaking is used with normal articulation and complete sentences (Foster, et al, 1989, p. 2028).

Maximize residual hearing; investigate the possible benefits of a hearing aid.

Hearing aids are designed to amplify sounds and are of greatest value in conductive hearing loss (Whaley and Wong, 1987, p. 1020).

Teach child and parents the need to avoid excessive noise pollution.

Excessive noise pollution is a well-established cause of sensorineural hearing loss (Whaley and Wong, 1987, p. 1017). Without more specific and intensive instruction to help children understand how and why hearing may be threatened by environmental noise and other factors, they cannot be expected to make intelligent decisions to protect their hearing (Frazer, 1986, p. 168).

# QUESTIONS FOR DISCUSSION

1. Identify the signs and symptoms of:
   a. Acute otitis media
   b. Chronic otitis media
2. Compare and contrast otitis media in childhood versus in adults.
3. What are the long-range complications of chronic otitis media?
4. What are the medications primarily used in the treatment of otitis media?
5. What would you want to teach the parents about these medications?
6. Discuss the importance of follow-up care for ear infections.
7. What special teaching is necessary for parents of children with chronic otitis media?
8. Discuss the following tests for hearing:
   a. Rinne test
   b. Weber test
   c. Audiometry test
9. What are some of the signs a child might exhibit who is having difficulty hearing?

10. Discuss other possible treatment modalities for otitis media.
11. When surgery is planned for chronic otitis media, what preoperative preparation should be considered for both parents and a child of this age?
    a. How long is the readjustment period after surgery?
12. Define cholesteatoma.
    a. How is a cholesteatoma treated?

# REFERENCES

Atkinson, L and Murray J: Fundamentals of Nursing. Macmillan, 1985.

Fischer, RG: Drug management of otitis media. Pediatr Nurs, November/December, 1985, p. 474.

Foster, R, et al: Family Centered Nursing Care of Children. WB Saunders, Philadelphia, 1989.

Frazer, M: Toward improved instruction in hearing health of the elementary school level. Journal of School Health 56(5):166, 1986.

Gettrust, KV: Applied Nursing Diagnosis. John Wiley & Sons, New York, 1985.

Mott, S: Nursing Care of Children and Families. Addison-Wesley, Menlo Park, Calif, 1985.

Servonsky, J, and Opas S: Nursing Management of Children. Jones and Bartlett Publishers, Boston, 1987.

Waechter, EH: Essentials of Pediatric Nursing. JB Lippincott, Philadelphia, 1985.

Whaley, L, and Wong, D: Nursing Care of Infants and Children. CV Mosby, St. Louis, 1987.

# BIBLIOGRAPHY

————. A quiet aftermath of otitis media. Emerg Med 16:71, 1984.

Bluestone, C: Recent advances in pathogenesis, diagnosis and management of otitis media. Pediatr Clin North Am 28(4):727, 1981.

Bueche, M, et al: The student with a hearing loss: Coping strategies. Nurs Educ 8(4):7, 1983.

Carpenito, LJ: Nursing Diagnosis. JB Lippincott, Philadelphia, 1983.

Castiglia, PT, et al: Focus: Nonsuppurative otitis media. Pediatr Nurse, November/December 1983, p 427.

Cunha, BA: Case studies in infectious disease: Otitis media. Emerg Med 20(9):164, 1988.

DiChiara, E: A sound method for testing children's hearing. Am J Nurs 84(9):1104, 1984.

Dyson, AJ et al: Speech characteristics of children after otitis media. J Pediatr Health Care, September-October 1987, p 261.

Eichenwald, HE: Otitis media in the child. Hosp Pract, 20(5):51, 1985.

Fireman, P: Newer concepts in otitis media. Hosp Pract 22:85, 1987.

Fria, L: Assessment of hearing. Pediatr Clin North Am 28(4):757, 1981.

Harrison, CJ: Tympanostomy tubes—To use or not to use. Consultant 27(3):143, 1987.

McDermott, JC: Physical and behavioral aspects of middle ear disease in children. J School Health, October 1983, p 463.

Mitchell, A, et al: Must children with tympanotomy tubes avoid swimming? Pediatr Alert 8(7):27, 1983.

Nurses Drug Manual. JB Lippincott, Philadelphia, 1985.

O'Shea, JS, et al: Childhood serous otitis media. Clin Pediatr 21:150, 1982.

Patlak, M: Children's all-too-common ear infections. FDA Consumer 21(10): December 1987–January 1988.

Servonsky, J, et al: Nursing Management of Children. Jones and Bartlett Publishers, Boston, 1987.

Stataloff, RT, et al: Otitis media: A common childhood infection. American J Nurs August 1981, p 1480.

Voke, J: Physiology of the ear. Nurs Times 80(33):29, 1984.

Voke, J: Functions of the cochlea. Nurs Times 80(33):60, 1984.

Wagner, JA, et al: Children and parents and otitis media. J Emerg Nurs, November/December 1982, p 306.

Wayoff, M: Surgical treatment of middle ear cholesteatoma. Advanced Otorhinolaryngology. 36:1–237, 1987.

Yon, T, et al: The effects of chronic otitis media on motor performance in 5 and 6 year old children. Am J Occup Ther 42(7):421, 1988.

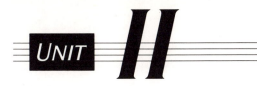

# THE PATIENT WITH ALTERATIONS IN PERFUSION

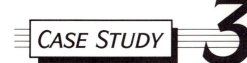

# A PATIENT WITH PERIPHERAL VASCULAR DISEASE

Dorothy Bagnell Kelliher, M.S., R.N.
Jean D'Meza Leuner, M.S., R.N.
Sharon P. Sullivan, M.S., R.N.

## ANATOMY AND PHYSIOLOGY OF THE PERIPHERAL VASCULAR SYSTEM

The peripheral vascular system refers to the arteries, veins, and lymphatics in the periphery of the body. The peripheral vessels are part of the systemic circulation and the pulmonary circulation, which form a closed system with the right and left sides of the heart. Arteries are the vessels that carry oxygenated blood from the left side of the heart to the tissues. Arteries consist of three layers: the innermost layer is referred to as the tunica interna or intima, the middle layer is the tunica media, and the outermost layer is the tunica externa or adventitia. The tunica media represents the thickest layer and is composed of elastic and collagenous fibers. These elastic and connective tissue fibers provide the vessel with strength and allow for constriction or dilation in response to the flow of blood. Arteries branch to smaller vessels, the arterioles, and the media in these vessels, unlike the larger arteries, consists primarily of smooth muscle.

Capillaries are microscopic blood vessels that connect arterioles to venules and in turn form larger vessels, the veins. The veins transport unoxygenated blood from tissues to the right side of the heart. Veins are analogous to arteries and consist of three layers. Veins, however, consist of less elastic and smooth muscle and contain more white fibrous tissue. The vein wall, while less muscular than the arterial wall, does allow for greater distensibility. Thus, approximately 75% of the total volume of blood in the body is contained in the venous system. The veins that transport blood flow in opposition to the force of gravity contain one-way valves to propel the blood toward the heart.

Lymphatic circulation originates within the tissues of the body. The peripheral lymphatic system consists of thin-walled capillaries that appear to be similar to blood capillaries except that the vessel walls have a greater permeability for large molecules. The peripheral lymph system branches into larger vessels as well as regional lymph nodes prior to joining the venous system. Lymph, a fluid similar to plasma, in conjunction with tissue fluids made up of smaller proteins, cells, and cellular debris, empty into the thoracic duct and the right lymphatic duct. Both of these ducts flow into the junction of the subclavian and internal jugular veins. Lymph vessels, like veins, contain one-way valves to direct the flow of lymph into the venous system.

# PATHOPHYSIOLOGY

## Peripheral Arterial Occlusive Disease

Peripheral arterial occlusive disease is a condition that results in a narrowing of arterial vessels or damage to the endothelial lining of arterial vessels. Peripheral arterial occlusive disease can be caused by the presence of arteriosclerosis, direct arterial trauma, arterial injury, peripheral emboli, thrombosis, inflammation, or autoimmunity.

Atherosclerosis is responsible for most of the pathogenic changes that are associated with peripheral arterial occlusive disease. It is considered a generalized disease of the arterial system and therefore can be observed in the peripheral vessels as well as within other vessels in the body. Atherosclerosis is a process characterized by changes in the intima of the arteries. Fatty substances, especially cholesterol and triglycerides, calcium, fibrous tissue (plaque), and blood components accumulate in the walls of medium and large-sized arteries. While the principle changes occur in the intima of the arterial vessel, secondary changes are seen in the tunica media. These changes occur in response to dilation of the vessel and localized aneurysm formation.

The lesions that have been identified as atherosclerotic in nature are the fatty streak, raised fibrous plaque, and complicated plaques. The fatty streak has been observed in people of all ages. It is yellow in color, smooth, and does not obstruct the flow of blood. The fatty lesion is made up of cholesterol and cholesterol esters that accumulate within smooth muscle cells in the intima of the artery to cause an irregular arterial surface. The raised fibrous plaque is yellow-gray in color and remains localized within the intima of the artery. This lesion has the ability to cause complete obstruction to the flow of blood in the artery. This plaque usually consists of a fibrous cap over a deep, central mass of lipid material combined with cellular debris and plasma proteins. This central portion of the plaque may be responsible for a tenacious yellow exudate (atheroma) that can be seen on autopsy. A complicated plaque is most often seen in people with advanced stages of disease. This lesion is a fibrous plaque with calcification, thrombus rupture, or hemorrhage into the plaque. The presence of this lesion is usually associated with signs and symptoms of arterial occlusion and significant sequelae.

Atherosclerosis has been called the disease of old age; however, the incidence in younger persons has been increasing. It is the most frequent cause of death in people over 65 years of age, and more than half of people ages 60–70 will die of some manifestation of this disease. The cause of atherosclerosis remains unknown. While many theories continue to be explored, only hypotheses surface (Fig. 3–1).

# RISK FACTORS

Several risk factors have been closely associated with atherosclerosis. A diet high in saturated fat has been positively correlated with an elevation in serum cholesterol and triglycerides, which results in the development of atherosclerosis. Additional risk factors include a sedentary lifestyle, emotional stress, obesity, cigarette smoking, diabetes mellitus, hypertension, and a family history of atherosclerosis. Caffeine and alcohol may contribute to the presence of atherosclerosis as well. While no one risk factor is considered the most significant contributor to the development of this disease, all risk factors should be considered together in an attempt to eliminate as many as possible for a preventative approach to this disease.

# COMMON CLINICAL FINDINGS

The changes that occur within the arterial system result in the narrowing of vessels. The extent of the stenosis present within the vessels accounts for the variability in the signs and symptoms a person may experience.

A significant manifestation of chronic arterial occlusive disease is the presence of intermittent claudication and pain at rest. Coldness or numbness may be evident in the extremities, and a marked change in the color of the affected limb may be observable. Skin and nail changes and muscle atrophy may occur. Bruits may be auscultated in stenosed vessels, and peripheral pulses may be diminished or absent.

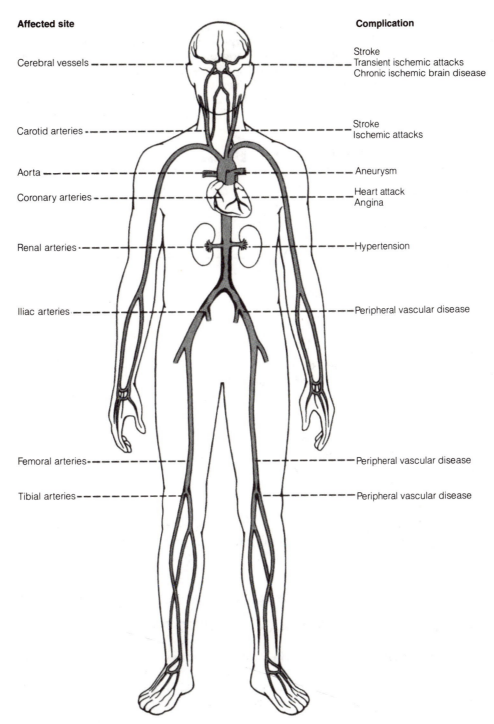

| Affected site | | Complication |

**FIGURE 3–1.** Major blood vessels that are affected by atherosclerosis and some complications of the process. (From Porth, CH: Pathophysiology Concepts of Altered Health States, ed 2. JB Lippincott, Philadelphia, 1986, p 206, with permission.)

## TREATMENT MODALITIES

A medical treatment plan for patients with peripheral arterial occlusive disease without the evidence of ischemia should include the treatment of hyperlipidemia, maintenance of skin integrity of the affected limbs, avoidance of tobacco smoking, and a carefully monitored exercise program. Drug therapy may be attempted with the use of anticoagulants and fibrinolytic agents. In the presence of ischemia or intermittent claudication that interferes with a patient's ability to function, surgical intervention is advisable. An endarterectomy may be performed on the stenosed vessel or a bypass operation may be considered using either a vein graft or a synthetic material. Percutaneous transluminal angioplasty is being used as an alternative to surgery. In this fluoroscopic procedure, the stenosed segment of the vessel is dilated by the inflation of a balloon within the affected vessel. A vessel suitable for this procedure has an intraluminal diameter of 2.5 mm and is not longer than 10 cm. An unsuccessful treatment plan for peripheral occlusive disease may result in an amputation.

# PATIENT ASSESSMENT DATA BASE

## Health History

**Client:**
Robert H. Holland

**Address:** 104 Maple Street, Milwaukee, WI
**Telephone:** 414-555-0762
**Contact:** Rose (wife)
**Address of contact:** Same
**Telephone of contact:** Same
**Age:** 55    **Sex:** Male    **Race:** Black
**Educational background:** High school graduate
**Religion:** Baptist    **Marital status:** Married
**Usual occupation:** Mail carrier
**Present occupation:** Same
**Source of income:** Disability insurance
**Insurance:** Blue Cross/Blue Shield
**Source of referral:** Self
**Source of history:** Self plus old chart
**Reliability of historian:** Reliable
**Date of interview:** 2/16/89
**Reason for visit/Chief complaint:** My doctor has been treating me with Trental but it's not working. I can hardly walk 20 steps without my left leg cramping. It even wakes me up at night out of a sound sleep. They are going to operate and put a graft in or something. I'm not really sure about the procedure."

## HEALTH PERCEPTION/HEALTH MANAGEMENT PATTERN

**Present Health Status**

Up until a few years ago Mr. Holland states that he was in good health. Then his left leg started to cramp up while he was doing his mail route, but once he rested it would be okay. He sought medical help 2 months ago due to the severity and frequency of the leg cramps.

**Past Health Status**

**General Health.** General health is described as good. On routine examination 4 years ago he was found to have elevated cholesterol and was advised to modify his diet. Recently, 2 months ago, his cholesterol level was found to be even higher requiring implementation of drug therapy, probucol (Lorelco). Mild hypertension was also diagnosed and chlorothiazide (Diuril) was prescribed.

**Prophylactic Medical/Dental Care.** Sees own physician every 6 months; has seen him more often this past year. Visits dentist about once a year; last visit about a year ago. Mr. Holland states, "I have some of my own teeth to hold in the partial plates."

***Childhood Illnesses.*** Can't remember. States "usual childhood illnesses"; does not think he had rheumatic fever.

***Immunizations.*** Last recollection was when he entered the service in 1952. "I had every shot possible and then some."

***Major Illnesses/Hospitalizations.*** Pneumonia (1978) — hospitalized 1 week.

### Current Medications

*Prescription:* Probucol (Lorelco): "A medicine for the cholesterol. I take 2 pills per day, 1 with my breakfast and 1 with my dinner." Does not recall dosage.

Pentoxifylline (Trental): "One pill at meal time."

Chlorothiazide sodium (Diuril): "One pill in the morning for my blood pressure." Does not recall dosage.

*Nonprescription:* Milk of magnesia (MOM) once in a while for constipation.

***Allergies.*** Penicillin: "I get hives."

### Habits

*Alcohol:* Has 1–2 beers a day.

*Caffeine:* Two cups of coffee in AM; 2 or 3 glasses of cola per day; 1 cup of tea with dinner; chocolate several times a day.

*Drugs:* None.

*Tobacco:* Two packs/day for 36 years. "My doctor told me to give them up. I would really like to. I've tried a few times to quit but I always go back."

### *Family Health History*

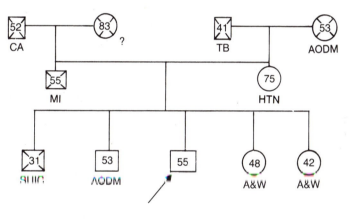

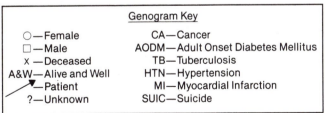

Genogram Key

| | |
|---|---|
| ○—Female | CA—Cancer |
| □—Male | AODM—Adult Onset Diabetes Mellitus |
| X—Deceased | TB—Tuberculosis |
| A&W—Alive and Well | HTN—Hypertension |
| ⬈—Patient | MI—Myocardial Infarction |
| ?—Unknown | SUIC—Suicide |

## NUTRITIONAL/METABOLIC PATTERN

*Nutritional*

Appetite is excellent; enjoys all types of foods. Wife cooks and prepares all meals. Mr. Holland follows no special diet, has bacon and eggs 3–4 times per week, loves pork and pork products, likes vegetables "loaded with butter," and does admit to having a "sweet tooth."

**Nutritional—Continued**

**Usual Daily Menu**
*Breakfast:* Two eggs, pork sausage (2 patties), 1 English muffin with butter, orange juice, 2 cups of coffee (cream, no sugar).
*Lunch:* One meat or fish sandwich, pickles, potato chips, 2 brownies, milk.
*Dinner:* Pork chops (2–3), gravy, mashed potatoes (lots of butter), green beans, applesauce (good-sized portions). "Then best of all," chocolate cake, a big wedge, with 2 glasses of milk. "I try not to use sugar and only a little salt."
*Snack:* Cola and chips.

**Metabolic**

Has gained 22 lb (10 kg) in last 18 months. Skin on lower extremities is dry and flaky.

## ELIMINATION PATTERN

**Bowel**

Normal bowel pattern in 1 bowel movement a day; soft, formed, medium-brown color. Approximately once a month uses laxatives, MOM, for problems with constipation.

**Bladder**

Urinates 4–6 times a day, light yellow in color, no odor; occasionally wakes to urinate once at night. Sometimes has trouble starting to urinate; has been told he has a somewhat enlarged prostate.

## ACTIVITY/EXERCISE PATTERN

**Activity/Exercise**

Within the last year it has become increasingly difficult for Mr. Holland to complete his daily mail route. Because of this he was transferred to a more sedentary job that involves mostly standing or sitting. At present he experiences calf and foot pain after walking 20–50 feet, and he has difficulty with climbing stairs. He is unable to engage in many of the activities he enjoyed doing in the past.

**Self-Care Ability**
Feeding—0
Bathing—0
Toileting—0
Bed mobility—0
Dressing—0

Grooming—0
General mobility—0
Cooking—0
Home maintenance—II
Shopping—0

**Functional Levels Code**
0—Full self-care
I—Requires use of equipment or device
II—Requires assistance or supervision from another person
III—Requires assistance or supervision from another person and equipment or device
IV—Is dependent and does not participate

**Oxygenation/Perfusion**

*Chest x-ray.* Last chest x-ray, 1980; Had x-ray this admission: no dyspnea at rest or on exertion. Patient denies chest pain or palpitations.

### Cardiac Risk Factors

|  | Positive | Negative |
|---|---|---|
| Sedentary life-style |  | X |
| Hyperlipidemia | X |  |
| Cigarette smoking | X |  |
| Diabetes |  | X |
| Obesity | X |  |
| Hypertension | X |  |
| Hypervigilant personality |  | X |
| Family history of heart disease | X |  |

## SLEEP/REST PATTERN

### Sleep/Rest

Usually sleeps 8 hours but over the past 2–3 months he has been awakened with increasing frequency because of severe leg cramps, which are relieved by standing. He occasionally awakes to void once during the night—returns to sleep easily. In spite of sleep disruptions, he usually feels rested upon awakening. Denies use of sleep aids.

## COGNITIVE/PERCEPTUAL PATTERN

### Hearing

Reports no difficulties with hearing. Denies earaches, vertigo, and ringing.

### Vision

Wears bifocals; his prescription was changed 1½ years ago. Denies other visual problems.

### Sensory Perception

Notices a decrease or change in sensation in his left leg. Frequent crampy pain in the calves of both legs; left leg is worse than right. Patient states that he thought he could tolerate pain, but realizes that he can't after experiencing this leg pain. "I don't want to be a baby, but this is rotten." Patient is right-handed.

### Learning Style

Learns best by demonstration and use of visual aids. Has noted no change in memory or concentration.

## SELF-PERCEPTION/SELF-CONCEPT PATTERN

### Self-Perception/Self-Concept

Describes himself as independent, good-natured, a hard worker, not a complainer. Says his illnesses of the past few months have made him feel old. Claims not to be uncomfortable expressing thoughts and feelings, but says "people don't want to hear about your trouble," so he tends to keep negative thoughts and feelings to himself. Not a "toucher," but doesn't mind being touched by others.

## ROLE/RELATIONSHIP PATTERN

### Role/Relationship

Patient lives in a 2-family home in a suburb of Milwaukee. This home is owned by the patient and his wife, who live on the second floor. Has been married for 25 years and has 3 children; 2 daughters live nearby and 1 son is away at college. Describes relationship with 2 daughters as very good. They are supportive of the patient and his wife. Sees son infrequently due to distance. They have a comfortable relationship and communicate regularly by phone.

*Role/Relationship—Continued*

Describes his relationship with his wife as "she's what keeps me going."

Considers neighborhood to be safe, but says, "It's really changed a lot in the past few years. People don't care about their property or each other the way they used to."

Has been primary wage earner in the family; however, does not anticipate major financial difficulties because of disability insurance and income from his wife's part-time job.

Has good relationship with downstairs neighbors: "They've helped out a lot when I haven't been well."

## SEXUALITY/REPRODUCTIVE PATTERN

*Sexuality/Reproductive*

Describes decreased desire for sexual activity during the last several months. Has had no problems with impotence. Feels very close to wife, thinks she understands his "lack of attention." He has 3 children.

## COPING/STRESS TOLERANCE PATTERN

*Coping/Stress Tolerance*

Walking used to take Mr. Holland's mind off his problems, but he is no longer able to do this. Has experienced loss of father and brother. His brother's suicide was especially traumatic; was supported through these losses by wife, children, and surviving brother and sisters. Feels he is overeating due to upset over his condition and inability to continue work. Copes by turning to God and asking for His help. Tries to be positive: "No sense in feeling sorry for yourself." Admits to being afraid of becoming a "burden to my family."

## VALUE/RELIEF PATTERN

*Value/Belief*

He is a Baptist and goes to church fairly often. He finds himself praying a little more intently since his illness. Also values independence and "work ethic."

# Physical Examination

*General Survey*

Fifty-five-year-old black male looking his stated age; alert, pleasant, very cooperative, oriented × 3. *Height*: 6 ft (183 cm). *Weight*: 240 lb (109 kg).

*Vital Signs*

*Temperature:* 97.6°F (36.4°C) (oral)
*Pulse:* 92 regular (apical)
*Respirations:* 20 regular
*BP:* 160/90 (right arm, sitting).

*Integument*

*Skin.* Skin on torso, arms, and head is moist, warm, supple, and without lesions or scarring. Skin on the left leg is shiny and thin with little evidence of hair below the knee. Skin color is dark brown, but lower left extremity appears to be mottled when dependent; this is difficult to assess due to the natural darkness of his skin. His left leg is significantly colder to the touch than the right leg, but the right leg is also cool to the touch.
*Mucous Membranes.* Smooth, moist, no inflammation or lesions noted.

*Nails.* Nails on hands are smooth. Toenails of both feet are thick, ridged, and brittle.

**HEENT**

*Head.* No palpable masses or tenderness. Hair is short, coarse, curly, black with some gray, neatly groomed. Scalp is clean and without lesions or scaling. Face is symmetrical, no droops or swelling, no tenderness on palpation. Temporomandibular joint (TMJ) is fully mobile without crepitation or pain.

*Eyes.* Pupils equal, round, reactive to light and accommodation (PERRLA). Visual fields equal to examiner; full range of extraocular movements (EOMs) without nystagmus. Visual acuity 20/25 on right eye and 20/30 on left eye using Rosenbaum chart with glasses in place.

*Ears.* Able to discern whisper test at 2 ft (62 cm); both ears symmetrically placed and equal in size and shape. *Rinne test:* Air conduction > bone conduction. *Weber test:* Lateralization of sound equal in both ears.

*Nose.* Nostrils are patent; no nasal deviation noted.

*Mouth/Throat.* Mucous membranes are dusky pink, smooth and moist; uvula is midline. Several teeth are missing. Tonsils present, not enlarged.

**Neck**

Trachea is midline; thyroid gland not enlarged or palpable. No nodes noted.

**Pulmonary**

Slight barrel chest; anteroposterior diameter less than 2:1. No abnormalities in rate or rhythm. Lungs clear to auscultation; resonance on percussion bilaterally.

**Breast**

Normal male breasts. Nipples dark brown, no exudate, no swelling, masses or tenderness.

**Cardiovascular**

$S_1$ and $S_2$, no $S_3$ or $S_4$, no murmurs; point of maximal intensity (PMI) identified at 5th intercostal space at left midclavicular line.

**Peripheral Vascular**

Pulses in upper extremities are normal. Pulses in lower extremities are diminished (see chart). Temperature of lower extremities is cool to the touch below the knees bilaterally. Left leg is significantly cooler from midshin to toes when compared with the right leg. Color seems dusky but is difficult to assess due to patient's natural dark color.

**Peripheral Pulses**
Temporal—4 bilaterally
Carotid—4 bilaterally
Brachial—4 bilaterally
Radial—4 bilaterally
Femoral—2 bilaterally
Popliteal—3 on right and 1 on left
Posterior tibialis—3 on right and 0 on left
Dorsalis pedis—3 on right and 0 on left

**Peripheral Pulse Scale**

| |
|---|
| 0—Absent |
| 1—Markedly diminished |
| 2—Moderately diminished |
| 3—Slightly diminished |
| 4—Normal |

*Abdomen*

Moderately rounded; active bowel sounds in all 4 quadrants; soft, no tenderness or masses noted. Liver size 8 cm (3 in.) percussed at right midclavicular line; liver not palpable.

*Musculoskeletal*

Full range of motion of upper extremities. Muscle strength of upper extremities is normal; no pain on movement. Limited range of motion in lower extremities due to pain on movement.

*Neurological*

***Mental Status.*** Alert, oriented × 3, cooperative, aware of condition, good historian.
***Cranial Nerves.*** I through XII intact.
***Sensory.*** Diminished response to light touch on left leg from knee to toes; right leg is within normal limits. Complains of numbness and tingling in lower left leg.

### *Deep Tendon Reflexes*

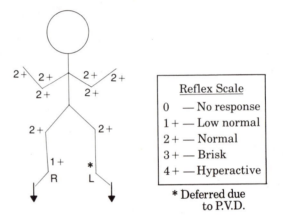

Reflex Scale

0  — No response
1 + — Low normal
2 + — Normal
3 + — Brisk
4 + — Hyperactive

\* Deferred due to P.V.D.

*Rectal*

Prostate 5 cm (2 in.), firm, smooth, no tenderness.

*Genitalia*

Penis nontender, no discharge. Testes nontender, no pitting.

## Laboratory Data/Diagnostic Studies

*Laboratory Data*

***Hemoglobin:*** 14 g/dl
***Hematocrit:*** 42%
***WBC:*** 6.8 mm³
***Na:*** 138 mEq/L
***K:*** 3.6 mEq/L
***Cl:*** 99 mEq/L

***CO₂:*** 23 mM/L
***BUN:*** 12 mg/dl
***Creatinine:*** 0.9 mg/dl
***Cholesterol:*** 275 mg/100 ml
***Triglycerides:*** 240/100 ml
***Blood sugar (fasting):*** 140 mg/dl

*Diagnostic Studies*

***Chest X-Ray.*** Slight flattening of diaphragm; otherwise within normal limits (WNL).
***Angiography.*** Demonstrates markedly decreased flow distal to the femoral popliteal segment of left leg.
***Doppler.*** Sounds of blood flow are slurred in the left lower extremity distal to the popliteal artery.
***Pulse Volume Recording (PVR).*** Prolonged and flattened.
***Electrocardiogram.*** Within normal limits.
***Ankle-Arm Index Pressure:*** < 0.5.

# COLLABORATIVE PLAN OF CARE

| | |
|---|---|
| *Diet* | Patient is on a 1500-calorie, low-fat, low-cholesterol, 2-g sodium diet. |
| *Medications* | Probucol (Lorelco) 500 mg PO bid.<br>Pentoxifylline (Trental) 400 mg PO bid.<br>Chlorothiazide sodium (Diuril) 500 mg PO qd.<br>Milk of magnesia (MOM) 30–60 ml PO qhs prn.<br>Oxycodone and acetaminophen (Percocet) 1–2 tabs PO q4h prn for pain.<br>Triazolam (Halcion) 0.125 mg PO qhs prn. |
| *Intravenous Therapy* | Does not apply. |
| *Therapeutic Measures* | Temperature, pulse, respirations (TPR) and blood pressure bid.<br>Monitor peripheral pulses in lower extremities q4h.<br>Weight once a week.<br>Out of bed as tolerated; encourage moderate activity.<br>Protect extremities from injury.<br>Keep extremities warm; avoid application of external heat.<br>Do not elevate legs when up in chair.<br>Keep foot of bed flat.<br>Special foot and skin care.<br>No smoking. |
| *Consults* | Nutrition consult. |
| *Preoperative Plan* | Begin preoperative teaching for femoral popliteal bypass graft surgery. |

# NURSING DIAGNOSES DEVELOPED IN CARE PLAN

Pain, p. 45
Potential Impaired Skin Integrity, p. 47
Altered Nutrition: More than Body Requirements, p. 48

# ADDITIONAL NURSING DIAGNOSES TO BE CONSIDERED

Activity Intolerance
Altered Sexuality Patterns
Altered Tissue Perfusion, Peripheral
Home Maintenance Management, Impaired
Knowledge Deficit
Sleep Pattern Disturbance

# NURSING CARE PLAN BASED ON IDENTIFIED NURSING DIAGNOSES

| | |
|---|---|
| *Pain* | ***Related to:*** Decreased tissue perfusion to lower extremities.<br>***Evidenced by:*** Complaints of leg pain at rest and with ambulation. |

| Desired Patient Outcomes | • The patient's pain will be minimized and/or controlled.<br>• The patient will be knowledgeable about pain relief measures. |
| --- | --- |
| Evaluation Criteria | *Prior to Surgery, the Patient Will:*<br>• Report increased comfort levels.<br>*After Instruction, the Patient Will:*<br>• Demonstrate use of relaxation techniques.<br>• Report decreased anxiety level.<br>• State methods used to promote circulation to lower extremities.<br>• Discuss the proper use of pain medications. |

## Interventions

Encourage patient to verbalize fears and feelings about pain.

Discuss the physiological causes of leg pain.

Identify with patient the methods to promote circulation and reduce pain. Some examples are:

• Place bed in reverse Trendelenburg position either by increasing the head of bed by 15 degrees or by using 6-in (15-cm) blocks, and sit with feet in a dependent position.
• Avoid crossing legs and sitting with knees bent for prolonged periods.

Maintain a warm environment without extremes of hot and cold.

Avoid constrictive clothing.

Discuss the effects of cigarette smoking and the importance of not smoking.

Discuss the availability of and rationale for pain medications.

Discuss the preventative approach to pain controls.

## Rationale

"Heightened anxiety is known to increase pain" (Turner, 1986, p. 238).

When the individual understands what is causing a particular bodily state, this understanding will reduce anxiety which, in turn, will reduce pain (Radwin, 1987, p. 260).

Dependent positioning of lower extremities while in bed will increase peripheral blood flow, thus decreasing pain (Luckmann and Sorensen, 1987, p. 1092).

Sitting for long periods with knees bent or crossed results in undue pressure on popliteal vessels, which decreases circulation to and from the area and causes leg swelling and pain (Kneisl and Ames, 1986, p. 851).

A warm environment is important because it causes vasodilatation, which in turn increases blood supply to the extremities (Kneisl and Ames, 1986, p. 851).

Constricted clothing may compromise circulation to already deficient areas (Kneisl and Ames, 1986, p. 851).

Smoking causes vasoconstriction of both small and large blood vessels and damages intimal cells (Kneisl and Ames, 1986, p. 842). Studies have found that smoking after arterial bypass surgery is associated with poorer graft patency rates (Turner, 1986, p. 235).

Analgesics may be used for symptomatic relief in the person with peripheral vascular disease (PVD). Analgesics are most effective if they are given before pain becomes severe (Heldrick and Perry, 1982, p. 1829).

See above.

## Interventions

Instruct the patient in relaxation and distraction techniques.

## Rationale

Relaxation training can reduce anxiety and be useful in pain management (Wells, 1982, p. 236). Distraction focuses on pleasant situations unrelated to pain that take the mind away from the experience of pain (Carrieri, Lindsey, and West, 1986, p. 260).

---

**Potential Impaired Skin Integrity**

*Related to:* Impaired circulation in the lower extremities. *Evidenced by:* Altered sensation in the left lower extremity. Temperature change in the lower extremity. Shiny, scaly, thin skin in the lower extremity.

**Desired Patient Outcomes**

• The patient's skin will remain intact.
• The patient will be knowledgeable about measures to maintain intact skin.

**Evaluation Criteria**

*During the Hospital Stay, the Patient Will:*
• Verbalize an understanding of foot care measures and perform self foot care.
• Protect the lower extremities from injury.
• Utilize pressure-relieving devices for the lower extremities.
• Discuss measures to prevent injury to the lower extremities while in the hospital and after discharge.

---

## Interventions

Assess the lower extremities for change in skin color, sensation, and skin breakdown.

Instruct the patient and perform daily foot care to include:

• Washing with warm water and mild soap.
• Pat area dry, especially between toes.
• Apply emollient cream to area.
• May place lambswool between toes.
• Inspection of toenails and referral to podiatrist if indicated.
• Use white cotton socks and loose-fitting shoes or slippers.

Teach the patient to use pressure-relieving devices for the lower extremities.

Avoid keeping the extremities in 1 position for a long period of time.

Keep the bed linen and any additional clothing that comes in contact with the patient dry.

## Rationale

Hygiene measures and prevention of injury are important to promote skin integrity in order to maintain the skin as the first line of defense (Turner, 1986, p. 724).

Foot care is an essential element for people with peripheral vascular disease; it is a way of life (Luckmann and Sorensen, 1987, p. 1096).

Pressure-relieving devices provide for more even distribution of weight over the body surface. Pressure over time will cause tissue breakdown (Fowler, 1987, p. 458).

Patients at high risk and immobile need to be moved as often as every 30–60 minutes to prevent tissue breakdown (Fowler, 1987, p. 459).

Moisture reduces the resistance of the skin to ulceration and infection. Wet epidermal tissue has decreased tensile strength and is easily macerated by compression and eroded by frictional forces (Maklebust, 1987, p. 369).

## Interventions

Teach the patient to avoid exposing his lower extremities to hot or cold temperatures (i.e., bath water, heating pad, cold weather).

Teach the patient to protect his lower extremities from injury (i.e., cuts, bruises, abrasions, tight-fitting shoes, walking barefoot).

## Rationale

A patient with decreased sensation will not perceive injurious temperature changes (Turner, 1986, p. 725).

Tissues that are poorly nourished are more susceptible to damage and bacterial invasion. Trauma to the extremities should be avoided. Constricting clothing and accessories will impede circulation (Brunner and Suddarth, 1988, p. 629).

---

### Altered Nutrition: More than Body Requirements

**Related to:** Dysfunctional eating patterns. Imbalance between food intake and energy expenditure.
**Evidenced by:** Weight 20% over ideal for height and frame. Elevated blood pressure. Diet pattern as presented by the patient. Sedentary activity level.

### Desired Patient/Family Outcomes

• The patient will understand his weight problem and related risk factors.
• The patient and wife will be knowledgeable about the patient's prescribed diet, meal planning, and food preparation techniques.

### Evaluation Criteria

**After Instruction, the Patient or Wife Will:**
• Choose and consume foods that are consistent with the diet prescription.
• Discuss the risk factors associated with obesity.
• Describe methods of meal planning and food preparation consistent with a weight reduction diet.
• Discuss becoming a member of a group that assists in maintaining weight control.

---

## Interventions

Review with the patient his diet history and focus on eating patterns and his emotions just prior to eating.

Discuss with the patient the fact that obesity is one of several risk factors associated with atherosclerosis. Additional risk factors include cigarette smoking, use of tobacco, hypertension, diabetes, and a high-fat, high-cholesterol diet. Discuss with the patient the fact that there is a positive relationship between body weight and blood pressure.

Invite the patient's wife to contribute to the discussions concerning the patient's diet and plans to modify the existing diet.

## Rationale

Food records as identified by the patient provide the best target for change (Simko, Cowell, and Gilbride, 1984, p. 127). As a first step in a behavior modification program, eating and activity patterns must be identified (Shils and Young, 1988, p. 810).

Specific risk factors have been associated with atherosclerosis. These factors include cigarette smoking, tobacco use, hypertension, diabetes, diets high in fat content and cholesterol, and a family history of atherosclerosis. Atherosclerosis as well as associated ischemic disorders are caused by the altered metabolism that accompanies obesity (Luckmann and Sorensen, 1987, pp. 1101, 1291). Weight reduction is an effective nonpharmacological modality to be used to reduce blood pressure. Research has demonstrated that when a person with high blood pressure loses weight, a reduction in blood pressure can be measured (Patrick, et al, 1986, p. 611). Reductions in both systolic and diastolic blood pressure have been demonstrated with a weight loss program (Cunningham, 1987, p. 19).

Weight loss efforts tend to be more successful if a supportive person or group of people can be of assistance (Suitor and Crowley, 1984, p. 470).

| Interventions | Rationale |
|---|---|

*Interventions*

Provide the patient and his wife with information/literature concerning sound nutritional practices:

- Lower intake of foods high in cholesterol and saturated fat.
- Reduce alcohol consumption.
- Restrict dietary sodium.
- Increase fiber content in the diet.
- Eat more fresh fruit and vegetables.
- Reduce intake of total calories.

Discuss a weight reduction diet with regard to the patient's individual food likes and dislikes.

Discuss with the patient and his wife food preparation techniques and meal planning.

Discuss the role of exercise in a weight reduction diet.

Discuss with the patient the usefulness of a support group and weight control group.

*Rationale*

The traditional means of helping clients lose weight is through the use of a balanced reducing diet (Suitor and Crowley, 1984, p. 467).

Since an obese person should be on a diet for a long period of time, the diet should be acceptable and fit the tastes and habits of the individual for eating at home and away from home (Shils and Young, 1988, p. 808).

Diet instruction should include information on menu planning, shopping, food preparation, and eating away from home (Suitor and Crowley, 1984, p. 500).

Exercise is a valuable adjunct in a weight reduction regimen. If energy expenditure can be increased by incremental physical activity and if food intake is kept constant, weight will drop (Shils and Young, 1988, p. 808).

Becoming an active participant in a weight reducing group helps many people lose weight (Suitor and Crowley, 1984, p. 470). A support group as a mode of intervention merges two perspectives, social support and small groups. Social support assists a person in coping with stressful events and in the maintenance of health (Bulechek and McCloskey, 1985, p. 186).

## QUESTIONS FOR DISCUSSION

1. Define intermittent claudication.
2. Compare and contrast the assessment findings for the patient with arterial vascular disease with those of a patient with venous insufficiency.
3. Discuss the treatment modalities for essential hypertension.
4. An angiography, a Doppler ultrasound, and a pulse volume recording (PVR) were performed as part of the vascular workup. Explain their purpose.
5. Mr. Holland asks you to explain the femoral popliteal bypass graft procedure again, saying his doctor went over it too fast. How would you explain this surgery? Why is an autograft preferable to a synthetic graft?
6. Postoperatively 2 important concerns are monitoring and maintaining the patency of the graft. Explain how you would do this. Identify signs and symptoms of a failing graft.

## REFERENCES

Brunner, LS and Suddarth, DS: Textbook of Medical-Surgical Nursing, ed 6. JB Lippincott, Philadelphia, 1988.

Bulechek, GM and McCloskey, JC: Nursing Interventions: Treatments for Nursing Diagnoses. WB Saunders, Philadelphia, 1985.

Carrieri, VK, Lindsey, AM, and West, CM: Pathophysiological Phenomena in Nursing: Human Responses to Illness. WB Saunders, Philadelphia, 1986.

Cunningham, SG: Nonpharmacologic management of high blood pressure. Cardiovasc Nurs 23:18, 1987.

Fowler, EM: Equipment and products used in management and treatment of pressure ulcers. Nurs Clin North Am 22:449, 1987.

Heldrick, G and Perry, S: Helping the patient in pain. Am J Nurs, 82:1829, 1982.

Kneisl, CR and Ames, SW: Adult Health Nursing: A Biopsychosocial Approach. Addison-Wesley, Menlo Park, Calif, 1986.

Luckmann, J and Sorensen, KC: Medical-Surgical Nursing: A Psychophysiologic Approach, ed 3. WB Saunders, Philadelphia, 1987.

Maklebust, J: Pressure Ulcers: Etiology and Prevention. Nurs Clin North Am 22:359, 1987.

Patrick, ML, et al: Medical Surgical Nursing: Pathophysiological Concepts. JB Lippincott, Philadelphia, 1986.

Radwin, LE: Autonomous nursing interventions for treating the patient in acute pain: A standard. Heart Lung 16:258, 1987.

Shils, EM and Young, VR: Modern Nutrition in Health and Disease, ed 7. Lea & Febiger, Philadelphia, 1988.

Simko, MD, Cowell, C, and Gilbride, JA: Nutrition Assessment: A Comprehensive Guide for Planning Intervention. Aspen Systems Corp, 1984.

Suitor, CW and Crowley, MF: Nutrition Principles and Application in Health Promotion. JB Lippincott, Philadelphia, 1984.

Turner, J: Nursing intervention and patients with peripheral vascular disease. Nurs Clin North Am 21:233, 1986.

Wells, N: The effect of relaxation on postoperative muscle tension and pain. Nurs Res 31:236, 1982.

# BIBLIOGRAPHY

Ameli, FM, et al: Etiology and management of aorto-femoral bypass graft failure. J Cardiovasc Surg 28:695, 1987.

Snetselaar, LG: Nutrition Counseling Skills Assessment, Treatment and Evaluation. Aspen Publishing, Rockville, Md, 1983.

Spies, ME: Vascular complications associated with diabetes mellitus. Nurs Clin North Am 18:721, 1983.

Ventura, MR, et al: Effectiveness of health promotion interventions. Nurs Res 33:162, 1984.

Warbinek, E and Wyness, MA: Designing nursing care for patients with peripheral arterial occlusive disease. Part 1: Update. Cardiovasc Nurs 22:1, 1986.

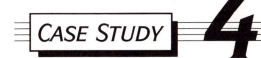

# A PATIENT WITH A MYOCARDIAL INFARCTION

Sharon P. Sullivan, M.S.,R.N.

## ANATOMY

### Structure of the Heart

The heart is a cone-shaped, muscular, 4-chambered pump located between the lungs in the mediastinal space of the intrathoracic cavity. The 4 cardiac chambers form right- and left-sided pumps composed of an upper chamber (atrium) and a lower chamber (ventricle). A muscular wall, the septum, separates the right and left chambers. The atria serve as reservoirs and entryways for blood flowing into the ventricles. The pumping action of the ventricle ejects blood into the lungs or the systemic circulation. The forward directional flow is controlled by the 2 atrioventricular and 2 semilunar valves.

The wall of the heart is composed of 3 layers: the outer layer, or epicardium; the muscular layer, or myocardium; and the innermost layer, or endocardium. The left ventricular wall is 2–3 times as thick as the right ventricle because the left ventricle pumps blood throughout the systemic circulation, a high-pressure system. In contrast, the right ventricle delivers blood into the low-pressure pulmonary circulation (Porth, 1986).

### Coronary Circulation

The blood supply for the heart is provided by the left main and right coronary arteries, which branch from the aorta in the region of the sinus of Valsalva. The coronary arteries extend over the surface of the heart and penetrate through the wall of the myocardium and branch further. The left main coronary artery divides into 2 main branches: the left anterior descending (LAD) artery and the left circumflex artery. The LAD artery supplies blood to the anterior wall of the left ventricle, the septum, and the apex of the heart. The left circumflex artery supplies blood to the left atrium and the lateral and posterior walls of the left ventricle. The right coronary artery supplies the right atrium, right ventricle, and the inferior wall of the left ventricle, as well as the sinoatrial (SA) node and the atrioventricular (AV) node (Fig. 4–1).

### Conduction System

The normal rhythmic excitation and contraction of the heart is initiated by specialized cells in the conduction system. Pacemaker cells generate the cardiac impulses that travel the conduction pathway. The structures of the conduction system are the SA node, the AV node, the bundle of His, right and left bundle branches, and the Purkinje fibers.

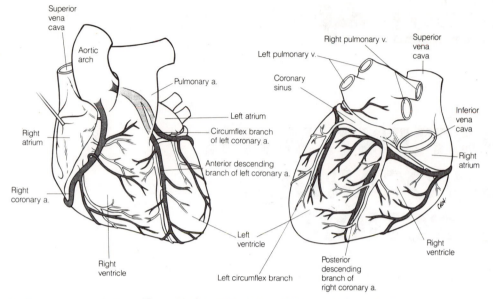

**FIGURE 4–1.** Coronary circulation. (From Hudak, CM, Gallo, BM, and Lohr, TS: Critical Care Nursing, ed 4. JB Lippincott, Philadelphia, p 221, 1986, with permission.)

# PHYSIOLOGY OF THE CORONARY CIRCULATION

The efficiency of the heart as a pump depends on a constant supply of oxygen and the availability of other nutrients for myocardial contraction. Since oxygen cannot be stored by myocardial tissue, a continuous supply is critical to ensure myocardial function. The oxygen supply is derived from blood in the coronary arteries.

The blood flow in the coronary arteries is regulated by the metabolic and oxygen demands of the myocardial tissue. If there is an increase in myocardial oxygen demands, the oxygen supply must also increase to meet the demand. To increase the supply of oxygen, coronary artery blood flow must increase since myocardial utilization of oxygen is maximal under normal conditions (Underhill, et al, 1982).

Myocardial oxygen demands are determined by 4 factors: the tension the heart must generate to pump blood, the stroke volume that is ejected, the contractile state, and the heart rate (Porth, 1986).

The flow of blood through coronary arteries can be affected by various factors. During systole, myocardial contraction compresses the coronary arteries and causes a reduction in blood flow. The major portion of coronary blood flow occurs during diastole. With increased heart rates, time spent in diastole is reduced and may affect coronary perfusion. Coronary circulation is autoregulated, which means that the heart has the ability to adjust vascular tone to maintain a constant flow of blood. Fibers from the autonomic nervous system innervate the coronary arteries and play a role in coronary blood flow by influencing vascular resistance; stimulation of the α-receptors produces vasoconstriction and that of β-receptors produces vasodilatation. Various substances released by myocardial tissue during periods of increased oxygen demand have been suggested as causing vasodilatation. Substances such as carbon dioxide, lactic acid, hydrogen ions, histamine, and others, as well as reduced oxygen tension, have been implicated as possible mediators (Porth, 1986).

Arteries that are diseased with atherosclerosis are unable to dilate, inhibiting the increase in blood flow necessary when there is an increased demand for oxygen delivery. When the oxygen demand exceeds the capacity of the vessel to supply oxygen, myocardial ischemia results (Price and Wilson, 1986).

# PATHOPHYSIOLOGY

Myocardial infarction (MI) results from "prolonged ischemia to the myocardium with irreversible cell damage and muscle death" (Porth, 1986, p. 248). It is usually accompanied by complete cessation of blood flow to the affected area.

The cause of myocardial infarction is commonly associated with atherosclerotic coronary artery disease (CAD). In this form of arteriosclerosis, fatty fibrous plaques progressively narrow the lumen of the coronary artery compromising the flow of blood to myocardial tissue. As the lumen narrows, the balance between myocardial oxygen supply and demand is threatened. Plaque formation becomes significant when it has progressed to obstructing more than 75% of the vessel lumen. Myocardial ischemia and dysfunction result.

Development and recruitment of collateral circulation to reroute blood flow may partially compensate for the compromised vessel and limit or delay infarction. In the person with severe CAD, this may be insufficient to prevent the ischemia or infarction.

In the final step leading to a total blockage of the vessel lumen and infarction, a number of possible events are thought to occur:
1. Progressive narrowing of the vessel lumen by plaque enlargement
2. Formation of a thrombus initiated by platelet aggregation
3. Embolization of a thrombus or plaque fragment
4. Hemorrhage into the plaque
5. Coronary artery spasm

Myocardial infarction almost always occurs in the left ventricle and can involve the full thickness of the wall (transmural) or some portion of the wall (subendocardial). The location of the infarct is described in terms of its location on the left ventricular wall, and it corresponds with a particular region of the coronary circulation. For example, an anterior infarction usually results from occlusion of the LAD coronary artery.

All infarcts have a core of necrotic tissue that is functionally dead, surrounded by a zone of ischemia. Ischemic zones are variable in size, supplied by a waxing and waning blood flow. The fate of these marginal zones will ultimately determine the size of the infarct (Underhill, et al, 1982).

Myocardial infarctions can significantly depress left ventricular function due to the loss of contractility in the necrotic tissue and the impaired contractility in ischemic areas. The larger the size of the infarct, the greater the effect on left ventricular function. The severity of the dysfunction depends not only on the size of the infarct, but also on its location. A transmural infarct has a greater impact than a subendocardial infarct because all the layers of the myocardial wall are involved. Additional factors to consider include the function of the uninvolved myocardium, the patency of collateral circulation, and the cardiovascular compensatory mechanism to preserve cardiac output and peripheral perfusion (Price and Wilson, 1986).

## RISK FACTORS

Multiple risk factors have been identified as increasing a person's susceptibility to the development of CAD. These factors probably interact to accelerate the atherosclerotic process. Modifying risk factors may slow the progress of the disease. CAD risk factors are divided into modifiable and nonmodifiable factors. The 4 nonmodifiable factors are age, sex (male), family history, and race. Modifiable risk factors include elevated serum lipid levels, hypertension, cigarette smoking, impaired glucose tolerance, stress, obesity, and sedentary lifestyle.

## COMMON CLINICAL FINDINGS

The majority of persons experiencing an MI complain of chest pain. Typically, the chest pain is severe and prolonged, located substernally with radiation to the neck, jaw, or left arm and accompanied by nausea, vomiting, sweating, and extreme anxiety. The chest pain signals the presence of myocardial ischemia, and if it lasts longer than 30–45 minutes, it causes irreversible damage and necrosis.

A diagnosis of MI is confirmed when laboratory studies reveal elevated cardiac enzyme levels. Electrocardiographic changes, ST and T wave changes, and a prolonged Q wave also show the evidence of an acute infarction.

The complications occurring after an MI and their severity relate to the extent and location of the infarct and the changes that take place within the infarcted area. The most common complications include recurrent chest pain, arrhythmias, pericarditis, congestive heart failure, pulmonary edema, and the lethal cardiogenic shock. Unusual but potentially fatal complications that can occur in the acute period are ventricular septal defect, rupture of the heart, and rupture of the papillary muscle.

## TREATMENT MODALITIES

The goals of treatment in the person with an MI are (1) management of the acute attack; (2) early detection and prevention of complications; and (3) rehabilitation and education.

In the early treatment of the acute attack, therapeutic measures are aimed at relieving chest pain, stabilizing heart rhythm, and reducing cardiac workload. Pain relief is achieved with the use of nitrates and calcium channel blockers by redistributing blood flow to ischemic areas and also with narcotics for both pain relief and sedation. Prophylactic use of antiarrhythmics may be given to prevent ventricular dysrhythmias. Supplemental oxygen maintains the oxygen content of blood perfusing coronary arteries. Drugs may also be needed to improve contractility and increase blood pressure. Rest is an important intervention, allowing time for the healing and recovery of damaged tissue and reducing cardiac workload.

More recent advances in the treatment of an acute MI are directed toward acute reperfusion of the newly occluded coronary artery in the attempt to limit the infarction. Current research indicates that thrombosis is responsible for part of the blockage in the coronary artery, and thrombolytic therapy with tissue plasminogen activator (TPA) dissolves or lyses the clot and reestablishes blood flow to the occluded artery. Angioplasty and anticoagulants may be indicated to reduce the risk of thrombosis (Price and Wilson, 1986).

Cardiac rehabilitation programs in the acute period aid the person in reaching an activity level required for self-care. In the long term, the goals are to provide cardiovascular conditioning, restore the individual to optimal health, and prevent or slow the progression of the disease process (Underhill, et al, 1982).

# PATIENT ASSESSMENT DATA BASE

## Health History

*Client:*
John Norton

*Address:* 34 No. Main St., Syracuse, NY
*Telephone:* 963-1234
*Contact:* Carol (wife)
*Address of contact:* Same as patient
*Telephone of contact:* Same as patient
*Age:* 50    *Sex:* Male    *Race:* White
*Educational background:* High school
*Religion:* Roman Catholic    *Marital status:* Married
*Usual occupation:* Contractor
*Present occupation:* Same
*Source of income:* Self-employed
*Insurance:* Blue Cross/Blue Shield
*Source of referral:* Self
*Source of history:* Patient
*Reliability of historian:* Reliable
*Date of interview:* 2/15/90
Reason for visit/Chief complaint: "While at work on Friday morning, I began having this ache in my chest and left arm. I thought it was just a muscle cramp, but after an hour, I began feeling pretty bad. The pain was the worst I've ever experienced—it was like something heavy was sitting on my chest. I was sweating and feeling sick to my stomach. I knew something wasn't right so I came to the hospital. They told me it was my heart."

# HEALTH PERCEPTION/HEALTH MANAGEMENT PATTERN

*Present Health Status*

Mr. Norton describes himself as being very healthy, "I have never been sick a day in my life, except for colds." Since his admission 2 days ago, he has had brief episodes of chest pain, "but not as bad as the pain that I came in with." He realizes that he has had a heart attack but states: "I can't understand why it happened to me when I've never had any heart problems before." He spent 2 days in the coronary care unit (CCU) and then moved to a step-down unit on 2/15.

**Past Health Status**

***General Health.*** General health has been excellent, with no major health problems.
***Prophylactic Medical/Dental Care.*** Sees a physician every 3–5 years for medical checkups. Annual dental visits.
***Childhood Illnesses.*** Unknown.
***Immunizations.*** All childhood immunizations; last tetanus shot in 1981.
***Major Illnesses/Hospitalizations.*** Appendectomy (age 11).

***Current Medications***
*Prescription:* None.
*Nonprescription:* Cold remedies prn.
***Allergies.*** Penicillin ("gets hives").

***Habits***
*Alcohol:* 1–2 beers usually about twice a week.
*Caffeine:* 5–6 cups of coffee a day.
*Drugs:* See Current Medications.
*Tobacco:* One pack of cigarettes a day for the last 30 years.

***Family Health History***

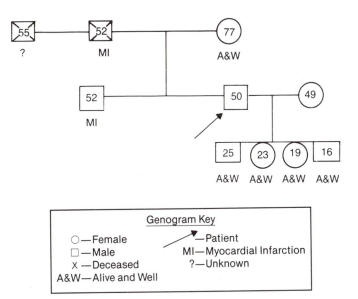

NUTRITIONAL/METABOLIC PATTERN

**Nutritional**

Mr. Norton follows no special diet; enjoys his wife's cooking. Began reducing the amount of cholesterol in his diet about 3 years ago. He uses margarine, drinks low-fat milk, and his wife uses corn oil for cooking. He doesn't add salt to his foods. Denies food allergies or intolerances.

***Usual Daily Menu***
*Breakfast:* Toast (2–3 slices) with margarine or muffin, 1 fried egg, 1 glass of juice, 2 cups of coffee with cream.
*Lunch:* Tuna fish or turkey sandwich, pickles, bag of chips, 1 slice of cake or pie, 1 cup of coffee with cream.
*Dinner:* Chicken breast, baked potato with margarine, small salad with creamy dressing, 1 dish of ice cream, 2 cups of coffee with cream.
Recently, his appetite has been only fair. "I'm eating, but not enjoying my food."

*Metabolic*

Weight has been stable at 200 lb (90 kg) for last 5–10 years.

## Elimination Pattern

*Bowel*

Normal bowel pattern is 1, soft-formed, brown stool every day, usually in AM and without use of laxatives. Stool softeners have been prescribed since admission. Last bowel movement was on the morning of admission. Denies feeling constipated.

*Bladder*

Urinates 4–6 times per day. Denies burning, urgency, or difficulty. Urine is clear and yellow in color.

## Activity/Exercise Pattern

*Activity/Exercise*

Job-related activities, that is, climbing, bending, and lifting. Occasionally plays basketball with his son. He also enjoys doing his own automotive work. Since admission, he has experienced 2 episodes of chest pain while washing up and 1 after eating dinner. He complains of being tired, "after doing nothing all day." Requires a brief nap in the afternoon.

### Self-Care Ability

| | |
|---|---|
| Feeding — 0 | Grooming — 0 |
| Bathing — 0 | General mobility — 0 |
| Toileting — 0 | Cooking — 0 |
| Bed mobility — 0 | Home maintenance — 0 |
| Dressing — 0 | Shopping — 0 |

> *Functional Levels Code*
> 0 — Full self-care
> I — Requires use of equipment or device
> II — Requires assistance or supervision from another person
> III — Requires assistance or supervision from another person and equipment or device
> IV — Is dependent and does not participate

*Oxygenation/Perfusion*

**Chest x-ray:** Had a chest x-ray this admission. Last chest x-ray (1981) was normal. Denies having dyspnea at rest or on exertion. Currently, uses oxygen only during episodes of chest pain.

### Cardiac Risk Factors

| | Positive | Negative |
|---|---|---|
| Sedentary life-style | | X |
| Hyperlipidemia | X | |
| Cigarette smoking | X | |
| Diabetes | | X |
| Obesity | | X |
| Hypertension | | X |
| Hypervigilant personality | | X |
| Family history of heart disease | X | |

## Sleep/Rest Pattern

*Sleep/Rest*

Usually sleeps 6–7 hours at night. He has no trouble falling asleep; frequently watches TV before bedtime. Uses no sleep aids.

At present, sleep is disturbed by pill taking, and he has been requesting a sleeping pill at night. Able to sleep flat, with 1 pillow.

## COGNITIVE/PERCEPTUAL PATTERN

| | |
|---|---|
| *Hearing* | Has no problem with hearing; no earaches, vertigo, or ringing in ears. |
| *Vision* | Wears glasses; prescription changed 2 years ago. |
| *Sensory Perception* | Mr. Norton gets anxious when he has chest pain: "I'm afraid something is wrong." He is right-hand dominant. |
| *Learning Style* | Learns best by use of written materials and audiovisual aids. |

## SELF-PERCEPTION/SELF-CONCEPT PATTERN

| | |
|---|---|
| *Self-Perception/Self-Concept* | Mr. Norton describes himself as being a very independent, hard-working family man. He sees himself as the outgoing type; he finds it easy to get along with others and enjoys being around other people. |

## ROLE/RELATIONSHIP PATTERN

| | |
|---|---|
| *Role/Relationship* | Mr. Norton lives in a 4-bedroom ranch style home in a suburban area. He married his high school sweetheart 28 years ago. They have 4 children, 2 daughters and 2 sons. The oldest son works for him, and they have a close relationship. His wife works part-time as a secretary now that their children are grown. |

## SEXUALITY/REPRODUCTIVE PATTERN

| | |
|---|---|
| *Sexuality/Reproductive* | He describes his relationship with his wife as being close and loving. Sexual relations have never been a problem with them. He doesn't anticipate that his sex life will be changed because of his heart attack. |

## COPING/STRESS TOLERANCE PATTERN

| | |
|---|---|
| *Coping/Stress Tolerance* | Mr. Norton feels that he has been able to cope with most stressors and problems in his life to his satisfaction. He finds that his contracting business can be stressful at times, and it is not always easy to schedule vacations. His oldest son has been a big help with running the business, and he is relying on him "to keep things going." Relaxes best by working with his hands. He admits that smoking is harmful, but finds it difficult to be without cigarettes, especially when he is tense. |

## VALUE/BELIEF PATTERN

| | |
|---|---|
| *Value/Belief* | Believes strongly in the work ethic: "You need to work for what you want." He was raised as a Catholic, but only attends church on "special" occasions. He has a strong belief in God and raised his family the same way. He has requested to see the hospital chaplain. |

# Physical Examination

| | |
|---|---|
| *General Survey* | Fifty-year-old man, appearing his stated age; pleasant, cooperative; in no distress. *Height:* 6 ft 1 in. (185 cm). *Weight:* 200 lb (91 kg). |

| | |
|---|---|
| **Vital Signs** | **Temperature:** 98.8°F (37.1°C) (oral)<br>**Pulse:** 90 regular (apical)<br>**Respirations:** 18<br>**BP:** 130/82 (right arm, sitting). |
| **Integument** | **Skin.** Tan color, warm, moist, normal thickness and turgor.<br>**Mucous Membranes.** Pink, moist, intact.<br>**Nails.** Beds smooth; no clubbing. |
| **HEENT** | **Head.** Hair—dark brown with gray streaks, straight. Scalp—no tenderness. Face is symmetrical. Temporomandibular joint (TMJ) without crepitations.<br>**Eyes.** Vision (not tested), corrected with glasses. Extraocular movements (EOMs) intact. Pupils equal, round, reactive to light and accommodation (PERRLA).<br>**Ears.** Auricles intact bilaterally; canals clear.<br>**Nose.** Passages patent.<br>**Mouth/Throat.** Membranes and pharynx pink and moist; teeth intact. |
| **Neck** | Full range of motion; no jugular venous distention (JVD); no enlarged nodes. |
| **Pulmonary** | Thorax is oval; anteroposterior (AP) diameter 2:1; lungs are resonant with bibasilar rales that clear with cough. |
| **Breast** | No lumps, pain, discharge. |
| **Cardiovascular** | Normal $S_1$, $S_2$; point of maximal impulse (PMI) at fifth intercostal space at left midclavicular line. |

**Peripheral Vascular**

| Peripheral Pulses | Peripheral Pulse Scale |
|---|---|
| Temporal—4 bilaterally<br>Carotid—4 bilaterally<br>Brachial—4 bilaterally<br>Radial—4 bilaterally<br>Femoral—4 bilaterally<br>Popliteal—4 bilaterally<br>Posterior tibial—4 bilaterally<br>Dorsalis pedis—4 bilaterally | 0—Absent<br>1—Markedly diminished<br>2—Moderately diminished<br>3—Slightly diminished<br>4—Normal |

| | |
|---|---|
| **Abdomen** | Active bowel sounds present in all 4 quadrants. Abdomen is soft; no tenderness or masses; liver, spleen, and kidney not palpated. |
| **Musculoskeletal** | Full range of joint motion in all extremities; muscle strength normal against resistance and gravity. Gait not tested. |
| **Neurological** | **Mental Status.** Alert; oriented × 3<br>**Cranial Nerves.** II through XII intact.<br>**Sensory.** Light touch, pain, and vibration to face, trunk, and extremities within normal limits. |

*Deep Tendon Reflexes*

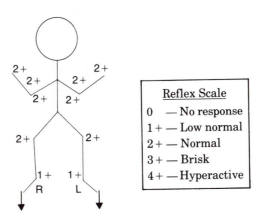

| Reflex Scale | |
|---|---|
| 0 | — No response |
| 1 + | — Low normal |
| 2 + | — Normal |
| 3 + | — Brisk |
| 4 + | — Hyperactive |

**Rectal**

Deferred.

**Genitalia**

Normal male.

# Laboratory Data/Diagnostic Studies

**Laboratory Data**

*Na:* 141 mEq/L
*K:* 4.1 mEq/L
*Cl:* 101 mEq/L
*Co₂* 27 mM/L
*BUN:* 12 mg/100 ml
*Creatinine:* 0.9 mg/100 ml

*Cholesterol:* 247 mg/100 ml ↑
*Triglycerides:* 209 mg/100 ml ↑
*Hct:* 41.7%
*Hgb:* 14.4 g/dl
*WBC:* 10.2 mm³ ↑

*February 13:*
*CK:* 71 U/L
*LDH:* 90 U/L
*SGOT:* 23 U/L

*February 14 (PM):*
*CK:* 472 U/L
*LDH:* 178 U/L
*SGOT:* 89 U/L
*CK-MB:* 20%

*February 14 (8 AM):*
*CK:* 370 U/L
*LDH:* 123 U/L
*SGOT:* 57 U/L
*CK-MB:* 19%

*February 15:*
*CK:* 204 U/L
*LDH:* 208 U/L
*SGOT:* 53 U/L
*CK-MB:* 15%

**Diagnostic Studies**

*ECG:* Anteroseptal MI.
*Chest X-Ray:* Clear lungs.

**Additional Data**

*Vital Signs for February 14*

| | HR | BP |
|---|---|---|
| At rest: | 88 | 128/78 |
| Eating: | 94 | 130/80 |
| Bath and linen change: | 96 | 136/84 |

HR, heart rate; BP, blood pressure.

### Chest Pain/Angina Log

| Date/Time | Location | Rating Scale (0–10) | Setting | Length | Treatment |
|---|---|---|---|---|---|
| February 14 9:00 AM | Midchest | 2–3 | After bath and turning side to side | 10 min | NTG SL × 2 |
| February 14 6:30 PM | Midchest | 2 | After eating | 5 min | NTG SL × 1 |
| February 15 10:00 AM | Midchest | 1 | During bath | 2 min | Stopped activity |

NTG, nitroglycerin; SL, sublingual.

# COLLABORATIVE PLAN OF CARE

**Diet**

Low cholesterol, no added salt.

**Medications**

Heparin 5000 units sc bid.
Propranolol (Inderal) 10 mg PO q6h.
Diltiazem 60 mg PO q6h.
Isosorbide dinitrate (Isordil) 20 mg PO q6h.
Docusate sodium (Colace) 100 mg PO tid.
Milk of magnesia (MOM) 30 ml PO qhs prn.
Lorazepam (Ativan) 1 mg PO qhs prn.
Acetaminophen (Tylenol) 650 mg PO q4h prn.

***Protocol for Chest Pain***
1. Obtain ECG.
2. Administer $O_2$ at 2 L via nasal prongs.
3. Administer nitroglycerin (NTG) 0.3 mg SL SOS × 2.

**Intravenous Therapy**

Intravenous catheter with injection cap. Flush with heparin flush solution every 8 hours.

**Therapeutic Measures**

Telemetry monitoring.
Obtain vital signs every 4 hours.
Record intake and output.
Daily weights.
Activity per cardiac rehabilitation protocol.
No smoking.

**Consults**

Nutritionist; cardiac rehabilitation nurse.

# NURSING DIAGNOSES DEVELOPED IN CARE PLAN

Pain, p. 61
Activity Intolerance, p. 62
Knowledge Deficit, p. 63

# ADDITIONAL NURSING DIAGNOSES TO BE CONSIDERED

Anxiety
Altered Health Maintenance
Constipation
Sleep Pattern Disturbance

# NURSING CARE PLAN BASED ON IDENTIFIED NURSING DIAGNOSES

| | |
|---|---|
| **Pain** | **Related to:** Inadequate blood flow to myocardial tissue.<br>**Evidenced by:** Complaints of chest pain. |
| **Desired Patient Outcomes** | • The patient's chest pain will be controlled and/or prevented.<br>• The patient will be knowledgeable about the cause, treatment, and management of chest pain. |
| **Evaluation Criteria** | **Throughout the Hospital Stay, the Patient Will:**<br>• Verbalize relief from or decrease in the severity and frequency of chest pain.<br><br>**After Instruction, the Patient Will:**<br>• Verbalize intent to report episodes of chest pain.<br>• Explain the cause of chest pain.<br>• Identify factors that may precipitate or aggravate chest pain.<br>• Describe how he will manage episodes of chest pain. |

## Interventions

Assess characteristics and description of each episode of chest pain, noting verbal and nonverbal responses.

Initiate the chest pain protocol:

• Obtain ECG.
• Administer oxygen as ordered.
• Administer nitroglycerin as ordered.

Auscultate breath and heart sounds. Monitor heart rate, blood pressure, and respiratory rate during and after chest pain and before and after administering medications and as indicated.

Relieve anxiety and offer reassurances.

## Rationale

An analysis of the characteristics of chest pain aids in determining the cause and effect of chest pain (Smith, 1988, p. 52) and will be used in comparing post-MI pain symptoms (Underhill, et al, 1982, p. 317).

ECG changes indicate the presence of myocardial ischemia.

Oxygen may reduce the hypoxia present in myocardial ischemia. Nitroglycerin is administered to increase blood flow and improve myocardial oxygen perfusion (Kneisl and Ames, 1986, p. 980).

Adventitious lung sounds (rales) may develop due to pulmonary congestion in the presence of cardiac dysfunction. Abnormal heart sounds ($S_3$, murmurs) may be indicative of cardiac decompensation (*Cardiovascular Care Handbook*, 1986, p. 36). Hemodynamic changes can result in response to drug administration and/or to cardiac dysfunction (Conti, 1986, p. 364).

A stress response is precipitated by fear and anxiety resulting in a release of and elevation in serum catecholamines that in turn raises myocardial oxygen consumption (Riegel, 1985, p. 251).

## Interventions

Provide a quiet, restful environment.

Provide physical comfort measures.

Instruct the patient to immediately report all episodes of chest pain.

Instruct the patient about chest pain:
• Cause
• Precipitating and aggravating factors
• Management

## Rationale

External stimuli may provoke/aggravate anxieties (Underhill, et al, 1982, p. 426).

Physical comfort will promote a sense of well-being and reduce anxiety (Underhill, et al, 1982, p. 317).

Episodes of angina must be identified and treated promptly to avoid complications from myocardial ischemia (Underhill, et al, 1982, p. 311).

The person who is able to acknowledge and understand the limitations imposed by his or her health problem can be helped to prevent future episodes of angina through teaching (Karch, 1981, p. 39).

---

### Activity Intolerance

*Related to:* Imbalance between oxygen supply and demand.
*Evidenced by:* Episodes of chest pain during activity. Complaints of fatigue after performing activities of daily living (ADLs).

### Desired Patient Outcomes

• The patient will be able to perform at his prescribed activity and exercise level without adverse responses.
• The patient's heart rate and blood pressure will be within acceptable parameters during and after activities.
• The patient will be knowledgeable about his prescribed activity and exercise program.
• The patient will be knowledgeable about the rationale for energy conservation methods.

### Evaluation Criteria

*Throughout the Hospital Stay, the Patient Will:*
• Participate in a progressive activity and exercise program.
• Have his heart rate and blood pressure within acceptable parameters during and after activities and exercise.
• Report the absence of any adverse responses to the activity and exercise program.

*After Instruction, the Patient Will:*
• Demonstrate the correct method for pulse taking.
• State safe limits for heart rate during activity performance.
• Employ energy conservation techniques.
• Discuss factors that may affect his level of performance.
• Identify the activities and exercises safe for him to perform.

---

## Interventions

Assess level of tolerance to specific activities.

Prescribe a progressive activity and exercise program for each phase of recov-

## Rationale

Assessment of the patient's responses to activities serves as a guide for planning an activity and exercise prescription appropriate to the patient and the phase of his recovery (Underhill, et al, 1982, p. 552).

Progressive activity and exercise combat anxiety, fatigue, depression, and prevent the hazards of bed rest (Winslow, 1985, p.

## Interventions

ery. Discuss factors affecting performance and outcomes of an activity and exercise program. Provide the patient with a chart listing energy costs of activities and exercises.

Monitor heart rate and blood pressure before, during, and after activity.

Ensure adequate sleep.

Instruct the patient about energy conservation and rest requirements.

Instruct and demonstrate the method for pulse taking. Identify the target heart rate.

Provide the patient with guidelines for safe performance of activities and exercise.

## Rationale

238). It also aids the individual in "attaining the level of cardiovascular functioning that will allow personal care and independent living at home" (Pollock and Schmidt, 1986, p. 408). Charts listing energy costs along with pictures of different types of activities and exercise aid patients in their progress by identifying the do's and don't's of exercise (Underhill, et al, 1982, p. 557).

Systolic blood pressure and heart rate increase during activity and are indirect measurements of myocardial oxygen consumption. In patients with CAD, this provides important information about the stress of a given activity or exercise (Underhill, et al, 1982, p. 553).

Quality sleep time has restorative power. It maintains emotional and mental well-being and replenishes energy stores (Sanford, 1983, p. 19).

Energy conservation measures allow the person to participate in more physical activities with less fatigue while reducing the possibility of adverse effects (Jones, Dunbar, and Jivorec, 1984, p. 993). Alternating activity with rest periods prevents fatigue (Pollock and Schmidt, 1986).

Heart rate can be used to monitor exercise and its intensity. The target heart rate range indicates safe limits of exercise performance (*Cardiovascular Care Handbook*, 1986, p. 454).

Symptoms indicating an adverse response to activity "serve as a warning signal of undue cardiovascular exertion" (Underhill, et al, 1982, p. 558).

---

| | |
|---|---|
| ***Knowledge Deficit*** | ***Related to:*** Lack of information about myocardial infarction, treatment regimen, risk factor modification, and cardiac rehabilitation. |
| | ***Evidenced by:*** Diagnosis of MI; patient's statements indicating lack of knowledge about heart disease and MI; presence of modifiable risk factors; and required period for cardiac rehabilitation. |
| ***Desired Patient Outcomes*** | ***The Patient Will Be Knowledgeable about:*** |
| | • Basic structure and function of the heart. |
| | • Myocardial infarction, its cause, signs and symptoms, treatment, and complications. |
| | • The rationale for and strategies employed to reduce cardiac risk factors. |
| | • All aspects of cardiac rehabilitation. |
| ***Evaluation Criteria*** | ***After Instruction/by Discharge, the Patient and/or Spouse Will:*** |
| | • Describe the structure and function of the heart. |
| | • Explain what an MI is, its cause, signs and symptoms, and treatment. |
| | • Discuss some of the emotional responses to an MI. |
| | • Verbalize an understanding of the relationship between his risk factors and CAD. |
| | • Identify the strategies employed and state intent to modify his risk factors. |

- Identify when sexual activity can be safely resumed.
- State the name, action, dose, frequency, and side effects of all prescribed medications.
- List signs and symptoms to be reported to his physician.
- State the importance of keeping follow-up visits with his physician.

| Interventions | Rationale |
|---|---|
| Establish goals for the teaching program. | "Learning is more effective when the content is relevant to the patient and his problem" (Underhill, et al, 1982, p. 582). |
| Develop a teaching plan to include the following content: | An overview of normal cardiac structure and function and information about CAD and myocardial infarction should be presented to enable the patient to understand the cardiac alterations that have occurred (Karch, 1981). |
| • Normal anatomy and physiology of the heart. | |
| • Myocardial infarction: its cause, manifestation, diagnosis, treatment, and risk factors. | |
| • Emotional reactions to MI. | Anxiety, denial, depression, and anger are commonly observed in persons suffering an acute MI (Underhill, et al, 1982, p. 573). |
| • Methods used for risk factor modification: stop-smoking program, diet modification, weight control, stress reduction, and activity/exercise program. | The educational goal is to provide the patient and family with the knowledge needed to understand and modify their lifestyles (Moynihan, 1984, p. 443). |
| • Sexual counseling. | The goal of sexual counseling is to return the patient to the level of sexual activity prior to infarction (Cohen, 1986, p. 22). |
| • Discharge planning: medications, signs and symptoms to be reported to the physician, and follow-up visits to physician. | Patients and their families need education and guidance in making the adjustments to living with CAD (Pinneo, 1984, p. 459). |
| Employ strategies to aid the teaching process: | The patient must understand what is being asked and what is being stated in order to cooperate fully (Byrne and Edeani, 1984, p. 178). "Retention of material learned is proportional to the number of senses involved in learning" (Underhill, et al, 1982, p. 583). |
| • Simplify the information. | |
| • Provide explicit instructions. | |
| • Provide written material. | |
| • Utilize audiovisual aids. | |
| • Encourage participation in group discussion. | Self-help groups are important sources of support for patients and family (Underhill, et al, 1982, p. 566). |
| • Encourage the patient's wife to participate. | The family has the potential for providing ongoing support in the home setting (Ballard, 1986, p. 57; Jillings, 1988, p. 77). |

# QUESTIONS FOR DISCUSSION

1. In the acute period after an MI, what are the priorities of care?
2. How is the diagnosis of an MI confirmed? Identify the specifics from the case study.
3. Identify the site of Mr. Norton's infarct and determine which coronary artery(ies) may be affected.
4. What are the dietary modifications needed during the acute phase of an MI? Why?
5. What is the rationale behind interventions to promote rest in the patient experiencing an MI?
6. On admission to your unit from the CCU, Mr. Norton asks you if he can take a shower. Discuss what your response might be.

7. Upon entering Mr. Norton's room, he tells you that he is experiencing chest pain. Identify the subjective characteristics to explore when assessing his chest pain.
8. What are the adverse reactions Mr. Norton could experience during an activity?

## REFERENCES

Ballard, N: Promoting compliance in rehabilitation of a patient with a myocardial infarction. Topics Clin Nurs 7:57, 1986.

Byrne, T and Edeani, D: Knowledge of medical terminology among hospital patients. Nurs Res 33:178, 1984.

Cardiovascular Care Handbook. Springhouse Corporation, Springhouse, Pa, 1986.

Cohen, C: Sexual counseling of the patient following myocardial infarction. Crit Care Nurse 6:18, 1986.

Conti, CR: Unstable angina before and after infarction: Thoughts on pathogenesis and therapeutic strategies. Heart Lung 15:361, 1986.

Jillings, CR: Cardiac Rehabilitation Nursing. Aspen Publishers, Inc., Rockville, Md, 1988.

Jones, B, Dunbar, C, and Jivorec, M: Medical-Surgical Nursing: A Conceptual Approach. McGraw-Hill, New York, 1984.

Karch, A: Cardiac Care: A Guide for Patient Education. Appleton-Century-Crofts, New York, 1981.

Kneisl, CR and Ames, SW: Adult Health Nursing. Addison-Wesley, Menlo Park, Calif, 1986.

Moynihan, M: Assessing the educational needs of post-myocardial infarction patients. Nurs Clin North Am 19:441, 1984.

Pinneo, R: Living with coronary artery disease. Nurs Clin North Am 19:459, 1984.

Pollock, M and Schmidt, D (eds): Heart Disease and Rehabilitation. John Wiley & Sons, New York, 1986.

Porth, CM: Pathophysiology. JB Lippincott, Philadelphia, 1986.

Price, SA and Wilson, LM: Pathophysiology. McGraw-Hill, New York, 1986.

Riegel, BJ: The role of nursing in limiting myocardial infarct size. Heart Lung 14:247, 1985.

Sanford, S: Sleep and the cardiac patient. Cardiovasc Nurs 19:19, 1983.

Smith, CE: Chest pain. Nursing '88 18:52, 1988.

Underhill, SL, et al: Cardiac Nursing. JB Lippincott, Philadelphia, 1982.

Winslow, EH: Cardiovascular consequences of bedrest. Heart Lung, 14:236, 1985.

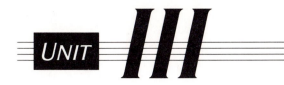

# THE PATIENT WITH ALTERATIONS IN NEUROLOGICAL FUNCTION

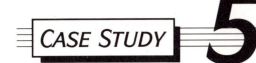

# A PATIENT WITH A CEREBROVASCULAR ACCIDENT

Anne Keiran Manton, M.S., R.N., CEN

Cerebrovascular accident, or stroke, can be described as a condition in which an area of the brain has become ischemic due to an interruption in perfusion. Such an interruption can be the result of an occlusion of the perfusing artery or result from hemorrhage of the artery. Both mechanisms lead to an inadequate blood supply to a specific part of the brain.

The significance of the problem of cerebrovascular accidents (CVA) is noteworthy. Statistics have shown CVAs to be the fourth leading cause of death in the United States, and the second leading cause of chronic disability. The National Stroke Survey, conducted in 1980, estimated the economic cost of CVAs to be more than $7 billion dollars per year. "In 1981, the American Heart Association estimated that there were 164,000 deaths attributable to stroke and 1,870,000 stroke survivors" (Gorelick, 1986, p. 275). Cerebrovascular accident is the fourth most common diagnosis for Medicare inpatients (Tellis-Nayack, 1986, p. 340).

## ANATOMY AND PHYSIOLOGY OF THE BRAIN

A brief review of the anatomy of the brain with regard to cerebrovascular accidents requires discussion of cerebral blood supply. Cerebral blood flow remains constant over a wide range of systemic blood pressures (approximately 150–60 mmHg). This phenomenon is due to cerebral autoregulation. When systemic blood pressure falls, there is a compensatory decrease in cerebral vascular resistance. When there is an elevation of blood pressure, there is an increase in cerebrovascular resistance. An increase in intracranial pressure also increases cerebrovascular resistance. The brain copes most effectively with changes that are gradual.

Blood supply to the brain is rich. The right and left common carotid arteries arise from the aorta and subsequently branch into the internal and external carotid arteries. Once the internal carotid arteries pass into the cranium, arteries branch off that supply most of the brain. There are 3 major branches: the middle cerebral arteries, the anterior cerebral arteries, and the posterior communicating arteries.

The two anterior cerebral arteries are joined by the anterior communicating artery and supply the medial aspect of the hemispheres. The lateral aspects of the hemispheres are supplied by the middle cerebral arteries.

The vertebral arteries, which arise from the right and left subclavian arteries, ascend through the foramen magnum and join to form the basilar artery. The medulla, pons, and cerebellum receive their blood supply from branches of the basilar artery.

The two posterior cerebral arteries result from the bifurcation of the basilar artery. The posterior cerebral arteries supply blood to the thalamus, hypothalamus, the posterior two thirds of the temporal area, the medial occipital area, and portions of the brain stem and cerebellum. The branches of the internal carotids and the vertebral-basilar system (the anterior and posterior systems) join to form the circle of Willis by way of the

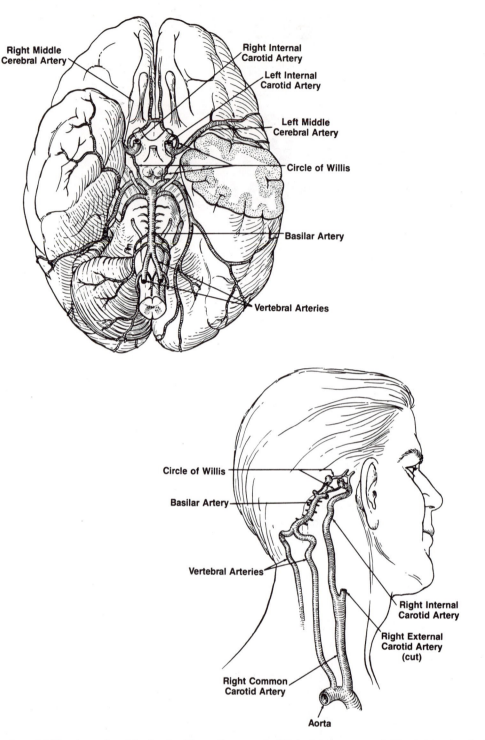

**FIGURE 5–1.** Arterial blood supply of the brain. (From Stewart, J: Clinical Anatomy and Physiology for the Frustrated and Angry Health Professional. Medmaster, Miami, p 76, 1986, with permission.)

anterior and posterior communicating arteries. In this way, a continuous blood supply is available to all parts of the brain even if one of the major vessels experiences a decrease in blood flow (Fig. 5–1).

It is essential that all parts of the brain receive an adequate blood supply because, although the brain accounts for only 2% of the total body weight, the adult brain requires 20% of the cardiac output and is responsible for the consumption of 20% of the oxygen and 70% of the glucose in the body.

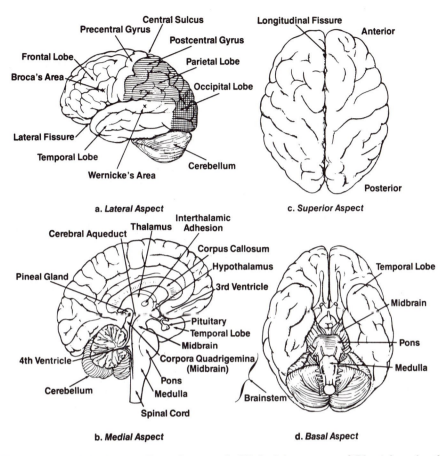

**FIGURE 5–2.** Four aspects of the brain. (From Stewart, J: Clinical Anatomy and Physiology for the Frustrated and Angry Health Professional. Medmaster, Miami, 1986, p 70 with permission.)

Although the brain functions as a whole, specific sequelae result from lesions according to their location in the hemispheres. Observation and investigation have demonstrated that persons with lesions of the left hemisphere will likely develop motor and/or sensory loss of the right side of the body and a variety of communication problems. The left hemisphere usually determines symbolic language. Those with lesions of the right hemisphere develop left-sided sensory or motor loss and neglect of the left side of the body. The right hemisphere governs spatial and perceptual information.

Each of the hemispheres can be thought of in terms of 4 lobes: the frontal lobe, the temporal lobe, the parietal lobe, and the occipital lobe. The prefrontal areas in the frontal lobe are concerned with what might be called the human being's truly higher functions: intellect, personality, and elaboration of thought. The precentral gyrus, also in the frontal lobe, is the major motor area, sending impulses down the pyramidal paths to effectors on the contralateral side of the body. Located at the base of this motor area in the dominant hemisphere is Broca's area, which controls the motor aspects of speech. The parietal lobe is the major area of perception, while the temporal lobe assumes responsibility for memory, auditory interpretation, and hearing. The temporal lobe of the dominant hemisphere also contains Wernicke's area, which is involved with the comprehension of language. Finally, the occipital lobe receives input through the visual sense and integrates and interprets these data (Stewart, 1986; Wallhagen, 1979) (Fig. 5–2).

## PATHOPHYSIOLOGY

The effects of ischemia resulting from interruption of blood supply to a portion of the brain are primarily determined by 3 factors. The first is the location of the decreased blood supply. This factor is of major concern because lasting sequelae, if there are any, will be determined by the location of the event. The other variables of concern are the cause of the decreased perfusion, for example, thrombus, embolus, hemorrhage, or trauma, and whether the diminished blood supply was of rapid or gradual onset. These factors may influence the eventual outcome, since they may indicate the likelihood of established collateral circulation that would decrease the impact of the vascular event. Collateral circulation may gradually develop when normal flow to a part is decreased. Most cerebral collateral circulation between major arteries is by way of the circle of Willis. The brain also has collateral circulation sites that function only when other routes are impaired, such as that between the external and internal carotid arteries by way of the ophthalmic artery. These communicating channels are capable, theoretically, of providing an adequate supply to all areas of the brain. In a practical sense this is often not the case. The variability of outcome from major vessel occlusion in different individuals is believed to be related to the state of the individual's collateral circulation. The cause of the interruption of blood supply is important in the determination of treatment plans.

The impact is significant when blood supply is markedly decreased or interrupted altogether because then the particular part of the brain receives insufficient oxygen and glucose for cells to survive. It is believed that if the lack of oxygen and glucose is corrected within 15 minutes, the ischemia is reversible. If, however, blood supply is not reestablished in 15 minutes, irreversible cell death occurs. With cell death or infarction, changes in the membrane permeability can result in edema and consequently increased intracranial pressure.

The most common cause of CVA is thrombosis, accounting for about 40% of all pathologically verified CVAs. Thrombosis is the result of cerebral atherosclerosis, which leads to a gradual narrowing and eventual occlusion of the affected artery. "In the cerebral circulation, atherosclerotic plaques are found most commonly at arterial bifurcations, branch points and curves. Common sites of predelection include the internal carotid artery origin, the junction of the basilar and vertebral arteries, the initial segment of the middle cerebral artery, and the proximal posterior cerebral artery" (Gorelick, 1986, p. 276). Because of its gradual development, this type of vascular compromise may have transient episodes that precede the major event. It is also more likely that collateral circulation will have been established.

A cerebral embolism is an example of a cause of decreased cerebral perfusion with rapid onset. The origin of the embolus is frequently cardiac, due either to valvular disease, myocardial infarction, or atrial fibrillation.

Cerebral hemorrhage accounts for about 15% of CVAs, according to the Framingham Study on Heart Disease. Causes of cerebral hemorrhage may be trauma, aneurysm, bleeding disorder, or rupture of the blood vessel due to hypertension and cerebral atherosclerosis.

# RISK FACTORS

Because of the cost of cerebrovascular accidents in terms of the quality of peoples' lives and in terms of the economic realities that ensue, it is important for health professionals to be vigilant in assisting the public to recognize and reduce the risk factors identified as contributing to the occurrence of CVA. Prevention is the best cure. Fortunately, many of these risk factors are amenable to treatment.

Hypertension is considered to be the major risk factor in CVA. Control of hypertension is an important determinant in the prevention of CVA and has been associated with a reduction in CVA-related mortality by approximately 20% (Kasuya and Holm, 1986, p. 294). Cardiac disease also places the patient at risk, especially for an embolic incident, as previously discussed. Patients known to have cardiac risk factors such as valvular disease or atrial fibrillation should be managed appropriately by their physician. The importance of compliance with the prescribed medical regimen in the prevention of CVA must also be stressed.

Both diabetes, probably because of its association with atherogenesis, and atherosclerotic disease of the intracranial and extracranial blood vessels are considered risk factors for CVAs. Hyperlipidemia, especially hypercholesterolemia, is a risk factor that is amenable to treatment by careful attention to diet and, if necessary, pharmacotherapy. Polycythemia (increased hematocrit levels) also is a risk factor for a cerebral embolic event. The medical literature reports that women over the age of 35 who take oral contraceptives may be at risk for a CVA. This risk is considerably increased if the woman has hypertension and is a cigarette smoker. These, too, are risk factors that can be readily reduced by attention to the patient's health history, appropriate medical management, and health education. Other risk factors include advanced age, family history of stroke, obesity, drug abuse, and alcohol consumption. Some of these risk factors also can be reduced.

# COMMON CLINICAL FINDINGS

Clinical manifestations of cerebrovascular accident vary according to the location and size of the area of inadequate perfusion. Findings are common, not to CVAs, but rather to the area of the brain affected by the decrease in perfusion. While keeping the awareness of the variability of findings in mind, some common clinical manifestations can be identified. These general findings may include headache, vomiting, seizures, loss of consciousness, change in blood pressure, confusion, disorientation, and other mental status changes. More location-specific clinical findings may include the following:

- Vertebral-basilar system: Manifestations are usually bilateral and may include extremity weakness, ataxia, dysphagia, dysarthria, dizziness, syncope, memory disturbances, stupor, coma, visual disturbances, numbness of face, increased tendon reflexes, and positive Babinski signs.
- Internal carotid artery: Manifestations are usually unilateral and may include monocular blindness, sensory and motor deficits of the contralateral extremities and face, and expressive aphasia if the area of decreased blood supply is in the dominant hemisphere.
- Anterior cerebral artery: The primary symptom is confusion; other manifestations include contralateral weakness (especially of the leg), contralateral sensory deficits, and dementia.
- Middle cerebral artery: If the dominant hemisphere is involved, all functions of speech and communication are disturbed (global aphasia); dysphasia, contralateral hemiparesis or monoparesis (of the arm), and occasionally contralateral hemianopsia may occur.
- Posterior cerebral artery: Manifestations may include contralateral hemiparesis, visual aphasia (word blindness), hemianopsia, and coma (Baxter, 1987; Kneisl and Ames, 1986, Chapter 37).

## TREATMENT MODALITIES

Treatment modalities vary with the clinical findings present and the cause of the stroke; however, initial treatment includes measures to protect the patient's airway and to maximize cerebral perfusion and oxygenation. The adequacy of the patient's airway, therefore, must be frequently assessed. Interventions such as endotracheal intubation, positioning, or suctioning may be needed to maintain the airway. Blood pressure also must be frequently monitored to ensure adequate cerebral perfusion. Measures must be undertaken if blood pressure is determined to be insufficient. Intravenous fluids and oxygen therapy also may be considered in the initial treatment of the stroke patient. "Because cerebral edema is the cause of early death from cerebral infarction, treatment with drugs is directed toward this. After the first four days, cerebral edema is gradually absorbed and for this reason, the critical stage is often the first week following the stroke. After this point, assessment of the amount of brain damage allows a prognosis to be made concerning the likely degree of immediate recovery and the eventual outcome in terms of functional ability" (Rose and Capildeo, 1981, p. 35). After the acute phase, treatment focuses on minimizing functional deficits and maximizing remaining functional abilities. During all phases of stroke recovery, prevention of complications is an important treatment consideration.

## PATIENT ASSESSMENT DATA BASE

## Health History

*Client:*
Mr. Arthur Todd

*Address:* 106 Pleasant St., Boston, MA 02116
*Telephone:* 555-1234
*Contact:* Mrs. Florence Todd (wife)
*Address of contact:* Same as client
*Telephone of contact:* Same as client
*Age:* 65    *Sex:* Male    *Race:* White
*Educational background:* High school graduate
*Religion:* Protestant    *Marital status:* Married
*Usual occupation:* Police officer
*Present occupation:* Retired
*Source of income:* Pension and Social Security
*Insurance:* Medicare, Medex
*Source of referral:* Department of Health and Hospitals (ambulance)
*Source of history:* Wife
*Reliability of historian:* Good reliability
*Date of interview:* 1/5/88
*Reason for visit/Chief complaint:* Confused speech and right-sided weakness.

## HEALTH PERCEPTION/HEALTH MANAGEMENT PATTERN

**Present Health Status**

Approximately 72 hours ago Mr. Todd awoke and on attempting to arise from bed fell to the floor. Mrs. Todd noted marked weakness of his right side and she was not able to understand his attempts to communicate. He was brought to the hospital by ambulance for evaluation and admission. Although he can be roused, she believes he has become more lethargic since admission. His speech remains unintelligible.

**Past Health Status**

*General Health.* Diagnosed as hypertensive 12 years ago, asymptomatic, first identified on routine police department physical. Initially treatment was limited to weight reduction and decreased sodium intake. His wife says that compliance with dietary recommendations was inconsistent and medication (chlorothiazide) was initiated about 10 years ago for blood pressure readings > 160/95. Mrs. Todd states that her husband occasionally will not take medications because of side effects. She relates that Mr. Todd has experienced several episodes of slurred speech and tingling on the right side during the past year. These occurrences passed spontaneously and therefore evaluation and treatment was not sought. She describes his health as otherwise good.

*Prophylactic Medical/Dental Care.* Mr. Todd had a routine physical examination about 6 months ago by primary care physician. His wife does not know whether this examination was precipitated by symptoms of concern to Mr. Todd; he told her at the time that it was "just routine." She observed no change in his treatment regimen as a result of the examination. He was seen by ophthalmologist for routine eye examination about 5 months ago. His last dental examination was many years ago; his wife cannot remember when. She states patient has had dentures for at least 15 years.

*Childhood Illnesses.* Wife thinks Mr. Todd had "most of them," but she does not think he had rheumatic fever or any illnesses that were "out of the ordinary".

*Immunizations.* Had tetanus shot 2 years ago, according to wife. Otherwise, immunization status unknown.

*Major Illnesses/Hospitalizations.* Wife states Mr. Todd has had no major illnesses. He was hospitalized about 20 years ago for herniorrhaphy; recovery was uncomplicated.

*Current Medications*
*Prescription:* Chlorothiazide (Diuril) once a day, usually in the morning. Clonidine hydrochloride (Catapres) also once a day. Wife is unsure of dosages of drugs; they will be checked with prescribing physician. No other prescription medications known.
*Nonprescription:* Occasional use of cold capsules, cough medicine, and acetaminophen. Fairly consistent use of milk of magnesia.
*Allergies.* None known.

*Habits.*
*Alcohol:* Approximately a 6-pack of beer per week.
*Caffeine:* Previously 6–8 cups of coffee per day; since retirement, usually coffee with breakfast and 1 cup by midmorning. Tea with lunch and dinner, rarely a cola drink.
*Drugs:* None.
*Tobacco:* Smokes 2 or 3 cigars per day.

## *Family Health History*

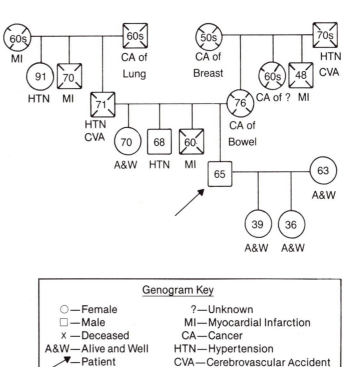

```
                        Genogram Key
          ○—Female              ?—Unknown
          □—Male                MI—Myocardial Infarction
          x —Deceased           CA—Cancer
          A&W—Alive and Well    HTN—Hypertension
          ▼—Patient             CVA—Cerebrovascular Accident
```

## NUTRITIONAL/METABOLIC PATTERN

*Nutritional*

Wife states Mr. Todd is a good eater; he enjoys all types of food and is a particularly big meat eater. He eats regularly, and she believes that he eats healthier foods since his retirement from the police force. She states he has gained weight since his retirement (about 15 lb [6.8 kg]), and she estimates his present weight to be about 200 lb (90.9 kg) and his height to be about 5 ft 10 in. (175 cm). He rarely eats dessert and does not use table salt, although he does not refrain from eating highly salted foods.

*Usual Daily Menu*
*Breakfast:* Two eggs, bacon (3–4 slices), toast, orange juice, coffee.
*Lunch:* Two sandwiches with mayonnaise and luncheon meat, tea.
*Dinner:* Meat (usually red meat), potatoes, vegetables, tea and occasionally some milk or fruit.
*Snack:* Does not snack daily, but several times per week may have some crackers and cheese or packaged cookies.
At present Mr. Todd has been maintained on a primarily liquid diet and intravenous fluids due to considerable difficulty swallowing even a soft diet. Attempts to feed him pureed foods have precipitated coughing or have been found to remain in his mouth.

*Metabolic*

Wife denies Mr. Todd has any metabolic problems. He has no difficulty with wound healing, with skin problems, or with extremes of hot or cold. Wife attributes weight gain to change in activity and diet since retirement.

## ELIMINATION PATTERN

### Bowel

Constipation is a chronic problem. Wife states that Mr. Todd takes milk of magnesia 3–4 times per week. He has not had a bowel movement since admission.

### Bladder

Wife knows of no problems with urination except that he arises 2 or 3 times per night to urinate. She does not believe he perceives this to be a problem. Since admission Mr. Todd has experienced frequent urinary incontinence.

## ACTIVITY/EXERCISE PATTERN

### Activity/Exercise

Since retiring 4 years ago Mr. Todd spends time reading, watching television, and working in the yard. His hobby is carving wood birds and painting them and this occupies much of his time. He also likes to attend craft shows and auctions. He has no regular exercise routine. Mrs. Todd believes that until this time he has had no limitations to self-care, and had sufficient energy for all desired and required activities.

#### Self-Care Ability

| | |
|---|---|
| Feeding—IV | Grooming—IV |
| Bathing—IV | General mobility—IV |
| Toileting—IV | Cooking—IV |
| Bed mobility—III | Home maintenance—IV |
| Dressing—IV | Shopping—IV |

---

**Functional Levels Code**
  0—Full self-care
  I—Requires use of equipment or device
 II—Requires assistance or supervision from another person
III—Requires assistance or supervision from another person and equipment or device
IV—Is dependent and does not participate

---

### Oxygenation/Perfusion

Wife states that in the past, Mr. Todd did not complain of dyspnea at rest or on exertion. She denies he had chronic cough or shortness of breath before the CVA. Mrs. Todd does not recall her husband ever complaining of chest pain, irregular heartbeats, or palpitations. She does not know date or findings of last chest x-ray or electrocardiogram.

#### Cardiac Risk Factors

| | Positive | Negative |
|---|---|---|
| Sedentary life-style | X | |
| Hyperlipidemia | X | |
| Cigarette smoking | | X |
| Diabetes | | X |
| Obesity | X | |
| Hypertension | X | |
| Hypervigilant personality | | X |
| Family history of heart disease | X | |

## SLEEP/REST PATTERN

*Sleep/Rest*

Mr. and Mrs. Todd retire about 10:00 PM each evening. Mr. Todd arises about 6:30 AM. Mrs. Todd is unaware of any sleep difficulties that Mr. Todd might have except awakening to urinate. She believes he has no trouble returning to sleep following these interruptions. They have no particular bedtime routine. She states Mr. Todd has never expressed a need to take sleeping medication.

## COGNITIVE/PERCEPTUAL PATTERN

*Hearing*

Usual function. No diagnosed hearing problem, although Mrs. Todd believes Mr. Todd may have slight hearing loss as evidenced by louder TV volume and asking her to repeat phrases spoken in a conversational tone.

*Vision*

Usual function. Has worn eyeglasses (bifocals) for many years. On a recent visit to ophthalmologist an early cataract was noted; no treatment was prescribed at that time.

*Sensory Perception*

Usual function. No previous sensory perceptual problems noted. At present, Mr. Todd does not respond to touch on the right arm or leg. Until present event, no changes were noted in memory or thought processes. Right hand is dominant. No chronic difficulties with pain or pain management.

*Learning Style*

Usual function unable to be determined.

*Present Function*

Mr. Todd is unable at present to communicate verbally. Speech is garbled and assessment of the level of patient's understanding is incomplete; however, he does nod yes and no appropriately most of the time. Hemiparesis of the right side in this right-handed man prevents adequate assessment of writing abilities at this time. Shows no interest in programs on TV in his room. Wife states he usually enjoys these programs.

## SELF-PERCEPTION/SELF-CONCEPT PATTERN

*Self-Perception/Self-Concept*

Mrs. Todd states that she believes that Mr. Todd has a very positive self-concept. Numerous accomplishments in his police career fostered a belief in his own abilities and allowed him to feel comfortable with himself. He has adjusted well to retirement and had expressed satisfaction with this stage of his life.

## ROLE/RELATIONSHIP PATTERN

*Role/Relationship*

Mr. and Mrs. Todd live alone in a house they have owned for 30 years. Although she states they have had some problems over the years, Mrs. Todd believes they have a stable marriage. They have been able to talk things out with each other comfortably for many years now, she says. Mr. Todd has a good relationship with their 2 adult daughters, but according to his wife, he may be hesitant to ask for their help. "He would never want to burden them," she says. Mr. Todd enjoys activities with his grandchildren and has a close relationship with his brother.

## SEXUALITY/REPRODUCTIVE PATTERN

*Sexuality/Reproductive*

Prior antihypertensive medications caused impotence. No problems with current medications. Wife believes Mr. Todd finds sex life satisfactory, and is comfortable with his own sexuality.

## COPING/STRESS TOLERANCE PATTERN

*Coping/Stress Tolerance*

Wife states patient has "a short fuse"; he blows up but gets over it quickly and doesn't hold grudges. "Once it's over, it's over with him," she says. Usually he tries to handle problems on his own, and dislikes having to ask for help. He becomes frustrated when he can't get things to work as expected; his wife says this is because usually he is able to manage everything so well that he becomes frustrated when he can't. Overall, he has handled losses well but did have a difficult time accepting the death of a brother with whom he had a close relationship.

## VALUE/BELIEF PATTERN

*Value/Belief*

Wife states Mr. Todd has no real religious preference, but occasionally accompanies her to services at the Protestant church that she attends and is active in. He believes in a higher power, but not a specific religion. He has no ethnic customs or beliefs that are important to him.

# Physical Examination

*General Survey*

Sixty-five-year-old male, looking stated age, moderately obese, eyes closed—right eyelid does not close completely. Right-sided facial drooping. Right arm is against the body and the right leg is externally rotated with the knee flexed.

*Vital Signs*

**Temperature:** 99.2°F (37.3°C) (per rectum)
**Pulse:** 88 per minute, regular (apical)
**Respirations:** 20 per minute, regular
**BP:** 160/90 (right arm, supine position).

*Integument*

**Skin.** Warm and dry, no lesions except for several moles on trunk.
**Mucous Membranes.** Pink, slightly dry.
**Nails.** No evidence of clubbing; no lesions.

*HEENT*

**Head.** Symmetrical, normal adult shape. Hair and scalp: Slightly balding, somewhat dry, gray hair; scalp clean, no flaking or lesions. Face: Facial structures symmetrical, but with right-sided drooping, and evidence of capillary dilatation on cheeks and nose. Temporomandibular joint was not evaluated.
**Eyes.** Pupils equal, round, reactive to light and accommodation (PERRLA). Is able to follow penlight with eyes. Right eyelid does not close completely.
**Ears.** Symmetrical, no visible lesions or drainage. Hearing was not tested, but patient does respond to verbal stimuli.
**Nose.** No lesions noted, no discharge; further assessment deferred.
**Mouth/Throat.** Gag reflex diminished, difficulty swallowing; tongue deviates to the right.

*Neck*

Audible bruits of carotids bilaterally.

**Pulmonary**

Anteroposterior (AP) diameter 2:1, symmetrical; slight rales noted at both bases.

**Breast**

No masses or tenderness noted.

**Cardiovascular**

No murmurs, rubs, or extra sounds noted. Point of maximal impulse (PMI) palpable at the 5th intercostal space; rhythm regular.

**Peripheral Vascular**

Skin warm, dry, with good capillary refill.

*Peripheral Pulses*
Temporal—3 bilaterally
Carotid—3 bilaterally
Brachial—4 bilaterally
Radial—4 bilaterally
Femoral—4 bilaterally
Popliteal—4 bilaterally
Posterior tibial—4 bilaterally
Dorsalis pedis—4 bilaterally

*Peripheral Pulse Scale*

| |
|---|
| 0—Absent |
| 1—Markedly diminished |
| 2—Moderately diminished |
| 3—Slightly diminished |
| 4—Normal |

**Abdomen**

Symmetrical, small right-sided scar from past herniorrhaphy. Bowel sounds normoactive in all 4 quadrants. No pain or tenderness noted on palpation. Dullness on percussion in left lower quadrant. Liver 10 cm (4 in.) at right midclavicular line and palpable at costal margin.

**Musculoskeletal**

Passive range of motion of all joints without difficulty or limitation. No apparent joint tenderness to palpation; no swelling at joints noted. Muscles are developed symmetrically; no muscle wasting noted.

**Neurological**

*Mental Status.* Lethargic; able to be aroused. Due to speech difficulties at present, unable to accurately assess patient's mental status more completely.

*Cranial Nerves*
CN I:      Deferred.
CN II:     Pupils constrict equally; visual acuity not tested.
CN III ⎫
CN IV  ⎬  Is able to follow penlight with eyes.
CN VI ⎭
CN V:      Corneal reflexes intact; decreased jaw strength.
CN VII:    Right-sided mouth and facial drooping.
CN VIII:   Not tested.
CN IX:     Gag reflex diminished.
CN X:      Uvula deviates to the left.
CN XI:     Not tested.
CN XII:    Tongue deviates to the right.

*Motor.* Unable to move right arm and leg; some spasticity of muscles of right limbs noted. Able to move left extremities.
*Sensory.* Absent response to pain and vibration on right side. Responds to pain and vibration on left side by withdrawal of limb and verbal utterance.

*Deep Tendon Reflexes*

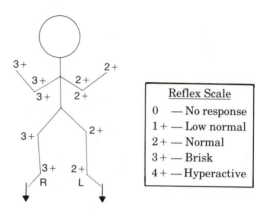

Rectal

Deferred.

Genitalia

Normal adult male.

## Laboratory Data/Diagnostic Studies

**Laboratory Data**

*Hemogloblin:* 14 g/100 ml
*Hematocrit:* 40%
*WBC:* 12,000/mm$^3$
*Na:* 140 mM/L
*K:* 3.5 mM/L
*Cl:* 102 mM/L
*CO$_2$:* 30 mM/L
*BUN:* 10 mg/dl

*Serum Cholesterol:* 312 mg/dl
*Serum triglycerides:* 220 mg/dl
*Arterial blood gases:*
*pH:* 7.39
*Po$_2$:* 92 mmHg
*Pco$_2$:* 38 mmHg
*Glucose:* 108 mg/dl

**Diagnostic Studies**

*Electrocardiogram: 12-Lead.* Sinus rhythm, left ventricular hypertrophy (LVH) noted; otherwise within normal limits.
*Chest X-Ray.* No abnormalities noted.
*Computed Tomography (CT) Scan.* Areas of infarction seen in left frontal parietal cortex with surrounding cerebral edema.
*Cerebral Angiography.* 70% occlusion in left carotid artery; 95% occlusion in left middle cerebral artery.

## COLLABORATIVE PLAN OF CARE

**Diet**

Soft solid diet as tolerated; pureed foods.

**Medications**

Dulcolax suppository prn.

**Intravenous Therapy**

1000 ml 5% D/W IV at 100 ml/hour today.

**Therapeutic Measures**

Head of bed elevated 30° if blood pressure is > 110/70.
Oxygen at 2 L/minute via nasal prongs.
Neurological vital signs including temperature q2h.
Notify physician if BP ≥ 180 systolic or ≥100 diastolic.
Suction prn.
Range of motion and reposition q2h.
Double egg-crate foam on bed.

Boots on both feet q2h.
Aspiration precautions.
Measure intake and output.
Elastic stockings.

*Consults*

Consult speech-language pathologist.
Consult physical therapy department.
Schedule modified barium swallow (sinefluorography).

## NURSING DIAGNOSES DEVELOPED IN CARE PLAN

Impaired Verbal Communication, p. 81
Potential for Injury, p. 82
Impaired Swallowing, p. 83

## ADDITIONAL NURSING DIAGNOSES TO BE CONSIDERED

Altered Cerebral Tissue Perfusion
Anticipatory Grieving
Anxiety
Body Image Disturbance
Bathing/Hygiene Self-Care Deficit
Constipation
Dressing/Grooming Self-Care Deficit
Impaired Physical Mobility
Ineffective Airway Clearance
Ineffective Individual Coping
Potential for Aspiration
Potential Impaired Skin Integrity
Sensory/Perceptual Alterations (Kinesthetic, Tactile)
Spiritual Distress
Toileting Self-Care Deficit
Total Incontinence

## NURSING CARE PLAN BASED ON IDENTIFIED NURSING DIAGNOSES

| | |
|---|---|
| ***Impaired Verbal Communication*** | ***Related to:*** Ischemic changes in the brain affecting communication centers.<br>***Evidenced by:*** Inappropriate verbalization; speaks or verbalizes with difficulty; unable to be understood; seems to understand incoming stimuli (as demonstrated by appropriate nodding of head and following simple commands). |
| ***Desired Patient Outcomes*** | The patient will be able to communicate needs and desires adequately, given limitations related to the disease process. |
| ***Evaluation Criteria*** | ***By the Time of Discharge, the Patient Will:***<br>• Have developed alternative methods of communications.<br>• Be able to communicate his needs.<br>• Be able to respond appropriately to verbalized communications. |

## Interventions

To the extent possible, have the patient's schedule consistent with regard to routines and repeated activities.

Be sensitive to the patient's reactions and needs. Treat him as an adult.

When speaking to the patient, make sure you have his attention; speak slowly and give only one instruction at a time.

When communicating with the patient, decrease other environmental stimuli.

Provide and/or utilize appropriate aids to communication, for example, related gestures, pictures, letter board.

Ask questions in a manner that only requires short answers or a nod of the head in response.

Give patient extra time to respond.

Make frequent rounds to ascertain the patient's needs.

Schedule rest periods prior to visiting hours or speech therapy sessions.

Do not pressure or tire the patient.

## Rationale

Helps patient to function in spite of deficit; helps memory and concentration (Brunner and Suddarth, 1988, p. 1447).

Fosters relationship conducive to communication (Brunner and Suddarth, 1988, p. 1447).

Helps patient to process what has been said (Brunner and Suddarth, 1988, p. 1447).

Patient can better concentrate on efforts to communicate (Ulrich, Canale, and Wendell, 1986, p. 135).

Facilitates communication (Ulrich, Canale, and Wendell, 1986, p. 135).

Decreases frustration and fatigue (Ulrich, Canale, and Wendell, 1986, p. 135).

There may be a lag time between when the patient is asked something and when he is able to respond (Pimental, 1986, p. 328).

Having needs consistently met can facilitate communication (Ulrich, Canale, and Wendell, 1986, p. 135) and helps in decreasing frustration when the patient is unable to adequately communicate desires (Doenges, Moorhouse, and Geissler, 1989, p. 250).

Allows for maximization of communication during that time (Ulrich, Canale, and Wendell, p. 135).

Symptoms of aphasia will worsen if the patient is fatigued, anxious, or upset (Pimental, 1986, p. 328).

---

**Potential for Injury**

*Related to:* Recent onset of right-sided hemiparesis, decreased ability to communicate, and potential for seizure activity.
*Evidenced by:* The presence of risk factors such as right-sided muscle weakness; mobility impairment; uncertainty with regard to patient's mental status, his ability to make judgments, and his ability to understand and follow directions; and signs and symptoms of central nervous system pathology.

**Desired Patient Outcomes**

Patient will remain injury free.

**Evaluation Criteria**

Throughout hospitalization and at time of discharge, Mr. Todd will be free of injury.

## Interventions

Keep bed in low position at all times, except during treatments, etc. Consider risk vs. benefit in determining position of side rails.

If possibility of seizure exists, keep side rails padded.

Have suction available at patient's bedside.

Have call light accessible to the patient and instruct regarding its use. Place it in a location accessible to the unaffected side.

Change patient's position frequently:

• Place in lateral or semiprone position.
• Limit the amount of time the patient spends on the affected side.
• Place the patient in prone position for 15–30 minutes several times per day.

## Rationale

Prevents falls if patient becomes confused or restless or minimizes likelihood of injury (Long and Phipps, 1985, p. 380). Use of side rails is a nursing decision. If a patient attempts to climb over side rails, he may have farther to fall (Phipps, Long, and Woods, 1987, p. 2038).

Minimizes injury in the event of seizure (Doenges, Moorhouse, and Geissler, 1989, p. 264).

Maintain airway and prevent aspiration in the event of seizure or increased salivation (Doenges, Moorhouse, and Geissler, 1989, p. 264) or swallowing disorder (Dudas, 1986, p. 349).

Allows patient to have assistance with needs rather than attempting to do for self (Kneisl and Ames, 1986), p. 1171).

Protects from aspiration of secretions.
May not be aware of pressure due to impaired sensation.

Helps prevent knee and hip flexion contractures, and helps drain bronchial secretions (Brunner and Suddarth, 1988, p. 1444).

---

| *Impaired Swallowing* | ***Related to:*** Sensory-motor impairment of the muscles of swallowing. <br> ***Evidenced by:*** Observed difficulty swallowing, coughing when eating, and food remaining in oral cavity after swallowing. |
|---|---|
| *Desired Patient Outcomes* | • Patient's nutritional needs will be met and the risk of aspiration minimized. <br> • Patient's swallowing will improve. |
| *Evaluation Criteria* | ***Throughout Hospitalization and at Time of Discharge:*** <br> • The patient will not experience signs and symptoms of nutritional deficit such as weight less than standard for height and body build, dehydration, anemia, or muscle wasting. <br> • The patient will not experience signs and symptoms of aspiration such as fever, productive cough, or pneumonia. <br> • By time of discharge, the patient will demonstrate improved ability to swallow. |

---

## Interventions

Keep accurate record of intake.

In accordance with the treatment prescribed by the speech therapist, rein-

## Rationale

Impaired swallowing may interfere with adequate nutrition. An alternate method of feeding may be required (Dudas, 1986, p. 349).

Radiographic studies provide the speech therapist with the data to determine the specific etiology of the swallowing disorder.

## Interventions

force exercises to improve oral motor control of the bolus and voluntary stage of swallowing, that is, exercises to increase range of motion of the tongue, bolus control exercises, and bolus propulsion exercises.

Give only small amounts of food at a time. Show the patient the amount of food as reassurance that it cannot obliterate his airway.

Have the patient in high Fowler's position for meals and for 30 minutes afterward.

Place food on the unaffected side and tilt head toward the unaffected side.

Be familiar with the patient's swallowing therapy instructions, which should be posted in the patient's room.

Check the patient's mouth frequently for food remaining after the swallowing attempt has been completed.

Have suction available.

When the patient is lying down, assure that he or she is in the lateral position.

Provide a quiet environment and refrain from distracting the patient during swallowing procedure.

Offer foods that are stimulating in temperature and texture.

Make note of foods that cause difficulty and convey this information to appropriate persons, for example, speech therapist, nurses, and physician.

## Rationale

Nurses are with the patient more than other professionals and so are important reinforcers of the patient's regular and correct practice of swallowing procedures (Logemann, 1983, pp. 132, 155).

Large amounts of food may cause aspiration or airway obstruction (Logemann, 1983, p. 139).

Assists in swallowing and prevents aspiration (Dudas, 1986, p. 349; Ulrich, Canale, and Wendell, 1986, p. 133).

Food may be better managed on the unaffected side (Logemann, 1983, p. 141).

Reinforcement and feedback are important in the total management of this patient problem (Logemann, 1983, p. 155).

The patient may not be aware of food pocketed on the affected side, which could pose a later danger (Dudas, 1986, p. 349).

The patient may not be able to handle secretions, food, and liquids (Dudas, 1986, p. 349).

Prevents aspiration (Brunner and Suddarth, 1988, p. 1414).

Swallowing for this patient requires intense concentration (Dudas, 1986, p. 349).

Such foods are often helpful in initiating the swallowing reflex (Dudas, 1986, p. 350).

Some foods may pose greater problems than others depending on the source of the dysfunction (Luckmann and Sorensen, p. 1425).

## QUESTIONS FOR DISCUSSION

1. List the 3 main causes of cerebrovascular accident, and identify in order of frequency of occurrence. Discuss similarities and dissimilarities in their presentation.
2. Who are the populations at risk for CVA and why? What role can nurses play in the prevention of CVAs?
3. In the early care of the patient who has had a CVA, what nursing actions are of greatest importance? How would you prioritize these?
4. What are important nursing interventions for the continued care of a patient who has had a CVA with regard to visual disturbances, elimination, dependency issues, and grieving?
5. Discuss concerns of immobility for the CVA patient, and nursing actions to prevent complications.

6. What information can you give to Mr. Todd's wife and family about his current situation and projected recovery? Include potential tests, treatments, therapies, and rehabilitation strategies.
7. Discuss discharge planning considerations for Mr. Todd.
8. List some outcome criteria by which the overall nursing care of Mr. Todd could be evaluated.

## REFERENCES

Baxter, D: Clinical syndromes associated with stroke. In Brandstater, ME, and Basmajian JV (eds): Stroke Rehabilitation. Baltimore, Williams & Wilkins, 1987, pp 36–54.

Brunner, LS and Suddarth, DS: Textbook of Medical-Surgical Nursing, ed 6. JB Lippincott, Philadelphia, 1988.

Doenges, ME, Moorhouse, MF, and Geissler, AC: Nursing Care Plans: Guidelines for Planning Patient Care. FA Davis, Philadelphia, 1989.

Dudas, S: Nursing diagnoses and interventions for the rehabilitation of the stroke patient. Nurs Clin North Am 21(2):347–357, 1986.

Gorelick, PB: Cerebrovascular disease: Pathophysiology and diagnosis. Nurs Clin North Am 21(2):275–288, 1986.

Kasuya, A and Holm, K: Pharmacologic approach to ischemic stroke management. Nurs Clin North Am 21(2):289–296, 1986.

Kneisl, CR and Ames, SW: Adult Health Nursing: A Biopsychosocial Approach. Addison-Wesley, Reading, Mass, 1986.

Logemann, JA: Evaluation and Treatment of Swallowing Disorders. College-Hill Press, San Diego, Calif, 1983.

Luckmann, J and Sorenson, KC: Medical-Surgical Nursing: A Psychophysiologic Approach, ed 2. WB Saunders, Philadelphia, 1980.

Phipps, WJ, Long, BC, and Woods, NF: Medical-Surgical Nursing Concepts and Clinical Practice. CV Mosby, St Louis, 1987.

Pimental, PA: Alterations in communication: Biopsychosocial aspects of aphasia, dysarthria, and right hemisphere syndromes in the stroke patient. Nurs Clin North Am 21(2):321–337, 1986.

Rose, FC and Capildeo R: Stroke: The Facts. Oxford University Press, New York, 1981.

Stewart, J: Clinical Anatomy and Physiology for the Frustrated and Angry Health Professional. MedMaster, Miami, 1986.

Tellis-Nayak, M: The challenge of the nursing role in the rehabilitation of the elderly stroke patient. Nurs Clin North Am 21(2):339–343, 1986.

Ulrich, SP, Canale, SW, and Wendell, SA: Nursing Care Planning Guides: A Nursing Diagnosis Approach. WB Saunders, Philadelphia, 1986.

Wallhagen, MI: The split brain: Implications for care and rehabilitation. Am J Nurs 79:2118–2125, 1979.

## BIBLIOGRAPHY

Barnett, HJM, et al (eds): Stroke Pathophysiology, Diagnosis and Management, Vols 1–2. Churchill Livingston, New York, 1986.

Brandstater, ME and Basmajian, JV (eds): Stroke Rehabilitation. Williams & Wilkins, Baltimore, 1987.

Goetter, W: Nursing diagnoses and interventions with the acute stroke patient. Nurs Clin North Am 21(2):309–319, 1986.

Mitchell, PH, et al: Neurological Assessment for Nursing Practice. Reston Publishing Co, Reston, Va, 1984.

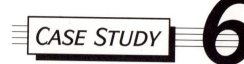

# A PATIENT WITH SPINAL CORD INJURY

Meg Doherty, M.S., R.N.

Approximately 10,000 cases of spinal cord injury are reported annually in the United States. It is one of the most devastating of all injuries because, in one instant, spinal cord injury creates lifelong physiological, emotional, social, and economic alterations in one's life and is an experience that affects not only the individual, but the entire family unit.

## ANATOMY AND PHYSIOLOGY OF THE SPINAL CORD

The spinal cord is a conduit for messages to and from the higher levels within the central nervous system and participates in reflex motor activities. It is continuous with the brain stem, beginning with the foramen magnum, descending through the vertebral canal, and terminating at the level of the first and second lumbar vertebra in a tapered cone, the conus medullaris. The very thin end of this cone extends downward as a connective tissue filament, the filum terminale, attached to the periosteum of the coccyx. The cord is protected by the bony vertebral column, dura mater, arachnoid, and pia mater, respectively. The area between the arachnoid and the pia mater is the subarachnoid space, which contains arteries, veins, and cerebrospinal fluid. Within the spinal cord denticulate ligaments join the pia mater with the arachnoid and dura mater, helping to stabilize the cord within the spinal canal.

Multiple arteries feed the spinal cord. The vessels join, forming a complex network that supplies the vertebrae, periosteum, and the dura mater. Branches supply the ventral and dorsal roots and penetrate deeply into the cord. Anterior and spinal arteries extending the length of the cord originate from the carotid and vertebral arteries. The venous system of the spinal cord is a rich network. The internal vertebral venous plexus is made up of anterior and posterior venous channels that extend from the skull to the sacral region. Thoracic, abdominal, and intercostal veins as well as the external vertebral plexus have connections with the internal vertebral plexus at each intervertebral space.

The spinal cord contains neuronal cell bodies, ascending sensory tracts, and descending motor tracts. A cross section of the spinal cord demonstrates an H formation of gray matter (nerve cell bodies), surrounded by white matter (nerve tracts and fibers). Within the center of the gray matter lies the central canal, which contains some cerebrospinal fluid and cellular debris.

The functions of the spinal cord include:

- The transmission of sensory impulses from the skin and viscera by way of afferent nerves through ascending tracts to the brain.
- The transmission of motor impulses from the brain by way of efferent pathways to the appropriate nerves supplying muscles, glands, and other body parts. Both motor and sensory pathways are located on either side of the cord.

- Reflex movements (automatic, stereotypic movements that do not require cortical functioning), by way of a reflex arc within the spinal cord. Sensory neurons relay impulses from sensory receptors to central neurons located within the cord. Central neurons then send impulses to motor neurons leading to glands and muscles. Reflex movements are initiated by various noxious stimuli such as pain, rapid stretch, and fear.

The *peripheral nervous system* is composed of cranial and spinal nerves (Fig. 6–1). These nerves may be afferent (carry impulses toward the central nervous system), efferent (carry impulses away from the central

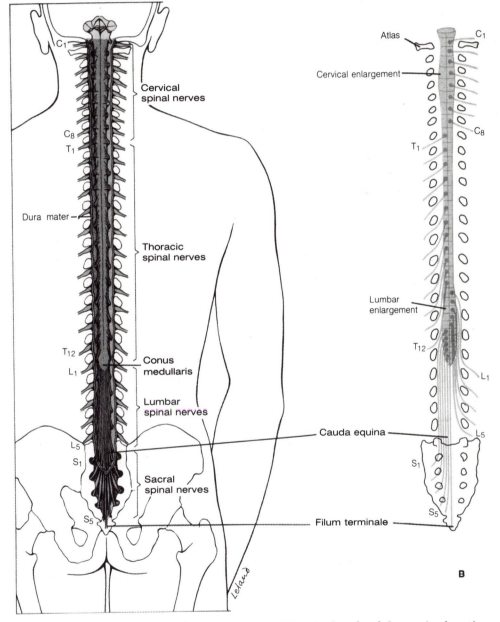

**FIGURE 6–1.** The spinal cord regions and principal nerves. (**A**) The spinal cord and the proximal portions of the spinal nerves in the normal positions, viewed with the neural arches of the vertebrae removed and the dura mater that surrounds the cord open. (**B**) The spinal cord and spinal nerves illustrating the cauda equina. The letters indicate specific spinal nerves. C = cervical; T = thoracic; L = lumbar; S = sacral. (From Spence, A P and Mason, E B: Human Anatomy and Physiology, ed 3. Benjamin/Cummings, Menlo Park, CA, 1987, p. 358, with permission.)

nervous system), or mixed (composed of both afferent and efferent fibers). There are 31 pairs of spinal nerves (8 cervical, 12 thoracic, 5 lumbar, 5 sacral, and 1 coccygeal). Each nerve is attached to the spinal cord by 2 roots: the dorsal root, which receives sensory input from sensory receptors throughout the body, and the ventral root, which contains a combination of motor fibers innervating glands and voluntary and involuntary muscles. Generally, each cord segment is named for the vertebral body below its exit point. Each spinal nerve branches into small posterior divisions and large anterior divisions at a short distance from the spinal cord. Anterior branches interweave, forming 3 major plexuses that branch out into body parts: the cervical, brachial, and lumbosacral plexuses. Smaller nerves emerge from these plexuses and continue to subdivide to innervate distal regions of the extremities.

The *autonomic nervous system* is composed of 2 subdivisions: the sympathetic nervous system and the parasympathetic nervous system. The sympathetic nervous system originates from the thoracic and lumbar areas of the spinal cord. It functions to accelerate some body processes in response to stress or emergencies, for example, it increases heart rate, dilates blood vessels, increases blood sugar, and increases secretion of epinephrine and norepinephrine. The parasympathetic nervous system originates in the 3rd, 6th, 9th, and 10th cranial nerves and in the sacral segment of the spinal cord. Parasympathetic action primarily maintains body functions under normal conditions. The overall function of the autonomic nervous system is that it provides a homeostatic internal state despite changing external conditions.

## PATHOPHYSIOLOGY

The neural elements of the spinal cord and spinal nerve roots are injured by the mechanisms of compression from bone and ligaments, disk herniation, and hematoma; edema following compression or concussion; overstretching or disruption of neural tissue; and disturbances in spinal circulation. Following an impact injury to the spinal cord, pathological changes occur (Fig. 6–2).

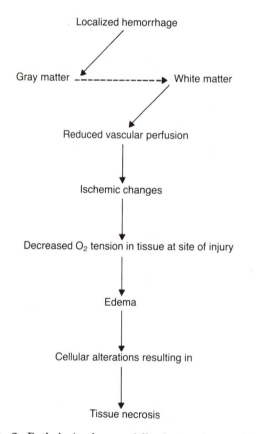

**FIGURE 6–2.** Pathologic changes following an impact injury to the spinal cord.

Several minutes after traumatic injury, microscopic hemorrhages appear in the central gray matter and in the pia-arachnoid. The small hemorrhages increase in size until the entire gray matter is hemorrhagic and necrotic. Hemorrhaging and peritraumatic edema progress transversely and longitudinally to the white matter, impairing the microcirculation to the spinal cord. Circulation in the white matter returns to normal within approximately 24 hours, but circulation in the gray matter remains altered. Within 36–48 hours after injury phagocytosis occurs around the necrotized area. Blood is gradually removed from the tissue by disintegration of red cells and reabsorption of hemorrhages. Macrophages engulf degenerating axons in the first 10 days after injury. By the third or fourth week after injury, injured segments of the spinal cord are replaced with acellular collagenous tissue, which connects the meninges to the cord and central canal. Scarring in the area of destruction consists mainly of thickened meninges and connective tissue.

Injury to the spine may involve the vertebral column, the surrounding ligaments, or the spinal cord. In general, injury to all 3 structures is usually the most serious. Injury to the cord and its roots may be caused by concussion, producing transient neurological symptoms that resolve within hours; contusion, producing changes within the cord itself and causing edema and surface hemorrhage; or by compression, producing edema and ischemia leading to necrosis. Deficits that follow contusion and compression may resolve slowly; some are permanent. Transection or severe interruption of spinal cord function results in complete paralysis and sensory loss below the level of injury.

## RISK FACTORS

There is a higher incidence of spinal cord injury among males, by approximately 82%. The mean age of injury is 33 years. The leading cause of injury is motor vehicle injury, followed by falls, gunshot wounds, diving and motorcycle accidents, and other types (including sports and occupational injuries). Cervical injuries are the most common of the spinal cord injuries and are usually related to flexion-extension maneuvers during a traumatic injury. Fracture-dislocations in the thoracic and lumbar areas usually arise from compression injuries, as in falls from high places. Fracture-dislocations can occur anywhere along the spine.

## COMMON CLINICAL FINDINGS

Symptoms reflect the specific area of cord damage and vary in severity depending on the amount of cord compression or cord transection.

*Cervical cord transection* results in quadriplegia with varying degrees of respiratory and arm paralysis, depending on the injury level. Cord transection of the thoracic spine through L-1 and L-2 causes paraplegia. There is absence of pain, pressure, and joint sensation below the level of injury.

Incomplete spinal cord injuries result in varying degrees of sensory and motor deficits, for example:

*Anterior cord syndrome,* usually caused by flexion injuries to the cervical spine, results in complete loss of sensation to pinprick below the level of injury, upper and lower extremity weakness, and preservation of deep pain, light touch, and joint sensation.

*Brown-Séquard syndrome,* resulting from hemitransection of the cord, causes loss of voluntary control of the upper and lower extremities on the same side as the injury and loss of pain and temperature on the opposite side.

*Central cord syndrome,* caused by damage in the central portion of the spinal cord, is manifested by decreased motor ability of the upper extremities, the lower extremities remaining less severely affected. There may be bilateral loss of pain and temperature sensation below the level of injury, and the bladder may also be affected.

**Spinal shock.** Spinal shock usually occurs within 30–60 minutes of spinal cord injury producing a complete loss of sensory, motor, autonomic, and reflex functioning below the level of injury. It is characterized by flaccid paralysis, flaccid sphincters, loss of sensation, absent deep-tendon reflexes, and profound hypotension associated with bradycardia. Spinal shock may last for days or months and ends with the return of reflex activity. Indications of recovery are the return of the anal reflex, flaccid paralysis becoming spastic, and gradual return of autonomic functions and of reflex bowel and urinary bladder contraction.

# TREATMENT MODALITIES

The acute phase of management focuses on both medical and bony stabilization. The airway and ventilation of the patient must be ensured. Approximately 20%–30% of patients with spinal cord injuries require some form of temporary ventilatory assistance. Approximately 2%–4% require continued mechanical ventilation. These patients have injury at the level of C-3 and above. Patients with lower cervical injuries demonstrating respiratory fatigue and a vital capacity of less than 1000 ml require immediate evaluation for supportive mechanical ventilation. The cardiovascular system is another major concern. There is an initial loss of sympathetic nervous system control, resulting in a loss of tone in the peripheral vasculature causing vasodilation and decreased arterial blood pressure. Because of parasympathetic nervous system dominance, bradycardia occurs. Interventions may include administration of intravenous (IV) vasopressors and when bradycardia is profound, IV atropine.

With evidence or suspicion of spinal instability, immobilization is essential. Patients with diagnosed cervical instability are treated with skeletal traction such as Gardner-Wells tongs applied in the emergency department. Maintenance of spinal stability is further enhanced by the use of specific immobilization beds. The two used most frequently are the Stryker frame and the Roto-Rest bed. The halo traction device is used to maintain immobilization of the cervical spine in the postoperative phase or to facilitate immobilization when surgery is not possible.

Determination of instability is confirmed by a lateral x-ray study of all 7 cervical vertebrae as well as subsequent additional views and by anteroposterior, oblique, and open-mouth odontoid films. The thoracic and the lumbar spine are studied by anteroposterior and lateral x-ray films. Other diagnostic studies that may be employed include computed tomography (CT) scan to determine spinal cord edema, magnetic resonance imaging to detect spinal cord edema and cord compression, and myelography to establish the presence of spinal block.

Surgical stabilization of the spine and spinal cord decompression during the initial management are controversial. Usually surgical intervention is indicated when there is a progressive neurological deficit, in order to preserve remaining function and prevent further damage; with compound fractures and penetrating wounds of the spine; in the presence of bone fragments in the spinal canal and in the presence of anterior cord syndrome. Spinal fusion and Harrington rod insertion for treatment of fracture instability facilitate early, active rehabilitation activities and help prevent complications of bed rest.

Investigational treatments of spinal cord injury include hypothermia produced by local perfusion with iced saline, hyperbaric oxygenation, and early surgical decompressive techniques. To date, no treatment has been shown to restore spinal cord function in complete injuries.

Corticosteriod therapy to reduce spinal cord edema during the acute stage of injury is frequently prescribed although its efficacy remains controversial.

## Rehabilitation

Rehabilitation for the spinal cord–injured patient begins on admission to the acute care facility and is an extensive care process. The biopsychosocial alterations that occur after a spinal cord injury demand an integrated and collaborative multidisciplinary approach. The focus of the plan is to prevent the secondary complications of immobility and altered body states and to educate the patient and family. The educational process strives to develop competence in all areas of self-care. The overall goal is the productive and self-fulfilling reintegration of the injured person into society (Hargrove and Reddy, 1986, p. 599).

To date, there are 14 federally designated Model Spinal Cord Injury Systems in the United States. This concept links together the services required by the spinal cord injured from the moment of injury through the initial medical-surgical management, blending into lifetime follow-up services providing appropriate medical-surgical health maintenance and crisis intervention (Metcalf, 1986, p. 589).

# PATIENT ASSESSMENT DATA BASE

## Health History

*Client:*
Caroline Griffin

*Address:* 7 Longwood Ave., Colorado Springs, CO 80906
*Telephone:* 303-555-8361
*Contacts:* (1) Philip Barry (boyfriend)
         (2) Thomas Griffin (father)
*Address of contacts:* 7 Longwood Ave., Colorado Springs, CO 80906 (boyfriend)
                        2 Puritan Ave., Denver, CO 80262 (father)
*Telephone of contacts:* 303-555-8361 (boyfriend); 303-555-5543 (father)
*Age:* 25    *Sex:* Female    *Race:* White
*Educational background:* Engineering student (Carson Military College)
*Religion:* Catholic    *Marital status:* Single
*Usual occupation:* Full-time student
*Present occupation:* Same
*Source of income:* None
*Insurance:* Prudential
*Source of referral:* Community Hospital, Colorado Springs
*Source of history:* Patient; patient record
*Reliability of historian:* Reliable
*Date of interview:* 2/1/90
*Reason for visit/Chief complaint:* Acute care; surgical exploration/stabilization of thoracic spine, and rehabilitation secondary to complete transection of the spinal cord at the T-4 level.

## HEALTH PERCEPTION/HEALTH MANAGEMENT PATTERN

### Present Health Status

This 25-year-old white female was injured in a motor vehicle accident on 1/7/90 at 8:30 AM and was found in a ditch about 25 ft (750 cm) from her car, immersed in water. The patient has no recollection of events surrounding the accident or of her transport to the local hospital. On admission to the local hospital she was found to have complete loss of motor and sensory function from the nipples down, was stabilized, and then transported to this facility. On admission the patient was found to have a T-4 fracture, subluxation of T-3, complete paraplegia, with absent deep tendon reflexes (DTRs) and plantar response in both lower extremities. She was placed in a Roto-Rest bed, begun on dexamethasone (Decadron) and spent 3 days in the intensive care unit. On 1/14/90 she underwent exploration of the thoracic spine and Harrington rod fusion of T1-6. Her postoperative course was uneventful and she began with rehabilitation activities (active) 2/1/90 on the rehabilitation unit.

### Past Health Status

*General Health.* General health was essentially excellent, without any major health problems. Patient states the only time she was ever injured or ill was in 1981 when she fell from her bike and dislocated her shoulder.
*Prophylactic Medical/Dental Care.* Caroline has visited physician only for physical examination required for school or to travel, when she needed "shots." She does, however, have annual gynecological examination and Pap smear. Teeth are in good

repair; she visits the dentist every 6 months and when she has a problem.

***Childhood Illnesses.*** "Routine"; she reports several episodes of strep throat treated with antibiotics, the last episode when she was age 18.

***Immunizations.*** All childhood immunizations and revaccinated to travel abroad in 1981. Last tetanus shot in 1980.

***Major Illnesses/Hospitalizations.*** None.

### Current Medications

*Prescription:* Oral contraceptives—1985–1990 (discontinued [d/c] on admission); probantheline bromide (Pro-Banthine), 15 mg PO bid; methenamine hippurate (Urex), 1 g PO bid; docusate sodium (Colace), 100 mg PO bid; vitamin C, 500 mg PO qid; glycerin suppository, 1 rectally qod; Senokot ii tabs PO qod hs.

*Nonprescription:* Occasional aspirin and cold medicines.

***Allergies.*** None to food or medications known.

### Habits

*Alcohol:* "Social only."
*Caffeine:* Caffeinated coffee in the morning; 2 cups/day.
*Drugs:* See Current Medications.
*Tobacco:* ½–1 pack per day for 5 years; d/c 2 years ago.

### *Family Health History*

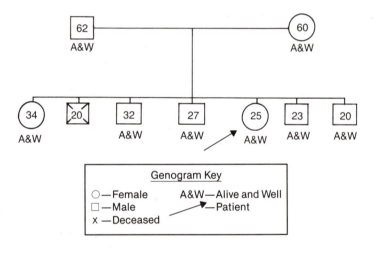

Family history includes, father "ulcers" and "stomach removed" at age 27; mother, rheumatoid arthritis, onset—age 43; brother, killed in an airplane crash, age 20.

## NUTRITIONAL/METABOLIC PATTERN

### *Nutritional*

The patient describes her nutritional status as usually well balanced and states that during the week at school it's usually "salads and fish or chicken."

### *Usual Daily Menu*

*Breakfast:* Juice; coffee; toast, muffin, or cereal.
*Lunch:* Yogurt, salad, sandwich or soup, and diet soda.
*Dinner:* Larger meal, usually consisting of meat, fish, salad, and a vegetable. "If the meal at school isn't good, I'll eat at Wendy's."

*Metabolic*

She states that her weight has been stable at 130 lb (59 kg) for the past 5 years, but "I would like to be thinner." "Usually when I make up my mind to diet, I don't have much of a problem sticking to it." Height is 5 ft 4 in. (162.5 cm). Appears well nourished. Excellent dentition.

## ELIMINATION PATTERN

*Bowel*

Prior to injury Caroline did not have any problems. "I never used laxatives"; "I had regular bowel movements every day." Patient now has neurogenic bowel and has begun instruction with bowel care. "At first I didn't quite believe them [about how bowel care was performed], but if this is what has to be done I'll learn." (At this time the patient cannot actively participate since she is still in a neck brace; her sister and boyfriend have been instructed).

*Bladder*

Prior to injury, patient denies any problem with urination. She has had 2 urinary tract infections "a few years ago, when I was in the Army; it was treated with Gantrisin [sulfisoxasole]." No problems since. Secondary to the injury, the patient has a neurogenic bladder. The Foley catheter is out and the patient is insistent to begin bladder training today (intermittent self-catheterization). "I don't know why, but I just don't want to be attached to a bag and prone to a lot of infections." "I am a very determined and conscientious person and I feel strongly that I can accomplish this." The staff demonstrates technique and explains while they perform the procedure since the patient will not be able to actively participate until the brace is removed.

## ACTIVITY/EXERCISE PATTERN

*Activity/Exercise*

The patient describes herself as extremely physically active. She attends Carson Military College, in which physical exercise (e.g., calisthenics and running) is "part of the daily routine." She and her boyfriend of 5 years run daily and participate in competitive races for enjoyment on their time off together. "We also run to keep our weight down," she adds. The patient describes herself as fairly disciplined about this: "Even when we vacation we bring along our running gear." Caroline and her boyfriend travel "somewhere" each year and are socially active. "We usually try new restaurants or attend plays and movies on weekends with friends or family members."

### Self-Care Ability

| | |
|---|---|
| Feeding—0 | Grooming—0 |
| Bathing—III | General mobility—III |
| Toileting—IV | Cooking—0 |
| Bed mobility—II | Home maintenance—IV |
| Dressing—III | Shopping—IV |

---

### *Functional Levels Code*

0—Full self-care
I—Requires use of equipment or device
II—Requires assistance or support from another person
III—Requires assistance or support from another person and equipment or device
IV—Is dependent and does not participate

Rehabilitation potential in all categories is estimated to be 0, except for General Mobility, which is estimated to be I prior to discharge.

**Oxygenation/Perfusion**

*Last Chest X-Ray:* 1/20/90 — Clear. No history of pulmonary problems; without respiratory difficulty since injury.
*Last ECG:* 1/13/90 — within normal limits (WNL).
*Sinus Rhythm:* Normal — rate = 72.

*1/22/90.* Patient experienced an episode of "feeling faint and dizzy" following a shower while waiting to be assisted into the wheelchair. Blood pressure was 70/52; patient was tilted back for a few minutes. Repeat blood pressure was 90/60. Orthostatic hypotensive episode was caused by blood pooling and rapid change of position. Patient was instructed re: slower position changes, necessity for elastic stockings, and physiological dynamics involved. Usual blood pressure is 120/64. Patient is at risk for deep vein thrombophlebitis secondary to effects of immobilization.

**Cardiac Risk Factors**

|  | Positive | Negative |
|---|---|---|
| Sedentary life-style |  | X |
| Hyperlipidemia |  | X |
| Cigarette smoking | X |  |
| Diabetes |  | X |
| Obesity |  | X |
| Hypertension |  | X |
| Hypervigilant personality |  | X |
| Family history of heart disease |  | X |

## SLEEP/REST PATTERN

**Sleep/Rest**

Patient denies any problem with sleeping: "I usually average 6–8 hours of sleep, waking early, around 6 AM, refreshed." She has never relied on sleep aids and does not require rest during the day; reports no problem with sleep since hospitalization. "I sleep like a log. They keep you pretty busy here during the day. By the time they help you shower and the OT [occupational therapist] helps with dressing, it's lunchtime; then after PT [physical therapy], meetings, and classes, you're pretty tired out at the end of the day."

## COGNITIVE/PERCEPTUAL PATTERN

**Hearing**

Patient denies problems with hearing.

**Vision**

"Perfect vision"; does not wear glasses or contacts.

**Sensory Perception**

Prior to injury, the patient experienced no problems; currently she describes loss of feeling "at nipple line on the left, slightly below the breast on the right, continuing downward including both lower extremities." The patient verbalizes understanding that she will feel no pain and that she will need daily skin inspection. The patient is right hand dominant.

**Learning Style**

Caroline learns best by explanation and demonstration. Describes herself as an "eager and quick learner." She denies difficulty with decision making and in fact describes herself as sometimes "being impulsive."

## SELF-PERCEPTION/SELF-CONCEPT PATTERN

### Self-Perception/Self-Concept

Caroline believes herself to be a very "up" person. "I'm not the type of person to dwell on things or worry too much about what other people may think. I'm usually very positive about myself and my abilities; I feel very secure." When asked about her usual emotional response to specific life situations, she responded, "In terms of anger, I consider it a flash in the pan; I maybe get upset for the moment but it's over and done with. I never hold a grudge." When asked specifically about her reaction to her injury, she said, "I knew when I couldn't feel anything that it was serious. When I was transferred here I asked immediately and the doctors and nurses were honest about my situation. I think if they had misled me even for a moment, it would have been much more difficult for me. I've had times of denial, periods of 'why me?' and difficult days. Sometimes I think that maybe something will happen and I will walk, but generally I realize that this is the situation I am faced with and have to do my best to live my life as normally as possible. I do have concerns about still being attractive. I asked my roommate [a spinal cord–injured man] about the impact of being in a wheelchair on my appearance and he replied, 'You have nothing to worry about'. That made me feel a little better."

"In general, I feel that I have a very positive attitude about myself and my future." During the interview she also included the following statement: "Crying is a wasted emotion. All it does is give me a headache and a red face, so why waste time on it. One year from now people will be so used to my being in a wheelchair that they probably won't even notice it."

## ROLE/RELATIONSHIP PATTERN

### Role/Relationship

The patient is a junior in Carson Military College, where she is an older student; she is 1 of 5 females in a class of 200 males. She resides in a mixed dormitory during the school week and with her boyfriend, Phil, on weekends. "I am concerned about returning to school; already some faculty have implied that I should consider transferring to another college. I don't want that and I'm willing to pursue every avenue to return. The dorm where I live is completely accessible and in fact, the first level is designed for the disabled. I have invested a lot of time and energy and all my friends are there."

"Phil is looking for a more accessible apartment for us when I get discharged. When I begin to go out for weekends I can stay at my sister's house, which is accessible, and my parents are having a ramp built so that I can visit there."

Caroline is one of 7 children in a very close family. "My brothers and sister visit all the time. My mother and father are extremely supportive and encouraging, although I know this has been very rough on them. They will do anything to help out. We had our usual family Thanksgiving, with relatives and friends and the entire dinner here in the PT room — tablecloth, centerpiece, and all."

The patient and her boyfriend have lived together for 5 years in a third-floor modern apartment. He is very supportive. Caroline states that "we're good for each other; he is older (34), has his own business, and economically we'll be ok until I can return to school." She describes herself as "friendly and outgoing; not at all shy about asking for what she needs or needs to know. I'm lucky to have so much great support . . . family and friends to count on. What I like is that most of my friends and my family don't treat me any differently."

## SEXUALITY/REPRODUCTIVE PATTERN

### Sexuality/Reproductive

The patient reports regular monthly periods that resumed 3 weeks after the injury. Her sexual relationship is a monogamous one, and she reports sexual relations as twice a week since the start of school. She feels her questions have been somewhat answered during her hospital stay, especially by a graduate nursing student who has had much experience in this area. "She has given me some printed materials and some resources for me to send for. Of course this is something I will have to do more reading about. I am concerned about how Phil will feel about all of this. It's something we'll just have to work out. When I approached the subject earlier in my hospitalization, Phil stated that 'we have more important things to worry about right now.'" The patient is aware that reproduction is still a possibility and that a change in birth control method needs to be addressed. Caroline has always felt satisfied with her sexuality.

## COPING/STRESS TOLERANCE PATTERN

### Coping/Stress Tolerance

Caroline reports: "I usually work out when I'm under stress and it has generally worked for me. I'm not usually afraid of a challenge, and can meet things head on. I have had and continue to have fears about certain aspects of my situation, for example, when I think of the future I worry a little about what might happen to me . . . Will I finish school? Will I ever be really totally independent? What if I develop arthritis like my mother, how would I get around?" Caroline reports that encouragement from the nurses about what she will be able to do is very helpful. "Just knowing that eventually I will be able to drive a car again, swim, participate in wheelchair sports, helps me to focus on the positive. I'm trying to take one day at a time; I admit, sometimes it is hard." Caroline states that she began to smoke again while hospitalized. "I'm sure it's related to stress; I don't even enjoy it, but most of the other patients here smoke and I've started again. I'm sure I'll be able to quit. The fact that I have good emotional support has helped me a lot. What I find most frustrating about my experience here is when I can't reach the things I need for showering and dressing; when I have to wait to put deodorant on or when I've forgotten to bring along my toothbrush to the bathroom and I have to wait for 20 minutes until someone comes back."

## VALUE/BELIEF PATTERN

### Value/Belief

Caroline states that life in general has been good for her, without major difficulties. She reports that she is a nonpracticing Catholic; that she believes in a God who is helpful and comforting in a time of need. She related, "When this first happened I thought, What did I do that God would punish me like this? I quickly replied to myself that God would not do this to anyone. I believe in being a good person and usually I try to be that person. I do believe that I have the strength to become independent again."

# Physical Examination

*General Survey*

Twenty-five-year-old attractive female, appearing stated age, in no apparent distress. She is neatly groomed, well dressed, sitting in a wheelchair in her room; alert and cooperative.

*Vital Signs*

***Temperature:*** 98°F (36.5°C) (oral)
***Pulse:*** 72, regular (apical)
***Respirations:*** 12, regular
***BP:*** 122/65 (right arm, sitting); 120/62 (left arm, sitting).

*Integument*

***Skin.*** Skin on head, arms, and torso is dry, warm, supple; no bruising, lesions or scarring. Skin on lower extremities is dry, warm, supple; no bruising, lesions, or scarring.
***Mucous Membranes.*** Pink, moist, and intact.
***Nails.*** Healthy in appearance and well groomed.

*HEENT*

***Head.*** Scale is normocephalic; no palpable masses noted. Hair is thick, neatly groomed. Face is symmetrical, without pain or crepitus on palpation; no bruises or scarring. Temporomandibular joint (TMJ) is fully mobile without pain or crepitation.
***Eyes.*** Pupils equal, round, reactive to light and accommodation (PERRLA). Extraoccular movements (EOMs) intact. Fundi are without edema, hemorrhage, or exudate. Gross visual acuity is intact.
***Ears.*** Able to hear whisper at 2 ft (60 cm). Ears are bilaterally symmetrical and equal in size and shape. Weber-Rinne test: air conduction > bone conduction. Canals are clear; no exudate. Tympanic membranes are intact, without scarring.
***Nose.*** Nostrils are pink and patent; no septal deviation.
***Mouth/Throat.*** Uvula is midline; excellent dentition. Tonsils are present; not enlarged.

*Neck*

Trachea is midline. Thyroid is nonpalpable. No palpable nodes; no rigidity; 17-cm surgical scar noted on the posterior aspect of the neck extending along the spine.

*Pulmonary*

Lungs are clear to auscultation with bilateral breath sounds; no abnormalities in rate or rhythm of breathing. Symmetrical, bilaterally diminished chest expansion.

*Breast*

Well-developed female breasts; nipples pink, without masses, swelling, tenderness, or exudate.

*Cardiovascular*

Apical pulse 72 and regular, no audible murmurs; $S_1$ and $S_2$ of good quality; no rub. Point of maximal impulse (PMI) at 5th intercostal space, midclavicular line; no carotid bruits heard.

*Peripheral Vascular*

Pulses in upper and lower extremities are within normal limits and are bilaterally equal. No edema noted.

***Peripheral Pulses***
Temporal—4 bilaterally
Carotid—4 bilaterally
Brachial—4 bilaterally
Radial—4 bilaterally
Femoral—4 bilaterally
Popliteal—4 bilaterally
Posterior tibial—4 bilaterally
Dorsalis pedis—4 bilaterally

***Peripheral Pulse Scale***

0—Absent
1—Markedly diminished
2—Moderately diminished
3—Slightly diminished
4—Normal

**Abdomen**

Active bowel sounds in all quadrants. Abdomen is nondistended, soft, and depressible. Nonpalpable liver, spleen, kidneys, without masses or bruits.

**Musculoskeletal**

Upper extremities are bilaterally equal with normal muscle tone, mass, and strength. No signs of joint inflammation, and no loss of motion. Lower extremities have no voluntary motion, with slightly increased tone and mild spasticity, bilaterally.

**Neurological**

*Mental Status.* Alert and oriented to time, place, and person.
*Cranial Nerves.* Intact.
*Motor.* Full range of motion in upper extremities; complete motor loss in lower extremities.
*Sensory.* Normal sensation to light touch in bilateral upper extremities. Complete loss of sensation from nipple line downward, including abdomen and lower extremities.

*Deep Tendon Reflexes*

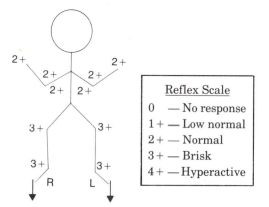

Reflex Scale
0 — No response
1+ — Low normal
2+ — Normal
3+ — Brisk
4+ — Hyperactive

**Rectal**

Loss of sphincter tone noted. Stool guaiac test is negative.

**Genitalia**

Normal external female genitalia; no bulging of the vaginal walls noted. No ulcerations, nodules, bleeding, or discharge from the cervix or vagina. Pap smear negative on 11/30/88.

# Laboratory Data/Diagnostic Studies

**Laboratory Data**

*1/9/90* CBC
*WBC:* 9.5/mm$^3$
*Hct:* 37.6%
*Hgb:* 12.2 g/dl

*1/20/90* CBC
*WBC:* 9.7/mm$^3$
*Hct:* 38%
*Hgb:* 12.5 g/dl
*PT:* 10.7/11.6
*PTT:* 33/30

*1/20/90 Urinalysis:*
*WBC:* 2–3/mm$^3$
*RBC:* 0
*Bacteria:* 0

*1/20/90 Urine Culture:*
No growth.

**Diagnostic Studies**

*Chest X-Ray:* *1/9/90:* Negative; *1/20/90:* Negative.
*Skull Film:* Negative.
*Intravenous Pyelogram:* No extravasation; normal kidneys.
*Thoracic Spine Film: 1/9/90:* Obvious burst fracture of T-4, subluxation of T-3; *1/20/90:* Normal kyphotic curve, Harrington rods extending from T1-7; no obvious scoliosis noted.

# COLLABORATIVE PLAN OF CARE

| | |
|---|---|
| *Diet* | Normal house diet. |
| *Medications* | Glycerin suppository 1 rectally qod.<br>Senokot ii tabs PO qod hs.<br>Pro-Banthine 15 mg PO bid.<br>Urex 1 g PO bid.<br>Colace 100 mg PO bid.<br>Vitamin C 500 mg PO qid. |
| *Activity* | Out-of-bed activities as tolerated. Passive participation in rehabilitation protocol until neck brace is removed (target date is 2/5/90). |
| *Therapeutic Measures* | ***Rehabilitation (PT):*** Passive range of motion (ROM) in lower extremities/active ROM in upper extremities qid.<br>***Bladder Training:*** Passive participation.<br>***Bowel Training:*** Passive participation.<br>Elastic stockings. |

# NURSING DIAGNOSES DEVELOPED IN CARE PLAN

Impaired Physical Mobility, p. 99
Altered Patterns of Urinary Elimination, p. 103
Potential Body Image Disturbance, p. 105

# ADDITIONAL NURSING DIAGNOSES TO BE CONSIDERED

Activity Intolerance
Altered Bowel Elimination
Altered Peripheral Tissue Perfusion
Dressing Self-Care Deficit
Fear
Knowledge Deficit (Self-Care)
Potential for Injury
Potential Impaired Skin Integrity
Potential Sexual Dysfunction
Sensory/Perceptual Alterations
Toileting Self-Care Deficit

# NURSING CARE PLAN BASED ON IDENTIFIED NURSING DIAGNOSES

| | |
|---|---|
| ***Impaired Physical Mobility*** | ***Related to:*** Paralysis, (spinal cord injury).<br>***Evidenced by:*** Complete loss of sensory/motor function below the level of injury (T-4 fracture; complete spinal cord transection; paraplegia). |

*Desired Patient Outcomes*

*The Patient Will:*
- Demonstrate independence with comprehensive mobilization (appropriate to level of injury), prior to discharge.
- Achieve an optimal level of independence in the activities of daily living, prior to discharge.
- Be aware of and able to prevent potential complications secondary to decreased mobility, prior to discharge.

*Evaluation Criteria*

*Upon Discharge, the Patient Will Be Able to Independently:*
- Transfer from bed to wheelchair/wheelchair to bed.
- Transfer from wheelchair to shower chair/shower chair to wheelchair.
- Transfer from wheelchair to floor/floor to wheelchair.
- Be independent in manual wheelchair indoors and outdoors, including curbs.
- Independently drive car with hand controls.
- Independently place wheelchair into car.
- Independently adhere to an exercise program for upper and lower extremities.
- Independently and routinely provide pressure relief.
- Independently perform AM care, shower, and dressing.
- Independently prepare meals.
- Identify risk factors associated with skin breakdown.
- Identify methods of prevention of skin breakdown.
- Demonstrate methods of skin inspection.
- Identify signs and symptoms of autonomic dysreflexia.
- Verbalize how, when, and where to seek medical attention if symptoms of autonomic dysreflexia occur.

## Interventions

Develop and coordinate a plan of progressive mobilization:

- Assure spinal stability.

- Establish mutual goal setting with the patient.
- Promote regularly scheduled interdisciplinary conferences (nursing, medicine, physical therapy, occupational therapy, social services) with patient, family, and significant others.

Assess and evaluate baseline vital signs prior to initiation of activities and reevaluate with increase in level of activity. If pulse increases >50 beats/minute reevaluate.

Observe for orthostatic hypotension with changing positions. If blood pressure drops or patient feels faint or dizzy, tilt chair back, elevate lower extremities, perform shoulder shrugs.

## Rationale

The nurse coordinates and integrates the multiple services of the total setting and develops and executes an individualized, comprehensive patient and family-centered care plan (Hargrove and Reddy, 1986, p. 599).

Once spinal stability is established, the elevation process and progressive mobilization can begin (Hargrove and Reddy, 1986, p. 600).
Mutual goal setting is a basic requisite for successful rehabilitation (King and Dudas, 1980, p. 228).
Regular interdisciplinary conferences that include the patient and the family are necessary since so many disciplines are involved in the rehabilitation program (King and Dudas, 1980, p. 229).

The process of mobilization must be gradual to avoid cardiovascular insult (Hargrove and Reddy, 1986, p. 600).

"Orthostatic hypotension occurs when the vasoconstrictor fibers of the sympathetic system are not stimulated in response to the decreased blood volume brought on by the change in position. To reduce the amount of blood that pools in the abdomen and the extremities, abdominal binders and elastic stockings should be

| Interventions | Rationale |
|---|---|
| | worn, head of bed raised gradually, or wheelchair should be tilted back and all position changes should be made slowly" (Metcalf, 1986, p. 595). |
| **2/1–2/15/90**<br>Initiate assistance with periods of dangling at the bedside up to 15 minutes, bid. | To promote balance, practice long-sitting at the bedside, sitting on side of the bed with assistance (Hargrove, 1986, p. 606). |
| Teach, assist with teaching, and reinforce transfer from bed to wheelchair with assistance bid, until independence with transfer is achieved. | A sliding board transfer may be used initially. The person needs good upper extremity strength to be able to slide buttocks from the bed to wheelchair (Carpenito, 1987, p. 269). |
| Instruct and supervise active range-of-motion exercises for upper extremities. Provide passive range-of-motion exercises to the lower extremities until the patient is able to perform them independently. | Range-of-motion exercises (qid) that concentrate on areas important to activities of daily living are essential (Hargrove and Reddy, 1987, p. 600). Passive range-of-motion exercises will keep muscles and joints limber (Carpenito, 1987, p. 267). Passive range-of-motion exercises can facilitate venous return (Metcalf, 1986, p. 595). |
| Increase wheelchair sittings from 1 hour to 2 hours, gradually increasing sittings until 8-hour wheelchair sitting is achieved. Provide for rest between sittings, decreasing rest periods as patient progresses. | Tolerance for activity gradually increases. Care must be taken not to fatigue the patient; periods of planned rest are important (Luckmann and Sorensen, 1987, p. 439). |
| Teach and reinforce weight shifting, wheelchair pushups, and leaning forward in wheelchair q30min until pressure relief is automatic behavior while sitting. | Prevention of pressure sores must continue whenever the patient is sitting (King and Dudas, 1980, p. 231). When sitting up in a wheelchair, a paralyzed person needs to shift body weight periodically and lift the body by pushing with the arms and hands against the chair arms or seat. This relieves pressure on the buttocks and prevents skin breakdown (Luckmann and Sorensen, 1987, p. 439). |
| Teach patient methods and areas for AM/PM skin inspection. | Decreased sensation, paralysis, and altered health states after a spinal cord injury increase the risk of skin breakdown. The client will need early prevention-oriented instruction to avoid skin breakdown and its sequelae of infection (Hargrove and Reddy, 1986, p. 602). |
| Initiate weight lifting, 5 lb (2.2 kg), each arm, increasing in 2-lb (0.9-kg) increments, qod as tolerated until 10 lb (4.5 kg) each arm for 10 minutes is achieved bid. | Increasing the muscular capability of nonaffected muscle groups supports greater motor ability. Initiation of weight lifting is a critical intervention. Upper extremity muscle strengthening will facilitate wheelchair mobilization and transfers (Hargrove and Reddy, 1986, p. 600). |
| Assess muscle strength daily. | Determination of muscle strength is achieved through daily grading and should be consistent with an accepted tool (Hargrove and Reddy, 1986, p. 600). |
| **2/15–Discharge (Target Date–1/20/91)**<br>Observe and evaluate independent transfer from wheelchair to shower chair; complete shower and transfer from wheelchair to bed for assist with dressing. | The nurse will provide practice in the activities of daily living and increase activity periods to the patient's tolerance (Hargrove and Reddy, 1986, p. 606). |

## Interventions

Assist occupational therapist with teaching and reinforcing shifting and weight-lifting techniques to facilitate dressing.

Assist patient with plans for 8-hour pass to family home.

Evaluate with patient and family members/significant other experiences and problems encountered during home visits. Assist with problem solving following each weekend pass.

Initiate and supervise advanced wheelchair transfer activities:

- Floor to chair
- Chair to floor

Assist with instructing, reinforcing, and evaluating patient with community mobility:

- "Curb wheelies"
- Hills
- Supermarket, use of pincers
- Restaurant
- Car transfer; independent wheelchair into car placement

Assist with supervision and evaluation of patient's ability to function in simulated kitchen:

- Use and safety with stove
- Use of assistive devices

Coordinate and assist with on-site home visit (physical therapy, occupational therapy) to patient and family, prior to discharge:

- Assess architectural barriers.
- Provide recommendations for alterations.
- Assess patient's ability to mobilize within the home (kitchen, bathroom, bedroom, and access).
- Provide written recommendations for renovations and assistive devices.

Assist patient with plans for initiation of driver's education, prior to discharge.

Provide information about services and resources for the spinal cord–injured patient, that is, National Spinal Cord Foundation, National Wheelchair Asso-

## Rationale

The nurse will work closely with the interdisciplinary team to determine the patient's individual learning/teaching needs. Sufficient time for dressing needs to be allocated (Hargrove and Reddy, 1986, p. 606; Carpenito, 1987, p. 386).

Weekly home visits by the patient are major steps in the preparation for discharge (King and Dudas, 1980, p. 242).

During home visits, the patient and family solve problems, face new experiences, and adapt what they have learned to a real life setting (King and Dudas, 1980, p. 242).

Transfers must include mastery of transfer to floor from wheelchair and from floor to wheelchair without assistance to promote safety and increase independence (Hargrove and Reddy, 1986, p. 608).

Mobilization in the home and to the community imposes definitive barriers. Comprehensive mobilization must include all possible situations a person may encounter (Hargrove and Reddy, 1986, p. 602).

The goal of rehabilitation of the person with a spinal cord injury is to enable the person to live successfully in the community. This implies that persons are prepared to care for themselves and are independent to the greatest extent possible. The nurse is a key provider and facilitator of patient adaptation (King and Dudas, 1980, p. 242).

A home visit by the staff prior to discharge is recommended. Rehabilitation and long-term care must be prevention-oriented, patient- and family-centered, and transcend all geographical boundaries (King and Dudas, 1980, p. 241).

Education about available resources and services is a part of any comprehensive retraining program (Hargrove and Reddy, 1986, p. 609).

Same as above.

## Interventions

ciation, The Regional Model Spinal Cord Injury Systems, and the National Institute on Handicapped Research.

Identify for the patient potentially serious complications and methods to reduce risks of:

• Skin breakdown

• Autonomic dysreflexia

## Rationale

The prevention of complications secondary to pressure requires the provision of pressure relief, close inspection of the skin, intelligent use of supportive devices, and education of the patient and family (King and Dudas, 1980, p. 231). Spinal cord injury increases the risk of skin breakdown. The patient will need instruction in good hygiene, nutrition, weight relief, and proper transfer (Hargrove and Reddy, 1986, p. 602).

Autonomic dysreflexia is an acute syndrome related to massive vasodilatation above the level of injury and vasoconstriction below it. Patients with spinal cord injuries at the T-6 level or above are at risk. When present, the situation is emergent and intervention must be immediate. Classic signs and symptoms include severe headache, reddened face, hypertension, a blood pressure reading significantly above the baseline for the individual, bradycardia, and diaphoresis above the level of injury. Common causes include bowel impactions, bladder overdistention, skin breakdown, infections, and severe spasms. The only definitive treatment is to find and remove the cause. The initial intervention is immediate elevation of the head to reduce blood pressure. If the cause cannot be immediately determined, antihypertensive medications can be used to lower blood pressure until the cause is determined (Metcalf, 1986, p. 595). The severe hypertension can result in cerebrovascular accident, seizures, or death. All patients with injuries to T-6 or above must be taught symptoms, causes, and treatment. An initial episode may occur months after injury; therefore, it is important to teach all patients who are likely to develop symptoms, rather than wait for an episode to occur. If a patient with severe, recurrent episodes is going home for weekends, the emergency room staff at the local community hospital should be informed of this condition and its appropriate treatment (King and Dudas, 1980, p. 239).

| *Altered Patterns of Urinary Elimination* | *Related to:* Neurogenic bladder.<br>*Evidenced by:* Decreased urinary output and distended bladder. |
|---|---|
| *Desired Patient Outcomes* | *Upon Discharge, the Patient Will Be:*<br>• Able to perform independent intermittent self-catheterization.<br>• Knowledgeable about basic anatomy and physiology of the urinary system.<br>• Able to prevent bladder distention.<br>• Knowledgeable about prevention of urinary tract infections. |
| *Evaluation Criteria* | *Upon Discharge, the Patient Will Be Able to:*<br>• Demonstrate independent, intermittent self-catharization using clean technique. |

- Verbalize basic understanding of the anatomy and physiology of the urinary system.
- Demonstrate a pattern of intermittent catheterization consistent with intake and avoidance of bladder distention.
- Adequately control urinary output without incontinence.
- Verbalize understanding of the relationship between bladder distention and infection.
- Verbalize understanding of the relationship between bladder distention and autonomic dysreflexia.
- Verbalize the importance of daily urological medications.
- Verbalize the need for continued urological follow-up.

## Interventions

Provide an overview of the bladder training program and rationale.

Outline patient commitment and the responsibilities and advantages of the program.

Provide slide-tape presentation of the anatomy and physiology of the bladder, urinary tract, and urinary meatus. Demonstrate the self-catheterization procedure, utilizing a model. Promote discussion and questions, and provide answers.

Initiate fluid intake and output profile, teaching patient to:

- Monitor and document his or her own intake and output.
- Restrict fluids.
- Avoid caffeinated drinks.

Instruct, assist with, and assess the patient's progress with self-catheterization:

- Sterile technique in the hospital.
- Clean procedure in the home.

- Initiate self-catheterization every 4 hours.

## Rationale

Patients with spinal cord injury have lost urinary sphincter control and the sensation of fullness. These result in the retention of urine or incontinence. Intermittent catheterization is aimed at prevention of bladder overdistention and the possibility of stimulating autonomic dysreflexia. Intermittent catheterization has replaced the indwelling catheter as the favored method of management for persons with spinal cord injuries. The major retraining goals are to control bladder functions and to avoid bacteriuric states (Hargrove and Reddy, 1986, p. 603).

The risk of urinary tract infections is reduced by the selection of patients for intermittent self-catheterization who are reliable in following regimens of care and are amenable to frequent reevaluation by the medical team (Hargrove and Reddy, 1986, p. 603).

The goal of education is to assist the person to implement positive choices about actions required to maintain health. For the patient to assume this increased responsibility, participation in goal setting, knowledge of the rationale for care measures, and specific teaching in all aspects of care are necessary (King and Dudas, 1980, p. 241).

Intakes and outputs are related; efforts are to avoid >400-ml volume in the bladder and overdistention. Fluids must be spaced to stimulate the bladder's reflex activity (Hargrove and Reddy, 1986, p. 604). Self-catheterization, adjustment of fluid intake, and intake and output documentation by the patient should be taught early in the program (King and Dudas, 1980, p. 253).
The use of coffee, tea, and alcohol should be limited because of their diuretic effect, which may affect predictability of voiding pattern (Carpenito, 1987, p. 192).

Clean technique has the same infection rate as sterile insertion methods for home catheterization (Luckmann and Sorensen, 1986, p. 438).
Periodic distention and relaxation of the bladder muscle facilitate early reflex activity of the bladder (Hargrove and Reddy, 1986, p. 604). Frequent catheterization decreases the chance of bacterial infection, since bladder overdistention causes stretching and fissure formation, predisposing to infection (Luckmann

## Interventions

- Emphasize success; deemphasize incontinence.

- Provide discharge education:

  ○ Explain appropriate use and rationale for urological medications.

  ○ Reemphasize the importance of avoiding overdistention of the bladder.

  ○ Provide information about urological follow-up.

## Rationale

and Sorensen, 1986, p. 435). Levels of residual urine will indicate the need for increasing or decreasing the frequency of catheterization (Hargrove and Reddy, 1986, p. 604).

Incontinence is a source of embarrassment, and success in the area of elimination is often perceived as progress in self-control (Hargrove and Reddy, 1986, p. 604).

Patient education is directed toward prevention of genitourinary complications by maintenance of an acid pH of urine, aseptic performance of procedures, avoidance of bladder distention, and use of urinary medications (King and Dudas, 1980, p. 235).

Urex contributes to the acidification of urine and provides weak antibacterial action (Govoni and Hayes, 1988, p. 758). Pro-Banthine is used to treat urinary bladder spasm. Expect dry mouth (Govoni and Hayes, 1988, p. 1001).

Frequent and complete emptying of the bladder is necessary; avoidance of accumulating over 300–400 ml of urine is the best method (King and Dudas, 1980, p. 235).

Yearly urological workup and cultures can be anticipated. Follow-up will be a lifelong process (Hargrove and Reddy, 1986, p. 604).

---

### Potential Body Image Disturbance

*Related to:* Physical change: paralysis.
*Evidenced by:* Questions of being attractive; cessation of the ability to physically engage in running; and the possibility of change in educational/career goals.

### Desired Patient Outcomes

*The Patient Will:*
- Maintain a positive, accepting, and realistic body image.
- Accept and incorporate the physical change into her body image and self-concept.

### Evaluation Criteria

*Upon Discharge, the Patient Will Be Able To:*
- Acknowledge her own strengths and abilities.
- Verbalize feelings and thoughts relating to paralysis and its effects on her lifestyle.
- Demonstrate an interest in learning about the body change and its effects on daily living and coping patterns.
- Effectively problem-solve.
- Demonstrate, behaviorally and verbally, an understanding of the limitations imposed by the body change.

---

## Interventions

Accurately assess the patient's concept of self, before and after disability.

## Rationale

The key to all steps of the nursing process is accurate assessment. Assessment of change requires information about the patient's previous status with regard to self-perception, social interactions, and behavioral patterns prior to the disability. The goal is to obtain reliable information about the psychosocial impact of the disability (Carlson, 1980, p. 317).

"If nurses have a framework for assessing patient's self-concept, they will be better able to predict potential problems in temporary or permanent adaptation to stressful situations. In addition, nurses would be better able to help patients use the strengths of their self-concept to cope with situations. In turn, nurses would be promoting the patient's adaptation skills" (Thompson, 1986, p. 814).

## *Interventions*

Assess the patient's self-perception:

- Assist the patient with identification of past/present, pleasing/not-pleasing physical aspects.
- Continually assess and evaluate patient references to physical self and all other self-evaluative statements.
- Observe the manner in which the patient treats himself or herself.
- Continually assess for verbal/nonverbal cues that may alter original assessments.

Assess social interactions:

- Discuss social interactions between patient and significant others prior to disability.
- Observe and assess behaviors of others in response to the patient.
- Validate interpretations of observed interactions with patient and significant others, when possible.

Assess behavioral patterns:

- Ask about previous coping behaviors in specific situations, for example, when patient has been frightened or anxious or when goals have been interfered with.

Assist patient to deal with and accept issues of self-concept related to body image.

Enhance improved and realistic patient self-perception:

- Acknowledge and provide positive reinforcement when patient enhances personal appearance (new clothing, makeup, etc).
- Provide time for and encourage those aspects of personal care that are important to the patient.
- Establish with the patient and emphasize her unique, positive strengths. Reinforce them when the opportunity arises.
- Focus on realistic, achievable goals, (i.e., wheelchair racing, driving).

## *Rationale*

Accurately assessing how a patient did or does perceive himself or herself is a complicated process. Until more precise measures are available, nurses should be cautious about the accuracy of their references and be observant for new information that would change their judgments. Self-perception must be inferred from what a person says and does. The way persons treat themselves provides clues to the value they place on themselves (Carlson, 1980, p. 318).

One of the major characteristics associated with self-concept is that it is inseparable from social life and develops out of experiences, particularly out of social interactions with significant others (Thompson, 1989, p. 1755). Significant others' responses may be most critical to the patient's self-assessment, self-esteem, self-concept, and body image (Carlson, 1980, p. 317). When assessing social perception and response the nurse is trying to learn how others perceive and behave in response to the patient. Retrospective information provides the baseline for assessing change and for setting goals that will help the patient return to baseline to whatever extent possible (Carlson, 1980, p. 318).

Coping patterns can be determined by asking questions about previous stressful situations, and about what the patient did at those times (Carlson, 1980, p. 317). The nurse must consider what patterns were present prior to the injury and attempt to determine the needs or goals that were served by the behaviors. One must determine which patterns can be reestablished and which potential behavioral patterns can be developed to replace former ones (Carlson, 1980, p. 319).

Helping patients with body-image disturbance requires a supportive approach. Being supportive also implies the ability to help the patient in more concrete ways, to look at strengths and capitalize on them and to assist with problem solving for the limitations or alterations caused by the body change (Kneisl and Ames, 1986, p. 59).

Through careful guidance, the patient can accept an altered body image and lifestyle. The major components of the plan are to establish a trusting relationship; be an active listener; reinforce positive feelings; clarify misconceptions; promote social interaction; and provide anticipatory guidance (Kneisl and Ames, 1986, p. 1857).

## Interventions

• Encourage verbalization of feelings, concerns, and fears about the body change.

Promote social interaction:

• Encourage verbalization of the impact of body change on assuming activities of daily living (family, school, social relationships).
• Encourage discussion and further exploration of attitudinal/behavioral responses of significant others.
• Provide information about "typical" social perceptions, misconceptions, and responses to disability (e.g., patient can do nothing for self; spinal cord–injured patients all want to commit suicide; patients in wheelchairs also have cognitive disabilities.
• Provide practice in handling social situations: role playing, alternative actions, and community encounters.
• Encourage the patient's assumption of normal social activities as soon as possible.

Assist patient to identify behavioral patterns necessary to meet needs and cope with stress:

• Assist patient to establish alternate methods of coping, if necessary (e.g., if running was a method of stress reduction, perhaps encourage wheelchair racing).
• Assist patient with setting realistic, achievable goals.
• Assist patient to utilize identified, positive behavioral patterns to achieve goals.
• Gently reinforce the reality of the permanency of the disability.

## Rationale

Patients may profit from an understanding of the behavioral patterns that will be encountered in social situations and why they tend to occur. Anticipation of unpleasant events may increase anxiety; however, anticipation allows time for preparation for those events. Practice in handling situations may be helpful (Carlson, 1980, p. 315). Although nurses can work to educate the public and change values, more immediately effective approaches are required to help patients learn ways to handle the pressures and processes of social interactions (Carlson, 1980, p. 319). Patients need to understand social phenomena, recognize behaviors associated with them, and demonstrate methods of responding to these tendencies in others (Carlson, 1980, p. 319).

Almost everyone has developed ways by which they meet everyday physical, psychological, and social needs. The spinal cord–injured patient requires major changes in the established patterns of living and even in methods of coping with the changes. Some changes occur as a direct consequence of injury, while others occur because of the effects the condition has on other people. Change, even when it involves improvement, adds stress. Neurological disabilities may severely limit the behavioral options available for coping attempts. Coping patterns that require physical strength and coordination may be disrupted; thus, the very methods used to handle stress are frequently unavailable (Carlson, 1980, p. 315).

## QUESTIONS FOR DISCUSSION

1. During the acute phase of spinal cord injury what physical parameters would indicate spinal shock? How do these differ from hypovolemic shock?
2. What critical intervention before arriving at the hospital and in the emergency department can significantly reduce the risk of life-threatening consequences for the cervical spine–injured patient?
3. What levels of injury would pose most threat to the respiratory system in the spinal cord–injured patient and why?
4. Discuss how you would respond to a patient with spinal cord injury in the acute phase who asks, "Will I ever walk again?"
5. What self-evaluation statements in this case study would lead you to believe that the patient will be successful with achieving an optimal level of independence?

6. Develop a prioritized list of nursing diagnoses that would relate to the acute phase of care for the spinal cord–injured patient.
7. Identify the signs and symptoms of autonomic dysreflexia.
8. Identify this patient's risk factors for developing deep vein thrombophlebitis.
9. Identify actual and potential safety problems associated with the sensory/perceptual deficits experienced by the patient in this case study.

# REFERENCES

Carlson, C: Psychosocial aspects of neurologic disability. Nurs Clin North Am 15:2, 1980.

Carpenito, L: Nursing Diagnosis: Application to Practice, ed 2. JB Lippincott, Philadelphia, 1987.

Hargrove, SD and Reddy, M: Rehabilitation of spinal cord injury. Nurs Clin North Am 21:4, 1986.

Govoni, L and Hayes, J: Drugs and Nursing Implications. Appleton-Century-Crofts, Norwalk, Conn, 1988.

King, R and Dudas, S: Rehabilitation of patients with spinal cord injury. Nurs Clin North Am 15:2, 1980.

Kneisl, C and Ames, S: Adult Health Nursing. Addison-Wesley, Reading, Mass, 1986.

Luckmann, J and Sorensen, K: Medical-Surgical Nursing: A Psychophysiologic Approach. WB Saunders, Philadelphia, 1987.

Metcalf, J: Acute phase management of persons with spinal cord injury: A nursing diagnosis perspective. Nurs Clin North Am 21:4, 1986.

Thompson, J, et al: Clinical Nursing. CV Mosby, St. Louis, 1986.

Thompson, J, et al: Clinical Nursing, ed 2. CV Mosby, St. Louis, 1988.

# BIBLIOGRAPHY

Cardona, V (ed): Trauma Reference Manual. Brady Communications, Bowie, Md, 1985.

Doenges, M, et al: Nursing Care Plans: Nursing Diagnosis in Planning Patient Care. FA Davis, Philadelphia, 1985.

Donovan, W and Bedrook, G: Comprehensive management of spinal cord injury. Clinical Symposia 34:1, 1982.

Fischbach, F: Manual of Laboratory Diagnostic Tests, ed 3. JB Lippincott, Philadelphia, 1988.

Gordon, M: Nursing Diagnosis: Process and Application, ed 2. McGraw-Hill, New York, 1987.

Guyton, A: Textbook of Medical Physiology. WB Saunders, Philadelphia, 1983.

Hickey, J: The Clinical Practice of Neurological and Neurosurgical Nursing, ed 2. JB Lippincott, Philadelphia, 1986.

MacKechnie, J: Regional spinal cord injury center nursing care: Prescription of the present and future. J Neurosurg Nurs 14:3, 1982.

Matthews, P and Carlson, C: Spinal Cord Injury: A Guide to Rehabilitation Nursing. Aspen Publications, Rockville, Md, 1987.

Mooney, T, et al: Sexual Options for Paraplegics and Quadriplegics. Little, Brown & Co, Boston, 1975.

Niederpruem, M: Autonomic dysreflexia. Rehabil Nurs vol 9, 1984.

Price, S and Wilson, L: Pathophysiology: Clinical Concepts of Disease Processes. McGraw-Hill, New York, 1986.

Richmond, T: A critical care challenge: The patient with cervical spinal cord injury. Focus Crit Care 12:2, 1985.

Romeo, JH: The critical minutes after spinal cord injury. RN, April, 1988.

Rudy, E: Advanced Neurological and Neurosurgical Nursing. CV Mosby, St. Louis, 1984.

Trafton, P: Spinal cord injuries. Surg Clin North Am 62:1, 1982.

Vermeer, M: Cervical spine immobilization: A sampling. J Emerg Nurs 9:3, 1983.

Woods, N: Human Sexuality in Health and Illness, ed 3. CV Mosby, St. Louis, 1984.

# UNIT IV

# THE PATIENT WITH ALTERATIONS IN THE RENAL SYSTEM

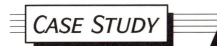

# A PATIENT WITH RENAL CALCULI

Jean D'Meza Leuner, M.S., R.N.

## ANATOMY AND PHYSIOLOGY OF THE KIDNEY

The two kidneys are located in the posterior abdominal area on either side of the lumbar spinal column at the region of the 12th thoracic and 3rd lumbar vertebrae (Fig. 7–1). The left kidney is positioned slightly higher than the right. While each kidney is partially protected by the ribs, the lower portions of both kidneys extend beyond the rib cage.

Each kidney is surrounded by a tough fibrinous capsule (Fig. 7–2). The capsule is smooth and transparent and serves as a barrier to trauma and infection. The cortex of the kidney lies below the fibrinous capsule. It extends to the inner medulla of the kidney with the renal pelvis located at the innermost aspect of the kidney. The renal pelvis is a sinus or open area into which the urine flows from the medulla. The hilus is the entrance to the renal pelvis. Blood, lymph vessels, and nerves communicate with the kidney through the hilus. Renal pyramids (8–18 cone-shaped masses) located in the medulla open into the renal pelvis. The end of each pyramid forms a papillae. Each papillae has 10–25 openings. Eight or more groups of papillae empty into a minor calix and several minor calices form a major calix. Major calices channel urine to the renal pelvis. The major calices and the renal pelvis can hold approximately 8 ml of urine.

The functional unit of the kidney is the nephron. Each kidney contains over 1 million nephron units. The nephron consists of a glomerular (Bowman's) capsule, proximal and distal tubules, and most of the loop of Henle. Nephrons are located in the cortical area with the descending loop of Henle and the collecting ducts in the medullary area.

At the hilum of the kidney, the renal nerves and blood supply enter the kidney. Arising from the abdominal aorta, the renal arteries emerge at the level of the second lumbar vertebra. The renal arteries branch into the interlobar, arcuate, and interlobular arteries. Blood leaves the kidney through interlobular veins followed by arcuate veins, interlobar veins, and finally into the renal vein. Ultimately the blood from the kidney empties into the inferior vena cava.

The nerve supply to the kidney arises from the renal plexus of the sympathetic division of the autonomic nervous system. The nerves are distributed to the vessels and have a vasomotor function. The circulation of blood within the kidney is regulated with arteriolar constriction or dilation.

The main function of the kidney is to maintain the volume and composition of the extracellular fluid. The excretory and nonexcretory functions of the kidney serve to regulate the constituents of plasma. Urine, a solution consisting of plasma waste products and other substances, is produced in the kidneys and transported by way of the ureters to the bladder and urethra and out of the body.

Urine is produced in the nephrons by 3 processes: filtration, reabsorption, and secretion. The filtration process produces approximately 90% water along with the excretion of several solutes, namely, sodium, potassium, calcium, magnesium, chloride, bicarbonate, phosphate, sulfate, and organic acids. The excretory functions of the kidney include excretion of urea, phosphates, sulfate, uric acid, nitrate, and phenols. These

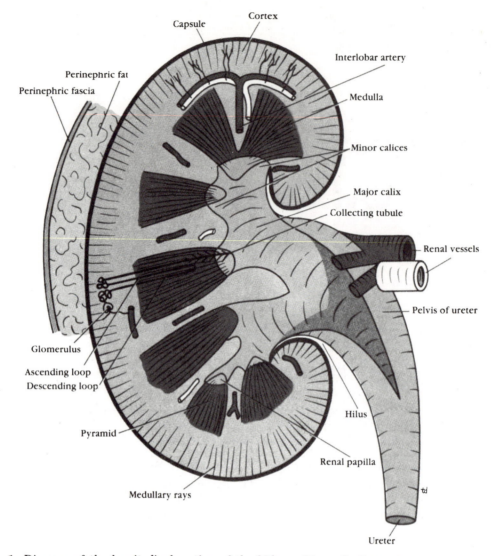

**FIGURE 7-1.** Diagram of the longitudinal section of the kidney. (From Snell, R: Clinical Anatomy for Medical Students, ed 2. Little, Brown & Co, Boston, 1981, with permission.)

are excreted during tubular reabsorption. The nonexcretory functions of the nephron include the secretion of renin, erythropoietin, kallikrein, and prostaglandins. Carbohydrates, lipids, plasma proteins, and peptide hormones are metabolized in the kidney and vitamin D metabolism is regulated as well.

# PATHOPHYSIOLOGY: UROLITHIASIS

Urolithiasis, or the presence of stones in the urinary tract, can occur anywhere within the urinary system. The most frequent site of stone formation is the kidney; however, stones can travel along the urinary tract and lodge in many different locations. The size of stones can vary from gravel-like particles to large masses that require surgical extraction. Calculi are more frequently seen in men than in women. While they have been identified in all age-groups, most are seen in persons between the ages of 20 and 55. Urinary calculi of the kidneys and ureters are more prevalent in developed countries of the world. The southeastern United States has been a location with a large number of persons afflicted with this problem. It has been hypothesized that this is due to a combination of 2 factors, soft water and consistent hot weather. The heat tends to lead to dehydration and the urine becomes more concentrated, thus producing an environment conducive to stone formation.

The etiology of stone formation is not clearly understood; however, several factors influence this process. Inhibitors are substances that have been identified through their ability to chelate stone constituents

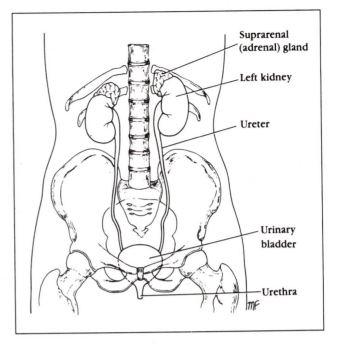

**FIGURE 7–2.** Diagram of the posterior abdominal wall showing the kidneys. (From Snell, R: Clinical Histology for Medical Students. Little, Brown & Co, Boston, 1984, with permission.)

rendering them nonsuitable for stone formation. Inhibitors include citrate, pyrophosphate, magnesium, and glycosaminoglycans that, when present in adequate quantities, inhibit crystal aggregation.

The presence of precipitators may predispose a person to crystal formation. Precipitators include protein matrix, which is predominantly mucoproteinaceous material, bacteria, and inflammatory elements. The presence of precipitators in the urine creates an environment that attracts crystallites and causes stone formation. An increase in urine concentration may predispose a person to stone formation. In addition, urine pH affects the ability of specific crystalline types to precipitate.

Kidney stones may be composed of a variety of elements. Approximately 65% of renal stones are composed of calcium and another substance. The substances that combine with calcium are typically phosphate or oxalate, or a combination of both. The remaining 35% of renal calculi are struvite (magnesium ammonium phosphate) (15%), uric acid (10%), and cystine (10%).

*Calcium stones* may vary in size from very fine gravel to large stones. The cause of calcium stone disease is multifactorial except for approximately 5% of patients who present with well-defined pathological conditions such as renal tubular acidosis, primary hyperparathyroidism, sarcoidosis, or inflammatory bowel disease.

Hypercalciuria or hyperuricosuria are two metabolic disorders commonly associated with calcium stone formation. Hypercalciuria is the hyperexcretion of calcium into the urine. An increase in urinary calcium can result from an increase in absorption of calcium from bone or intestine or an impairment in renal tubular absorption. Medications such as furosemide, exogenous steroids, ammonium chloride, acetazolamide, excessive thyroid hormone, and excessive intake of vitamin D are known to cause hypercalciuria.

Hyperuricosuria, or increased levels of uric acid in the urine, is mainly attributed to an excessive intake of dietary purines. Patients with hyperuricosuria have a lower urine pH that predisposes to uric acid crystallization.

Hyperoxaluria is associated with stone formation. Severe calcium restrictions, an excessive intake of ascorbic acid, or methoxyflurane anesthetic can result in hyperoxaluria. Patients with inflammatory bowel disease or small bowel bypass surgery are at risk for an increase in absorption of oxalate and the development of renal calculi.

Calcium stones are opaque and can be visualized on x-ray examination. Calcium phosphate stones are usually yellow or brown in color and are found in varying degrees of hardness. Calcium oxalate stones are dark in color and are small, hard, and rough in texture.

Hyperuricuria or an increase in the excretion of urate results in the formation of uric acid stones. An increase in the formation of uric acid within the body can be observed with gout or myeloproliferative disease. In addition, a diet rich in purines or the administration of uricosuric agents can also contribute to the formation of *uric acid stones*. Uric acid stones are typically nonopaque. They are usually present bilaterally and are multiple in number.

*Cystine stones* result from an inherited autosomal recessive disorder. If this disorder is present, it is seen in young children and adolescents. It is rarely observed in adults. Cystine stones are light yellow in color. Usually more than 1 stone is present at a time. These stones are opaque and difficult to visualize on x-ray examination.

Triple phosphate or *struvite stones* occur in the presence of a bacterium, usually *Proteus*, which contains the enzyme urease. Urease splits urea in half to form 2 ammonia molecules, thus raising the pH of the urine. Struvite stones are characteristically hard and form staghorn calculi. The presence of bacteria in the center of this stone formation makes it difficult to treat and reinfection is often common. Struvite stones are yellow in color, opaque, and easy to visualize on x-ray examination.

# RISK FACTORS

Persons who are at a high risk for the development of urolithiasis are those with problems resulting in immobility, urinary tract infections, dehydration, gout, malignant neoplasms, and disorders of the endocrine system. Patients with a familial history or a medical history suggestive of problems of the genitourinary tract should be carefully assessed.

# COMMON CLINICAL FINDINGS

Patients with renal calculi, irrespective of the type of stone, exhibit similar signs and symptoms. The presence of pain is described most often in patients with renal calculi. Pain may be very severe with a sudden onset. This pain is often referred to as renal colic or ureteral colic. Pain can be intermittent or continuous and may be accompanied by nausea, vomiting, and diarrhea. In contrast, patients may describe their discomfort as an ache in the flank or abdominal area.

Patients may complain of urinary frequency and urgency. An obstruction to the flow of urine may occur and infections may result. Tissue trauma has been seen in persons with renal calculi, and hemorrhage may occur as well.

# TREATMENT MODALITIES

The treatment plan for a patient with renal calculi is developed with the careful consideration of several factors. The size and location of the stone(s) must be ascertained. Renal structure and function must be evaluated along with the presence or absence of infection and the degree of pain the patient is experiencing.

Medical management includes maintenance of adequate hydration, the use of pharmacological agents, and dietary restrictions. Chemolysis can be employed to dissolve stones, in particular struvite, uric acid, and cystine stones. This would require the surgical placement of a nephrostomy tube.

Surgical intervention is performed with an open approach to the anatomical area harboring the calculi or a percutaneous approach to allow for the extraction and/or evacuation of the calculi. Stone disintegration may be achieved with the use of an ultrasound transducer. High frequency vibrations from this transducer reduce the stone mechanically.

Extracorporeal shock wave lithotripsy (ESWL) is a noninvasive procedure that is used to crush calculi with the use of shock waves. To perform this procedure, the patient's trunk is submerged in a tank of water. An underwater electrode is positioned to generate a spark. Water is vaporized from the spark to create a shock wave in the water. The shock wave moves in a spherical pattern as it is reflected from an ellipsoid portion of the tank to the site of the stone location. The shock waves are automatically discharged on the R wave of an EKG monitor to avoid a disruption in the patient's cardiac rhythm. The gravel that is produced by this procedure is then eliminated with urination.

# PATIENT ASSESSMENT DATA BASE

## Health History

*Client:*
Ms. Ruth Greene

*Address:* Atlanta, Georgia
*Telephone:* 404-555-1200
*Contact:* Allison (daughter, a student in college)
*Address of contact:* Atlanta, Georgia
*Telephone of contact:* 404-555-7231
*Age:* 52    *Sex:* Female    *Race:* Black
*Educational background:* Ph.D. from Georgetown University
*Religion:* Baptist    *Marital status:* Divorced
*Usual occupation:* College professor at Emory University
*Source of income:* Self
*Insurance:* Master Health Plus
*Source of referral:* Self and Dr. Carter
*Source of history:* Patient and daughter
*Reliability of historian:* Reliable, but questioning is limited due to acuity of symptoms. Old chart is available and daughter is able to provide information. (Additional information gathered after admission.)
*Date of interview:* 1/12/90
*Reason for visit/Chief complaint:* Fever of 101.4° (38.5°C), sudden sharp severe pain in the left flank area radiating to the left diaphragm and the left lower abdomen and groin area. "Please don't touch me, the pain is excruciating."

## HEALTH PERCEPTION/HEALTH MANAGEMENT PATTERN

*Present Health Status*

Pain began insidiously 1 day ago, first noted while Ms. Greene was sitting at her desk trying to prepare a class lecture. During the evening she began to feel chilly and nauseated. Also noticed she had diarrhea. "I was perspiring all night long." Temperature was 100.2°F (38°C), then 101°F (38.3°C). She started to try to increase her fluid intake but the nausea wouldn't go away. It was a very restless night. Temperature rose to 101.4°F (38.5°C) this morning. She called her physician, who advised immediate admission to the hospital. Accompanied by daughter on admission.

*Past Health Status*

**General Health.**   General health has been good. Occasional urinary tract infections that resolve with a course of medication. One year ago she had the last episode of renal colic. At that time, she increased her fluid consumption and spontaneously passed the stone. Had 1 other episode of pain due to a kidney stone 4 years ago, which required hospitalization. "I was on intravenous fluids, pain medications, and I passed the stone without surgery."
**Prophylactic Medical/Dental Care.** Ms. Greene sees her physician annually for an examination; more often if the need arises. Sees the dental hygienist every 6 months.
**Childhood Illnesses.** Had chickenpox, mumps, measles, and German measles. "Can't recall dates."
**Immunizations.** Last tetanus shot 1 year ago when she stepped on a nail at the beach.
**Major Illnesses/Hospitalizations.** Appendectomy (age 22). Kidney stone (1986); she was hospitalized and passed the stone spontaneously. "I wasn't this sick then."

### Current Medications
*Prescription:* None.
*Nonprescription:* Aspirin or Bufferin for cold or headache. Usually takes 2 tabs qid prn. Daily multivitamin, daily Vitamin C in time-release capsules.
**Allergies.** None.

### Habits
*Alcohol:* Usually 1 glass of white wine in the evening daily. Never more than 2–3 glasses of wine when out socially.
*Caffeine:* 3–4 cups of coffee a day; 1 cup of tea a day and on a hot day she will have a few glasses of iced tea.
*Drugs:* None.
*Tobacco:* Quit smoking cigarettes at age 26.

### Family Health History

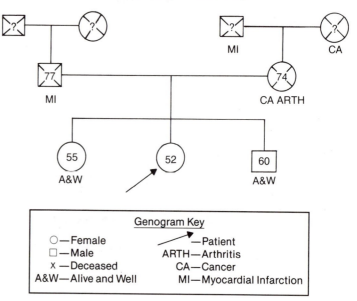

Genogram Key

○—Female          ↗—Patient
□—Male            ARTH—Arthritis
x —Deceased       CA—Cancer
A&W—Alive and Well    MI—Myocardial Infarction

## NUTRITIONAL/METABOLIC PATTERN

### Nutritional

Tries to follow a low-calorie diet to keep her weight down. "I love some of the foods I should avoid, so I occasionally cheat. With my erratic schedule, I can't always plan my meals. Some days I just eat and run. I would imagine that there is a specific diet I should follow to stop the stones from forming but I don't know what it is."

#### Usual Daily Menu
*Breakfast:* Juice, coffee, toast or bran cereal, 1–2 glasses of water.
*Lunch:* Soup or a sandwich, occasionally a salad, coffee, cookies or a piece of fruit, 1 glass of water.
*Dinner:* Fish, chicken, or occasionally meat; green or yellow vegetable (broccoli, peas, cauliflower, corn); potato or pasta on occasion; tea or coffee (usually 1 or 2 cups); ice cream (a small serving) or fruit; 2 glasses of water.

### Metabolic

*Weight:* 148 lb (67.3 kg). *Height:* 5 ft 5 in. (165.1 cm). No problems with chewing or swallowing and is unaware of any healing or bruising problems.

## ELIMINATION PATTERN

### Bowel

Three to 5 loose stools/day for the past 48 hours; light brown in color. Normally, 1 brown semiformed stool every other day. She has never used laxatives. Bran cereal in the morning does help with bowel regularity.

### Bladder

During the last few days she reports feeling as though she had to urinate all day long. When she did urinate it was in small amounts. Patient noted that the urine was pink-red in color. Prior to the recent problem, she would experience occasional pain and burning on urination. For this she would call the physician who would prescribe nitrofurantoin (Macrodantin, Furadantin) 4 times a day. When a urinary tract infection was present she tried to drink more fluids, especially water.

## ACTIVITY/EXERCISE PATTERN

### Activity Exercise

Daily activities of Ms. Greene include a combination of walking and sitting depending on her class/lecture schedule. Minimal daily physical activities. Minimal leisure time with work schedule. Any free time is spent reading, sitting by the pool, or on an infrequent golf game. Does have sufficient energy for activities.

#### Self-Care Ability

| | |
|---|---|
| Feeding — 0 | Grooming — 0 |
| Bathing — 0 | General mobility — 0 |
| Toileting — 0 | Cooking — 0 |
| Bed mobility — 0 | Home maintenance — 0 |
| Dressing — 0 | Shopping — 0 |

> #### Functional Levels Code
> 0 — Full self-care
> I — Requires use of equipment or device
> II — Requires assistance or supervision from another person
> III — Requires assistance or supervision from another person and equipment or device
> IV — Is dependent and does not participate

### Oxygenation/Perfusion

Last chest x-ray and ECG were done 1 year ago. Patient denies shortness of breath, wheezing, cough, sputum production or bronchitis, asthma, or respiratory infections. Denies palpitations, rapid heartbeat, irregular rhythm, or pain in her chest.

#### Cardiac Risk Factors

| | Positive | Negative |
|---|---|---|
| Sedentary life-style | | X |
| Hyperlipidemia | | X |
| Cigarette smoking | | X |
| Diabetes | | X |
| Obesity | | X |
| Hypertension | | X |
| Hypervigilant personality | | X |
| Family history of heart disease | X | |

## SLEEP/REST PATTERN

*Sleep/Rest*

Usually sleeps 6–8 hours per night. Awakens rested unless it has been a bad week with late meetings and long hours. Occasionally she awakens to use the bathroom. Has no difficulty returning to sleep. Never used any medications for sleep. "An occasional warm drink at bedtime is sometimes relaxing."

## COGNITIVE/PERCEPTUAL PATTERN

*Hearing*

Reports no difficulties with hearing. Denies earaches or vertigo.

*Vision*

Has worn bifocals for last 10 years. Sees ophthalmologist annually to check her eyes and the prescription. "My vision is very important to me; I take very good care of it."

*Sensory Perception*

Denies any problems with taste or smell. "I try to use distraction when I have pain. I am a busy woman and I try not to let any discomforts affect me too much. This kidney pain is unbearable; I need some medication to help with the pain." The patient is right-hand dominant.

*Learning Style*

Learns best by reading relevant information followed by the opportunity to ask questions for clarification.

## SELF-PERCEPTION/SELF-CONCEPT PATTERN

*Self-Perception/Self-Concept*

Ms. Greene describes herself as independent, lucky to have a wonderful daughter. Feels good about her life in general. Illness is "aggravating," making her fall behind in her work and she becomes more dependent on others than she would like. Claims to have no discomfort expressing her thoughts and feelings. Considers herself to be a good listener. "I listen to students and colleagues constantly. I'm always anxious to learn something or be challenged." Does not mind being touched, but does not engage in touching usually.

## ROLE/RELATIONSHIP PATTERN

*Role/Relationship*

Ms. Greene lives in a 3-bedroom condominium in a suburb of Atlanta. The condominium allows her to have a home with minimal maintenance worries. "I can always call the maintenance people when I have a problem. No lawn to mow, or house to paint. It is perfect for me."

Daughter lives with patient although her daughter's college life keeps her very busy and their schedules seldom match. "We, my daughter and I, have a very pleasant relationship. We enjoy each other's company and respect each other's privacy."

The patient's brother lives in the area and he is helpful. "I try not to bother him and his family unless it is appropriate. We do see each other for an occasional Sunday dinner or a holiday celebration." Patient's sister lives across the country and they seldom see each other but talk on the phone almost weekly.

She has no financial concerns. "My ex-husband has been supportive and I make a decent living as a professor. I'll never be rich, but I'm comfortable."

## SEXUALITY/REPRODUCTIVE PATTERN

*Sexuality/Reproductive*

Denies use of contraceptives. Has been divorced for 12 years now. Occasionally sees a male friend and has a pleasant sexual relationship with this man.

Menarche at age 13, menopause at age 45. Denies postmenopausal bleeding. Has an annual Pap smear. To date, results have been negative. Does not practice self–breast examination (SBE); unsure of how to do it and when to do it.

Gravida 1 and para 1; spontaneous vaginal delivery; uncomplicated pregnancy.

## COPING/STRESS TOLERANCE PATTERN

*Coping/Stress*

"My divorce was one of the most stressful events of my life. It was unpleasant to watch a relationship fall apart." Ms. Greene recalls that friends and family were supportive and staying busy with her job was crucial. "At times it was difficult to concentrate but I had to keep busy." She states that when she is stressed, she tries to put things into perspective. She tries to prioritize her problems and deal with the smaller issues rather than the larger concerns. "I have some wonderful friends, and an occasional lunch or dinner with friends takes my mind off my problems. My male friend is a good listener, and I am glad to have his company."

## VALUE/BELIEF PATTERN

*Value/Belief*

Patient states that she is a Baptist. Religion is an important part of her life even though she can't always attend church. "When my daughter was small, we always attended church and she had Bible study classes each week." Denies following any specific cultural customs.

# Physical Examination

*General Survey*

Fifty-two-year-old black female, as pleasant as can be expected and cooperative, while in acute distress splinting her left flank area. She is diaphoretic and restless.

*Vital Signs*

*Temperature:* 101.8°F (38.7°C) orally
*Pulse:* 110 regular (apical)
*Respirations:* 20 regular
*BP:* 152/78, right arm; 150/80, left arm, taken lying down.

*Integument*

*Skin.* Skin is warm and moist. Diaphoretic and without lesions or scarring.
*Mucous Membranes.* Mucous membranes are pink, moist, and smooth.
*Nails.* Nails on her hands are smooth; no clubbing noted.

*HEENT*

*Head.* Normocephalic, no palpable masses. Scalp appears dry; patches of eczema noted. Hair is coarse, curly, and slightly disheveled. Face is symmetrical; no droops or swelling; no tenderness on palpation. Temporomandibular joint (TMJ) is fully mobile, without crepitation or pain.
*Eyes.* Eyes have an equal gaze. Eyebrows are equal and lift symmetrically. Lacrimal gland is nontender; conjunctivae are clear, light pink in color. Pupils equal, round, reactive to light

and accommodation (PERRLA). Visual fields are equal. Full range of extraocular movements. No signs of nystagmus. Visual acuity: 20/20 with glasses using the hand-held eye chart.

*Ears.* Symmetrical, equal in size and shape. No pain in external auricles. Able to discern whisper at 1 ft with both ears. Weber test: Patient hears tuning fork equally in both ears. Rinne test: Positive with air conduction greater than bone conduction.

*Nose.* Nostrils are patent; mucosa pink and without drainage. No septal deviation noted.

*Mouth/Throat.* Mucous membranes are pink and moist. Uvula is midline. Tongue is fully mobile; no presence of lesions. Teeth with good dentition. No pain when tapping the teeth.

**Neck**

Neck is symmetrical; equal strength with sternocleidomastoid and trapezius muscles. No nodes palpated. Trachea is midline. Thyroid gland is not enlarged; no carotid bruits auscultated.

**Pulmonary**

Anteroposterior chest diameter 2:1. Respirations shallow and rapid. Chest excursion is symmetrical. Tactile fremitus is symmetrical. Lungs are clear on auscultation. Resonance noted on percussion.

**Breast**

No nodes palpable. Left breast slightly larger than the right. Symmetrical at rest and with movement. No masses or lesions noted and no dimpling. Nipples are without discharge.

**Cardiovascular**

No obvious jugular vein pulsations in a sitting position. Carotid pulses are strong and regular bilaterally; no bruits auscultated. No $S_3$ or $S_4$; no murmurs heard. Point of maximal impulse (PMI) identified at the fifth intercostal space, midclavicular line.

**Peripheral Vascular**

Extremities slightly diaphoretic with good skin turgor. Peripheral pulses equal and strong.

*Peripheral Pulses*
Temporal—4 bilaterally
Carotid—4 bilaterally
Brachial—4 bilaterally
Radial—4 bilaterally
Femoral—4 bilaterally
Popliteal—4 bilaterally
Posterior tibialis—4 bilaterally
Dorsalis pedis—4 bilaterally

*Peripheral Pulse Scale*

| |
|---|
| 0—Absent |
| 1—Markedly diminished |
| 2—Moderately diminished |
| 3—Slightly diminished |
| 4—Normal |

**Abdomen**

No obvious lesions or masses. Healed right lower quadrant (RLQ) scar (appendectomy). Abdomen tense; unable to palpate due to pain and splinting of left lower abdomen. No abdominal bruits auscultated. Patient restless, pain radiating from costovertebral angle to abdomen near umbilicus and into groin area. Peristaltic sounds present upon auscultation. Slight abdominal distention.

**Musculoskeletal**

Muscular development and mass appear normal for age. Patient states that she has full range of motion. Difficult to assess at this time due to level of discomfort.

**Neurological**

*Mental Status.* Patient is fully conscious; responds without difficulty to questions.

*Cranial Nerves.* CN I–XII intact; no problems elicited.

*Sensory.* Light touch, pain, and vibration to the face and extremities are normal and symmetrical. Patient states she walks without coordination difficulties. Not assessed at this time by examiner.

### *Deep Tendon Reflexes*

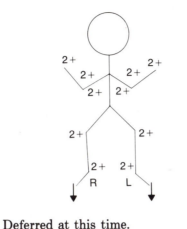

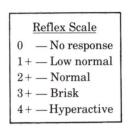

Reflex Scale

0 — No response
1+ — Low normal
2+ — Normal
3+ — Brisk
4+ — Hyperactive

| Rectal | Deferred at this time. |
|---|---|
| Genitalia | Deferred at this time. |

## Laboratory Data/Diagnostic Studies

**Laboratory Data**

*Hgb:* 14.0 g/100 ml
*Hct:* 36%
*Na:* 142mM/L
*K:* 4.0 mM/L
*Cl:* 104 mM/L
*CO₂:* 27 mM/L
*Ca:* 9.4 mg/dl
*Phosphorus:* 3.5 mg/100 ml
*BUN:* 24 mg/dl
*Creatinine:* 1.2 mg/dl
*PT:* 10.6/10.8

*Urinalysis*
*Urine:* Yellow, slightly turbulent; pH 7

*WBC screen:* positive
*Specific gravity:* 1.018
*Urobilinogen:* negative
*Nitrite:* negative
*Protein:* trace
*Bile:* negative
*Blood:* positive
*Crystals:* present
*Creatinine clearance:* 550 mg/24 hr
*Sodium:* 160 mEq/L/24 hr
*Calcium:* 360 mg/24 hr

**Diagnostic Studies**

*Chest X-Ray.* Lungs are clear.
*ECG.* Regular rate and rhythm; Normal sinus rhythm — rate 96.
*KUB and Upright Film.* Film showed long, approximately 1.5- cm calcification in area corresponding to left kidney calix.
*Intravenous pyelogram (IVP).* Hydronephrosis on the left collecting system down to the lower ureter. No clear stone seen.

## COLLABORATIVE PLAN OF CARE

**Diet**

Diet as tolerated (on admission).

**Medications**

Morphine sulfate 5–10 mg IM/SQ q3h prn for pain.
Flurazepam hydrochlorate (Dalmane) 15 mg PO prn hs.
Acetaminophen (Tylenol) 650 mg PO or rectally q4h for temperature over 101°F (38.3°C).

**Intravenous Therapy**

Begin IV with dextrose 5% and 0.45 sodium chloride at 100 ml/hr.

| | |
|---|---|
| **Therapeutic Measures** | Does not apply. |
| **Consults** | Does not apply. |
| **Preoperative Plan** | Soapsuds enema night before surgery. NPO after midnight (night before surgery). Cefazolin sodium (Ancef) 1 g/150 ml normal saline IV on call to OR. |

**Postsurgical Plan of Care**

### DIET

Diet as tolerated.

### MEDICATIONS

Morphine sulfate 5–10 mg IM/SQ q3h prn for pain or Percocet 1–2 tabs PO q3h prn for pain.
Dalmane 30 mg PO qhs prn for sleep.
Milk of magnesia (MOM) 30 ml PO prn.
Docusate sodium (Colace) 100 mg PO tid.
Trimethoprim/sulfamethoxasole (Bactrim DS) 1 tab PO bid.
Bisacodyl (Dulcolax) suppositories 1 rectally prn.
Ancef 3 g/250 ml 5% D/W. Give 83 ml IV q8h.

### INTRAVENOUS THERAPY

Dextrose 5% and Ringer's lactate solution at 125 ml/hr. IV can be converted to a heparin lock when fluid intake is greater than 1000 ml PO within 24 hours.

### THERAPEUTIC MEASURES

Measure intake and output.
Strain all urine.
Out of bed.
Maintain a dry sterile dressing at nephrostomy tube site.

**Additional Information**

The patient underwent surgery and had a percutaneous stone extraction by placement of a percutaneous nephrostomy tube. An ultrasonic lithotripsy was performed to facilitate the removal of the stone. Intermittent fluoroscopic monitoring occurred during the procedure and an x-ray was taken on completion of the procedure to ensure the removal of stone fragments. The patient left the operating room with a nephrostomy tube in place, as well as a Foley catheter drainage tube. The patient was in stable condition and encountered no complications during the procedure.

# NURSING DIAGNOSES DEVELOPED IN CARE PLAN

# ADDITIONAL NURSING DIAGNOSES TO BE CONSIDERED

Activity Intolerance
Altered Patterns of Urinary Elimination
Anxiety
Body Image Disturbance
Fear
Fluid Volume Deficit
Impaired Skin Integrity
Knowledge Deficit Regarding Self–Breast Examination

# NURSING CARE PLAN BASED ON IDENTIFIED NURSING DIAGNOSES

| *Pain* | ***Related to:*** Ineffective management of pain secondary to the presence of renal calculi.<br>***Evidenced by:*** Patient writhing in pain; verbalizing feelings of discomfort; diaphoresis and guarding the lower abdominal area. |
|---|---|
| ***Desired Patient Outcomes*** | ***The Patient Will:***<br>• Relate that she is experiencing a decrease in pain.<br>• Demonstrate the use of pain relief measures that are nonpharmacological in nature. |
| ***Evaluation Criteria*** | ***During the Hospital Stay, the Patient Will:***<br>• Assess her level of discomfort using a pain flow chart.<br>• Identify her level of discomfort as lessened.<br>• Verbalize an understanding of around-the-clock (ATC) pain medication administration.<br>• Have all her questions answered about pain relief measures.<br>• Demonstrate use of specific nonpharmacological pain relief measures.<br>• Plan activities to occur at the time of optimal pain relief. |

## Interventions

Reassure the patient that her pain is real and that you are interested in working with her to develop a plan to minimize the discomfort she is experiencing.

Teach the patient to evaluate her level of discomfort with the use of a pain assessment scale and flow sheet. Plan medication dosages with the patient based on the information on the pain assessment sheet.

## Rationale

A supportive nurse-patient relationship is integral to the successful management of pain by reducing the patient's anxiety about whether he or she will receive needed pain medication and by providing an emotional climate of caring and a sense of security that individual pain needs will be met. The nursing assessment of a patient in pain can justifiably rely on what the patient says (Carrieri et al, 1986, pp. 247, 253).

In order to assess pain effectively, the nurse should select a valid and reliable tool that is appropriate for the patient population and use it to evaluate pain over time (Carrieri et al, 1986, p. 251).

## Interventions

Explain to the patient why there is a need to administer pain medication on an ATC basis.

Answer all the patient's questions concerning the administration of pain medications. Stay with the patient and be sure that the patient knows you are committed to decreasing her level of discomfort.

Discuss with the patient the need to plan activities, scheduling tests to coincide with the maximum effectiveness of the pain medication.

Teach alternative pain control techniques to the patient that are non-pharmacological. The techniques should include distraction and relaxation techniques, contralateral stimulation, application of hot and cold, and guided imagery.

## Rationale

By encouraging the patient to take pain medication before the pain becomes unbearable, the nurse assists the patient to achieve relief and effective control of pain. Around-the-clock scheduling of pain medication prevents the pain from becoming too severe (Atkinson and Murray, 1985, p. 667).

Adequate doses of narcotics should be administered to the patient with renal colic without fear of narcotic addiction (Patrick et al, 1986, p. 825). Presence is the nurse's physical being there and being with a patient for the purpose of meeting the patient's health care needs. It is a dynamic, conscious, and interactive process of nursing care (Bulechek and McCloskey, 1985, p. 317).

Pharmacological management of pain is a shared responsibility between the physician and the nurse in collaboration with the patient. Mutually agreed-on strategies of administration will enhance the ability to care for the patient effectively (Carrieri et al, 1986, p. 258).

The use of a nonpharmacological approach to pain control takes into account the gate control theory of pain. The interaction between cognitive, motivational-affective, and sensory stimuli results in the perception of pain. The manipulation of any one of these components influences the person's perception of pain (Carrieri et al, 1986, p. 259). Using nonpharmacological pain relief methods involves the patients' active participation in making decisions about what will relieve the pain. This has been identified as a significant determinant of pain relief (Peric-Knowlton, 1984, p. 138).

---

**Potential for Infection**

*Related to:* The placement of a percutaneous nephrostomy tube and an indwelling urinary drainage tube.
*Evidenced by:* Not applicable; presence of signs and symptoms establishes an actual diagnosis.

**Desired Patient Outcomes**

*The Patient Will:*
• Be free from an infection of the urinary tract.
• Be knowledgeable about the signs and symptoms of a urinary tract infection.

**Evaluation Criteria**

*During the Hospital Stay, the Patient Will:*
• Verbalize an understanding of the signs and symptoms of a urinary tract infection.
• Be free from the signs and symptoms of a urinary tract infection.
• Consume at least 4000 ml of fluid every 24 hours.
• Maintain a closed urinary drainage system that is free of kinks or problems that would cause an infection to occur.
• Verbalize an understanding of the importance of ambulation and will develop a plan of progressive ambulation.

---

## Interventions

Assess the patient's knowledge about the signs and symptoms of a urinary tract infection. Teach the patient the

## Rationale

Sepsis is an inherent risk with any urological manipulation (Cohen and Persky, 1983, p. 705). Physicians and other health care professionals play a significant role in educating patients at

## Interventions

signs and symptoms of a urinary tract infection or reinforce the patient's existing knowledge. Teaching should include the following changes that would occur with the presence of an infection:

- A rise in temperature
- An increase in pulse rate
- Chills
- Flank pain
- Malaise
- A change in the characteristics of the urine

Assess the characteristics of the drainage from the urinary tract. Assess the quantity, color, and consistency every 4 hours. Report deviations from the baseline.

Using sterile technique, the dressing at the nephrostomy tube insertion site will be changed every shift or as ordered.

Provide the patient with fluid intake of at least 4000 ml/24 hr to enhance constant urinary output.

Explain to the patient the techniques used to care for the urinary drainage tubes. The following principles should be reviewed: avoid restrictions on the tubing with careful positioning and anchoring of the tubes, keep the drainage bag below the level of the site of entrance into the body, drain the bag each shift or more frequently as needed into the patient's individual drainage container, avoid touching the dressing at the drainage tube insertion site.

Assist/encourage the patient to ambulate frequently. A plan for progressive ambulation should be developed with the patient.

## Rationale

risk for a urinary tract infection. One must take care to prevent an infection when a nephrostomy tube is in place, for renal damage could occur (Patrick et al, 1986, pp. 796, 826).

The characteristics of the drainage from the urinary tract can indicate if an infection is present (Patrick et al, 1986, p. 824).

The nephrostomy tube goes directly into the renal pelvis to drain urine. Care should be used to prevent the introduction of microorganisms into this area (Patrick et al, 1986, p. 826).

Forcing fluids prevents urinary stasis and provides a means of flushing bacteria from the urinary tract (Young, 1986, p. 39). Fluids are usually increased to above 4000 ml/24 hr to produce urine that is more dilute than extracellular fluid (Patrick et al, 1986, p. 822).

Careful handling of the urinary drainage system is necessary to avoid an infection (Patrick et al, 1986, p. 826). The use of a closed urinary drainage system is essential to reduce contamination of the system and infection. The practice of strict asepsis helps prevent infection. Adequate drainage prevents obstruction and infection (Brunner and Suddarth, 1988, p. 1028).

Frequent ambulation may assist the movement of any stones in the system and prevent obstruction (Brunner and Suddarth, 1988, p. 1057).

| **Knowledge Deficit** | **Related to:** Dietary requirements that will aid in preventing a recurrence of renal calculi.<br>**Evidenced by:** Patient's verbalization that she was not aware of a diet that would help prevent stone recurrence. |
|---|---|
| **Desired Patient Outcomes** | **The Patient Will:**<br>• Be aware of the elements of a dietary regimen to prevent renal calculi.<br>• Discuss ways in which she can integrate this dietary regimen into her lifestyle. |

## Evaluation Criteria

*During the Hospital Stay, the Patient Will:*
- Discuss specific information concerning a diet plan to aid in the prevention of stone formation.
- Discuss her lifestyle and food preferences to enable her to integrate a diet regimen into her daily routine.
- Demonstrate the procedure to test urine for pH level with Nitrazine, pH paper.
- Verbalize an understanding of the significance of testing the urine for pH level.
- Demonstrate an understanding of the fact that drug therapy is usually suggested with a diet regimen to decrease stone formation.

## Interventions

Discuss with the patient her previous knowledge concerning stone formation and diet therapy.

Discuss with the patient the elements of a diet that will aid in preventing the recurrence of renal stones.

Provide the patient with written guidelines for a calcium and phosphate restricted diet. Discuss the importance of adequate hydration. Include the following principles in the teaching plan: calcium and phosphorus restrictions, reduction of animal proteins, avoidance of vitamin C and D supplements, avoidance of foods high in oxalate content, avoidance of foods high in sodium content.

Discuss with the patient her specific lifestyle as well as food likes and dislikes and food preparation techniques.

Teach the patient how to evaluate her urinary pH with the use of Nitrazine, pH paper.

Discuss with the patient the fact that a diet regimen is often suggested in conjunction with drug therapy to prevent the formation of renal calculi.

## Rationale

Patient education should be focused on problem solving with the patient, incorporating environment, altering his or her regimen, exploring the patient's feelings and attributions, and allowing the patient the freedom to approach the behavior change in his or her own way (Bulechek and McCloskey, 1985, p. 164).

Diet restriction has been a major aspect in preventive programs for renal stone disease (Menon and Krishnan, 1983, p. 605).

A diet low in calcium and phosphate will decrease urinary calcium excretion. To counteract the hyperoxaluric effects of a low-calcium diet, oxalates should be restricted. The ingestion of purine-rich foods, such as meat, has been associated with hyperuricosuric calcium oxalate stone formation (Menon and Krishnan, 1983, pp. 605–606). Excessive intake of vitamin D should be avoided to prevent parathyroid hormone production; large doses of vitamin C increase oxalate excretion; a low-sodium diet will decrease calcium excretion, and a large fluid intake will decrease the concentration of solutes in urine (Luckmann and Sorensen, 1987, p. 1213).

A patient's dietary pattern, fluid intake, and assessment concerning high-risk status for renal calculi should be evaluated to plan patient-specific teaching needs (Patrick et al, 1986, p. 823).

Determining urine to have a pH below 6 prevents possible calcium and triple phosphate or struvite stone formation (Luckmann and Sorensen, 1987, p. 1214).

Medical management is focused on decreasing the concentration of crystals that precipitate out of solution to form stones when concentrations approach saturation levels. To this end, dietary management and pharmacological agents are useful (Patrick et al, 1986, p. 822).

Frequently prescribed medications include a calcium binding resin, for example, sodium cellulose phosphate; thiazide therapy, for example, hydrochlorothiazide; phosphate therapy, specifically neutral or alkaline forms; allopurinol therapy; magnesium preparations and long-term antibiotics (Menon and Krishnan, 1983, pp. 606–611).

# QUESTIONS FOR DISCUSSION

1. Discuss the factors in Ruth Greene's history that predispose her to renal stone formation.
2. Why is the finding of hydronephrosis on the intravenous pyelogram not an unusual finding for a patient with renal stones?
3. Discuss the alternative treatment for renal calculi, extracorporeal shock wave lithotripsy (ESWL).
4. What are the advantages/disadvantages of performing an ESWL as a treatment for renal stones?
5. Discuss the nursing care for a patient who has undergone an ESWL.
6. Prepare a diet plan for Ms. Greene that includes all of the elements of a diet to aid in the prevention of renal calculi.
7. Stone dissolution is a treatment alternative for specific patients. Discuss when this treatment modality is indicated and what the procedure entails.
8. Patients often experience a recurrence of renal calculi. Discuss how your discharge teaching plan might address this issue.

# REFERENCES

Atkinson, LD and Murray, M: Fundamentals of Nursing: A Nursing Process Approach. Macmillan, New York, 1985.

Brunner, LS and Suddarth, DS: Textbook of Medical-Surgical Nursing, ed 6. JB Lippincott, Philadelphia, 1988.

Bulechek, GM and McCloskey, JC: Nursing Interventions: Treatments for Nursing Diagnoses. WB Saunders, Philadelphia, 1985.

Carrieri, VK, Lindsay, AM, and West, CM: Pathophysiological Phenomena in Nursing: Human Responses to Illness. WB Saunders, Philadelphia, 1986.

Cohen, JD and Persky, L: Ureteral stones. Urol Clin North Am 10:4, 1983.

Luckmann, J and Sorensen, KC: Medical-Surgical Nursing: A Psychophysiologic Approach, ed 3. WB Saunders, Philadelphia, 1987.

Menon, M and Krishnan, CS: Evaluation and medical management of the patient with calcium stone disease. Urol Clin North Am 10:4, 1983.

Patrick, ML, et al: Medical-Surgical Nursing: Pathophysiological Concepts. JB Lippincott, Philadelphia, 1986.

Peric-Knowlton, W: The Understanding and management of acute pain in adults: The nursing contribution. Int J Nurs Stud 21:131, 1984.

Young, M: Lithotripsy: A revolutionary technique with implications for nursing care. J Nephrol Nurs, p 34, January/February, 1986.

# BIBLIOGRAPHY

Charton, M, et al: Urinary tract infection in percutaneous surgery for renal calculi. J Urol 135:15, January 1986.

Coe, FL and Parks, JH: Recurrent renal calculi: Causes and prevention. Hosp Pract 21(3A):49, March 30, 1986.

Goldwasser, B, Weinerth, J, and Carson, CC: Calcium stone disease: An overview. J Urol 135:1, January 1986.

Harwood, CT: Pulverizing kidney stones: What you should know about lithotripsy. RN p 32, July 1985.

Latham, E and Marden, W: Percutaneous nephrolithotripsy. Nurs Times, June 18, 1986.

Metheny, N: Renal stones and urinary pH. Am J Nurs 82:1372.

Plumb, RT, et al: Managing urinary calculi. Patient Care 18:37, November 15, 1984.

Streem, SB, et al: Percutaneous extraction of renal calculi. Urol Clin North Am 12:381, May 1985.

Wells, N: Responses to acute pain and the nursing implications. J Adv Nurs 9:51, 1984.

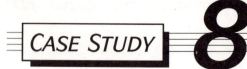

# A PATIENT WITH CHRONIC RENAL FAILURE

Dorothy Bagnell Kelliher, M.S., R.N.

## ANATOMY AND PHYSIOLOGY OF THE KIDNEY

For kidney anatomy and physiology, see Case Study 7, A Patient With Renal Calculi, p. 111.

## PATHOPHYSIOLOGY OF CHRONIC RENAL FAILURE

Chronic renal failure (CRF) is the slow gradual loss of renal function over a period of years or months. Renal failure requires *bilateral* kidney damage. CRF leads to the body's inability to maintain metabolic and fluid and electrolyte balance resulting in uremia that is fatal. Uremia is diagnosed by findings of elevations of nitrogenous wastes in the blood. This finding is called azotemia. Uremia affects all organ systems of the body.

Some of the different causes of CRF are related to chronic glomerulonephritis, traumatic loss of kidney tissue, congenital absence of kidney tissue, congenital polycystic disease, urinary tract obstruction by renal stones, pyelonephritis, and diseases of the renal vasculature. Other causes of CRF may be due to drug reactions, contact with toxic agents, and systemic infections.

## RISK FACTORS

Chronic renal failure remains a significant health care problem in the United States. More than 60,000 deaths occur each year as a result of renal failure. As far back as 1984, 80,000 people were being treated with dialysis and this number represents a 12% increase over the previous year.

Persons who are most at risk are those who have had recurrent nephritis, obstruction of the urinary tract, diabetes mellitus, with its destruction of blood vessels, and long-standing hypertension. Age and sex have no special significance in this disease.

Prevention or reduction in the incidence of CRF can be effected through increasing attention to general health promotion. Yearly physical examination can uncover problems with blood pressure, urinalysis may reveal the presence of sugar, and health histories may elicit problems with urinary tract pain or obstruction. This type of early detection can possibly reduce the number of people who progress from renal insufficiency into frank renal failure.

# COMMON CLINICAL FINDINGS

Independent of underlying disease, the major clinical manifestations of CRF result from disturbances in electrolyte and fluid imbalance, elimination of metabolic wastes and other toxins, erythropoietin production, and blood pressure control.

The problems of fluid and electrolytes lead to hyperkalemia, volume overload, hypocalcemia, hyperphosphatemia, and metabolic acidosis. Moderate renal insufficiency leads to problems with urine concentration; therefore, patients drink and excrete more water than normal to handle the same solute load. This results in polydipsia, polyuria, and nocturia. The ability to dilute urine is further impaired as insufficiency increases and eventually manifests itself in an oliguric stage. The situation is similar with sodium: the moderate renal insufficiency produces mild salt wasting. In later stages, sodium excretion becomes limited, salt retention develops, and edema is manifested.

Potassium excretion is usually not affected until late in CRF. This retention of potassium is seen when oliguria develops and the ability of the distal tubules to secrete potassium is disturbed. Phosphate retention, secondary hypocalcemia, and secondary hyperparathyroidism are evidenced as renal function continues to decrease. Decreased intestinal absorption of calcium secondary to impaired hydroxylation of vitamin D also contributes to hypocalcemia.

Acidosis results from the compromised kidneys' decreased excretion of acid resulting primarily from the inability of the tubules to secrete ammonia and to reabsorb sodium bicarbonate. Vomiting or diarrhea can intensify this metabolic acidosis by causing sodium and water depletion.

Impairment of the kidneys' endocrine function leads to anemia, hypertension, and congestive failure that in turn further compromises renal function. When the kidneys are unable to secrete the substance erythropoietin, which stimulates the bone marrow to produce red blood cells, this eventually results in a mild to moderate normochromic normocytic anemia. If platelet adhesiveness is impaired causing hemolysis and bleeding, anemia is further aggravated. An increase in renin levels causes moderate hypertension and fluid retention.

The signs and symptoms that appear early in renal failure are anorexia, lassitude, fatigability, and weakness. As renal insufficiency increases, pruritus, nausea, vomiting, constipation, or diarrhea are noted. Shortness of breath may be secondary to coronary failure and fluid overload. Late in the disease process edema, hypertension, and pericarditis are common developments; the development of uremic frost also is possible. Uremia is a white, powdery substance composed chiefly of urates that appears on the skin. The final neurological manifestations are drowsiness, lethargy, peripheral myopathy, seizures, coma, and death.

# TREATMENT MODALITIES

The goals of treatment intervention are aimed at preserving renal function, improving body chemistries, alleviating extrarenal manifestations, and providing the optimal quality of life for the person and his or her significant others.

Nutrition must be regulated to monitor protein, sodium, potassium, and fluid intake. The diet should also be high in calories to prevent wasting and in vitamins to offset any protein restriction. The proteins that are allowed should be complete proteins and should contain essential amino acids that are necessary for growth and cell repair. Fluid intake should not be greater than 500 to 600 ml more than the 24-hour output.

Sodium and potassium intake is determined by the levels of these electrolytes in serum and urine. Phosphorus levels are controlled by giving aluminum hydroxide, which binds phosphorus in the intestinal tract.

Hypertension is controlled by the use of antihypertensive medications and preventing intravascular fluid overload by control of fluid intake and use of diuretics.

When renal failure has progressed to the point that the kidneys are no longer able to remove unwanted fluid and waste products from the body, the patient must be dialyzed. There are several methods of dialysis: hemodialysis (Fig. 8–1), hemofiltration, and peritoneal dialysis. Although dialysis can prolong life indefinitely, it does not cure or treat the underlying kidney disease process.

The ultimate treatment for chronic renal failure is kidney transplantation. Transplantation may be from a living donor (usually a relative) or a cadaver. This procedure allows the patient to resume a more normal life but it must be emphasized that follow-up care after a transplantation is a lifelong necessity.

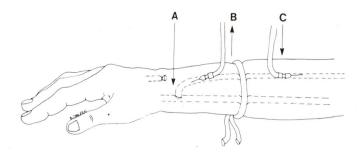

**FIGURE 8–1.** Internal arteriovenous fistula. (*A*) By a surgical procedure, an artery is anastamosed to a vein. (*B*) Venous access to hemodialyzer. (*C*) Arterial access FROM hemodialyzer. Note—Fistulas take 2–6 weeks to mature before they can be used. Peritoneal dialysis or an external arteriovenous shunt may be used during this time (Art Courtesy of B. Chalfin, student MGH Institute of Health Professions, Boston, Mass).

# PATIENT ASSESSMENT DATA BASE

## Health History

*Client:*
Mr. Brian C. Sheppard

*Address:* 76 Pinecone Lane, Forestdale, NH
*Telephone:* 603-424-5678
*Contact:* Heather (wife)
*Telephone of contact:* Same
*Age:* 44   *Sex:* Male   *Race:* White
*Educational background:* MBA from Harvard University
*Religion:* Christian Scientist   *Marital status:* Married
*Usual occupation:* Executive (own company)
*Present occupation:* Same
*Source of income:* Salary
*Insurance:* Blue Cross/Blue Shield
*Source of referral:* Dr. J. Browne (Renal Clinic)
*Source of history:* Patient
*Reliability of historian:* Reliable
*Date of interview:* 3/12/90
*Reason for visit/Chief complaint:* Chronic renal failure. Now admitted for living-related renal transplant (from brother).

### HEALTH PERCEPTION/HEALTH MANAGEMENT PATTERN

*Present Health Status*

Mr. Sheppard states: "I am in irreversible renal failure. My doctor calls it ESRD (end stage renal disease). I have been on hemodialysis 3 times per week for the last 4 months. I don't feel well. It takes so much time—I really cannot work too much—and I always get a terrific headache toward the end of the treatment. I know I have to have the dialysis but I hate it. I'll be so glad to have the transplant surgery. Thank God my brother's kidney matched and he was willing to donate it to me."

**Past Health**

*General Health.* Was diagnosed 24 years ago (1966 — age 20) with insulin-dependent diabetes. He states he has always been pretty good about adhering to his diabetic regimen but even with good health practices he has suffered some problems (retinopathy and renal failure). Feels infection is always a risk; had repeated episodes of boils a year or 2 ago, several of which had to be incised and drained. He has not "felt well for a long time." He suffers with frequent nausea, vomiting, and fatigue.

He was first diagnosed with renal insufficiency 2 years ago when he went for a physical checkup. Until he was 20 years of age everything was fine. Once diagnosed with diabetes, he has had his ups and downs with health. Usually he felt quite fine but over last 6–8 years different things have "popped up" — first retinopathy and now kidney failure.

*Prophylactic Medical/Dental Care.* Mr. Sheppard has been going to the renal clinic "every couple of weeks" for the last year or so. He does have a primary care physician who is in contact with the renal clinic. Has been going for dialysis 3 times per week for 4 months. Sees dentist twice a year — more often if necessary; reports no current dental problems.

*Childhood Illnesses.* Only remembers mumps and chickenpox. Occasional earaches and sore throats.

*Immunizations.* "All the usual, I guess." He remembers smallpox vaccination. Had tetanus booster last year after cutting foot.

*Major Illnesses/Hospitalizations*
Diagnosed with diabetes at age 20. Frequent hospitalizations for complications of diabetes, retinopathy, renal failure, and hypertension.

*November 1987:* Arteriovenous (AV) fistula in left arm to facilitate dialysis treatment.

*June 1982:* Laser surgery for retinopathy on right eye.

*Current Medications*
*Prescription:* 44 units NPH insulin SC 8 AM; 10 units CZI insulin SC 8 AM; methyldopa (Aldomet) 500 mg PO 8 AM and 9 PM.

*Nonprescription:* Aluminum hydroxide gel (Amphojel) 300 mg after meals; folate ẗ tab 8 AM; multivitamin ẗ tab 8 AM; psyllium hydrophilic mucilloid (Metamucil) 1 packet 3 times per day.

*Allergies.* None known.

*Habits*
*Alcohol:* No.
*Caffeine:* 2–3 cans diet cola per day.
Drugs: No.
Tobacco: Has never smoked.

## Family Health History

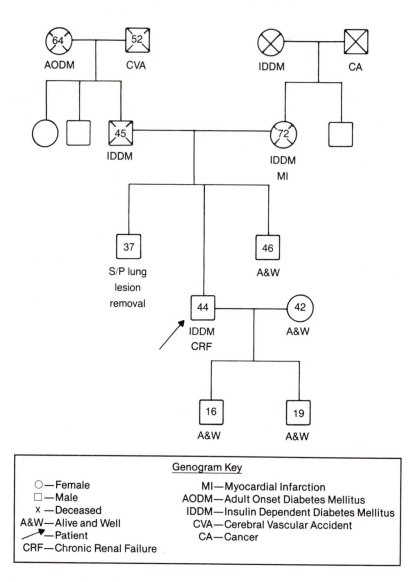

Genogram Key

○—Female
□—Male
x —Deceased
A&W—Alive and Well
⬈—Patient
CRF—Chronic Renal Failure

MI—Myocardial Infarction
AODM—Adult Onset Diabetes Mellitus
IDDM—Insulin Dependent Diabetes Mellitus
CVA—Cerebral Vascular Accident
CA—Cancer

## NUTRITIONAL METABOLIC PATTERN

### Nutritional

Reports some difficulty complying with renal diet — "everything tasty has sodium or potassium in it!" Able to state foods high in potassium and sodium. Occasionally craves sweets. "All those diet restrictions make me feel so down." Compliant with 1000 ml/day fluid restriction. His usual weight gain between dialysis is 2–3 lb (0.9–1.35 kg). Normal weight is 185 lb (84.9 kg) but he has lost 20 lb (9 kg) over the past 4 months. He attributes this to inadequate caloric intake due to nausea and occasional vomiting prior to dialysis.

### Usual Daily Menu*

*Breakfast:* One orange (slices), 2 cups of coffee with cream and 2 sugar substitutes.
*Lunch:* Three-ounce meat sandwich, 1 can of diet cola.

*Admits he has not been eating all of this food for the last several months.

|            |                                                                 |
|------------|-----------------------------------------------------------------|
| *Afternoon snack:* | One apple, 2 or 3 cookies or crackers.                   |
| *Dinner:*  | Baked chicken (3 oz), 1 cup of yellow vegetable, medium baked potato, ½ cup fresh fruit, 1 can of diet cola. |

**Metabolic**

*Height:* 6 ft 2 in. (188 cm). *Weight:* 165 lb (75 kg). Skin integrity: General dry skin; extremities have dry, flaking skin, but no breaks in skin are noted. No history of lesions at corner of mouth or mucous membranes. Does engage in daily diabetic foot care. Has not experienced pruritus.

## ELIMINATION PATTERN

**Bowel**

Has a black, hard stool about every 3–4 days. Claims he has to "really strain" to have a movement. Feels this irregularity is due to Amphojel, and a decrease in activity and fluid intake. He takes Metamucil, docusate sodium (Colace), and sometimes resorts to a Fleet enema to overcome constipation. Feels his constipation is becoming an increasing problem and is not sure what to do about it. Has noted a small amount of blood in his stool from time to time and feels it might be from his hemorrhoids.

**Bladder**

Has been anuric for the past 3–4 months; he denies past or recent urinary tract infections.

## ACTIVITY/EXERCISE PATTERN

**Activity/Exercise**

Independent in activities of daily living (ADLs). States prior to dialysis he experiences more fatigue/decreased activity tolerance, and anorexia and nausea. States he doesn't feel like bathing or eating after morning dialysis treatments. "Sleeps a lot" after dialysis. Ambulates independently except after dialysis, when he needs assistance due to weakness/fatigue. Prior to illness he enjoyed sailing and downhill skiing. States he is no longer able to work full-time, and unable to actively participate in sailing and skiing. Relates chronic fatigue and inability to function at desirable level.

*Self-Care Ability*

| | |
|---|---|
| Feeding—0 | Grooming—0 |
| Bathing—0 | General mobility—0 |
| Toileting—0 | Cooking—II |
| Bed mobility—0 | Home maintenance—II |
| Dressing—0 | Shopping—IV |

> *Functional Levels Code*
>   0—Full self-care
>   I—Requires use of equipment or device
>   II—Requires assistance or supervision from another person
>   III—Requires assistance or supervision from another person
>        and equipment or device
>   IV—Is dependent and does not participate

**Oxygenation/Perfusion**

**Chest X-Ray:** Had chest x-ray on this admission. No difficulty breathing in recumbent position; no paroxysmal nocturnal dyspnea (PND); slight to moderate dyspnea on climbing stairs.
**ECG:** Two weeks ago; no abnormal changes. Has left forearm

fistula for hemodialysis. Mild peripheral edema. No congestive heart failure noted.

### Cardiac Risk Factors

|  | Positive | Negative |
|---|---|---|
| Sedentary life-style | X | |
| Hyperlipidemia | | X |
| Cigarette smoking | | X |
| Diabetes | X | |
| Obesity | | X |
| Hypertension | X | |
| Hypervigilant personality | X | |
| Family history of heart disease | X | |

## SLEEP/REST PATTERN

### Sleep/Rest

Usual sleep pattern: retires at 11:00 PM and awakes at 8:00 AM. States "seldom feels rested after sleep." Naps in morning and afternoon due to chronic fatigue and decreased activity. Usually sleeps after dialysis. States he awakens in the morning many times thinking about dialysis. Denies use of sleeping medications. States he will read or listen to radio to help him fall back to sleep.

## COGNITIVE/PERCEPTUAL PATTERN

### Hearing

No difficulty.

### Vision

Sight corrected with contact lenses. Diabetic retinopathy was treated with laser beam 6 years ago.

### Sensory Perception

No change in taste or smell. Complains of "numbness" and "coldness" in his toes and states he "bumps" into objects as he walks. Is right hand dominant. English is native language. Handles pain by thinking of cool, peaceful places, like the ocean.

### Learning Style

Mr. Sheppard learns best by reading and discussion. He has an MBA from Harvard. Adequate knowledge base of renal disease and diabetes. Fair knowledge base of transplantation. Understands function and need for hemodialysis, medication, and diet regimen. Compliance to regimen has been difficult for him.

## SELF-PERCEPTION/SELF-CONCEPT PATTERN

### Self-Perception/Self-Concept

States his life has progressively deteriorated in past 3 years due to his diabetes. He now thinks of himself as a sick person. States he is unable to function at a desirable level, but he hopes his life will change and go back to "normal" after a successful transplant. States his illness has changed his lifestyle dramatically. "I can't do the things that make me feel good—sailing, skiing, and actively working." States weight loss makes him appear "sickly." He now realizes how much his friends care for him since he has been ill, and that knowledge helps him when he is down.

## ROLE/RELATIONSHIP PATTERN

### Role/Relationship

Has been married for 20 years and has 2 sons (ages 16 and 19). He lives with his family in a 2-story home in a local suburb. Wife is unemployed and primarily at home. Younger son lives at home, and older son is a freshman in college. Describes his family as "close and supportive." Reports his friends and 2 brothers have also been supportive since his illness began. He has only, with much effort, been able to work 4–5 hours each day. States he is concerned he may have to sell his company in the future, but currently co-workers are managing the business. Reports he would like to discuss financial concerns with his social worker at the renal clinic.

## SEXUALITY/REPRODUCTIVE PATTERN

### *Sexuality/Reproductive*

States "everything has changed" in the past 2–3 years. He felt this was a problem for him and his wife but right now the real priority is getting the kidney transplant. He hopes once this is accomplished his "sex life" will get better; if not, this could be a serious concern. Usual sexual activity pattern has changed due to decreased libido, impotence (documented in chart), and decreased activity tolerance. Usual method of contraception: wife uses diaphragm.

## COPING/STRESS TOLERANCE PATTERN

### *Coping/Stress Tolerance*

Feels tense while on dialysis and unable to relax. Denies tension while at work. States he copes by not focusing on the fact that "things might go wrong. I take events as they come." In the past, he would usually "explode" under stress, but religion has made him "calm" and helped him work out his problems. He usually doesn't talk things over with his wife, but copes independently. Life changes: Father died 1 year ago; major lifestyle changes due to chronic renal failure and diabetes.

## VALUE/BELIEF PATTERN

### *Value/Belief*

Mr. Sheppard describes his faith as a major component in his life. He has been a practicing Christian Scientist for over 2 years and feels it gives him a "calmness" within himself. Denies any conflicts with religious beliefs and current medical regimen. Goal of major importance is to return to previous level of work and family life.

# Physical Examination

### *General Survey*

A 44-year-old white male who appears somewhat older than stated age, in bed in hospital attire. Speaks directly to interviewer. He is trying to be positive but appears slightly anxious and depressed.

### *Vital Signs*

*Temperature:* 99.2°F (37.3°C) (oral)
*Pulse:* 94 regular (apical)
*Respirations:* 20 regular
*BP:* 150/90 (right arm, supine).

### *Integument*

*Skin.* Skin integrity is intact; it is generally dry, flaky; right forearm fistula for dialysis; no itching and no other problems.
*Mucous Membranes.* Smooth, pink, moderately dry.
*Nails.* Well trimmed on hands and toenails; some yellowing, slightly thickened.

**HEENT**

*Head.* Symmetrical, somewhat balding; scalp is smooth, no lesions; facial features symmetrical.

*Eyes.* Pupils equal, round, reactive to light and accommodation (PERRLA). Extraocular movements (EOMs) intact. Peripheral vision equal to that of examiner. Visual acuity is 20/30 in left eye and 20/40 in right eye with contact lenses in place. Conjunctiva pale, pink, and moist.

*Ears.* Can hear whispered word at 2 ft (60 cm).

*Nose.* Symmetrical, patent bilaterally; mucous membranes are slightly dry.

*Mouth/Throat.* Mucous membrane is pink, somewhat dry. Teeth are in good repair—no dentures. Uvula is midline; active gag reflex. No areas of irritation or erosion noted in oral cavity.

**Neck**

Trachea is midline; no palpable nodes. Thyroid not palpable; full range of motion.

**Pulmonary**

Anteroposterior (AP) diameter of thorax 1:2. Expansion equal bilaterally. Lungs clear to percussion and auscultation. Respirations 22, regular.

**Breast**

No masses or tenderness noted; normal male configuration.

**Cardiovascular**

Point of maximal impulse (PMI) palpable at 5th intercostal space in midclavicular line. Apical pulse 88 regular. Blood pressure: 150/90. $S_2$ loudest at base, $S_1$ loudest at apex; no extra heart sounds; no murmurs noted.

**Peripheral Vascular**

Mild edema of both lower extremities. Extremities cool, no mottling. Capillary return slow to normal.

*Peripheral Pulses*
Temporal—4 bilaterally
Carotid—4 bilaterally
Brachial—4 bilaterally
Radial—4 bilaterally
Femoral—4 bilaterally
Popliteal—Unable to palpate bilaterally
Posterior tibialis—2 bilaterally
Dorsalis pedis—2 bilaterally

*Peripheral Pulse Scale*

| |
|---|
| 0—Absent |
| 1—Markedly diminished |
| 2—Moderately diminished |
| 3—Slightly diminished |
| 4—Normal |

**Abdomen**

Low, somewhat infrequent bowel sounds in all 4 quadrants. No masses, no tenderness on palpation. Dullness noted in left lower quadrant (LLQ) on percussion; no bruits.

**Musculoskeletal**

Equal strength bilaterally, but some muscle wasting noted in all 4 extremities. Full range of motion in all extremities. Gait is even but lacks energy. No joint pain or tenderness. Spine has full range of motion; no abnormal curvature noted.

**Neurological**

*Mental Status.* Alert, oriented, pleasant. Fully aware of his condition; anxious about transplantation but very positive and hopeful.

*Cranial Nerves.* Cranial nerves I through XII intact.

*Sensory.* Feels and identifies correct location of soft touch bilaterally; decreased sensation noted on feet.

**Deep Tendon Reflexes**

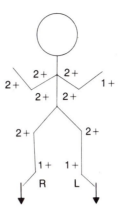

| Rectal | No masses or lesions noted. A few moderate to large hemorrhoids. Slight tenderness on palpation. Hard black stool, positive for occult blood. |
|---|---|
| *Genitalia* | Normal male genitalia; no lesions or discharge noted. Negative for inguinal and femoral hernias bilaterally. |

## Laboratory Data/Diagnostic Studies

**Laboratory Data**

*Hgb:* 12 g/100 ml
*Hct:* 27%
*K:* 5.9 mEq/L
*Serum Creatinine:* 4.2 mg/dl
*Fasting Glucose:* 182 mg/dl
*Serum Calcium:* 4.0 mEq/L

*BUN:* 78 mg/dl
*Na:* 135 mEq/L
*Cl:* 100 mEq/L
*Serum P:* 6.0 mg/dl
*Uric Acid:* 7.0 mg/dl
*Cholesterol:* 200 mg/dl

**Diagnostic Studies**

Chest x-ray, coagulation studies, blood typing and cross matching, tissue compatibility testing with human leukocyte antigen (HLA) and mixed lymphocyte culture (MLC), cystogram.

**Additional Data**

Mr. Sheppard is scheduled to receive a kidney from his brother on March 15th. He will have his last dialysis treatment late in the afternoon preceding the surgery.

## COLLABORATIVE PLAN OF CARE

**Diet**

40-gram protein, 1000-mg sodium, low-phosphate diabetic diet. Fluid restricted to 1000 ml/day.

**Medications**

*Prescription:* Aldomet 500 mg PO bid; 44 units NPH insulin SC 8 AM; 10 units CZI insulin SC 8 AM.
*Nonprescription:* Aluminum hydroxide 300 mg PO after meals; calcium supplement (Os-Cal) tab PO tid; sodium bicarbonate 325 mg PO qid; ferrous sulfate 325 mgm PO qd; vitamin D 400 units PO qd; Colace i cap PO tid; Metamucil 1 packet in water PO tid.

**Intravenous Therapy**

Does not apply.

| | |
|---|---|
| *Therapeutic Measures* | Out of bed (OOB) ad lib.<br>Weigh daily at 8 AM.<br>TPR and BP q8h; *no BP* on left arm (AV fistula).<br>Special foot care.<br>Preoperative teaching for transplant surgery on 3/14/90.<br>Monitor emotional and mental status. |
| *Consults* | Does not apply. |
| *Preoperative Plan* | To dialysis afternoon of 3/14/90.<br>Azathioprine (Imuran) 15 mg PO on night before transplant.<br>Wide abdominal, bilateral flank, and perineum, including scrotum (anterior) preparation with povidone-iodine (Betadine) the night before surgery.<br>Elastic stockings.<br>Place tape on the left extremity with fistula (*no BP* or venipuncture on this arm). |

# NURSING DIAGNOSES DEVELOPED IN CARE PLAN

# ADDITIONAL NURSING DIAGNOSES TO BE CONSIDERED

Activity Intolerance: Level I
Altered Nutrition: Less Than Body Requirements
Fatigue
Fluid volume deficit, Actual (1) (Regulatory Failure)
Knowledge Deficit: Transplantation and Management
Pain
Potential for Infection
Self-Esteem Disturbance
Tissue Perfusion, Altered: Renal

# NURSING CARE PLAN BASED ON IDENTIFIED NURSING DIAGNOSES

| | |
|---|---|
| **Constipation** | **Related to:** Low fluid intake; decreased activity.<br>**Evidenced by:** Hard-formed stool and decreased frequency of defecation. |
| **Desired Patient Outcomes** | The patient will evacuate a soft-formed stool without undo straining at least every third day. |
| **Evaluation Criteria** | By the second hospital day, the patient will have a soft bowel movement.<br><br>**By the Time of Discharge, the Patient Will:**<br>• Experience a soft-formed stool every 2 days.<br>• Verbalize an understanding of the role of diet and exercise in preventing constipation. |

## Interventions

Encourage regular activity within limits.

Teach abdominal muscle toning exercises.

Provide time for patient to verbalize his anxiety.

Encourage bran intake at least once per day.

Monitor the frequency and consistency of the stool.

## Rationale

Activity stimulates peristalsis in the gastrointestinal tract, promoting the passage of fluid and gas and thus helping to prevent abdominal distention, gas pains, and constipation (Phipps et al, 1987, p. 515).

Good abdominal muscle tone aids in defecation (Brunner and Suddarth, 1988, p. 802).

Anxiety often finds its chief expression in indigestion, anorexia, or motor disturbances of the intestines, producing diarrhea or constipation (Brunner and Suddarth, 1988, p. 743).

Fiber is important in the diet because it provides roughage and bulk and aids in preventing constipation (Brunner and Suddarth, 1988, p. 906).

Aluminum hydroxide is very constipating and stool softeners or laxatives may have to be given to prevent constipation (Phipps et al, 1987, p. 1665).

---

**Sexual Dysfunction**

**Desired Patient/Wife Outcomes**

**Evaluation Criteria**

*Related to:* Disease process and anxiety.
*Evidenced by:* Impotence and expressed fears of future limitations on sexual performance.

• Patient will be able to verbalize the cause and contributing factors for the problem.
• Patient and wife will verbalize confidence in ability to resume satisfying sexual activity.

*By the Time of Discharge, the Patient and His Wife Will Be Able to:*
• Explain factors contributing to impotence.
• Verbalize an understanding of this sexual dysfunction as it relates to organic disease and medication.
• Indicate that they feel positive about developing a satisfactory sexual relationship after surgery.

---

## Interventions

Create a trusting relationship.

Take a sexual history including past and present functioning.

## Rationale

Patients may experience anxiety, guilt, and embarrassment during a sexual assessment. Comfort and privacy without interruption, as well as verbal and nonverbal assurances of confidentiality are essential to establishing and maintaining rapport (Brunner and Suddarth, 1988, p. 202).

A detailed sexual history and physical examination are necessary to determine if the sexual dysfunction is due to antihypertensive medication, other medication, other organic causes (i.e., diabetes), or psychological factors (Brunner and Suddarth, 1988, p. 202). Estimates of sexual dysfunction among dialysis patients run as high as 80% to 90%. Many believe that the beginning of treatment means the end of their sex lives. (Solomon, 1986, p. 41).

| *Interventions* | *Rationale* |
|---|---|
| Explore alteration of sexual activity with patient and wife. | In a marital relationship an unexplained decrease in sexual activity owing to illness, lack of communication, or negative body image usually results in conflict, frustration, and irritability. The sexual partner may withdraw for fear sexual intercourse may harm the patient (Brunner and Suddarth, 1988, p. 204). |
| Review with patient and wife the causes of temporary impotence. | Transient impotence can occasionally be reversed with diabetic control (Brunner and Suddarth, 1988, p. 207). A person experiencing sexual dysfunction as a result of antihypertensive drugs should be counseled that the problem is reversible and that alternative medications are available (Brunner and Suddarth, 1988, p. 207). |
| Help patient and wife to evaluate alternative ways of expression. | Intercourse is just one part of the range of human sexual expressions (Gettrust et al, 1985, p. 147). Sex can be a fulfilling experience even if vaginal penetration is not possible. Patients and their partners can concentrate on emotional closeness — holding hands, touching, or sharing laughter, instead of erections or orgasms (Solomon, 1986, p. 43). |

---

| *Powerlessness* | *Related to:* Chronic disease process.<br>*Evidenced by:* Expressions of frustration over deterioration of health despite compliance with regimens and not being able to perform normal activities. |
|---|---|
| *Desired Patient Outcomes* | *The Patient Will:*<br>• Understand that compliance with past regimens cannot always prevent a deteriorating disease situation.<br>• Become more involved in activities surrounding his upcoming renal transplant.<br>• Realize that he does have control over some aspects of a positive recovery. |
| *Evaluation Criteria* | • Before surgery the patient will attend educational sessions regarding his upcoming transplant surgery.<br>• After surgery and before discharge the patient will have an understanding of his medications, diet, and exercise regimen necessary for recovery from transplant surgery and living with a transplanted kidney.<br>• Before discharge, the patient will verbalize that he now feels more in control of his life. |

---

| *Interventions* | *Rationale* |
|---|---|
| Encourage the patient to verbalize feelings of powerlessness. | Adaptation to a chronic illness is a lengthy and continuous process. Patients are often torn between living within their limitations or pushing for more (Brunner and Suddarth, 1988, p. 171). |
| Help the patient to express concerns over upcoming surgery. | Threats to body image and hence to self-esteem must be recognized. Organ transplant is another development that raises questions about body image. What does it mean to have another person's organ in your body? (Brunner and Suddarth, 1988, p. 173). |

## Interventions

Have the patient become involved with planning for new medical regimens following transplant surgery.

## Rationale

When a person comes to the hospital he or she struggles with the need to control. The rules of a hospital may take away the person's usual decision-making capacity. Nursing interventions that help the patient to assume responsibility *early* for making decisions about his or her own care contribute to restoring control (Brunner and Suddarth, 1988, p. 172).

Assist the patient to participate actively in learning about the new regimen.

Patients and their families are often relieved by information about illness, the self-care treatment possible, and the course the illness is expected to take. This provides a framework in which plans can be made and effective action taken. Informed patients are better able to participate in their own treatment (Brunner and Suddarth, 1988, p. 183).

Involve patient in planning care and daily routine.

Decision control can help prevent powerlessness in the hospitalized patient. Patients need to be expected to be an active decision maker in the nursing process (Fuchs, 1987, p. 12).

Help the patient to develop additional adaptive/coping skills to deal with the frustration of chronic illness.

Chronic illness or disability imposes additional adaptive tasks. These tasks include the prevention of medical crisis, control of ongoing symptoms, carrying out treatment regimens, adjustment to changes in the disease course, obtaining funds for survival and ongoing treatment, adapting to or preventing social isolation, normalizing relationships with others, and confronting psychological, marital, and family problems (Phipps et al, 1987, p. 135).

# QUESTIONS FOR DISCUSSION

1. Discuss the systemic effects of ESRD (end stage renal disease).
   a. Gastrointestinal
   b. Cardiovascular
   c. Dermatological
   d. Hematological
   e. Musculoskeletal
   f. Neurological
   g. Metabolic
   h. Reproductive
   i. Endocrine
2. Discuss dietary considerations and interventions for the chronic renal failure patient.
3. Identify factors that contribute to "alteration in bowel elimination in the dialysis patient." Suggest interventions and strategies.
4. Compare and contrast the 3 methods of dialysis: hemodialysis, peritoneal dialysis, and continuous ambulatory peritoneal dialysis.
5. Mr. Sheppard had an arteriovenous fistula put in his left arm to facilitate hemodialysis treatments. Describe an AV fistula and explain how it differs from an AV shunt or graft.
6. Why does Mr. Sheppard take Amphojel?
7. Comment on laboratory data in the ESRD patient. Identify abnormal values and the pathophysiological process that they represent.
8. Identify nursing diagnoses that are common to the renal failure/dialysis population.
9. Design a nursing care plan for Mr. Sheppard. Include desired patient outcomes, nursing strategies and rationale for those strategies selected, and evaluation criteria.

# REFERENCES

Brunner, L and Suddarth, D: Medical-Surgical Nursing. JB Lippincott, Philadelphia, 1988.

Fuchs, J: Use of decisional control to combat powerlessness — The patient with end stage renal disease on dialysis. ANNA 14(1):11, 1987

Gettrust, K, Ryan, S, and Engelman, D: Applied Nursing Diagnosis. John Wiley & Sons, New York, 1985.

Phipps, WJ, Long, B, and Woods, N: Medical-Surgical Nursing. CV Mosby, St. Louis, 1987.

Solomon, J: "Does renal failure mean sexual dysfunction," RN, August 1986, p 41.

# BIBLIOGRAPHY

Carbone, V and Bonato, J: Nursing implications in the case of the chronic hemodialysis patient in the critical care setting. Heart Lung 14:570, 1985.

Chambers, JK: Bowel management in dialysis patients. AJN 83(7): 1051, 1983.

Coleman, E: When the kidneys fail. RN, July 1986, p 28.

Freeman, R: Treatment of chronic renal failure: An update. New Eng J Med 312:577, 1985.

Harum, P: Renal nutrition for the renal nurse. ANNA J, 11(5):38, 1984.

Higley, R: Independence vs. dependence, whose decision? ANNA J 13(5):286, 1986.

Johnson, D: Pathophysiology of renal failure. Crit Care Nurse 5(4):18, 1985.

Kasch, CR: Communication, adaptation and the restoration of psychosocial competence: Helping patients cope with chronic renal failure. ANNA J, 11(4):14, 1984.

Lewis, SM: Pathophysiology of chronic renal failure. Nurs Clin North Am 16(3):501, 1981.

Luckmann, J and Sorensen, K: Medical-Surgical Nursing. WB Saunders, Philadelphia, 1987.

Mann, LM: A group approach to teaching and support in a renal transplant unit. ANNA J 12(2):102, 1985.

Rodriguez, DL and Hunter VM: Nutritional interventions in the treatment of chronic renal failure. Nurs Clin North Am 16(3):573, 1981.

Stephenson, T and Hayes CJ: Toward personalized education for adult ESRD patients. AANNT J, 9(1):39, 1982.

Taylor D: Renal hypertension: Physiology, signs and symptoms. Nursing '83, 13:44, October 1983.

Whitson, SE: Nursing care of the chronic renal failure patient with sexual dysfunction. AANNT J, 9(6):48, 1982.

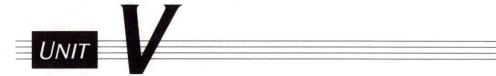

# THE PATIENT WITH ALTERATIONS IN OXYGENATION

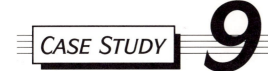

# CASE STUDY 9

# A PATIENT WITH CHRONIC OBSTRUCTIVE PULMONARY DISEASE

Sharon P. Sullivan, M.S., R.N.

## ANATOMY OF THE RESPIRATORY SYSTEM

The structure of the respiratory system consists of the thoracic cage, the lungs, and the conducting airways.

### Thoracic Cage

The thoracic or chest cage is formed by the 12 pairs of ribs, sternum, thoracic vertebrae, and the intercostal muscles (Fig. 9–1). The upper boundary of this compartment or cavity is the neck muscles and the lower boundary is the diaphragm, which separates the thoracic cavity from the abdominal cavity. A thin, double-layered serous membrane, known as the pleura, lines the thoracic cavity (parietal pleura) and surrounds the lungs (visceral pleura).

### Lungs

The lungs are elastic, cone-shaped organs, situated next to each other in the thoracic cavity and separated by the mediastinum. Each lung is composed of lobes, 3 on the right side and 2 on the left side. The lobes are further divided into lung segments; the right lung has 10 and the left lung has 8 segments. The lung segments are subdivided into smaller divisions called lobules.

### Conducting Airways

The conducting airways are the network of pathways that bring inspired air to the gas exchanging regions of the lung. Typically, the conducting airway system is divided into upper and lower airways. The upper airway consists of the nose, pharynx, epiglottis, and larynx. The lower airway, the tracheobronchial tree, is composed of the trachea, right and left mainstem bronchi, segmental and subsegmental bronchi, and terminal bronchioles, which are the smallest airways. Beyond the terminal bronchiole is the primary lobule, which forms an anatomical unit that is also called the acinus. The primary lobule consists of a respiratory bronchiole (which may have alveoli along its wall) and alveolar ducts and sacs that are lined with alveoli. The alveolated regions are the site for gas exchange (West, 1985, p. 2).

**145**

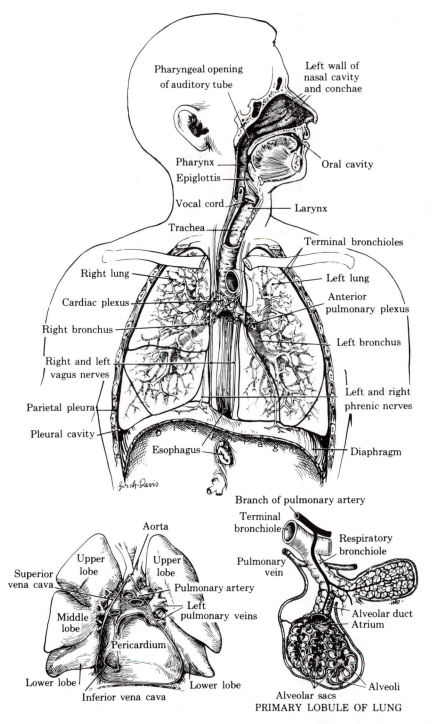

**FIGURE 9–1.** Organs of the respiratory system. (From Dorland's Illustrated Medical Dictionary, ed 27. WB Saunders, Philadelphia, 1988, p. 1654, with permission.)

## Blood Supply

The lung has dual blood supplies, the bronchial and the pulmonary circulations. The bronchial circulation arises from either the aorta or upper intercostal arteries and nourishes the trachea, the airways from the mainstem bronchi to the terminal bronchiole, and the lungs' supporting structure. Since bronchial circulation does not participate in gas exchange, it does not normally supply blood to the alveolar wall and respiratory bronchiole.

The second blood supply to the lungs is the pulmonary circulation, which begins at the pulmonary artery as it receives blood from the right ventricle. The pulmonary arteries follow the bronchial branching as far as the terminal bronchioles and then break up to form a capillary bed that surrounds the alveoli. The pulmonary veins return the blood to the left atrium.

# PHYSIOLOGY OF THE RESPIRATORY SYSTEM

The structure of the respiratory system provides the body with a means for respiration or the exchange of gases both with the environment and at the cellular level. Respiration is divided into 3 interdependent, functional parts (Porth, 1986, p. 334):

1. Ventilation
2. Perfusion or flow of blood in the pulmonary circulation
3. Diffusion of gases between the alveoli and the blood in the pulmonary circulation

## Ventilation

Ventilation is concerned with the bulk movement of gases into and out of the lung. The respiratory muscles, diaphragm, and intercostal and accessory muscles alter the size of the chest cage allowing the volume of air in the lungs to change with inspiration and expiration. The air moves through the conducting airways, which branch and become smaller and more numerous, toward the terminal bronchiole and the gas exchanging structure, the alveoli. The amount of air inspired into the lung is dependent on the distensibility of the lung and the factors that govern the movement of air through the conducting airways (West, 1985, p. 114).

Ventilation is controlled by neurons located in the pons and medulla, referred to as the respiratory center. Both automatic and voluntary components control the breathing process. Automatic regulation is controlled by two types of receptors: lung receptors, which serve to protect lung structures, and chemoreceptors, which respond to the chemical composition of the blood or fluid around it, thus adjusting ventilation to maintain a normal range in arterial blood gas (ABG) values. Voluntary control can override automatic breathing as seen with breath holding and voluntary hyperventilation (West, 1985, p. 114).

## Perfusion

The primary function of the pulmonary circulation is to move blood to and from the alveoli so that gas exchange can occur. The pulmonary circulation begins at the main pulmonary artery, which receives the mixed venous blood from the right ventricle. The pulmonary artery then branches and accompanies the bronchi and branching airways down to the terminal bronchiole. At the level of the alveoli, a pulmonary capillary bed forms a dense network in the alveolar wall where the exchange of gases takes place. The oxygenated blood is carried by way of smaller and then larger pulmonary veins to drain into the left atrium. Pulmonary hemodynamics regulate the behavior of blood flow as it rapidly flows through the pulmonary circulation (Murray, 1986, p. 116).

## Gas Exchange

The gas exchange properties of the lung are dependent on the alveoli receiving both air and blood so that ventilation and perfusion are matched. In the alveoli, oxygen diffuses into the capillary membrane for transport and carbon dioxide diffuses out of the capillary membrane to the alveoli for elimination. This passive diffusion of gases across the alveolar capillary membrane is influenced by 4 factors (Porth, 1986, p. 348):

1. The surface area available for diffusion
2. The difference in the gas partial pressure between the 2 sides of the membrane
3. The thickness of the membrane
4. The properties of the gas

The overall effectiveness of the process is reflected in arterial blood gas values.

# PATHOPHYSIOLOGY OF CHRONIC OBSTRUCTIVE PULMONARY DISEASE

Chronic obstructive pulmonary disease (COPD) refers to a group of diseases characterized by chronic obstruction to airflow within the lungs. Chronic bronchitis, pulmonary emphysema, and asthma are the 3 diseases that are commonly included in this group. Pulmonary emphysema is the most common chronic pulmonary disease, and it is frequently classified with chronic bronchitis because they are closely related and often coexist. For purposes of understanding this case study, only pulmonary emphysema is discussed.

Emphysema is a pathological process that is insidious and develops slowly over a long period of time. The pathological changes that occur are caused by injury and damage to the elastin and fiber network of the alveoli and airways. This results in a loss of alveolar walls along with their capillary beds, and destruction and narrowing of small airways. The loss of supportive structure and alveolar destruction greatly affect both the compliance and elastic recoil of lung tissue. Lung compliance increases, making the lungs more distensible. Elastic recoil is reduced and reflects the loss of elastic tissue caused by destruction of the alveolar walls (West, 1987, p. 72). Since recoil pressure influences the dimensions of airways, a reduction in recoil pressure contributes to the premature collapse or narrowing of the airways and slowing of expiratory airflow. The air trapped by the collapsed airways causes the remaining alveoli to enlarge and permanently dilate. Formation of blebs and bullae is common (Hodgkin and Petty, 1987, p. 54). The loss of alveolar walls affects gas exchange by reducing the area available for gas exchange.

## Pathogenesis

The exact mechanism responsible for the changes that occur in the emphysematous lung has not been clearly identified. Hodgkin and Petty (1987) reviewed the current research, which proposes an enzyme-inhibitor hypothesis to explain how emphysema occurs. In the normal lung, the presence of a serum protein called $\alpha_1$-antitrypsin inhibits and prevents proteolytic enzymes from injuring and damaging the lung's connective tissue, elastin. In pulmonary emphysema, an imbalance between the inhibitors and the proteolytic enzymes exists that favors the enzymes.

Substances in cigarette smoke known as oxidants play a critical role in the injury to the elastic network of the lung and the subsequent development of emphysema. The effects of cigarette smoking are multiple. It suppresses the function of $\alpha_1$-antitrypsin while producing an inflammatory response that causes the release of the proteolytic enzymes. Smoking may inhibit the synthesis of lung elastin needed for repair of injured lung tissue. Stimulation of excess mucus production, loss of ciliary function, and chronic pulmonary inflammations also occur in response to cigarette smoking.

## Types of Emphysema

The different types of emphysema are classified according to the anatomical area affected. Two major types have been described. Centrilobular emphysema (CLE) predominantly affects the central part of the lobule. In this type, the respiratory bronchioles become enlarged and are destroyed, and fenestrations develop in the walls. The peripheral alveolar ducts and alveoli may escape damage. CLE occurs most commonly in the upper portions of the lungs. It is more often seen in men and is usually associated with chronic bronchitis; it is seldom found in nonsmokers.

Panlobular emphysema (PLE) involves the lobule, in which the alveoli distal to the terminal bronchiole enlarge and are destroyed. With progression of the disease, there is a gradual loss of components of the lobule until all that remains are thin strands of tissue. PLE can occur throughout the lung but tends to involve the lower zones of the lung. It is equally common in men and women and is not usually associated with chronic bronchitis (Price and Wilson, 1986, p. 524.)

# RISK FACTORS

The relationship between emphysema and cigarette smoking is firmly established. The risk of developing emphysema increases with a history of prolonged cigarette smoking. Another known cause is an inherited deficiency of $\alpha_1$-antitrypsin in which there is an early onset of symptoms, usually by the age of 40. Environmental air pollution and occupational exposure have also been associated with emphysema (Fishman, 1988, p. 1209).

## COMMON CLINICAL FINDINGS

The chief symptom of emphysema is dyspnea; in the early stages, dyspnea occurs with exertion and is aggravated by exposure to cold air and infection. Dyspnea progresses in severity until regular daily activities or minimal exercise produces severe breathlessness. With the increased respiratory effort, malaise and easy fatigability occur, and eating is often difficult. As a result, general nourishment is below normal and weight loss is common. A chronic cough may be present with expectoration of small amounts of mucoid sputum. The typical barrel-chested appearance seen in these persons is a result of severe hyperinflation of the lungs. Dorsal kyphosis, a prominent anterior chest, and elevated ribs all give rise to this appearance. The accessory muscles of respiration are employed to raise the anterior chest on inspiration, and the abdominal muscles develop to aid in expelling the air during expiration. Breath sounds are diminished, and the expiratory phase is prolonged and may be accomplished through pursed lips. Pulmonary function tests show a reduced forced expiratory volume in 1 second (FEV), reduced vital capacity (VC), and lower expiratory flow rates that reflect the airway obstruction.

In the late stages of disease, hypoxia can develop, resulting in clubbing, cyanosis, and polycythemia. In response to alveolar hypoxia, vasoconstriction of the pulmonary vasculature occurs, imposing a heavy load on the right ventricle causing it to hypertrophy and fail, producing the clinical picture of cor pulmonale (Thompson and Hales, 1986, p. 457). Acute and chronic respiratory failure develops when the person can no longer maintain normal ABG levels because of the increasing amount of work required by the respiratory system. This results in a significantly limited lifestyle and reduced survival.

## TREATMENT MODALITIES

The major emphasis in the care and treatment of those afflicted with chronic obstructive pulmonary disease is to prevent exacerbations, eliminate factors that can cause progression of the disease process, and assist the patient and family in coping with the disease. A variety of factors, such as the severity of the disease, any coexisting medical problems, social support, and motivation, first need to be considered when planning the individualized pulmonary rehabilitation program because they influence the management and outcome. The patient and family must also be involved in the plan of care and educated concerning the reasons for and benefits of treatments (Traver, 1982, p. 327). Certain general guidelines of care are used and provide the basis for designing a pulmonary rehabilitation program that considers the unique needs of the individual. These guidelines include (1) prompt treatment and prevention of respiratory infections; (2) maintaining adequate nutritional status and fluid intake; (3) avoidance of smoking and air pollutants; (4) medications to treat respiratory infections, to reverse bronchospasms, and to promote mucociliary clearance; (5) low-flow oxygen to treat hypoxia; (6) physical conditioning to improve exercise tolerance; (7) breathing exercises; and (8) psychosocial rehabilitation to help the person return to a role that is as self-sufficient and useful as possible (Hodgkin and Petty, 1987, p. 68).

# PATIENT ASSESSMENT DATA BASE

## Health History

*Client:*
Sarah Lawson

*Address:* 18 Hill Road, Madison, Wisconsin
*Telephone:* 608-555-4321
*Contact:* John Lawson (son)
*Address of contact:* 112 River Street, Madison, Wisconsin
*Telephone of contact:* 608-555-9876
*Age:* 70   *Sex:* Female   *Race:* White
*Educational background:* Business School
*Religion:* Roman Catholic   *Marital status:* Widow
*Usual occupation:* Retired
*Present occupation:* Retired
*Source of income:* Social Security/pension
*Insurance:* Medicare
*Source of referral:* Patient
*Source of history:* Patient and son
*Reliability of historian:* Reliable
*Date of interview:* 2/21/90
*Reason for visit/Chief complaint:* Mrs. Lawson began having flulike symptoms 4 days ago. She complained of a slight fever, listlessness, and a productive cough with small amounts of loose yellow sputum. Two days ago she called her physician when symptoms worsened and she was more short of breath. Her physician prescribed ampicillin, which she has taken for the last 24 hours. Early this morning (2:00 AM), she awoke diaphoretic and extremely short of breath and was having difficulty raising sputum that was a thick yellow. She also complained of weakness, dizziness, and palpitations, and she was unable to get out of bed. Mrs. Lawson called her son and he brought her to the emergency department.

## HEALTH PERCEPTION/HEALTH MANAGEMENT PATTERN

*Present Health Status*

Mrs. Lawson was diagnosed with emphysema several years ago. She has been feeling well and managing over the past year. No recent respiratory infections developed but dyspnea remains a problem, interfering with most activities. Oxygen was prescribed initially because of increasing episodes of shortness of breath.

Recently (3 months ago), she was told she had a hiatal hernia.

*Past Health Status*

*General Health.* Describes health as always being good. She exercised and was always active. Home oxygen was initially used on a prn basis but for the last 1½ years she has been using an oxygen delivery system continuously.
*Prophylactic Medical/Dental Care.* Medical visits every 3–4 months; Dental — she wears dentures.
*Childhood Illnesses.* Measles, mumps.
*Immunizations.* All childhood. Did not receive flu vaccine.

*Major Illnesses/Hospitalizations*
*1942 and 1945:* Vaginal delivery.
*1972:* Hemorrhoidectomy.
*1984:* Pneumonia.
*1986:* Phlebitis.

### Current Medications
*Prescription:* Procainamide (Procan) 500 mg PO qid; Theophylline (Theo-Dur) 200 mg PO bid; Ranitidine (Zantac) 150 mg PO bid; Alprazolam (Xanax) 0.5 mg PO tid prn.
*Nonprescription:* None.
**Allergies.** None.

### Habits
*Alcohol:* One beer at bedtime.
*Caffeine:* Three–4 cups tea/day.
*Drugs:* See Current Medications.
*Tobacco:* Two packs cigarettes/day for 45 years; she quit smoking 7 years ago.

### Family Health History

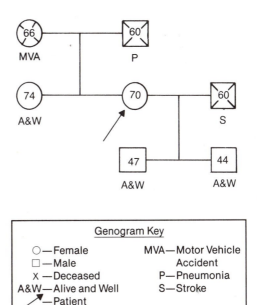

```
Genogram Key
○—Female            MVA—Motor Vehicle
□—Male                       Accident
X—Deceased          P—Pneumonia
A&W—Alive and Well  S—Stroke
╱—Patient
```

## NUTRITIONAL/METABOLIC PATTERN

### Nutritional

Follows a low-salt, bland diet. She enjoys most foods but fried and spicy foods give her indigestion. In the past, she has had problems with a poor appetite because the time required for food preparation caused her to become overtired. Since her son purchased her a microwave oven, food preparation is easier and less fatiguing and her appetite is much improved, that is, 4 on a scale of 1–5 (1 = poor; 5 = excellent). Generally, she eats meals that are easily prepared and purchases many foods that are frozen. Describes her diet as well balanced.

### Usual Daily Menu
*Breakfast:* Six-ounce glass of juice, oatmeal with milk and sugar, 1 cup of tea with milk.
*Lunch:* Macaroni with cheese (1 serving), 1 cup of tea with milk.
*Dinner:* Meatloaf (1 serving), baked potato with butter, carrots with butter (small portion), 1 dish sherbet, 1 cup of tea with milk.
Total fluid intake: 6–8 8-oz glasses.

*Metabolic*

*Weight* has been stable at 90 lb (41 kg) for the last 2 years. Usual weight is 110 lb (50 kg), with the weight loss occurring because of her "breathing problem." *Height:* 5 ft 2 in. (157 cm).

## Elimination Pattern

*Bowel*

Normal bowel pattern is 1 soft-formed, brown stool daily. On occasion, she experiences constipation, which usually responds to having prunes at breakfast.

*Bladder*

Urinates about 6–8 times a day. Denies burning, urgency, or difficulty. Urine is clear and yellow in color.

## Activity/Exercise Pattern

*Activity/Exercise*

Mrs. Lawson is able to perform most self-care activities using energy conservation techniques to minimize dyspnea and fatigue. She alternates rest periods with activity and schedules most appointments for late morning. She performs no regular exercise program.

She drives and has handicapped plates on her car. Outdoor activities are dependent on the weather conditions. She is house-bound when it is cold, windy, or humid. Any activity away from home requires the use of portable oxygen tanks. A homemaker is employed on a twice-weekly basis for housekeeping chores.

*Self-Care Ability*

| | |
|---|---|
| Feeding—I | Grooming—I |
| Bathing—I | General mobility—I |
| Toileting—I | Cooking—I |
| Bed mobility—I | Home maintenance—III |
| Dressing—I | Shopping—II–III |

---

*Functional Levels Code*
  0—Full self-care
  I—Requires use of equipment or device
 II—Requires assistance or supervision from another person
III—Requires assistance or supervision from another person
      and equipment or device
 IV—Is dependent and does not participate

---

*Oxygenation/Perfusion*

Uses oxygen at 2 L via nasal prongs at all times. She has become progressively more dyspneic over the past year; she is now dyspneic with minimal exertion. Daily sputum production of 1–2 teaspoons of clear secretions in AM. Denies any colds or flu in the past 2 years. Last chest x-ray was clear about 1 year ago. Describes episodes of palpitations in the past for which her doctor prescribed Procan. Denies chest pain. Dyspnea index = grade 3.

---

*Dyspnea Index**
*Grade Description*

0—No unusual shortness of breath compared to other persons of
    the same age, height, and sex
1—More short of breath than a person of the same age when
    walking up hills or hurrying on level ground
2—Short of breath while walking on level ground
3—Short of breath at rest or while dressing

*From Carrieri et al, 1984, p. 441.

---

### Cardiac Risk Factors

|  | Positive | Negative |
|---|:---:|:---:|
| Sedentary life-style | X | |
| Hyperlipidemia | | X |
| Cigarette smoking | | X |
| Diabetes | | X |
| Obesity | | X |
| Hypertension | | X |
| Hypervigilant personality | | X |
| Family history of heart disease | | X |

## SLEEP/REST PATTERN

### Sleep/Rest

Usually sleeps 6–8 hours a night. Retires to bed about 11 PM and sleeps until 7 AM. Her usual routine is to have 1 can of beer before going to sleep. "It helps to relax me and it is better than a sleeping pill." Sleeps almost in an upright position with 3 pillows. Uses a humidifier in the bedroom. Awakes feeling well rested.

## COGNITIVE/PERCEPTUAL PATTERN

### Hearing

Has no problem with hearing; no earaches, vertigo, or ringing in ears.

### Vision

Wears glasses for reading and close work; her prescription was changed 1 year ago.

### Sensory Perception

Becomes tense and nervous when anticipating any painful procedure. She is right-hand dominant.

### Learning Style

Learns best by demonstration and use of written materials.

## SELF-PERCEPTION/SELF-CONCEPT PATTERN

### Self-Perception/Self-Concept

She describes herself as an independent woman who enjoys life and takes pride in her family. She sees herself as a quiet, reserved person who enjoys having family and friends around her.

## ROLE/RELATIONSHIP PATTERN

### Role/Relationship

Mrs. Lawson lives alone in a 4-room, 2-bedroom duplex in a suburban community. Both bedrooms and bath are on the second floor. She rents the other half of her house to a married couple who are close friends.

She has been a widow for 8 years, having been married for 40 years. Two married sons and 7 grandchildren live in nearby communities and they visit her regularly. She is especially close to her eldest granddaughter, who visits at least twice a week.

## SEXUALITY/REPRODUCTIVE PATTERN

### Sexuality/Reproductive

Discusses married life and her husband with fond memories. "We had a wonderful life together, and I miss his company." No longer sexually active. Does not perform self-breast examinations.

## Coping/Stress Tolerance Pattern

*Coping/Stress Tolerance*

Mrs. Lawson feels that she is managing well with her lung disease. She has been able to cope with the changes in her lifestyle without too much difficulty. At times, she feels lonely and depressed, especially when weather restricts her outings. "I take each day as it comes and do what must be done. Fortunately I have my friends and family to keep me going."

## Value/Belief Pattern

*Value/Belief*

She is a practicing Catholic who attends Mass regularly. "Being able to go to church and pray has always helped me through the bad times in my life."

# Physical Examination

*General Survey*

A 70-year-old thin, frail-looking elderly woman, anxious and in acute respiratory distress, seated in upright position, speaking 1–2 words between breaths.

*Vital Signs*

**Temperature:** 100.6°F (38.1°C) (rectal)
**Pulse:** 112 irregular (apical)
**Respirations:** 40 labored
**BP:** 148/88 (right arm, lying down).

*Integument*

**Skin.** Pale color, cool, dry, normal thickness for age.
**Mucous Membranes.** Pale pink, dry, intact.
**Nails.** Beds smooth, no clubbing.

*HEENT*

**Head.** Hair is white, evenly distributed over scalp; scalp shows no tenderness. Face is symmetrical; temporomandibular joint (TMJ) is without pain.
**Eyes.** Pupils equal, round, reactive to light and accommodation (PERRLA). Extraocular movements (EOMs) intact. Vision not tested; focuses on objects; conjunctivae clear.
**Ears.** Auricles are intact; cerumen present.
**Nose.** Passages are patent.
**Mouth/Throat.** Membranes and pharynx are pale pink and dry; she wears upper and lower dentures; lips are dry.

*Neck*

Full range of motion; jugular venous pressure 6 cm at 45°; no enlarged nodes.

*Pulmonary*

Thorax is barrel-chested; anteroposterior (AP) diameter is enlarged; bilateral chest excursions; positive use of accessory muscles. Lungs with diffuse wheezes and a prolonged expiratory phase; hyperresonance to percussion; fremitus diminished.

*Breast*

Small in size; right breast is slightly larger than left; otherwise symmetrical; no redness, skin retractions, or dimpling noted; no lumps, pain, or nipple discharge.

*Cardiovascular*

Right ventricular lift; point of maximal impulse (PMI) at fifth left intercostal space at midclavicular line. $S_1$, $S_2$; no murmurs; rate rapid and irregular.

| *Peripheral Vascular* | *Peripheral Pulses* | *Peripheral Pulse Scale* |
|---|---|---|

*Peripheral Pulses*
Temporal — 4 bilateral
Carotid — 4 bilateral
Brachial — 4 bilateral
Radial — 4 bilateral
Femoral — 4 bilateral
Popliteal — 4 bilateral
Posterior tibialis — 3 bilateral
Dorsalis pedis — 3 bilateral

*Peripheral Pulse Scale*

| |
|---|
| 0 — Absent |
| 1 — Markedly diminished |
| 2 — Moderately diminished |
| 3 — Slightly diminished |
| 4 — Normal |

**Abdomen**

Contour is flat; active bowel sounds in all 4 quadrants; soft; no tenderness or masses. Liver, spleen, and kidneys not palpable.

**Musculoskeletal**

Full range of motion in all extremities; muscle strength normal for age.

**Neurological**

*Mental Status.* Alert; oriented to time, place, and person.
*Cranial Nerves.* II–XII are intact.
*Sensory.* Light touch, pain, and vibration to face, trunk, and extremities are within normal limits.

*Deep Tendon Reflexes*

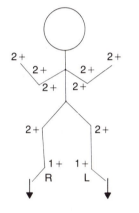

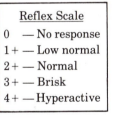

| Reflex Scale | |
|---|---|
| 0 | — No response |
| 1+ | — Low normal |
| 2+ | — Normal |
| 3+ | — Brisk |
| 4+ | — Hyperactive |

**Genitalia**

Normal elderly female.

**Rectal**

Deferred.

## Laboratory Data/Diagnostic Studies

**Laboratory Data**

*Na:* 129 mEq/L
*K:* 3.4 mEq/L
*Cl:* 93 mEq/L
*$CO_2$:* 27 mM/L
*BUN:* 12 mg/dl
*Creatinine:* 1.0 mg/dl
*WBC:* 10.3/mm³
*Hct:* 42.7%
*Hgb:* 14.8 g/100 ml
*Platelets:* 429,000/mm³

*Theophylline level:* 10.6 µg/ml (therapeutic level 10–20 µg/ml).
*Procainamide Level:* 4.0 µg/ml (therapeutic level 4–8 µg/ml).
*30% Face Mask Mask $O_2$ Saturation:* 90%.
*Sputum Gram Stain.* Moderate polys; few mixed flora; mouth flora present.
*Sputum Culture.* Pending.
*ABGs on Admission:* $O_2$ at 2 L $Pao_2$ 56 $Paco_2$ 67 pH 7.26

**Diagnostic Studies**

**Chest X-Ray.** Flattened diaphragm; hyperinflated lungs; no infiltrates.
**ECG.** Sinus tachycardia with frequent premature atrial contractions (PACs) and multifocal premature ventricular contractions (PVCs).

# COLLABORATIVE PLAN OF CARE

**Diet**

Keep NPO.

**Medications**

Heparin 5000 units SC bid.
Ampicillin 1 g IV q6h.
Zantac 50 mg IV q8h.
Metaproternol sulfate (Alupent) 0.3 ml in 2.5 ml normal saline via nebulizer q2h.
Aminophylline 500 mg and hydrocortisone sodium succinate (Solu-Cortef) 500 mg in 500 ml in 5% D/W at 20 mg/hour.
Lidocaine 2 g in 250 ml 5% D/W at 1 mg/minute.
Acetaminophen (Tylenol) 650 mg PR q4h prn for temperature >100°F (37.7°C).
Morphine sulfate 1–2 mg IV q2–4h prn.

**Intravenous Therapy**

Normal saline with 40 mEq KCl/L at 100 ml an hour.

**Therapeutic Measures**

Admit to Intermediate Care Unit.
Cardiac monitor.
Vital signs every 2 hours.
Record intake and output.
Daily weights.
Bed rest.
Chest physiotherapy every 2–4h.
Deep endotracheal suctioning if indicated.
Oxygen via face mask at 30%.
Pulse oximeter to monitor $O_2$ saturation.
Chest x-ray.

**Consults**

Chest physiotherapy.

# NURSING DIAGNOSES DEVELOPED IN CARE PLAN

Impaired Gas Exchange, p. 157
Ineffective Airway Clearance, p. 158
Potential for Decreased Cardiac Output, p. 160

# ADDITIONAL NURSING DIAGNOSES TO BE CONSIDERED

Activity Intolerance
Altered Nutrition: Less than Body Requirements
Anxiety
Bathing/Hygiene Self-Care Deficit
Impaired Home Maintenance Management
Ineffective Breathing Pattern
Powerlessness

Sleep Pattern Disturbance
Toileting Self-Care Deficit

# NURSING CARE PLAN BASED ON IDENTIFIED NURSING DIAGNOSIS

| *Impaired Gas Exchange* | ***Related to:*** Ventilation-perfusion mismatch<br>***Evidenced by:*** Abnormal ABG values, tachypnea (a respiratory rate of 40), restlessness, and complaints of shortness of breath. |
|---|---|
| *Desired Patient/Family Outcomes* | ***The Patient Will:***<br>• Maintain adequate gas exchange with $PaO_2 \geq 60$ mm Hg and $PaCO_2$ 35–45 mm Hg.<br>• Be free of signs and symptoms of respiratory distress.<br><br>***The Patient/Family Will:***<br>• Be knowledgeable about the purpose for and safe use of supplemental oxygen.<br>• Be knowledgeable about the early signs and symptoms of impaired gas exchange and steps taken if present. |
| *Evaluation Criteria* | ***After Instruction, the Patient and/or Family Will:***<br>• Wear an oxygen delivery device at all times.<br>• State the purpose, hazards, and side effects of oxygen therapy.<br>• Explain the steps used in safe administration of oxygen in the home.<br>• Identify signs and symptoms of impaired gas exchange and steps taken if present.<br><br>***During the Hospital Stay, the Patient Will:***<br>• Be alert and oriented to self and environment.<br>• Report a decrease in dyspnea.<br>• Have a respiratory rate normal for patient.<br>• Have ABG/oxygen saturation levels normal for patient. |

## Interventions

Assess respiratory effort, rate, breathing patterns, and use of accessory muscles. Observe for signs of respiratory distress.

Auscultate breath sounds.

Monitor ABG values and/or oxygen saturation ($Sao_2$) levels while awake and during sleep. Note trends.

## Rationale

A change in the patient's condition may signal illness progression. Close observation for any changes in breathing patterns, dyspnea, and increased respiratory rate are required, since these have been noted in patients with respiratory muscle fatigue and acute respiratory failure (Lareau and Larson, 1987, p. 179).

Auscultation of the lungs provides information about airflow through the tracheobronchial tree (Traver, 1982, p. 228).

ABGs are used to evaluate overall adequacy of lung function in maintaining effective gas exchange (Jones, Dunbar, and Jirovec, 1984, p. 887). $Sao_2$ is closely related to $Pao_2$. By measuring $Sao_2$, a close estimate of the $Pao_2$ can be obtained (Luckmann and Sorensen, 1987, p. 659).

Sleep is frequently punctuated by episodes of arterial oxygen desaturation. In many patients with COPD nocturnal desaturation leads to transient hypoxemia (Block, 1981, p. 94; Parkosewich, 1986, p. 60).

| Interventions | Rationale |
|---|---|
| Assess for signs and symptoms of hypoxemia. | Hypoxemia is dangerous because it causes tissue hypoxia. Deleterious effects are seen in the central nervous system, cardiovascular system, and renal system (West, 1987, p. 160). |
| Anticipate the need for intubation and ventilatory assistance. | Intubation and assisted ventilation may be indicated when inadequate ventilation is accompanied by fatigue, decreased mental status, and acidosis (Jones, Dunbar, and Jirovec, 1982, p. 898). |
| Position patient:<br>• Fowler's position<br>• Comfort<br>• Ease of respiratory effort<br>• Optimal matching of ventilation-perfusion | Severely dyspneic patients often need to sit completely upright to promote expansion of the lungs and respiratory muscles (Luckmann and Sorensen, 1987, p. 681).<br>Patients will usually assume the position of most comfort and physiological benefit to their breathing (Lareau and Larson, 1987, p. 188).<br>The distribution of blood flow and ventilation is greatly affected by body position and diseases of the heart and lung (Traver, 1982, pp. 86, 186). |
| Reduce the potential for increased oxygen consumption by:<br>• Reducing fever<br>• Allaying anxieties<br>• Limiting activities to within patient tolerance | The oxyhemoglobin curve shifts to the right with fever, acidosis, and increased $Paco_2$, which reflects increased metabolic needs of the tissue (Porth, 1986, p. 351).<br>Increased levels of anxiety are associated with increased ventilation, increased energy expenditure, increased oxygen consumption, and increased muscle tension (Hodgkin and Petty, 1987, p. 106).<br>Oxygen demand increases with activity. During an acute exacerbation, the patient's exercise workload should be minimized to prevent a fall in $Pao_2$ (Traver, 1982, p. 186). |
| Administer oxygen at prescribed level. | Supplemental oxygen corrects hypoxemia and alleviates symptoms (Traver, 1982, p. 87), and in patients with COPD, it limits systemic consequences and lowers mortality (Nocturnal Oxygen Therapy Trial Group, 1980, p. 391). |
| Administer sedatives and narcotics with caution. | Drugs that depress the respiratory center may cause impairment of ventilation by causing a decrease in respiratory drive (Porth, 1986, p. 398). |
| Instruct the patient and family about oxygen, its purpose, safe use in the home, and side effects. | Home use of oxygen has both risks and benefits. Patient teaching can prevent any hazardous consequences (Openbrier, Fuoss, and Mall, 1988, p. 198). |
| Teach the patient and family early signs and symptoms of impaired gas exchange, actions taken if present, and the available emergency resources. | If acute exacerbations are to be recognized early and treatment initiated, the patient and family must be educated to recognize early warning signs (Traver, 1982, p. 344). |

| | |
|---|---|
| **Ineffective Airway Clearance** | **Related to:** Thick secretions and tracheobronchial infection.<br>**Evidenced by:** Weak, ineffective cough, sputum that is thick and not easily expectorated, respiratory rate of 40, and adventitious breath sounds. |
| **Desired Patient Outcomes** | **The Patient Will:**<br>• Maintain a patent airway.<br>• Be knowledgeable about measures to promote secretion clearance and maintain a patent airway. |

- Be knowledgeable about signs and symptoms of infection, methods to prevent infection, and steps to be taken if infection is present/suspected.

**Evaluation Criteria**

*After Instruction, the Patient Will:*
- Perform and state rationale for coughing and breathing maneuvers.
- Ingest a minimum of 2 L of fluid per day.
- State importance of an adequate fluid intake.
- List 3 recommended fluids.
- State signs and symptoms of infection.
- Describe 3 measures to prevent infections.
- Identify steps to be taken if infection is present/ suspected.

*During the Hospital Stay, the Patient Will:*
- Have sputum that is thin, loose, and easily expectorated.
- Have clear lungs, a normal respiratory rate for the patient, and respirations of a normal depth and pattern for patient.

## Interventions

Monitor sputum characteristics: amount, color, odor, and consistency.

Auscultate breath sounds before and after bronchial hygiene measures. Document any changes in breath sounds.

Administer bronchodilators prior to and/or during bronchial hygiene measures.

Perform bronchial hygiene measures according to patient tolerance:
- Postural drainage
- Percussion and vibration

Perform endotracheal suctioning if indicated. Provide oxygen before, during, and after procedure.

Instruct and demonstrate coughing and controlled breathing maneuvers.

Instruct the patient to increase fluid intake to 2 L per day. Provide a list of recommended fluids. Monitor daily fluid intake.

Teach the patient signs and symptoms of infection, measures to prevent infection, and steps to be taken if infection is present/suspected.

## Rationale

Sputum characteristics may change with infection of the respiratory tract, frequently increasing in amount and containing infecting organisms and inflammatory debris (Porth, 1986, p. 351).

Auscultation of breath sounds "helps to evaluate the adequacy of ventilation. By establishing a baseline of findings before treatments, the nurse can assess for changes that occur during or that result from treatments" (Zadai, 1981, p. 1747).

Bronchodilators are used to dilate airways, lessen resistance to airflow, and aid in mobilization of secretions (Traver, 1982, p. 332; Petty, 1987, p. 180).

The aim of chest physiotherapy is "to loosen any inspissated secretions and mucus plugs and when combined with postural drainage, bring them into the larger airways where they can be coughed up" (Cosenza and Norton, 1986, p. 30).

The goal of suctioning is to remove secretions and to stimulate a productive cough without causing complications (Luckmann and Sorensen, 1987, p. 704).

In respiratory infections, coughing is a primary mechanism for airway clearance (Hanley and Tyler, 1987, p. 143). Performing breathing exercises in patients with infection "prevents closure of airways and the entrapment of secretions distal to the obstruction" (Hanley and Tyler, 1987, p. 142).

The rationale behind hydration therapy is "to prevent the drying of secretions and to increase the water content of the mucus and reduce its viscosity, thereby allowing easier clearance from the respiratory tract" (Cosenza and Norton, 1986, p. 25).

Early detection and treatment of infections "will diminish the severity of an acute exacerbation." Measures directed at bronchodilation and drainage of secretions will reduce the potential for retention of secretions and infections (O'Donahue, 1984, p. 231).

| Interventions | Rationale |
|---|---|
| Consult the chest physiotherapist. | The chest physiotherapist plays a major role in rehabilitation of patients for breathing exercises and breathing retraining (O'Donahue, 1984, p. 229). |

| | |
|---|---|
| ***Potential for Decreased Cardiac Output*** | ***Related to:*** Cardiac arrhythmias.<br>***Evidenced by:*** Reported history of arrhythmias and palpitations; documentation of atrial and ventricular arrhythmias on ECG; and the presence of predisposing conditions. |
| ***Desired Patient Outcomes*** | ***The Patient Will:***<br>• Maintain hemodynamic stability.<br>• Have an absence of or stability of arrhythmia. |
| ***Evaluation Criteria*** | ***During the Hospital Stay, the Patient Will:***<br>• Return to baseline rhythm.<br>• Have blood pressure >90/60 mmHg and heart rate 60–100 beats per minute. |

| Interventions | Rationale |
|---|---|
| Monitor heart/pulse rate and rhythm. Document and report arrhythmias noted. | Early detection of arrhythmias allows initiation of therapy and may prevent the occurrence of lethal arrhythmias (Underhill et al, 1982, p. 333). |
| Monitor blood pressure, urine output, and mentation. | Arrhythmias can result in reduced cardiac output, decreased perfusion to vital organs, "increased myocardial oxygen consumption, and predispose to lethal arrhythmias" (Underhill et al, 1982, p. 329). |
| Monitor potassium levels. | Cardiac muscle is vulnerable to changes in potassium levels (Underhill et al, 1982, p. 94). |
| Monitor ABG/oxygen saturation levels, and serum drug levels. | "Hypoxemia, acidosis, alkalosis and concurrent drug toxicity or subtherapeutic drug levels can cause arrhythmias and conduction disturbances" (Underhill et al, 1982, p. 334). |
| Assess for the presence of other predisposing conditions or precipitating factors. | Interventions to treat arrhythmias must be directed toward prevention by recognizing and controlling those predisposing conditions (Underhill et al, 1982, p. 329). |

## QUESTIONS FOR DISCUSSION

1. Define the following terms: dyspnea, hypoxia, hypoxemia, and hypercapnia.
2. Identify the signs and symptoms of hypoxemia.
3. What is cyanosis? What does it indicate?
4. Discuss the principles behind positioning to improve gas exchange.
5. Identify some contraindications to the use of chest physiotherapy.
6. Why is it important for patients with COPD to avoid respiratory infections? What information would you give Mrs. Lawson that will help her to avoid infection?
7. What is the rationale behind the chronic use of oxygen therapy in those persons afflicted with COPD? Why is a low-flow oxygen setting necessary?
8. What are the beneficial effects of pursed-lip breathing?
9. From the case study, list the specific factors that predispose Mrs. Lawson to developing cardiac arrhythmias.

# REFERENCES

Block, AJ: Respiratory disorders during sleep. Part II. Heart Lung 10:90, 1981.

Carrieri, V, Janson-Bjerklie, S, and Jacobs, S: The sensation of dyspnea: A review. Heart Lung 13:436, 1984.

Cosenza, J and Norton, L: Secretion clearance: State of the art from a nursing perspective. Crit Care Nurse 6:23, 1986.

Fishman, AP: Pulmonary Disease and Disorders, vol 2. McGraw-Hill, New York, 1988.

Hanley, M and Tyler M: Ineffective airway clearance related to airway infection. Nurs Clin North Am 22:135, 1987.

Hodgkin, JE and Petty, TL: Chronic Obstructive Pulmonary Disease: Current Concepts. WB Saunders, Philadelphia, 1987.

Jones, D, Dunbar, C, and Jirovec, M: Medical-Surgical Nursing: A Conceptual Approach. McGraw-Hill, New York, 1984.

Lareau, S and Larson, J: Ineffective breathing pattern related to airflow limitation. Nurs Clin North Am 22:179, 1987.

Luckmann, J and Sorensen, KC: Medical-Surgical Nursing: A Psychophysiologic Approach. WB Saunders, Philadelphia, 1987.

Murray, JF: The Normal Lung: The Basis for Diagnosis and Treatment of Pulmonary Disease. WB Saunders, Philadelphia, 1986.

Nocturnal Oxygen Therapy Trial Group: Continuous or nocturnal oxygen therapy in hypoxemic chronic obstructive lung disease. Ann Intern Med 93:391, 1980.

O'Donahue, W (ed): Current Advances in Respiratory Care. American College of Chest Physicians, Park Ridge, Ill, 1984.

Openbrier, DR, Fuoss, C, and Mall, CC: What patients on home oxygen therapy want to know. Am J Nurs 88:198, 1988.

Parkosewich, J: Sleep-disordered breathing: A common problem in chronic obstructive pulmonary disease. Crit Care Nurse 6:60, 1986.

Petty, TL: Drug Strategies for airflow obstruction. Am J Nurs 87:180, 1987.

Porth, C: Pathophysiology. JB Lippincott, Philadelphia, 1986.

Price, SA and Wilson, LM: Pathophysiology. McGraw-Hill, New York, 1986.

Thompson, BT and Hales, C: Hypoxic pulmonary hypertension: Acute and chronic. Heart Lung, 15:457, 1986.

Traver, G (ed): Respiratory Nursing: The Science and the Art. John Wiley & Sons, New York, 1982.

Underhill, SL, et al: Cardiac Nursing. JB Lippincott, Philadelphia, 1982.

West, JB: Pulmonary Pathophysiology. Williams & Wilkins, Baltimore, 1987.

West JB: Respiratory Physiology. Williams & Wilkins, Baltimore, 1985.

Zadai, CC: Physical therapy for the acutely ill medical patient. Phys Ther 61:1746, 1981.

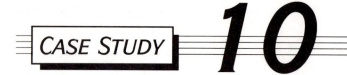
# A PATIENT WITH CANCER OF THE LUNG AND LOBECTOMY

Meg Doherty, M.S., R.N.

## DISTRIBUTION OF LUNG CANCER

From 76%–80% of all lung tumors are categorized as non–small cell lung cancer. Included in this category are the following:

*Epidermoid carcinoma*, or *squamous cell carcinoma*, the most common type, which accounts for about 40% of lung tumors. It most often appears as a small (approximately 1–2 cm), centrally located, hilar lesion that tends to spread by direct extension to the hilar lymph nodes, chest wall, and mediastinum.

The *adenocarcinomas* account for approximately 25% of lung cancers and tend to arise in the peripheral segmental bronchi. The tumor may be quite large when discovered and frequently demonstrates as a pleural effusion. These lesions often spread by way of the bloodstream with early metastasis to the central nervous system.

*Large cell cancers* tend to appear as large peripheral masses, are less well defined than the other cell types, and are highly metastatic by way of the lymphatic and blood circulation systems. Large cell cancer accounts for about 10% of lung cancer.

Twenty-five percent of lung cancers are attributed to *small cell carcinoma*. This type has the poorest prognosis because of its rapid growth rate and tendency toward early metastasis to the central nervous system by way of the lymphatics and bloodstream.

More than 90% of all lung cancers belong to the group called *bronchogenic carcinoma*, meaning that the cancer originates in the bronchi or bronchioles. Generally, lung cancers occur primarily in the segmental bronchi or beyond and have a preference for the upper lobes of the lung. About 50% of the lesions arise centrally in the hilar area and the first few orders of the bronchi; the others have a more peripheral origin in the terminal bronchioles.

The lung is a common site for secondary deposits of cancer originating from other organs because blood-borne microscopic tumor emboli are likely to become entrapped in the pulmonary bed. The most common cancers associated with *pulmonary metastasis* are carcinoma of the breast, male and female genital tract cancers, gastrointestinal and kidney carcinomas, and melanomas (Fig. 10–1).

## PATHOPHYSIOLOGY

The pathogenesis of primary lung cancer is not well understood; however, bronchogenic lung lesions are slow-growing. It usually takes 8–10 years for a tumor to reach 1 cm in size. The specific pathological alterations in the bronchial system are nonspecific inflammatory changes with hypersecretion of mucus, desquamation of cells, reactive hyperplasia of the basal cells, and metaplasia of normal respiratory epithelium.

*162*

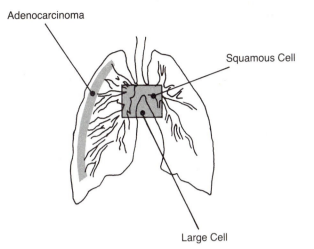

**FIGURE 10–1.** Anatomic distribution of lung cancer; 50% is located centrally while the other 50% is peripheral. (Adapted and reproduced with permission from: Price, SA and Wilson, LM: Pathophysiology: Clinical Concepts of Disease Processes, ed 3. McGraw-Hill, New York, 1986; copyright by CV Mosby, St. Louis.)

Primary lung cancers metastasize primarily by direct extension, by blood circulation, and by way of the lymph system. The common sites for metastatic growth are the scalene lymph nodes, liver, brain, adrenal glands, and the bones.

The "paraneoplastic syndrome" caused by the release of hormones, enzymes, and antigens produced by certain tumor cells results in cognitive, behavioral, and/or affective changes as well as various other systemic manifestations. Some examples include Cushing's syndrome, inappropriate secretion of antidiuretic hormone (ADH), hypercalcemia, gynecomastia, peripheral neuropathy, anemia, thrombophlebitis, nonbacterial endocarditis, and nonspecific arthralgias.

Some of the symptoms of paraneoplastic syndrome have been erroneously attributed to psychiatric illness. Mental status changes, depression, and manic psychosis in lung cancer patients have been associated with ectopically produced psychoactive substances such as parathormone, vasopressin, adrenocorticotropic hormone (ACTH), and β-endorphins, indicating the need for early identification of biological factors.

## RISK FACTORS

Lung cancer is recognized as a worldwide problem that commonly occurs in both sexes and in industrialized as well as in developing nations. The highest incidence is observed in men in the United Kingdom (89.5 per 100,000 age-adjusted population).

In the United States, the incidence of lung cancer is also high, increasing by 13% between 1973 and 1981. The mortality rate during the same period demonstrated a similar trend. Since the 1950s the death rate for men has exceeded that of any other cancer. It is only within the last decade that the steep incline in lung cancer mortality was observed among women. Although the absolute level is not as high as in men, the rate of increase for lung cancer mortality among women has been accelerating more rapidly than in men. In 1987, of all cancer deaths in men, 36% are due to lung cancer and in women, 20% are due to lung cancer.

The primary risk factor associated with lung cancer is cigarette smoking. Of the 35 retrospective studies conducted between 1939 and 1970 on the relationship of cigarette smoking and lung cancer, 19 demonstrated that the relative risk of lung cancer was over 5 times greater among smokers than nonsmokers. The risk of developing lung cancer is directly related to total exposure to cigarette smoke measured by total number of cigarettes smoked in a lifetime, depth of inhalation, and tar and nicotine content of the cigarettes smoked.

Current data suggest a positive association between passive smoking and lung cancer. Studies are exploring spouses' smoking habits, passive smoking pollution in the workplace, and early life exposure.

Certain high-risk groups have been identified with respect to occupation and exposure of inhaled carcinogens. Some of these include asbestos, nickel, iron, uranium, chromates, arsenic, and air pollution. The synergistic effect of cigarette smoking and an occupational environment at high risk for lung cancer has been demonstrated in several worker groups including shipyard workers and asbestos and uranium workers.

The association between vitamin A deficiency and lung cancer has been identified by a number of investigators. The increased risk has been found for squamous cell and small cell carcinoma in men. The role of this dietary factor in women is not confirmed. No other dietary factor to date has been found to have an etiological role in lung cancer.

Other possible risk factors include preexisting pulmonary diseases such as tuberculosis, pulmonary fibrosis, bronchiectasis, chronic obstructive pulmonary disease (COPD), as well as exposure to identified and unidentified air pollutants and irritants.

# COMMON CLINICAL FINDINGS

Most frequently, victims of lung cancer present with nonspecific symptoms of cough, shortness of breath, chest pain, hemoptysis, weight loss, and recurrent episodes of bronchitis or pneumonia. The diagnosis is often made following chest radiography performed for some unrelated reason and frequently there is extensive metastasis before symptoms become apparent.

One of the most significant symptoms, and often the one reported first, is a persistent cough that is productive of sputum. Blood-tinged sputum may be produced due to bleeding of the malignancy, but hemoptysis is not a common early presenting symptom. Chest pain may be present and localized or unilateral, ranging from mild to severe. Dyspnea and an auscultatory wheeze may be present if there is bronchial obstruction. The progression of respiratory symptoms may go unreported for long periods of time in the smoking population. A change in the character of a chronic cough is the most typical presenting symptom of disease.

Later manifestations may include nonspecific systemic symptoms such as anorexia, fatigue, weight loss, nausea, and vomiting. There may be palpable lymph nodes in the neck or axilla. Mediastinal involvement may lead to pericardial effusion, cardiac tamponade, and dysrhythmias.

Because the lung is a frequent site of metastasis with other malignancies, the diagnosis of lung cancer requires histological confirmation. This may involve bronchoscopy, percutaneous lung biopsy, mediastinoscopy, scalene node biopsy, and occasionally, open lung biopsy. The histological diagnosis, along with staging information, directs treatment.

Staging signifies the extent of the disease and minimally for non–small cell lung cancer includes a thorough history and physical examination, chest film, complete blood count (CBC), blood chemistries, and chest computed tomography (CT) scan, extending to the level of the adrenals. At the completion of these, a number of patients will be staged and found not to be surgical candidates by virtue of such findings as skin tumor nodules, rib erosion, or pleural effusion. No further staging workup is indicated in these patients. In the presence of symptoms of weight loss, bone pain, or elevated alkaline phosphatase, serum glutamic oxaloacetic transaminase (SGOT), bilirubin, or calcium levels, a bone scan is indicated. The treatment of non–small cell lung cancer depends primarily on the stage of the disease and includes surgery, radiotherapy, and chemotherapy.

The staging system for small cell lung cancer is more extensive because of its propensity for dissemination, its high proliferative rate, and its correlative responsiveness to cytotoxic drugs. Also included in the staging workup are CT scans of the liver and brain, bone scan, and bilateral bone marrow aspirates and biopsies. Most patients receive combination chemotherapy regardless of stage; however, the additional information is helpful in assessing individual prognosis, the ability to undergo treatment, and in identifying disease sites that can be assessed for response.

# TREATMENT MODALITIES

In general, treatment for limited-disease small cell lung cancer usually includes aggressive combination chemotherapy and radiation therapy. The role of the surgical approach for selected patients with limited disease is currently under investigation. Treatment for extensive-disease small cell lung cancer is usually palliative therapy consisting of combination chemotherapy, or chemotherapy combined with wide-field radiation therapy. The long-term survival rate for small cell lung cancer is still low.

The medical treatment for patients with lung cancer depends on the tumor type, cancer staging, and the patient's underlying condition. Interventions include immunotherapy, radiotherapy, and chemotherapy. Chemotherapy and radiotherapy are often used in combination, improving the survival rate of patients with some tumors.

The primary aim of surgical intervention for lung cancer is to completely remove the tumor. Surgical excision is often done for Stage I or Stage II cancers. Surgery is generally not helpful and causes unnecessary risk and stress for patients with metastasis. The least amount of lung tissue possible is excised depending on the area of malignancy and underlying pulmonary pathology. Patients with preexisting pulmonary disease may not be able to tolerate extensive lung resection. Consideration of such postoperative pulmonary effects is essential before surgery is performed to ensure the best possible quality of life. Surgical survival rates (over 5 years) range from 50% for Stage I disease to 15% for Stage III disease.

# PATIENT ASSESSMENT DATA BASE

## Health History

> **Client:**
> Janice Adams

**Address:** 200 St. James Street, St. Louis, Missouri, 63104
**Telephone:** 314-555-5102
**Contact:** Janice Slocum (mother)
**Address of contact:** 200 St. James Street, St. Louis, Missouri, 63104
**Telephone of contact:** 314-555-5102
**Age:** 44    **Sex:** Female    **Race:** White
**Educational background:** BA in Psychology
**Religion:** Roman Catholic    **Marital status:** Single
**Usual occupation:** Counselor, Crisis Intervention, Women's Center
**Present occupation:** Same as above
**Source of income:** Self
**Insurance:** Blue Cross/Blue Shield of Missouri
**Source of referral:** Gary Norman, M.D.
**Source of history:** Patient, patient record
**Reliability of historian:** Reliable
**Date of interview:** 12/9/89
**Reason for visit/Chief complaint:** "I'm here to have my lung operated on. I have lung cancer."

## HEALTH PERCEPTION/HEALTH MANAGEMENT PATTERN

*Present Health Status*

Early 9/89, the patient developed pain over the left scapula and described an occasional pain "radiating down the surface of my left arm and chest area, like a muscle ache." More recently the patient relates "tingling" in the ring and middle finger of the left hand. She further states the development of a cough for a few weeks but "it's gone now." She denies hemoptysis and attributed the left arm and scapula pain to musculoskeletal strain but ultimately sought medical attention on 9/15/89. Chest films at the local hospital revealed a "density" in the left apex. A needle biopsy was performed 9/28/89 demonstrating large cell carcinoma. On physical examination, a questionable palpable, nonenlarged lymph node was found in the left supraclavicular region. On the basis of suspected chest wall involvement, the last medical doctor felt the situation inoperable and recommended referral for palliative radiation therapy.

The patient was admitted to Strong Memorial for evaluation, staging, and therapeutic plan. Admission chest film revealed a 5-cm (2-in.) lesion in the left apex. Oblique views demonstrated nonadherence to the spine.

### Staging Report
*10/6/89:* Mediastinoscopy—negative
*10/6/89:* Fiberoptic bronchoscopy—positive
*10/7/89:* Liver, bone, brain CT—negative
*10/8/89:* Scalene lymph node biopsy—negative
***10/9/89 Diagnosis:*** Large cell carcinoma, Stage II, left upper lobe, superior sulcus invasion.
***Treatment:*** Local radiation therapy (6000 rad, total) on outpatient basis. Has returned now for left upper lobectomy (12/11/89).

## Past Health Status

***General Health.*** General health was "excellent, until this . . . I've never really been sick before."

***Prophylactic Medical/Dental Care.*** Has always, since adulthood, had annual medical and dental examinations.

***Childhood Illnesses.*** Patient reports "rheumatic fever as a child. I think I had a heart murmur too." No restriction in activity following the illness.

***Immunizations.*** "My records indicate all childhood vaccinations. I was revaccinated for travel in 1968. Last tetanus shot: "I can't recall."

***Major Illnesses/Hospitalizations.*** None prior to 9/89. "I was in the hospital for childbirth in 1965 and 1967." Reported normal vaginal deliveries.

### Current Medications
*Prescription:* Percocet 1 tab PO q3h prn for pain.
*Nonprescription:* "Iron tablet," every day. "I never take pills that are not prescribed."

***Allergies.*** None to food or drugs known.

### Habits
*Alcohol:* "Socially I'll have a highball; usually I have a glass of wine each day with dinner."
*Caffeine:* Six–8 cups of caffeinated coffee each day.
*Drugs:* See Current Medications; takes no over-the-counter medications.
*Tobacco:* Three packs per day for 20 years (60 pack-years). Reports smoking until office visit with surgeon on 10/2/89. "I've cut down to 3–4 cigarettes per day since."

No history of chemical or asbestos exposure, hemoptysis, recurrent pneumonia, tuberculosis, weight loss, anorexia, or malaise.

### Family Health History

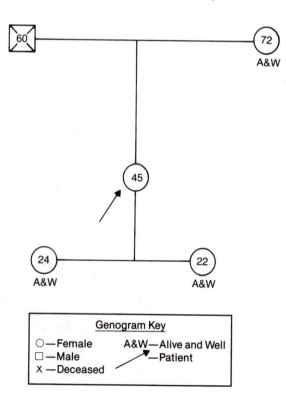

Genogram Key
○—Female   A&W—Alive and Well
□—Male   ➤—Patient
X—Deceased

## NUTRITIONAL/METABOLIC PATTERN

### Nutritional

The patient states that she usually eats 3 well-balanced meals a day but has a tendency to "oversnack." "All my life I've had a 10–20 lb (4.5–9 kg) weight problem." Denies any significant weight loss since diagnosis. "We are always trying to cut calories and we have eliminated salt since my mother's diagnosis of hypertension."

#### Usual Daily Menu
*Breakfast:* Tomato juice (4 oz), 2 slices wheat toast with salt-free margarine, ½ cup cornflakes with milk, 2 cups of coffee.

*Lunch:* Peanut butter and banana sandwich, 2 cups of coffee, cookies.

*Dinner:* Four–6 oz meat or chicken, baked potato, 1 tbsp margarine, green beans, 2 cups of coffee, fruit or cake.

### Metabolic

Patient reports weight as 135 lb (61.3 kg); she is 5 ft 4 in. (163 cm) tall; appears well nourished and denies problems with dentition.

## ELIMINATION PATTERN

### Bowel

The patient does not report any problems. She has regular bowel movements each day, which are brown in color and have moderately firm consistency. Has never relied on laxatives and denies any change, pain, or bleeding associated with bowel movement.

### Bladder

Janice describes voiding frequently during the day and denies changes in color, amount, burning, or other difficulty with urination.

## ACTIVITY/EXERCISE PATTERN

### Activity/Exercise

The patient describes herself as very active. "I work long hours. Sometimes the work can be quite emotionally draining, but I pamper myself with enjoying my many hobbies. I'm very involved in community activities and I have developed many and varied friendships. I enjoy playing bridge and I'm also active in my church." The patient does not schedule regular physical activity. "I always mean to but I really don't have much time for a physical routine with all my other activities."

#### Self-Care Ability
| | |
|---|---|
| Feeding—0 | Grooming—0 |
| Bathing—0 | General mobility—0 |
| Toileting—0 | Cooking—0 |
| Bed mobility—0 | Home maintenance—0 |
| Dressing—0 | Shopping—0 |

> #### Functional Levels Code
> 0—Full self-care
> I—Requires use of equipment or device
> II—Requires assistance or support from another person
> III—Requires assistance or support from another person and equipment or device
> IV—Is dependent and does not participate

**Oxygenation/Perfusion**

*Last Chest X-Ray:* As reported in Present Health Status.
*Last ECG:* 10/6/89—within normal limits. Normal sinus rhythm with a rate of 80.

***Cardiac Risk Factors***

|  | Positive | Negative |
|---|---|---|
| Sedentary life-style | X |  |
| Hyperlipidemia |  | X |
| Cigarette smoking | X |  |
| Diabetes |  | X |
| Obesity |  | X |
| Hypertension | X |  |
| Hypervigilant personality |  | X |
| Family history of heart disease | X |  |

## Sleep/Rest Pattern

**Sleep/Rest**

Janice routinely requires 5 hours of sleep a night. "I've never needed more than 5 hours." Describes being rested on awakening, usually around 6 AM, and does not require rest during the day. Has never required sleep aids nor had difficulty getting to sleep.

## Cognitive/Perceptual Pattern

**Hearing**

The patient denies problems with hearing.

**Vision**

She also denies problems with vision; does not wear glasses or contacts. Last eye examination: "Last May."

**Sensory/Perception**

Reports intact sense of taste, touch, and smell and denies any changes in memory. The patient is right hand dominant. She describes herself as being a person who "has never relied on medications for pain, except for what the doctor has recently prescribed for me." Janice reports current pain medication as "1 Percocet tablet every 4 hours for the pain in my left chest and arm. I usually wait until the pain really bothers me before I will take the pill."

**Learning Style**

"Usually I learn by following instructions, either written or verbal, but sometimes it's better if I see how to do it, too. I can quickly make decisions, weighing all my options, and don't have much difficulty once I know what they are."

## Self-Perception/Self-Concept Pattern

**Self-Perception/Self-Concept**

Janice describes a strong sense of self, knows "who I am and where I am going, both personally and professionally." She reports that she is very independent; makes her own decisions about things; and is able to accept "things as they are. I am very optimistic about this procedure. Since my diagnosis, I have kept myself together and I feel that I am both a very strong and positive person."

When asked to describe how she handled anger she replied, "I am a judicious person. If I feel it would be better to blow off steam, I do, yet there are times when I have to keep things to myself. I am well able to decide when to remain silent about my feelings and usually feel good about my decision in retrospect."

## ROLE/RELATIONSHIP PATTERN

### Role/Relationship

The patient describes a very loving, caring, and close-knit home environment. Janice's mother is very active, performing most of the household chores and the cooking. "The girls also pitch in; we all share and help each other." Both daughters attend college and hold part-time jobs. Janice has been divorced for many years; whereabouts of her husband is unknown. "He deserted the family when the children were young (ages 3 and 5). I am very fortunate to have family and good friends who are caring and supportive." She reports a rewarding, close relationship with a male friend. "I've known him since high school . . . he's a true friend and lover." The patient states that she will never remarry. "I enjoy my independence too much . . . but our relationship has withstood the test of time. We travel together and share each other's good and bad times."

## SEXUALITY/REPRODUCTIVE PATTERN

### Sexuality/Reproductive

Age of menarche is reported at 11 years of age, and she is still menstruating regularly without problems. The patient performs self–breast examinations (SBE) monthly and has a Pap smear and vaginal examination annually. The patient is gravida 2, para 2, with uncomplicated vaginal deliveries. Janice is sexually active, describing her relationship as "mutually satisfying" and without problems. Contraception is achieved with the use of a diaphragm.

## COPING/STRESS TOLERANCE PATTERN

### Coping/Stress Tolerance

The patient verbalizes concerns openly. She describes herself as a person who "does not agonize or internalize but rather confronts problems squarely. When I was first diagnosed with cancer, I immediately sought counseling, which I did not find helpful. I felt I was being patronized and that made me anxious. When I was hospitalized in October for the workup, I found the support I needed from another patient who had already undergone the same surgery I'll be having now. She really helped me. I'm anxious to have the surgery so that I can get back to the business of living. I'd prefer not to confront the role cigarettes have played in helping with stress, but let's face it, I've smoked a lot for quite some time. Being able to cut down like this has helped me see just how well I can do without them. I will ultimately quit."

## VALUE/BELIEF PATTERN

### Value/Belief

Janice described her divorce as "difficult" for her, in view of her beliefs and values, but "after 7 years without a trace of him, I secured a divorce on the grounds of desertion. I have deep faith and am strengthened by my religion. I believe that with faith in God you can attain anything."

# Physical Examination

### General Survey

Forty-four-year old, slightly overweight female, appearing stated age. Sitting in bed, in no apparent distress, neatly groomed, talkative, and friendly.

**Vital Signs**

*Temperature:* 99.6°F (37.5°C) (oral)
*Pulse:* 80 regular (apical)
*Respirations:* 16 regular
*BP:* 110/65 (right arm), 120/62 (left arm), seated.

**Integument**

*Skin.* Skin on head, torso, and extremities (both upper and lower) is dry, warm, and supple without bruising, lesions, or scarring.
*Mucous Membranes.* Pink, moist, and intact.
*Nails.* Well groomed, short, and healthy-appearing.

**HEENT**

*Head.* Hair is thick, of normal consistency, and neat. Scalp is normocephalic without palpable masses. Face is symmetrical without swelling, tenderness, or crepitus on palpation. No bruises or scarring noted.
*Eyes.* Pupils equal, round, reactive to light and accommodation (PERRLA). Extraocular movements (EOMs) are intact. Fundi are without edema, exudate, or hemorrhage. Gross visual acuity by Snellen chart is 20/20.
*Ears.* Ears are bilaterally symmetrical in size and shape. Canals are clear. Tympanic membranes are intact; no scarring noted.
*Nose.* Nostrils are patent, without deformity or inflammation.
*Mouth/Throat.* Mucosa is pink and moist; uvula is midline; teeth are in good repair; tonsils are visible and nonenlarged.

**Neck**

Trachea is midline. The thyroid is nonpalpable and a small left supraclavicular node, soft and freely movable, is noted. Carotids are 4+ without bruits.

**Pulmonary**

Breath sounds are slightly diminished at the left apex and are otherwise clear throughout. The rate and rhythm of breathing are within normal limits and there is symmetrical chest excursion.

**Breast**

Well-developed female breasts, symmetrical in size and shape, without masses or swelling. Moderate tenderness of left breast superiorly in both inner and outer quadrants. Tenderness is described as deep, in chest wall. Nipples are pink and without exudate.

**Cardiovascular**

Apical pulse is 80 and regular. A slight murmur is heard in the aortic area. $S_1$ and $S_2$ are of good quality; no rub heard; point of maximal impulse (PMI) at the fifth intercostal space, midclavicular line.

**Peripheral Vascular**

Pulses in the upper and lower extremities are within normal limits and are bilaterally equal. No edema is noted.

*Peripheral Pulses*
Temporal—4 bilaterally
Carotid—4 bilaterally
Brachial—4 bilaterally
Radial—4 bilaterally
Femoral—4 bilaterally
Popliteal—4 bilaterally
Posterior tibialis—4 bilaterally
Dorsalis pedis—4 bilaterally

*Peripheral Pulse Scale*

0—Absent
1—Markedly diminished
2—Moderately diminished
3—Slightly diminished
4—Normal

**Abdomen**

Active bowel sounds in all quadrants. Abdomen soft, nontender and depressible; nonpalpable liver, kidneys, and spleen; and without bruits.

**Musculoskeletal**

Upper and lower extremities are without edema, cyanosis, or deformity. Muscle mass, tone, and strength are within normal limits and are bilaterally equal. There is no apparent joint inflammation or crepitus. Normal joint range of motion (ROM).

**Neurological**

***Mental Status.*** Alert and oriented to time, place, and person.
***Cranial Nerves.*** I–XII intact.
***Motor.*** Full range of motion in upper and lower extremities. Muscle strength is grossly normal.
***Sensory.*** Normal sensation to light touch in upper and lower extremities.

***Deep Tendon Reflexes***

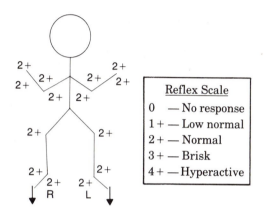

| Reflex Scale | |
|---|---|
| 0 | — No response |
| 1+ | — Low normal |
| 2+ | — Normal |
| 3+ | — Brisk |
| 4+ | — Hyperactive |

**Rectal**

Normal sphincter tone. Rectal examination negative for lesions, nodules, or tenderness. Stool test for occult blood, negative.

**Genitalia**

Pelvic examination deferred due to menstruation.

# Laboratory Data/Diagnostic Studies

**Laboratory Data**

***10/8/89 CBC***
***WBC:*** 10.3/mm$^3$      ***RBC:*** 3.51 mil/$\mu$l
***Hct:*** 28.6%      ***Hgb:*** 9.6 g/100 ml

***12/11/89 CBC***
***WBC:*** 10.0/mm$^3$      ***RBC:*** 4.0 mil/$\mu$l
***Hct:*** 33.0%      ***Hgb:*** 11.2 g/100 ml

***12/11/89***
***K:*** 4.0 mEq/L      ***Na:*** 136 mEq/L
***Blood Sugar:*** 118 mg/dl
(nonfasting)

***12/12/89 Postoperative Day #1 Arterial Blood Gases***
35% $O_2$ via face mask:
pH — 7.38 $PaCO_2$ — 44 mm Hg $PO_2$ — 104 mm Hg

28% $O_2$ via face mask:
pH — 7.39 $PaCO_2$ — 47 mm Hg $PO_2$ — 77 mm Hg

Room air (10 minutes):
pH — 7.41 $PaCO_2$ — 43 mm Hg $PO_2$ — 49 mm Hg

**Diagnostic Studies**

As outlined in the Staging Report on p. 165.

**Additional Data**

*Operative note 12/12/89:* 3-cm hard mass in periphery of left upper lobe, adherent to ribs 2 and 3. Left upper lobe entirely removed with en bloc chest wall resection (ribs 1, 2, 3, 4). T-1

**Additional Data—Continued**

nerve root had to be divided and taken with specimen. Remainder of brachial plexus and subclavian artery was well away from tumor.

*Operative findings:* All borders negative for tumor, ribs negative for tumor, nodes clinically negative.

## COLLABORATIVE PLAN OF CARE

### Postoperative Day #2—Return to Floor From Respiratory Intensive Care Unit

**Diet**

Clear liquids.

**Medications**

• Morphine Sulfate 5–20 mg IM q3h prn for pain; discontinued on postoperative day #3, then
• Codeine 30–60 mg PO q3h for pain *OR* Percocet ii tabs PO q3–4h for pain.

**Therapeutic Measures**

Vital signs q1h until stable then q4h.
Central venous pressure q 8°
D5 ½ normal saline IV at 80 ml/hr.
Humidified $O_2$ at 28% via face mask.
ABGs q8h and as necessary.
Chest tubes to 15 cm $H_2O$ suction.
Elastic stockings.
Ambulate as tolerated.

## NURSING DIAGNOSES DEVELOPED IN CARE PLAN

Impaired Gas Exchange, p. 172
Pain, p. 174
Potential for Impaired Physical Mobility, p. 176

## ADDITIONAL NURSING DIAGNOSES TO BE CONSIDERED

Impaired Tissue Integrity
Potential Activity Intolerance
Potential Altered Cardiopulmonary Tissue Perfusion
Potential Anxiety
Potential Decreased Cardiac Output
Potential Fear
Potential Fluid Volume Deficit
Potential for Altered Family Processes
Potential for Infection
Potential Ineffective Breathing Patterns

## NURSING CARE PLAN BASED ON IDENTIFIED NURSING DIAGNOSES

**Impaired Gas Exchange**

*Related to:* Left upper lobectomy.
*Evidenced by:* Alterations in arterial blood gases.

**Desired Patient Outcomes**

*The Patient Will:*
• Maintain patent airways.

*Evaluation Criteria*

- Develop and maintain optimal ventilation
- Maintain adequate tissue oxygenation.
- Avoid symptoms of respiratory distress.

- Arterial blood gases are within normal limits.
- The chest is clear on auscultation.
- Vital signs are within normal limits.

**The Patient:**
- Demonstrates stable and effective ventilatory patterns.
- Is able to mobilize secretions.

## Interventions

Assess preoperative baseline respiratory status.

Assess and evaluate skin color peripherally (nailbeds) and centrally (circumoral, mucous membranes, general duskiness).

Assess and evaluate respirations:

- Rate, depth, quality, and use of accessory muscles.
- Tidal volume measurements.

- Auscultate breath sounds.

Observe for early signs of respiratory insufficiency:
- Restlessness, anxiety, alteration in mental status, drowsiness, and depression.
- Increased, irregular pulse and increased blood pressure.

- Dyspnea

## Rationale

Past medical history of preexistent lung disease, smoking, sputum production, exercise tolerance, and preexistent cardiovascular, renal, and metabolic disease must be evaluated. Patterns of ventilation, auscultatory findings of the chest, complete pulmonary function studies, and a blood gas measurement will help identify the client at risk for developing pulmonary complications following thoracic surgery (Shapiro et al, 1982, p. 465).

Although cyanosis is not always a reliable index of hypoxia, when accompanied by other abnormal respiratory indicators it is considered serious since the $O_2$ saturation must be below 75% in persons with normal hemoglobin before it is detected. This finding needs to be correlated with arterial blood gases (Price and Wilson, 1986, p. 417).

The ventilatory pattern must be serially assessed and compared with blood gas measurements; respiratory rate and tidal volume measurements will also assist with assessment of the physiological efficiency of ventilation and the work of breathing (Shapiro et al, 1982, p. 467). Asymmetrical breathing may result from pain or guarding resulting in decreased ventilation. Decreased movement on the operative side of the chest during inspiration is one indication of possible pneumothorax (Luckmann and Sorensen, 1987, p. 828). Accessory muscles are not normally active during resting ventilation. When in obvious use, this compensatory mechanism improves the efficiency of diaphragmatic movement; however, it indicates increased respiratory effort and $O_2$ consumption (Shapiro et al, 1982, p. 238).
Crackles may indicate the development of pulmonary edema. Decreased or absent breath sounds over the remaining lung fields indicate atelectasis (Luckmann and Sorensen, 1987, pp. 2004–2005).

Clinical manifestations of hypoxemia affect the central nervous system first because the brain is the organ most sensitive to $O_2$ deprivation (Kneisl and Ames, 1986, p. 645).
The 4 most common signs of acute respiratory failure are headache, restlessness, confusion, and tachycardia. The effects on the cardiovascular system (of acute respiratory failure) are tachycardia, hypertension, and dysrhythmias (Kneisl and Ames, 1986, p. 645).

Sudden onset of dyspnea is indicative of acute respiratory failure (Kneisl and Ames, 1986, p. 645).

| Interventions | Rationale |
|---|---|
| Assess and evaluate circulation by obtaining vital signs, urinary output, and chest tube drainage. | Decreased blood pressure, and increased pulse and respirations are indicative of circulatory failure. Circulatory insufficiency may result from hypovolemia by blood loss or fluid depletion, producing hypoxia, acidosis, and ischemia of vital organs (Thompson et al, 1986, pp. 226–227). |
| Provide and promote frequent position change and turning; encourage ambulation. | Following lobectomy it is generally permissible to use full lateral turning on both sides. This permits expansion of lung tissue on both the operated and the unoperated side. Frequent turning will mobilize and promote drainage of secretions. Allowing the patient to remain in one position for too long predisposes to thrombus formation and may cause inadequate aeration of lung parts (Luckmann and Sorensen, 1987, pp. 829–830). Ambulation, with assistance, is allowed as soon as possible following surgery in accord with the patient's tolerance (Thompson et al, 1986, p. 251). |
| Provide coughing and deep breathing regimen. | Following chest surgery, coughing and deep breathing are important because they help to move tracheobronchial secretions out of the lung, assist with expanding the lung, improve pulmonary circulation, prevent stiffness of the lung, and help to force air and fluid out of the pleural space through the chest drainage tubes. Coughing loosens secretions and forces them into the upper respiratory tract, from which they may be expectorated or suctioned. Deep breathing dilates the airways, stimulates surfactant production, and expands lung tissue surface, thus increasing the area for respiratory gas exchange (Luckmann and Sorensen, 1987, p. 830). |
| Provide and monitor $O_2$ therapy. | The goal of $O_2$ therapy is to provide sufficient amounts of oxygen to the tissues at the lowest $FIo_2$, and to maintain a $Pao_2$ of at least 55 mmHg. Evaluation of the adequacy and effectiveness of $O_2$ therapy includes a basic, thorough physical assessment of the cardiopulmonary system and arterial blood gas measurements (Shapiro et al, 1982, p. 133). |

| | |
|---|---|
| **Pain** | **Related to:** Thoracic surgery/chest tube placement.<br>**Evidenced by:** Patient complaints of pain; patient's ability to actively participate in postoperative care. |
| **Desired Patient Outcomes** | • Resting comfort will be maximized.<br>• Pain will be relieved with minimal side effects.<br>• Fear and anxiety will be minimized.<br><br>**The Patient Will:**<br>• Be able to actively and progressively participate in essential postoperative activities.<br>• Maintain an effective breathing pattern. |
| **Evaluation Criteria** | **While Hospitalized:**<br>• Physiological parameters of pain are within normal limits: vital signs, level of consciousness, mobility, and pupils.<br>• Sleep/rest patterns are maximized.<br><br>**The Patient:**<br>• Verbalizes less time in pain.<br>• Verbalizes adequacy of pain relief utilizing rating scale.<br>• Requests pain medication with onset of pain. |

- Is able to actively participate in progressive exercise activities with minimal/decreasing discomfort.
- Progresses toward independence in exercise/activities of daily living (ADLs) without anxiety and with decreasing discomfort.

## Interventions

Anticipate the need for adequate and appropriate pain management.

Provide medication with a "preventive approach" by teaching the patient to request pain medication as soon as pain occurs. (Ms. Adams has used pain medication preoperatively for intolerable pain.)

Teach the patient that chest surgery *requires* preventive pain-relieving measures.

Assess and adjust to effectiveness the medication and dosage.

- Assess respiratory status after administering narcotics.

- Teach patient how to rate pain on a scale of 1 to 10 before and after administration of pain reliever.

- Plan medication doses with the patient utilizing the pain rating scale.

Schedule activities essential for recovery when pain medications are having maximum effect.

Splint the patient's chest; teach the patient splinting technique as soon as possible.

Teach the patient alternative/adjunct pain relief and relaxation techniques.

## Rationale

Unless the thoracic surgical patient is adequately medicated, the extreme pain and discomfort of the first few postoperative days may result in complications.

Following thoracic surgery the patient's chest is often extremely painful not only because of surgery but because of the presence of large chest drainage tubes (Luckmann and Sorensen, 1987, p. 832).

Medications should be administered as soon as pain begins and before it gets out of control. The patient is less anxious about the return of pain; there is decreased concern about obtaining relief when needed (McCaffrey, 1985, p. 18). The nurse assists the patient to achieve relief and effective control of pain by encouraging him or her to take pain medication before the pain becomes unbearable (Atkinson and Murray, 1985, p. 667).

Some patients hesitate to take pain-relieving measures routinely for fear of becoming addicted (Luckmann and Sorensen, 1987, p. 189).

Smaller, more frequent doses of narcotics are sometimes used so that the respiratory center is not depressed (Luckmann and Sorensen, 1987, p. 832).

The pain-relieving intervention must be evaluated and not merely assumed successful. With successful intervention the number assigned to the pain is lower after the intervention than before it was performed (Luckmann and Sorensen, 1987, p. 189).

Carefully monitoring the patient during the first 2–3 dose intervals helps gauge the efficacy and duration of the analgesic effect as well as adverse side effects (Kneisl and Ames, 1986, p. 107).

A person in severe pain breathes shallowly and rapidly and tries to avoid chest or other movements. Consequently secretions are retained and the lung on the operative side does not reexpand properly. Atelectasis and pneumonia develop (Luckmann and Sorensen, 1987, p. 832).

Chest splinting after chest surgery reduces discomfort when the patient coughs and deep-breathes, and decreases stretching the chest incision (Luckmann and Sorensen, 1987, p. 832).

Touch, massage, breathing techniques, repositioning, explanation, and teaching are also helpful in relieving pain. When the patient is receiving analgesic medications, nursing activities involving touch, explanation, and listening enhance the effect of the drug (Kneisl and Ames, 1986, pp. 106–107).

| | |
|---|---|
| **Potential for Impaired Physical Mobility** | **Evidenced by:** Impaired mobility of shoulder joint on operative side.<br>**Related to:** Surgical trauma to nerve and muscle tissue and potential for development of postoperative adhesions. |
| **Desired Patient Outcomes** | **The Patient Will:**<br>• Be able to regain shoulder ROM consistent with preoperative abilities.<br>• Avoid "dysfunction syndrome" of the shoulder joint. |
| **Evaluation Criteria** | • By the third postoperative day the patient is able to actively participate in shoulder ROM exercises.<br><br>**By Discharge, the Patient:**<br>• Has achieved preoperative ROM abilities.<br>• Is able to fully perform self-care utilizing affected shoulder/arm with minimal discomfort. |

## Interventions

Passively move affected arm and shoulder through full ROM 2 times q4–6h for first 24 hours after recovery from anesthesia.

Initiate active ROM exercises as soon as possible.

Provide preplanned and adequate pain control prior to initiation of exercise. Describe the expected discomfort to the patient.

Assess and evaluate exercise tolerance and abilities.

Inspect the integrity of the suture line before and after exercises.

Promote the use of the affected arm and shoulder in ADLs throughout the postoperative period.

## Rationale

Arm and shoulder exercises specifically help prevent adhesion formation between the muscles that are surgically incised.

Active participation often begins on the first or second postoperative day (Luckmann and Sorensen, 1987, p. 833).

Anticipatory fears prior to and in expectation of pain-producing stimuli can be minimized by an explanation of what to expect and by reassurance that pain control will be provided beforehand. Adequate pain management is essential for success (Luckmann and Sorensen, 1987, p. 188; Kneisl and Ames, 1986, p. 647).

Restrict or modify activities if the patient develops shortness of breath or dyspnea or becomes fatigued. Exercises should not be progressed beyond the point of pain (Luckmann and Sorensen, 1987, p. 833).

This is especially important during the first 24 hours postoperatively (Luckmann and Sorensen, 1987, p. 834).

Painful, permanent contractures must be avoided. Encouragement to reach with the affected arm and utilize affected muscle groups for ADLs are effective methods of increasing strength and mobility (Luckmann and Sorensen, 1987, p. 834).

## QUESTIONS FOR DISCUSSION

1. Mrs. Adams expresses a desire to ultimately stop smoking. How would you assist her in obtaining this goal?
2. Identify the actual and potential nursing diagnoses and defining characteristics related to the postoperative care of Mrs. Adams.
3. On the second postoperative day, you notice an increase of greater than 100 ml/hr of chest tube drainage. What nursing interventions are indicated?
4. In order to maintain the integrity of the closed chest drainage system, what nursing observations/assessments/interventions are involved?

5. Under what conditions would "stripping" the chest tube be indicated?
6. In order to provide adequate pain control for Mrs. Adams, what data in the case study would assist you in your needs assessment? Outline a preoperative teaching plan for postoperative pain control, utilizing the identified data.
7. Mrs. Adams identifies support from others in a similar situation as helpful with coping. Identify resources that may be helpful with regard to her diagnosis and with smoking cessation following discharge.
8. On the day before discharge, Mrs. Adams begins to cry and expresses concerns about dying. Based on what you know about her diagnosis, what nursing actions would you take?

# REFERENCES

Atkinson, L and Murray, M: Fundamentals of Nursing: A Nursing Process Approach. Macmillan, New York, 1985.

Kneisl, C and Ames, S: Adult Health Nursing. Addison-Wesley, Reading, Mass, 1986.

Luckmann, J and Sorensen K: Medical-Surgical Nursing: A Psychophysiological Approach. WB Saunders, Philadelphia, 1987.

McCaffrey, M: Newer uses of NSAIDS. Am J Nurs 85(7):781, 1985.

Price, S and Wilson, L: Pathophysiology: Clinical Concepts of Disease Processes. McGraw-Hill, New York, 1986.

Shapiro, B, et al: Clinical Application of Respiratory Care. Year Book Medical Publishers, Chicago, 1982.

Thompson, J, et al: Clinical Nursing. CV Mosby, St. Louis, 1986.

# BIBLIOGRAPHY

American Cancer Society: Cancer Facts and Figures. American Cancer Society, New York, 1987.

Carpenito, L: Nursing Diagnosis: Application to Clinical Practice. JB Lippincott, Philadelphia, 1987.

Carroll, PF: The ins and outs of chest drainage systems. Nursing '86 16(12):26, 1986.

Coomis, R and Martin, G: Small cell carcinoma of the lung: An overview. Semin Oncol Nurs 3(3):174, 1987.

Doenges, M, et al: Nursing Care Plans. FA Davis, Philadelphia, 1989.

Doenges, M and Moorhouse, SM: Nursing Diagnoses With Interventions. FA Davis, Philadelphia, 1988.

Donovan, M: Cancer pain: You can help! Nurs Clin North Am 17(4):713, 1982.

Duncan, W (ed): Recent Results in Cancer Research: Lung Cancer. Springer-Verlag, Berlin, 1984.

Erikson, R: Mastering the ins and outs of chest drainage, part 1. Nursing 89 19(5):36, May 1989.

Knaus, P: Chest tube stripping—Is it necessary? Focus Crit Care 12(6):41, 1986.

Krumm, S: Psychosocial adaptation of the adult with cancer. Semin Oncol Nurs 3(3):729, 1987.

McCaffery, M and Beebe A: Pain: Clinical Manual for Nursing Practice. CV Mosby, St. Louis, 1989.

McNaull, F: Radiation therapy for lung cancer: Nursing considerations. Semin Oncol Nurs 3(3):194, 1987.

Oleske, D: The epidemiology of lung cancer: An overview. Semin Oncol Nurs 3(3):165, 1987.

Ryan, L: Lung cancer: Psychosocial implications. Semin Oncol Nurs 3(3):222, 1987.

Silverberg, E and Lubera, J: Cancer statistics, 1987. Ca 7:2, 1987.

Thompson, J, et al: Clinical Nursing. CV Mosby, St. Louis, 1986.

vanSlater, HK: Non-small cell lung cancer: Issues in diagnosis, staging and treatment. Semin Oncol Nurs 3(3):183, 1987.

Watson, P: Patient education: The adult with cancer. Nurs Clin North Am 17(4):739, 1982.

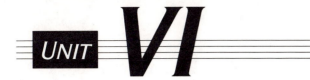

# THE PATIENT WITH ALTERATIONS IN METABOLISM RELATED TO THE GASTROINTESTINAL SYSTEM

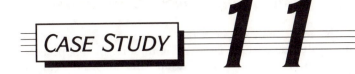
# A PATIENT WITH CROHN'S DISEASE

Jean D'Meza Leuner, M.S., R.N.

## ANATOMY AND PHYSIOLOGY OF THE GASTROINTESTINAL SYSTEM

The gastrointestinal (GI) tract, also known as the alimentary canal, consists of a series of organs (mouth, pharynx, esophagus, stomach, small intestine, and large intestine), and several accessory organs (teeth, tongue, salivary glands, liver, gallbladder, and pancreas) that extend from the mouth to the anus. The main functions of the GI system are to break down the nutrients into their smallest molecules for digestion, to absorb these molecules into the bloodstream, and to eliminate the by-products of digestion and other waste products from the body.

Digestion, absorption, and metabolism occur within the GI tract. Food is transported through the GI tract with the assistance of sequential rhythmic muscular contractions known as peristalsis. The existence of sphincters within the tract serves to regulate the passage of foodstuffs.

Digestion begins in the mouth. Saliva is produced to aid in mastication as well as to lubricate food for swallowing. Food passes through the esophagus with the assistance of mucus to lubricate it further, and then reaches the stomach.

The stomach acts as a reservoir for foodstuffs. Gastric secretions alter the composition of ingested material. Gastric juice is highly acidic due to the secretion of hydrochloric acid by the glands of the stomach. In addition, the enzyme pepsin is present for the digestion of proteins. The intrinsic factor produced by the parietal cells of the stomach is necessary for vitamin $B_{12}$ absorption to occur in the terminal ileum of the small intestine. Peristaltic motion in the stomach and contraction of the pyloric sphincter allow the liquefied material called chyme to enter the duodenum of the small intestine.

The function of the small intestine is to complete digestion and absorption. The waste products of digestion are then transported to the colon. The small intestine comprises three areas: the duodenum, jejunum, and ileum. The surface area available for the secretion and the absorption of various substances is extensive due to the characteristic circular folds of mucosa and submucosa as well as the presence of villi and microvilli in the small bowel. Digestion of lipids, carbohydrates, and proteins occurs within the small bowel. The products of digestion are absorbed with water and electrolytes through the processes of diffusion and active transport.

The terminal ileum, or distal portion of the small intestine, joins the colon at the site of the ileocecal valve. Absorption of water and electrolytes occurs in the colon. Fecal matter is stored in the distal portion of the colon and the rectum until defecation occurs as a result of the defecation reflex. Movement within the colon is less active than in the small intestine and consists of mixing and propulsive motions. The mixing, or haustral motion, aids the process of absorption by exposing the fecal matter to the colonic mucosal surface.

Bacterial formation in the colon assists with the movement of feces due to the emission of gases. Intestinal bacteria also transforms the substance urea into ammonium salts and ammonia. In this process, additional nutrients such as folic acid, riboflavin, vitamin K, vitamin $B_{12}$, thiamine, and nicotinic acid are synthesized and absorbed. The decomposition of bilirubin by bacteria in the colon gives feces their characteristic brown color.

The formation of mucus within the large intestine serves to protect the wall of the colon against abrasion from the fecal mass. In addition, the alkalinity of the mucus counteracts the acid created from the presence of bacteria in the colon and assists with the formation of a fecal mass.

# PATHOPHYSIOLOGY OF CROHN'S DISEASE

Chronic inflammatory bowel disease is the general term used to refer to disorders that involve the GI tract from the mouth to the anus. Regional enteritis or Crohn's disease and ulcerative colitis are the 2 most common inflammatory bowel diseases. Their presenting signs and symptoms are similar and therefore require a careful differential diagnosis to assist in developing treatment plans.

The etiology of Crohn's disease is presently unknown. A familial predisposition has been identified, and it is more prevalent among Jews than non-Jews and among whites than nonwhites. Crohn's disease may occur at any age; however, it is seen predominantly in both sexes between the ages of 20 and 30.

Crohn's disease is an ulcerative disease that can affect any segment of the GI tract with exacerbations and remissions. The inflammatory process occurs segmentally and extends through the layers of the intestinal wall. The invasive extension of this disease, or transmural involvement, is responsible for the formation of fistulas, fissures, and abscesses. Characteristic lesions called skip lesions occur in a noncontinuous fashion with normal intestinal mucosa in between the diseased areas. Crohn's disease most often affects the distal small intestine, perianal area, and colon. In Crohn's disease, the rectum is often spared, whereas rectal involvement often occurs in ulcerative colitis.

Crohn's disease may present in a mild form or as an acute, severe, debilitating disease. The presenting symptoms may strongly suggest that the disease is present; however, a definitive diagnosis can only be made based on microscopic analysis.

The following changes can be seen in the intestine to confirm a diagnosis: transmural inflammation, mucosal ulcerations, submucosal thickening and fibrosis, fissure formation, and the presence of abscess formation. Narrowing of the lumen may occur, as well as stenosis. Changes may also occur in the lymphatic system. Enlarged lymphatic vessels and mesenteric nodes may be seen.

The complications that are associated with Crohn's disease fall into two categories: intestinal changes, and systemic or extraintestinal complications. The complications that occur as a result of intestinal changes are the presence of obstructions, toxic megacolon, abscess formation, perforation, and malabsorption syndrome. Complications that are systemic in nature include hepatic disease, renal disorders leading to hydronephrosis and/or obstruction, arthritis, ocular changes, oral lesions, and inflammatory disorders of the skin.

# RISK FACTORS

To date, no clear relationship has been identified between specific risk factors and the presence of Crohn's disease. It can be stated, however, that certain conditions predispose a person with Crohn's disease to have an exacerbation of the illness. Exacerbations have been related to the presence of stress and dietary indiscretions. The ingestion of foods that stimulate the bowel can cause abdominal cramping and diarrhea. Lactose intolerance is often prevalent in persons with Crohn's disease. Persons with an allergic response to the ingestion of milk and milk products should be closely monitored.

The presence of chronic inflammatory bowel disease is associated with an increased risk of developing colorectal cancer. The length of time that a person has been afflicted with bowel disease will increase his or her chances of developing cancer of the small intestine or colon.

# COMMON CLINICAL FINDINGS

Crohn's disease is characterized by the presence of exacerbations and remissions. The onset of the disease is either inconspicuous or gradual and the presenting disease state may range from mildly active to severe.

Patients with a mild form of this disease present with abdominal tenderness, right lower quadrant discomfort, a change in bowel pattern, and a measurable weight loss due to nutritional deficits. These patients may be managed symptomatically or on an outpatient basis.

Patients with a severe form of the disease typically have grossly bloody diarrhea mixed with pus and mucus, greater than 6 stools in 24 hours, fever, nausea, and vomitus with colicky or persistent right lower quadrant abdominal pain. These patients are acutely ill and are often hospitalized for stabilization and treatment. Pain, identified in the periumbilical area or right lower quadrant, is consistent with involvement of the terminal ileum, whereas pain in the left upper middle abdomen can be attributed to involvement of the jejunum.

## TREATMENT MODALITIES

The medical management of Crohn's disease is focused on reducing the inflammation and infection and alleviating the associated symptoms causing distress. Pharmacological intervention is usually instituted with the administration of antibiotics, immunosuppressive agents, and anti-inflammatory agents. In addition, medications may be necessary for symptomatic relief.

Surgery is usually indicated for approximately 10% of patients. Surgical resection of the bowel is often performed, a proctocolectomy may be necessary, and a permanent ileostomy is created. Surgical intervention may be indicated when complications arise as a result of Crohn's disease. Some of the complications encountered are hemorrhage, obstruction, or fistula formation.

## PATIENT ASSESSMENT DATA BASE

## Health History

*Client:*
Ms. Sonia Silver

*Address:* 120 Main Street, Montclair, NJ 07043
*Telephone:* 555-7315
*Contact:* Mr. John Wellesley (boyfriend)
*Address of contact:* 120 Main Street, Montclair, NJ 07043
*Telephone of contact:* 555-7315
*Age:* 25    *Sex:* Female    *Race:* White
*Educational background:* High school graduate and 2 years of junior college
*Religion:* Jewish    *Marital status:* Single
*Usual occupation:* Clerk in a gift shop
*Present occupation:* Not able to work due to illness
*Source of income:* When working, weekly income
*Insurance:* None at the present time
*Source of referral:* Self
*Source of history:* Self
*Reliability of historian:* Reliable
*Date of interview:* 3/28/90
*Reason for visit/chief complaint:* Increased right lower quadrant pain, 7–10 loose, blood-streaked stools of small volume in the last 24 hours. Nausea, vomiting, persistent rectal discharge, and malaise. The patient relates that she is afraid to stand up; she feels "weak and miserable."

### HEALTH PERCEPTION/HEALTH MANAGEMENT PATTERN

*Present Health Status*

Until 2 weeks ago Sonia felt well. She took daily medications, maintained strict diet, and walked to work for exercise enjoying the spring weather. Crampy abdominal pain started to become bothersome and the frequency of stools made it impossible to go to work. Nausea and vomiting have continued and the patient states, "I feel too weak to be out of bed."

## Past Health Status

**General Health.** Diagnosed at age 15 as having regional enteritis (Crohn's disease) after a lengthy workup that included several hospitalizations. Maintained on drug and diet therapy until the present time. Saw physician approximately 1 month ago when patient thought she might be experiencing a flare-up of Crohn's disease. At that time prednisone dosage was increased from 20–40 mg/day and the patient began taking ampicillin. The symptoms have persisted and the patient is seen at the present time in acute distress.

**Prophylactic Medical/Dental Care.** Used to see physician every 6 months and more frequently if necessary. "I'm glad my doctor knows me and understands my history. This disease is very frightening and embarrassing. I have no medical insurance right now, and I am really afraid to run up a medical bill I can't afford." She has an annual visit to the dental hygienist.

**Childhood Illnesses.** Chickenpox, measles, and German measles. "That's all I can remember."

**Immunizations.** Tetanus shot about 5 years ago.

**Major Illnesses/Hospitalizations.** Admitted 3 times at age 15–16 to diagnose Crohn's disease and provide dietary supplementation and medication stabilization.

### Current Medications

*Prescription:* Sulfasalazine (Azulfidine) 5 g daily in divided doses; ampicillin 2 g daily PO; prednisone 40 mg PO OD; diphenoxylate hydrochloride/atropine (Lomotil) 5 mg PO tid; ferrous sulfate 30 mg PO daily.

*Nonprescription:* Multivitamin 1 tablet daily; calcium supplement 1 tablet daily; acetylsalicylic acid (A.S.A.) 2 tabs qid for joint pain prn.

**Allergies.** No known allergies.

### Habits

*Alcohol:* A few beers each week.

*Caffeine:* Occasionally has a cup of tea or coffee or coke after work.

*Drugs:* See Current Medications.

*Tobacco:* Two packs per day for 3 years (6 pack-years).

### *Family Health History*

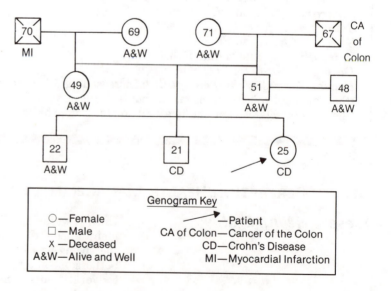

## NUTRITIONAL/METABOLIC PATTERN

### Nutritional

Sonia has tried to follow a specific diet that would help prevent a recurrence of symptoms associated with Crohn's disease. She is aware that the diet should be high in calories and vitamins and that it should have an adequate amount of protein. She avoids raw fruits and vegetables. Avoids milk and milk products as much as she can tolerate. Tries to eat 3 balanced meals a day. "The foods that I should eat are very expensive. I know I am not really consistent with my diet, if I have to tell the truth."

#### Usual Daily Menu

*Breakfast:* Small glass of powdered juice, toast, margarine, 1 egg scrambled or fried.
*Lunch:* Sandwich and/or clear soups, diet soda, cookies or pastry.
*Snack:* High-protein drink.
*Dinner:* Chicken, fish, meat (usually hamburger, chop, or steak), cooked vegetable (prefers carrots, broccoli, peas, green beans), potatoes (usually french fries), roll and margarine.
*Before bed:* High-protein drink. Occasionally a cup of hot tea. Shopping and food preparation usually done by patient. Does not have a large appetite.

### Metabolic

*Height:* 5 ft 3½ in. (161.3 cm). *Weight:* 90 lb (41 kg). Has lost 10 lb (4.5 kg) in last 2 weeks. Skin is dry and itchy at times. Denies difficulty with chewing.

## ELIMINATION PATTERN

### Bowel

Until 2 weeks ago, Sonia had occasional diarrhea, 2–4 loose stools a day with constipation at infrequent intervals. She states that she increased her intake of water and ate an additional piece of fruit daily when constipation recurred. Presently she is experiencing 7–10 loose, bloody stools with lower abdominal cramps. Small quantity with each stool. Acknowledges the use of anti-diarrheal medications as prescribed. "I'm tired of the diarrhea; it physically exhausts me and ruins my life."

### Bladder

Occasional strong odor to urine with urgency, frequency, and pain on urination. Awakens at night to void, usually twice each night.

## ACTIVITY EXERCISE PATTERN

### Activity/Exercise

Until recently, Sonia worked as a clerk in a gift shop. It required minimal activity and when it was not busy (most of the time) she could sit to do paperwork or straighten the shelves. She would walk to work (about 15–20 minutes) when there was nice weather. At present, she enjoys a more sedentary life-style (TV, movies, reading) due to the illness. She states, "I'm happy to be at home near the bathroom now; I know this could become very boring. I do miss getting around." Complains of mild joint pain and relies on her boyfriend to assist with the cleaning and shopping.

**Activity/Exercise — Continued**

**Self-Care Ability**

| | |
|---|---|
| Feeding — 0 | Grooming — 0 |
| Bathing — 0 | General mobility — 0 |
| Toileting — 0 | Cooking — 0 |
| Bed mobility — 0 | Home maintenance — 0 |
| Dressing — 0 | Shopping — 0 |

---

**Functional Levels Code**

0 — Full self-care
I — Requires use of equipment or device
II — Requires assistance or supervision from another person
III — Requires assistance or supervision from another person and equipment or device
IV — Is dependent and does not participate

---

**Oxygenation/Perfusion**

Could recall that she had previously had a chest x-ray but was unsure of date: "probably a year or so ago." Could not recall if she had a previous ECG. Denies evidence of palpitations, rapid heartbeat, irregular heart rhythm, or pain in the chest area. Denies any special problems such as shortness of breath, wheezing, cough, asthma, bronchitis, or respiratory infections.

**Cardiac Risk Factors**

| | Positive | Negative |
|---|---|---|
| Sedentary life-style | X | |
| Hyperlipidemia | | X |
| Cigarette smoking | X | |
| Diabetes | | X |
| Obesity | | X |
| Hypertension | | X |
| Hypervigilant personality | | X |
| Family history of heart disease | X | |

## SLEEP/REST PATTERN

**Sleep/Rest**

Needs 6–8 hours of sleep a night. Frequently has difficulty falling asleep after being awakened. Has not felt rested in a long time. "The diarrhea has me up all hours of the day and night." Tries to nap during the day whenever possible. Denies use of sedatives or sleep medications. "I'm afraid to take any more medications."

## COGNITIVE/PERCEPTUAL PATTERN

**Hearing**

Denies any problems with hearing.

**Vision**

Occasionally experiences eye pain and blurring of vision. Attributes this to being exhausted lately and feeling bad. Does not wear glasses. Can't remember ever having eyes checked by an ophthalmologist.

**Sensory Perception**

Has not noticed a change in sensation. She is right-hand dominant. No notable change in ability to concentrate. "I try to manage my pain to the best of my ability with my medications. I hate to complain although at times that is all that I seem to do."

**Learning Style**

Learns best with visual aids and clear explanation and working with someone she likes. "People who don't know me may think I am stupid. If I know the person I am talking to and that person knows me for who I am, I can do very well."

## SELF-PERCEPTION/SELF-CONCEPT PATTERN

*Self-Perception/Self-Concept*

"I would like to consider myself an easygoing person although I can be hyper at times. I often want things my own way, and I lack patience when I am focusing on my needs. I enjoy being around others; I try not to be too demanding. Lately I know I've been unpleasant and at times nasty. I keep thinking about my body and how it has ruined my life. I don't know if I'll be able to look at myself once I have had the surgery. Yes, I want to have it done, but what will I end up with? I'm at the point where I'll do anything to settle this problem down so I can regain my life and the person I used to be."

"Sometimes I have difficulty expressing my needs and feelings and other times I get so angry and frustrated that I let it all out. I don't mind being touched although I rarely touch others. My disease makes me feel alone and different when it flares up and I never know when it will escalate. Will I want to be touched by John after the surgery is another question." States she is a good listener when she wants to be and is probably considered an extrovert.

## Role/Relationship Pattern

**Role/Relationship**

Sonia lives in a 3-room modern apartment building with her boyfriend who is 16 years her senior. They have lived together for 3 years. He is divorced with 1 child, age 12, who visits infrequently (2–3 times a year). Her relationship with the child is "guarded. I feel imposed upon when the child comes to visit . . . ours is a fairly private life."

She describes her relationship with her boyfriend as good. "The only real solid relationship I've ever had." Patient states: "My mother who is divorced didn't want me and I don't get along with my father." She was close to her grandmother who now lives in California. She stresses her concern about the impact of impending surgery on her relationship with her boyfriend. "He's all I really have."

## SEXUALITY/REPRODUCTIVE PATTERN

*Sexuality/Reproductive*

Sonia states, "I have no problems with my sexual life." She has used birth control pills in the past and the couple now rely on condoms. "If I need surgery and have a 'bag' I don't know what it will do to my sexual relationship with my boyfriend. Will he even look at me, want to touch me? I guess I am really scared."

Menarche at age 13. Regular menstrual cycles every 26–28 days. Annual Pap smears have been negative. Gravida–0. "I try to remember to check my breasts monthly with a self-breast examination. I think I'm doing it correctly." Denies any vaginal discharge, itch, or venereal disease.

## COPING/STRESS TOLERANCE PATTERN

*Coping/Stress Tolerance*

Major concern of Sonia is her illness and what lies in the future. She tries to manage her disease alone and be independent. Hates to burden her boyfriend with the illness but she feels alone and

**Coping/Stress Tolerance— Continued**

afraid this time. Handles personal losses by surviving through them and then not thinking about them. Having a brother with the same disease gives her someone else to talk to, although she hates to bother him. "He has had his own problems to deal with in the past few years." Recently she has felt very depressed when the diarrhea wouldn't stop and she felt weaker by the day. "I wanted to lie in bed and cry."

## VALUE/BELIEF PATTERN

*Value/Belief*

Patient states she is not a very religious person. She recognizes the major Jewish holy days and occasionally goes to temple. As a child she attended a few years of Hebrew school because her friends were there and she was expected to go as well.

# Physical Examination

## General Survey

A 25-year-old white female appearing older than stated age. She is pale and thin and appears to be moderately anxious and in a moderate amount of discomfort. Has a cushingoid appearance secondary to prednisone use.

## Vital Signs

*Temperature:* 100.6°F (38.1°C) (oral)
*Pulse:* 92 regular (apical)
*Respirations:* 18 regular
*BP:* 90/60 (right arm), 88/60 (left arm), sitting.

## Integument

*Skin.* Skin is warm, pale in color, and without lesions or scarring.
*Mucous Membranes.* Smooth; appear dry with no inflammation or lesions noted.
*Nails.* Nails are rough and dry. No clubbing noted.

## HEENT

*Head.* Symmetrical, no palpable masses. Hair is curly brown, fine texture. No scalp lesions noted. Face is symmetrical with cushingoid appearance. No tenderness on palpation. Round face with cheeks appearing red. Temporomandibular joint (TMJ) is fully mobile without crepitation or pain.
*Eyes.* Pupils equal, round, reactive to light and accommodation (PERRLA). No tenderness or discharge noted at puncta. Visual fields appear equal on examination. Extraocular eye movements (EOMs) tested without nystagmus. Visual acuity is 20/20 in both eyes using hand-held chart. Does not wear glasses.
*Ears.* Ears are symmetrically placed, equal in size and shape, without lesions or nodules. Able to hear whisper and watch tick at 1 ft with both ears. *Weber test:* vibration heard equally well in both ears. *Rinne test:* Air conduction twice as long as bone conduction.
*Nose.* Nostrils are patent; no drainage; no septal deviation noted.
*Mouth/Throat.* Oral mucosa appears pink and dry. Tongue is midline without limited movement. Uvula is midline with rise of soft palate on saying "ah." Positive gag reflex. Floor of the mouth is without lesions or soreness. Teeth are in good repair. Tonsils are present, not enlarged.

## Neck

Trachea is midline; thyroid is not enlarged or palpable. No nodes palpated. Neck muscles (sternocleidomastoid and trapezius) are symmetrical, without masses or swelling with active range of motion of head and equal muscle strength against resistance.

**Pulmonary**

Anteroposterior diameter of thorax is 1:2. No difficulties with respiratory rate or rhythm. No clubbing noted; nailbeds pink. Fremitus is equal bilaterally. No crepitus noted. Lungs clear to auscultation. Resonance noted on percussion.

**Breast**

Breasts are symmetrical; nipples without discharge or lesions. Breasts without lumps; slight tenderness on palpation. Axilla without palpable lumps or lesions.

**Cardiovascular**

Apical pulse is 92 regular. Point of maximal impulse (PMI) at midclavicular line of fifth intercostal space. No $S_3$ or $S_4$ sounds or murmurs noted on auscultation. No visible jugular venous pulsations in a sitting position. Carotid pulse is bounding, strong, and without bruits.

**Peripheral Vascular**

Upper extremities appear symmetrically pale with pulses normal. Lower extremities appear symmetrically pale with pulses normal. No edema noted in extremities.

***Peripheral Pulses***
Temporal—4 bilaterally
Carotid—4 bilaterally
Brachial—4 bilaterally
Radial—4 bilaterally
Femoral—4 bilaterally
Popliteal—4 bilaterally
Posterior tibialis—4 bilaterally
Dorsalis pedis—4 bilaterally

***Peripheral Pulse Scale***

| |
| --- |
| 0—Absent |
| 1—Markedly diminished |
| 2—Moderately diminished |
| 3—Slightly diminished |
| 4—Normal |

**Abdomen**

Slightly rounded; no lesions or scars noted. Active bowel sounds heard in all 4 quadrants, high-pitched and rushing in nature. No audible bruits; tympany noted over most of the abdomen. Liver size is 6 cm ($2\frac{2}{5}$ in.) at midclavicular line. Abdomen is tender on light palpation; deep palpation not performed.

**Musculoskeletal**

Full range of motion noted in all extremities. Muscle strength is normal bilaterally when tested against resistance. Patient is unstable out of bed at this time due to generalized weakness.

**Neurological**

***Mental Status.*** Alert, oriented to time, place, and person. Cooperative young woman.
***Cranial Nerves.*** I–XII intact with no problems noted.
***Sensory.*** No difficulty discriminating light touch and deep touch. Appropriate discrimination of temperature and vibration.

***Deep Tendon Reflexes***

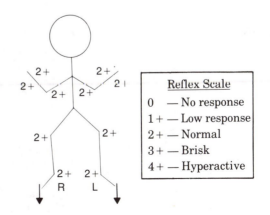

| Reflex Scale | |
| --- | --- |
| 0 | — No response |
| 1+ | — Low response |
| 2+ | — Normal |
| 3+ | — Brisk |
| 4+ | — Hyperactive |

| | |
|---|---|
| *Rectal* | Deferred. |
| *Genitalia* | Deferred. |

## Laboratory Data/Diagnostic Studies

*Laboratory Data*

*Na:* 141 mEq/L
*K:* 3.7 mEq/L
*Cl:* 105 mEq/L
*CO$_2$:* 26 mM/L
*Ca:* 9 mg/dl
*BUN:* 9 mg/dl
*Creatinine:* 0.7 mg/dl
*Glucose:* 104 mg/dl
*Triglycerides:* 118 mg/dl
*Hct:* 34.8%
*Hgb:* 12.0 g/100 ml
*WBC:* 7.6 $10^3$/mm$^3$

*RBC:* 3.9 $10^6$/mm$^3$
*Platelet Count:* 250,000/mm$^3$
*Alk Phos:* 26 U/L
*Serum Albumin:* 3.2 g/100 ml
*Serum Cobalamin:* 150 pg/ml
*Folic Acid:* 2.4 ng/ml
*Urine:* Colorless; ketones—negative; pH 7. Specific gravity—1.019. Protein—negative for occult blood. Bile—negative.
*Guaiac Test:* Positive.

*Diagnostic Studies*

**ECG.** Sinus rhythm; no ectopic activity; rate 90.
**Chest X-Ray.** Posteroanterior (PA) and lateral—clear.
**Proctosigmoidoscopy.** Multiple areas of transmural thickening; inflammation and granulomatous lesions throughout.
**Bowel Biopsy.** Examination revealed noncaseating granulomas with focal abscesses.
**Barium Enema.** Test revealed skip lesions in the terminal ileum and the colon.

*Additional Data*

Following diagnostic studies and stabilization of diarrhea and nutritional status, the patient was scheduled for a total colectomy and permanent ileostomy. At the time of surgery an incidental appendectomy was performed as well.

# COLLABORATIVE PLAN OF CARE

*Diet*

NPO except medications with a sip of water.

*Medications*

Erythromycin 1 g PO.
Neomycin 1 g PO tid.
Lomotil 5 mg q8h prn for diarrhea.
Phytonadione (AquaMEPHYTON) 10 mg IM once a week.
Meperidine hydrochloride (Demerol) 50–75 mg IM q4h prn for pain.

*Intravenous Therapy*

Insert a central venous access line with a total parenteral nutrition (TPN) solution of dextrose 25%, amino acids 41 g, nitrogen 6.5 g, potassium 35 mEq, sodium 50 mEq, calcium 10 mEq, phosphate 10 mM, magnesium 8 mEq, zinc 1 mg, copper 0.4 mg, manganese 0.1 mg, chromium .005 mg, selenium .015 mg. Add vitamins to the first bottle only. Give 125 ml/hr.

*Therapeutic Measures*

Daily weight.
Measure intake and output.
Test urinary sugar and acetone q6h.

*Consults*

Physician will mark the area for placement of the ostomy on the abdomen.

## Preoperative Plan

Soapsuds enema.
Wide abdominal and perianal preparation.
Set up 2 units of packed red blood cells for the OR.
NPO after midnight.
Diazepam (Valium) 5 mg PO with sip of water the night before surgery.
Morphine sulfate 5 mg IM on call to OR.
Cefazolin sodium (Ancef) 500 mg IM on call to OR.
Methylprednisone 20 mg IV in OR.

# Postoperative Collaborative Plan of Care

### Diet

NPO; advance to sips of clear liquids when bowel sounds are present.

### Medications

IV Ancef 3 g in 250 ml of 5% D/W to give 83 ml q8h.
IV hydrocortisone sodium succinate (Solu-Cortef) 50 mg/day.
When takings fluids:
  Prednisone 30 mg PO qd.
  Azulfidine 1.5 g PO tid.
  Valium 2 or 5 mg PO hs.

### Intravenous Therapy

TPN solution via central venous access line: dextrose 25%, amino acids 41 g, nitrogen 6.5 g, potassium 35 mEq, sodium 50 mEq, calcium 10 mEq, phosphate 10 mM, magnesium 8 mEq, zinc 1 mg, copper 0.4 mg, manganese 0.1 mg, chromium .005 mg, and selenium .015 mg. Give 125 ml/hr.
Peripheral IV line maintained with 5% D/W and .45 NaCl at 80 ml/hr.

### Therapeutic Measures

Test urinary sugar and acetone q6h. Encourage out of bed (OOB) tid with ambulation.
Monitor intake and output.
Daily weight.
Jackson-Pratt drainage monitored.
Change dressing at Jackson-Pratt site prn.
Clean abdominal suture line with ½ strength hydrogen peroxide prn and cover with a dry sterile dressing.
Nasogastric tube attached to 1.5 lb of suction. Irrigate with 30 ml normal saline q2h prn.

### Consults

Consult with ostomy nurse prn.

# NURSING DIAGNOSES DEVELOPED IN CARE PLAN

# ADDITIONAL NURSING DIAGNOSES TO BE CONSIDERED

Altered Family Processes
Altered Oral Mucous Membrane
Altered Role Performance
Diversional Activity Deficit
Dysfunctional Grieving

Fatigue
Fear
Ineffective Individual Coping
Pain
Potential for Infection
Sexual Dysfunction
Sleep Pattern Disturbance
Social Isolation

# NURSING CARE PLAN BASED ON IDENTIFIED NURSING DIAGNOSES

| | |
|---|---|
| *Body Image Disturbance* | *Related to:* Physical changes in body structures.<br>*Evidenced by:* Patient stating that she is concerned about a change in her appearance as a result of the ileostomy. |
| *Desired Patient Outcomes* | *The Patient Will:*<br>• Explore her feelings related to an alteration in her body structure and boundaries.<br>• Acknowledge the change in her body's appearance.<br>• Develop plans to integrate the change in her body structure into her daily routine.<br>• Develop strategies to cope with her negative feelings. |
| *Evaluation Criteria* | *During this Hospital Stay, the Patient Will:*<br>• Discuss her feelings concerning the change in her body structure.<br>• Develop a plan to care for her ileostomy that is directed toward independence.<br>• Be able to identify relevant support groups.<br>• Identify strategies that may help her increase her self-concept.<br>• Discuss inviting her significant other and/or family members to the discussions concerning her postoperative recovery. |

## Interventions

Encourage the patient to discuss her feelings concerning the change in her bodily appearance. Be accepting of the patient's possible feelings of resentment, anger, rejection, depression, fear, grief, and loss.

Encourage the patient to talk about how she viewed her life prior to the surgery. Discuss the creation of the ileostomy as a means of stabilizing the patient's life.

Develop a plan to care for the ileostomy that includes the patient. Gradually increase the patient's involvement in caring for the ileostomy to encourage independence on the part of the patient.

## Rationale

Gradually the bereaved patient comes to recognize and admit that a loss has occurred. Most people do resolve their feelings of loss and begin to construct a new social identity. Postoperative counseling by the ileostomist should aim to help the patient work through his or her grief. Grief work includes acceptance, and with acceptance the patient can begin to resolve his or her life (Kelly, 1985, pp. 523–524).

When an ostomy is created to cure a disease, the improved lifestyle may allow the patient to view the ostomy in a more positive manner (Shipes, 1987 p. 293).

When patients are emotionally ready, they will become involved in care of their ostomy and look at their stoma. (Patrick et al, 1986 p. 1178). The incorporation of an ostomy into a new body image is a long process. The proficiency in stoma care, a healthy adjustment, sound coping skills, and positive reactions from others are helpful for this adjustment (Shipes, 1987, p. 292).

## Interventions

Discuss with the patient the purpose of support groups. Provide her with information concerning local ostomy support groups. Introduce the patient to support groups and/or services in the area that can serve as reference groups.

Discuss with the patient her activities of daily living and self-care needs. Encourage the patient to discuss self-concept and the influence it has on self-care behaviors.

Discuss with the patient strategies to affect a change in her body image. Some ideas might include a change in clothing style, makeup, hair style, and integrating exercise into daily activities. Discuss with the patient an interest in becoming involved in community activities or a desire to take a class in a particular area of interest.

Focus on the normal aspects of the patient's life rather than the sick role. Support the patient's efforts to discuss her life as normal.

Discuss with the patient the inclusion of her significant other or family members in discussions of the patient's care.

## Rationale

Counselors knowledgeable of the postoperative concerns of the patient can be a major source of strength (Kelly, 1985 p. 522). Support groups with similar concerns are often helpful in identifying ways to manage long-term illness. They also provide companionship and reassurance of personal worth (Tilden and Weinert, 1987 p. 618).

Self-concept is a basic determinant of self-care activities directly and through its impact on perceptions of past, present, and future events (Connelly, 1987, p. 621).

Persons who believe in taking control over their own health attribute physical health to taking good care of themselves and they believe they have the power to make themselves well and have a higher quality of life (Pollock, 1987, p. 638).

In a healthy state, a person has a set of rights and obligations that could be jeopardized if he or she is defined as sick. Inflammatory bowel disease patients prefer to focus on normalcy (Joachim and Milne, 1985, p. 40).

Patients have been found to adapt better and feel less isolated when family members are included in teaching and care (Shipes, 1987, p. 297).

---

| **Potential Impaired Skin Integrity** | **Related to:** The presence of excretions on the skin. **Evidenced by:** (Not applicable; presence of signs and symptoms establishes an actual diagnosis.) |
|---|---|
| **Desired Patient Outcomes** | **The Patient Will:** <br>• Be aware of interventions to keep the skin intact. <br>• Be aware of the factors that indicate a change in skin integrity. |
| **Evaluation Criteria** | **While in the Hospital, the Patient Will:** <br>• Verbalize an understanding of the signs and symptoms that occur when the peristomal skin integrity is compromised. <br>• Demonstrate the procedure to change an ostomy appliance to minimize skin abrasion. <br>• Describe a diet that is consistent with principles to minimize abrasion of the skin at the peristomal site. |

---

## Interventions

Discuss with the patient the signs and symptoms that accompany an alteration in skin integrity in the peristomal area. Peristomal skin irritation may include any of the following:

## Rationale

To prevent skin breakdown persons need to be instructed in all the steps necessary to protect the skin. The instruction should include teaching the patient and family the early signs and symptoms of potential skin breakdown (Broadwell, 1987, p. 331).

## Interventions

- Erythema, edema, and erosion
- Ulceration and bleeding
- A change in pigmentation
- The presence of fluid-filled elevations on the skin
- Pain or the presence of fever

Teach the patient to prepare the appliance so that a close fit can be observed with the stoma. A protective skin barrier should be used with the pouch.

Teach the patient to empty the appliance when it is approximately one-third to one-half full.

Instruct the patient to use stoma bags that can be drained easily.

Discuss with the patient the significance of evaluating the peristomal skin with each bag change.

Reinforce with the patient the fact that skin irritants should be avoided. Avoid the use of soap in the peristomal area.

Teach the patient to use the least amount of tape on the skin necessary to keep the pouch intact.

Discuss with the patient the need to wear loosely fitting clothing. Avoid the use of a belt at the peristomal region.

Teach the patient to be aware of the type of foods she is consuming. Certain foods may be more difficult to tolerate and result in gas and/or diarrhea. Foods high in roughage should be consumed with caution.

## Rationale

The skin protector and appliance are fitted close to the stoma to prevent the high enzymatic content of the ileal effluent from damaging the skin (Rideout, 1987, pp. 257–258).

Emptying the pouch before it becomes full prevents the weight of the bag from breaking the seal with the skin and cause the leakage of excretions onto the skin (Rideout, 1987, p. 257).

A pouch that can be drained easily prevents frequent bag changes leading to skin irritation (Rideout, 1987, p. 257).

When the pouch is being changed, the skin should be carefully inspected for any signs of erosion (Rideout, 1987, p. 258). Total pouch removal and thorough cleansing and skin inspection are recommended once a week because stool may seep beneath the skin barrier and not be obvious (Erickson, 1987, p. 314).

Peristomal skin can be damaged due to the use of soaps, detergents, and chemical agents (Broadwell, 1987, p. 327).

The overuse of adhesive tape is associated with mechanical trauma to the skin (Broadwell, 1987, p. 324).

Tight clothing and equipment may exert pressure on the skin that can cause erythema and erosion (Broadwell, 1987, p. 325).

A low-residue diet will reduce the bulk of the stool and slow down the process of elimination (Dudek, 1987, p. 369).

---

## Altered Nutrition: Less than Body Requirements

*Related to:* Inability to absorb nutrients.
*Evidenced by:* Recent weight loss, weight 20% below ideal for height and frame, and the presence of diarrhea, vomiting, and fatigue.

## Desired Patient Outcomes

*The Patient Will:*
- Progress toward ideal body weight.
- Be knowledgeable about the administration of total parenteral nutrition (TPN) and related procedures as they pertain to improving nutritional status.
- Understand the nutritional principles that should be considered with Crohn's disease.

***Evaluation Criteria***

***While in the Hospital, the Patient Will:***
- Verbalize that she understands why she is receiving TPN.
- Verbalize that she understands the reasons why she will be closely monitored during TPN administration.
- Be knowledgeable about the need to have the intravenous equipment unoccluded and intact.
- Perform oral care at frequent intervals.
- Not lose any additional weight.
- Verbalize an understanding of the dietary principles that should be considered when she resumes eating.

## Interventions

Explain to the patient the reason for the administration of TPN and the need to monitor her frequently during the treatment.

Discuss with the patient the importance of maintaining an unoccluded TPN line that continues to deliver the prescribed solution.

Teach the patient not to touch the central intravenous catheter insertion site.

Explain to the patient the need to check the infusion rate frequently (every $\frac{1}{2}$–1 hour) and be alert to the alarm sounding on the infusion pump.

Explain to the patient the need to weigh herself daily at the same time each day and with similar clothing on each day.

Explain to the patient the need to monitor her urine glucose and acetone levels every 4–6 hours.

Instruct the patient to perform oral care frequently during TPN administration. Oral care may include the use of mouthwash, lip gloss, and hard candies. The patient may be permitted to use a humidifier at the bedside if the air is dry.

Discuss with the patient the fact that she should watch her diet carefully. Dietary bulk and fat intake should be monitored. Lactose intolerance should be respected. Dietary supplements may be necessary. Daily caloric intake should be calculated.

## Rationale

TPN provides a means of restoring positive nitrogen balance, but it is a complicated and potentially hazardous procedure. Patients are selected carefully for this treatment. Careful monitoring and conscientious care reduces the risk of complications (Brunner and Suddarth, 1988, pp. 766–767).

An occluded catheter can cause an increase in pressure created by the infusion pump and result in a separation of the IV tubing (Atkins and Oakley, 1986, p. 24).

Sepsis can be caused by contamination of the catheter or TPN solution. The TPN solution is an ideal culture medium for bacterial and fungal growth. The central venous catheter provides a port of entry for microorganisms to enter the system (Lee, 1987, p. 35).

A continuous, uniform infusion of TPN is desired. Too rapid a rate causes hyperosmolar diuresis and an infusion that is too slow does not allow the patient to receive the maximum benefit of caloric intake and nitrogen (Brunner and Suddarth, 1988, p. 769).

Daily weights under similar circumstances validate the expected weight gain on TPN of 0.11–0.45 kg (.24 lb–.99 lb) daily of lean body tissue (Brunner and Suddarth, 1988, p. 769).

Urine monitoring assists in determining the patient's requirements for insulin, fluids, glucose tolerance, and if there is a decrease in renal function or the presence of sepsis (Atkins and Oakley, 1986, p. 24).

Mouth care measures prevent dryness and discomfort that often accompany TPN administration while the patient remains NPO (Atkins and Oakley, 1986, p. 24).

Crohn's disease puts a person at risk for nutritional deficits due to an inadequate diet, restrictive diet, and malabsorption. Protein loss and malabsorption of calories, fat, and fat-soluble vitamins are often noted. Fat malabsorption is directly related to the presence of diarrhea. A diet for a person with Crohn's disease should contain adequate protein, calories, vitamins, and minerals to restore and maintain adequate body weight and well-being (Alexander-Williams and Haynes, 1987, p. 247).

## QUESTIONS FOR DISCUSSION

1. Discuss the systematic complications of inflammatory bowel disease.
2. Your female patient asks, "Can a patient with Crohn's disease become pregnant?" How would you answer her and what is the rationale for your answer?
3. Compare and contrast the signs and symptoms and differential diagnosis for a patient with Crohn's disease and a patient with ulcerative colitis.
4. Outline the steps you would use in teaching your patient how to care for an ileostomy.
5. Your patient states, "How can I have sexual intercourse with this bag?" How would you answer him or her, and discuss some suggestions you could offer to make sexual intercourse more pleasant.
6. What is a continent ileal reservoir?
7. What kinds of reactions could you expect from your patient who has just had an ileostomy?
8. Discuss preoperative teaching for the patient who is scheduled for an ileostomy.

## REFERENCES

Alexander-Williams, J and Haynes, IG: Up-to-date management of small-bowel Crohn's disease. Adv Surg 20:245, 1987.

Atkins, JM and Oakley, CW: A Nurse's Guide to TPN. RN, June 1986, p 21.

Broadwell DC: Peristomal skin integrity. Nurs Clin North Am 22:321, 1987

Brunner, LS and Suddarth, DS: Textbook of Medical-Surgical Nursing, ed 6. JB Lippincott, Philadelphia, 1988.

Connelly, CE: Self-care and the chronically ill patient. Nurs Clin North Am 22:621, 1987.

Dudek, SG: Nutrition Handbook for Nursing Practice. JB Lippincott, Philadelphia, 1987.

Erickson, PJ: Ostomies: The art of pouching. Nurs Clin North Am 22:311, 1987.

Joachim, G and Milne, B: The effects of inflammatory bowel disease on lifestyle. The Canadian Nurse, November 1985, p 38.

Kelly, MP: Loss and grief reactions as responses to surgery. J Adv Nurs 10:517, 1985.

Lee, B: Total parenteral nutrition. Nurs Times, Jan 7, 1987, p 32.

Patrick, ML, et al: Medical-Surgical Nursing: Pathophysiological Concepts. JB Lippincott, Philadelphia, 1986.

Pollock, SE: Adaptation to chronic illness: Analysis of nursing research. Nurs Clin North Am 22:631, 1987.

Rideout, BW: The patient with an ileostomy. Nurs Clin North Am 22:253, 1987.

Shipes, E: Psychosocial issues: The person with an ostomy. Nurs Clin North Am 22:291, 1987.

Tilden, VP and Weinert, C: Social support and the chronically ill individual. Nurs Clin North Am 22:613, 1987.

## BIBLIOGRAPHY

Baillie, J and Soltis, RD: Systemic complications of inflammatory bowel disease. Geriatrics: 40:53, 1985.

Butler, C: Supporting the patient with Crohn's disease. Nursing '83, November 1983, p 46.

Donaldson, RM: Management of medical problems in pregnancy–inflammatory bowel disease. New Engl J Med 312:1616, 1985.

Falchuk, ZM: Crohn's disease or ulcerative colitis? Patient Care, July 15, 1981, p 105.

Hively-Petillo, M: Psychologic factors and inflammatory bowel disease: A review of the literature. Journal of Enterostomal Therapy 12:214, 1985.

Jones, VA, et al: Crohn's disease: Maintenance of remission by diet. Lancet, July 27, 1985, p 177.

Scully, RE, Mark, EJ, and McNeely, BU: Case 41-1985, Case records of the Massachusetts General Hospital. Weekly clinicopathological exercises. New Engl J Med 15:943, 1985.

Spencer, MM and Barnett, WO: The continent ileal reservoir (Kock pouch): A new approach. Journal of Enterostomal Therapy: 9:8, 1982.

Thompson, WG: Gastrointestinal symptoms in the irritable bowel compared with peptic ulcer and inflammatory bowel disease. Gut 25:1089, 1984.

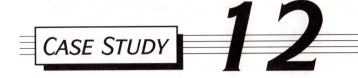

# A PATIENT WITH CIRRHOSIS OF THE LIVER

Anne Keiran Manton, M.S., R.N., CEN

The fifth leading cause of death among adults between the ages of 45 and 64 is cirrhosis of the liver. The association between chronic alcoholism and cirrhosis of the liver has been well established in the literature that addresses clinical, pathological, and experimental factors. Although there are other possible causes of cirrhosis, such as hepatitis or biliary obstruction, the majority of cases of cirrhosis are related to alcohol (Lieber, 1982). Statistics show that the 5-year survival rate for those people with cirrhosis who abstain from alcohol and eat properly is about 60%. Nurses can be influential in prevention of cirrhosis by advocating responsible alcohol use and proper dietary practices. Nurses can also positively influence the outcome for those patients already diagnosed with cirrhosis. By reinforcing the need for abstinence from alcohol, by providing assistance with motivation and problem solving, by teaching and encouraging healthy diet habits, and by referral to appropriate community resources, the nurse can improve the likelihood of the patient's 5-year survival. Thus, cirrhosis and the issues and problems that accompany it should be of significant concern to nursing.

## ANATOMY OF THE LIVER

The liver is the largest organ in the body. It is located in the right upper quadrant of the abdomen and is usually protected by the right rib cage. The liver is divided into 2 lobes with the right lobe markedly larger than the left. The falciform ligament marks the division of the two lobes. The 2 main lobes, in turn, may be divided into posterior, anterior, medial, and lateral segments.

The liver has a double blood supply. The portal vein, which results from the joining of the mesenteric and splenic veins, brings blood with nutrients, metabolic substances, and also toxins from the gastrointestinal tract (stomach and intestines). The other source of blood supply is the hepatic artery, which supplies oxygenated blood to the liver. Approximately two thirds of the incoming blood is venous, coming from the portal vein, and one third is arterial blood from the hepatic artery. Each minute, approximately 1400 ml of blood flows through the liver sinusoids; about 1000 ml is from the portal vein and about 400 ml is from the hepatic artery. Outflow of blood from the liver is by way of the three major hepatic veins (right, middle, and left), which flow into the inferior vena cava. In addition to the three major hepatic veins, there are various smaller veins that also empty into the inferior vena cava.

Processes that damage or alter blood flow through or out of the liver result in congestion of the portal venous system, or portal hypertension. In the presence of such increased pressure, collateral vessels form to divert some of the congestion from the liver. Two such collateral channels are significant. The first is in the upper stomach and lower esophagus where venous dilatations (varices) are produced. The other important collateral circulation is between the superior and inferior hemorrhoidal veins.

The functional unit of the liver is the liver lobule. The lobule is composed of many hepatic cellular plates (hepatocytes) that are arranged radially around a central vein by which the lobule is drained. Between the cellular plates are capillaries called sinusoids, which are branches of the portal vein and the hepatic artery.

The walls of the sinusoids are lined with endothelial cells and Kupffer cells. Kupffer cells are reticuloendothelial cells that function as phagocytes, engulfing bacteria and other foreign matter that may be present in the blood.

# PHYSIOLOGY OF THE LIVER

The functions of the liver can be classified into 3 primary categories: filtration and storage functions, secretory functions, and metabolic functions. A brief discussion of the liver's functions will assist in clarifying the importance of this organ and in understanding the signs and symptoms associated with liver disease.

The liver is considered to be a blood reservoir. It is capable of storing up to about 400 ml of blood if the pressure in the veins that drain the liver increases. An example of such an instance is right-sided heart failure. The liver also is able to release blood into the circulation in the instance of volume depletion such as occurs with hemorrhage. In this event, blood in the liver sinusoids drains into the general circulation to help replace lost blood.

In addition to blood storage, the liver stores vitamins and minerals. The fat-soluble vitamins (A, D, E, K) and vitamin $B_{12}$ are stored in large quantities in the liver. Vitamin K is required for the formation of prothrombin and other blood clotting factors. Iron, too, is stored in the liver in the form of ferritin.

The filtration function of the liver is performed by the phagocytic Kupffer cells, which make the liver 1 of the principal organs in the body's defense against bacteria and other foreign matter. Kupffer cells are responsible for removal of 99% of the bacteria from the portal venous blood as it passes through the liver sinusoids. Because it comes to the liver from the intestines, the portal venous blood contains a number of colon bacilli that are subsequently phagocytized by the Kupffer cells. When increased quantities of particulate matter or debris are present in the blood, the number of Kupffer cells increases. The importance of the filtration function of the liver is readily apparent.

A major function of the liver is the secretion and excretion of bile. Bile is composed of water, bile salts, bilirubin, cholesterol, lecithin, and the usual electrolytes of plasma. The liver secretes about 1 L of bile a day. As the bile is stored in the gallbladder, water and electrolytes are reabsorbed by the gallbladder mucosa so that bile becomes a concentration of its other constituents, such as bile salts, bilirubin, and cholesterol. Bile salts are necessary for the digestion and absorption of fats and fat-soluble vitamins from the intestinal tract.

The liver is responsible for numerous metabolic functions. In the small intestine, carbohydrates are broken down into monosaccharides (glucose, fructose, and galactose), absorbed through the intestinal mucosa, and transported to the liver by way of the portal vein. In the liver, the monosaccharides are converted into glycogen and stored in the hepatocytes. As needed, glycogen is converted back into glucose by the process of glycogenolysis and released into the blood to maintain normal glucose levels. By a process called gluconeogenesis, the liver is also able to synthesize glucose from proteins and fat. The liver is responsible for a major role in the metabolism of fats. In addition, the liver is able to convert large quantities of carbohydrates and proteins to fat, which is then transported in the lipoproteins to the adipose tissue to be stored.

The role of the liver in protein metabolism is essential. Functions of the liver with regard to protein metabolism are (1) the formation of plasma proteins including albumin, prothrombin, fibrinogen, and other clotting factors, (2) the deamination of amino acids, and (3) the formation of urea for the removal of ammonia. Ammonia formed by intestinal bacteria is also converted to urea by the liver, and subsequently excreted by the kidneys and intestines.

A large proportion of the substances important to the coagulation process are formed by the liver. These are factors I (fibrinogen), II (prothrombin), V, VII, VIII, IX, and X. Vitamin K is necessary for the synthesis of factors II, V, IX, and X.

The role of the liver in the process of detoxification is a critical one. Liver enzymes oxidize, hydrolyze, reduce, or conjugate many potentially harmful substances, thus making them nontoxic. Alcohol is detoxified in the liver by oxidation.

# PATHOPHYSIOLOGY

As the very important functions of the liver are reviewed, the systemically devastating effects of liver disease can be appreciated. Cirrhosis of the liver, then, has some predictable and potentially life-threatening sequelae.

The majority of instances of cirrhosis of the liver follow 1 of 3 characteristic forms: Laennec's cirrhosis (also called alcoholic cirrhosis), postnecrotic cirrhosis, and biliary cirrhosis. The most common type of cirrhosis is Laennec's. While the specific relationship between Laennec's cirrhosis and chronic alcohol abuse has not been determined, there is ample evidence to state unequivocally that the two are associated. "From studies of clinical and autopsy series, it can be stated that a majority of cases of cirrhosis are due to alcohol" (Lieber, 1982, p. 259).

Liver changes that can ultimately result in Laennec's cirrhosis are classified into 3 levels: fatty liver (hepatic steatosis), alcoholic hepatitis, and finally cirrhosis. In discussing the etiology of fatty liver, Lieber (1982) suggests that when alcohol (ethanol) is present, it becomes a preferred fuel for the liver and displaces fat as a source of energy. This contributes to an accumulation of fat within the liver cells. The fatty infiltrates cause decreased liver function. The contribution of inadequate nutrition to the development of fatty liver is unclear. It is known, however, that low-protein intake depresses the activity of alcohol dehydrogenase, which is the principal enzyme in the metabolism of alcohol. The fatty liver is enlarged, hepatomegaly being the most common clinical sign. Most often, patients with uncomplicated fatty liver are virtually asymptomatic. Degeneration resulting from fatty liver is reversible if the patient eliminates alcohol intake and maintains adequate nutrition.

Alcoholic hepatitis is regarded as a precursor of cirrhosis. Lieber (1982) states that while fatty liver is very common in alcoholics, alcoholic hepatitis develops in only a portion of chronic heavy drinkers. This inflammation of the liver may be acute or chronic and develops in response to hepatocellular damage resulting from alcohol abuse. Diagnosis of alcoholic hepatitis is confirmed by liver biopsy. Histological characteristics of alcoholic hepatitis include ballooning and great disarray of hepatocytes, parenchymal and portal infiltration with polymorphonuclear leukocytes, and varying degrees of fatty degeneration, necrosis, fibrosis, and cholestasis (Lieber, 1982). Patients with alcoholic hepatitis are usually symptomatic. Signs and symptoms include anorexia, fatigue, fever, right epigastric pain, and hepatomegaly. In more severe cases, signs and symptoms may also include jaundice, ascites, edema of the lower extremities, or even coma. There is a correlation between the histological features of alcoholic hepatitis and the degree of hepatomegaly and leukocytosis, as well as the intensity of signs and symptoms.

Cirrhosis occurs, it is believed, as a result of degeneration of hepatocytes, proliferation of connective tissue (scarring), and irregular regeneration of hepatocytes. Because of the connective-tissue scarring and the nodular regeneration of hepatocytes, the normal lobular structure of the liver is changed and the blood supply altered and obstructed. The increasing difficulty with which blood can flow throughout the liver leads to venous engorgement, dilatation, and subsequently to portal hypertension. The decreased circulation, increased cellular compromise, and fibrotic scarring result in an inability of the liver to perform vital functions.

One of the consequences of cirrhosis of the liver is the development of ascites, which is the intraperitoneal accumulation of a watery fluid of variable protein content (usually less than 3 g/dl) (Matheny, 1987). As Starling suggested in 1896, it is the balance between the capillary blood pressure, forcing fluid into the tissue spaces, and the osmotic pressure of the plasma proteins, retaining fluid in the vascular compartment, that controls the interchange of fluid between the blood and tissue spaces. Thus, there are two important factors in the formation of ascites, the portal venous pressure and the plasma colloid osmotic pressure (Sherlock, 1985). In the cirrhotic liver, albumin synthesis is decreased, and thus plasma colloid osmotic pressure is reduced. The decreased colloid oncotic pressure, combined with the increased capillary pressure as a result of portal hypertension, allows fluid to shift into the peritoneal cavity. Portal venous hypertension and increased liver sinusoidal pressure are consequences of the blockage of hepatic venous outflow from the cirrhotic liver and result in markedly increased hepatic lymph production. This protein-containing fluid leaks from the liver into the peritoneal space.

An important consequence of cirrhosis is hematological disorders. The hypersplenism that results from portal hypertension leads to increased red blood cell destruction. The anemia resulting from the destruction of red blood cells may be accompanied by a megaloblastic anemia related to folate deficiency. The possibility of chronic blood loss from the gastrointestinal tract must also be considered in the evaluation of anemia in the patient with cirrhosis.

Disturbances of blood coagulation are also common in patients with liver cirrhosis. Most of the clotting factors are produced in the liver. If the cirrhotic liver is unable to secrete bile salts sufficient to ensure adequate absorption of vitamin K (a fat-soluble vitamin) from the intestine, the synthesis of many essential clotting factors is greatly reduced. The clotting factors most affected are those dependent on vitamin K for their synthesis, that is, factors II (prothrombin), VII, IX, and X. In addition, synthesis of factor V and fibrinogen may be diminished. The liver is also concerned with fibrinolysis; antiplasmin is produced by the liver and plasmin activator is probably cleared by the liver.

As the collateral channels develop resultant to portal hypertension, more blood bypasses the liver. While this mechanism decreases to some extent the congestion in the hepatic circulation, some of the vital functions of the liver such as metabolism and detoxification are not performed on a portion of the circulating blood. The result of this shunting of blood is a neuropsychiatric syndrome referred to as hepatic encephalopathy. Hepatic encephalopathy is characterized by mental confusion, muscle tremors, and a flapping tremor called asterixis. The cause of hepatic encephalopathy is most often attributed to the effect on the brain of the breakdown products of protein metabolism produced by bacterial action in the intestine. Ammonia, which under normal circumstances is converted to urea in the liver, is one of the toxic substances identified with hepatic encephalopathy.

Postnecrotic cirrhosis accounts for about 20% of the cases of cirrhosis. Because about 25% of these patients have a prior history of viral hepatitis, and many more have positive test results for the hepatitis B antibody, chronic active hepatitis may be an important preceding event. Poisons and chemicals are believed to be precipitants in a small number of cases. Postnecrotic cirrhosis results in degenerative nodules of varying size that are surrounded and partitioned by scar tissue and are interspersed with normal liver parenchyma.

The most common etiology of biliary cirrhosis is posthepatic biliary obstruction. With outflow of bile obstructed, bile accumulates within the liver and results in destruction of liver cells. Liver cell destruction is found around the bile ducts. Fibrous bands form around the periphery of the liver lobules. The result is an enlarged, firm liver.

Cirrhosis is a relatively late stage of liver disease. The pathological changes of cirrhosis progress slowly, over a period of years, until the appearance of symptoms makes the diagnosis apparent.

## RISK FACTORS

Alcohol intake and poor or inadequate nutrition are the primary risk factors for Laennec's cirrhosis. The amount of alcohol needed to place a person at risk for Laennec's cirrhosis is not known at this time and it has been suggested that a genetic predisposition may exist in some instances. The characteristics of being male, nonwhite, and between the ages of 40 and 60 are associated with a higher incidence of the disease; however, these categories cannot in themselves be considered risk factors without attention being given to the lifestyle variables that these characteristics may represent. Another cause of cirrhosis is toxins, which may have as risk factors exposure to such chemicals as carbon tetrachloride. In addition, infectious processes can lead to cirrhosis and, therefore, exposure to infectious disease such as may be the case with health care personnel or intravenous drug abusers, must also be considered as risk factors.

## COMMON CLINICAL FINDINGS

Because of the importance of the liver in the overall functioning of the body, cirrhosis gives rise to numerous clinical findings. Common observable findings include fatigability, edema of the lower extremities, spider telangiectasias on the face and trunk, gynecomastia, changes in secondary sex characteristics such as decreased chest hair and testicular atrophy, muscle wasting particularly of the lower extremities, jaundice, ascites, and mental status changes. The patient may report chronic indigestion, anorexia, and bowel changes (either constipation or diarrhea). Abdominal pain may or may not be present, although it is more often reported earlier in the course of the disease. Because of the congestion in the venous system and the resulting pressure on the vessels, bleeding must always be a concern. Common findings that are determined by means other than history or observation include occult bleeding, anemia, vitamin deficiency, chronic gastritis, and electrolyte imbalance.

## TREATMENT MODALITIES

Treatment modalities include vitamin and nutritional supplements, potassium-sparing diuretics, and absolute avoidance of alcohol. Other treatment is according to the patient's symptoms and physiological needs, for example, antacids for chronic gastritis or lactulose for high ammonia levels.

# PATIENT ASSESSMENT DATA BASE

## Health History

---

*Client:*
Mr. Richard Barr

*Address:* 15 Lake Shore Dr, Cleveland, OH 44110
*Telephone:* 555-0987
*Contact:* Ms. Suzie Lincoln (friend)
*Address of contact:* 275 Riverview Ave, Cleveland, OH 44116
*Telephone of contact:* 555-5432
*Age:* 53     *Sex:* Male     *Race:* White
*Educational background:* Some high school (about 10th grade)
*Religion:* None     *Marital status:* Divorced
*Usual occupation:* Bartender
*Present occupation:* Same (recently on sick leave)
*Source of income:* Employment (salary and tips)
*Insurance:* Traveler's
*Source of referral:* Neighborhood health clinic
*Source of history:* Patient
*Reliability of historian:* Fair
*Date of interview:* 2/17/89
*Reason for visit/Chief complaint:* "Swollen belly and weakness and fatigue."

---

### HEALTH PERCEPTION/HEALTH MANAGEMENT PATTERN

*Present Health Status*

Swelling of Mr. Barr's abdomen has increased markedly in the past month and a half. He is no longer able to wear his usual trousers belt, and some of his trousers are too uncomfortable to wear. He has noted increased fatigue and shortness of breath. Position of comfort is sitting or high Fowler's.

*Past Health Status*

*General Health.* Mr. Barr was told several years ago that he had liver disease and should abstain from alcohol. He made a brief but unsuccessful attempt to stop drinking. Has not tried to stop drinking since that time. Occasionally has "stomach problems" that he relates to overindulgence of alcohol. Treated in the past with cimetidine (Tagamet) and an antacid preparation (Maalox) with good results. Able to work steadily until recently, but states he hasn't felt well for a long time. Patient describes general health as "not so good, I can't remember when I felt anything but lousy."

*Prophylactic Medical/Dental Care.* Does not have a family doctor. Uses neighborhood health clinic for episodic illnesses like gastrointestinal (GI) complaints in 1984, flu in 1986. Has not sought dental care since fitted for dentures following upper and lower teeth extractions in 1981.
*Childhood Illnesses.* Measles, mumps, chickenpox, scarlet fever.
*Immunizations.* Does not remember any shots; has a smallpox vaccination scar on upper left arm.

**Past Health Status — Continued**

### Major Illnesses/Hospitalizations

Mr. Barr was treated for a broken wrist about 20 years ago. Only hospitalization occurred in 1978, during a period of heavy drinking. Diagnosed at that time as trouble with his liver, gallbladder, and pancreas. Refused surgery and was discharged on a low-fat diet.

### Current Medications

*Prescription:* Has taken Tagamet in the past but none recently.
*Nonprescription:* Takes Maalox or calcium carbonate tablets (Tums) for indigestion; states fair relief; occasional aspirin or acetaminophen for headache or other aches and pains.

### Allergies. None known.

### Habits

*Alcohol:* Mr. Barr drinks "about 2 6-packs daily"; also has hard liquor, "maybe a pint every couple of days." He has maintained this pattern for 20 or 30 years. Describes occasional binges in the past, during which intake of alcohol would increase markedly for several days. Present symptoms have made him decrease alcohol intake within the past month. Has occasionally tried to quit before, but has never remained dry for more than a few days at a time.
*Caffeine:* Three or 4 cups of coffee per day when feeling well. Decreases when GI symptoms are present.
*Drugs:* Denies use of recreational drugs. See also Current Medications.
*Tobacco:* Mr. Barr has smoked 2 or more packs per day since a teenager (approximately 80 pack-years). He tends to smoke more when drinking. Has smoked less lately. Believes morning cough and short-windedness are probably the results of smoking but until now, neither has bothered him enough to try quitting.

### Family Health History

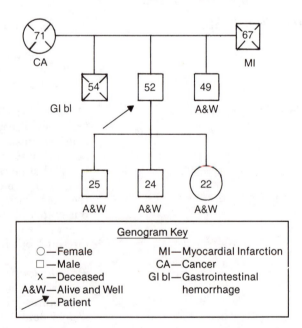

Genogram Key

○—Female                     MI—Myocardial Infarction
□—Male                       CA—Cancer
x—Deceased                   GI bl—Gastrointestinal
A&W—Alive and Well                   hemorrhage
↗—Patient

## NUTRITIONAL/METABOLIC PATTERN

**Nutritional**

**Usual Pattern:** Patient has no set timetable for his meals, usually gets by on 1 meal a day, but he prefers to eat it over time in small portions. "I get a full feeling fast." Likes Italian food, "but sometimes it gives me trouble." Avoids fresh fruit and meats (except hamburgers) because they are difficult to eat (dentures often slip), and tend to make him feel full or give him heartburn. He sometimes "forgets to eat" when appetite is down.

***Pattern During Past Month:*** As swelling in abdomen has increased, Mr. Barr's appetite has lessened. He is limited to small portions of food at a time, which he takes without feeling really hungry. He frequently feels nauseated after eating but does not vomit unless he has been drinking.

***Usual Daily Menu***

*Breakfast:* Coffee with milk and sugar, maybe a piece of toast.
*Lunch:* Couple of beers, maybe some crackers.
*Dinner:* One or 2 tablespoons of hamburger meat, 1 or 2 tablespoons of mashed potatoes.
*Other:* Occasionally a small amount of canned soup, several beers throughout the day and evening.

## *Metabolic*

States his skin is "always itchy." Some scratch marks on extremities and abdomen. Has several ecchymotic areas on arms that he says are usual. Believes he does not heal well from injuries, for example, lacerations (even small ones) seem to take a long time to heal. *Weight:* His usual weight is around 175 lb (79.5 kg); weight on admission was 156 lb (70.9 kg). *Height:* 5 ft 10 in. (177.8 cm).

# ELIMINATION PATTERN

## *Bowel*

Stools are medium brown in color, although 2 weeks ago they were unusually light-colored for a few days. He has had 1 episode, a few months ago, when his stools were darker than usual, "practically black" he states. This cleared spontaneously. He sometimes has 2 or 3 days of diarrhea that seems to subside on its own.

## *Bladder*

Recently urine has been darker than usual with a strong odor. He believes amount of urine per day has decreased lately, but attributes this to drinking less. Is occasionally incontinent; however, this is associated primarily with bouts of heavy drinking.

# ACTIVITY/EXERCISE PATTERN

## *Activity/Exercise*

Mr. Barr has worked off and on, putting in 8-hour days when feeling well. He has no regular exercise. Socializes with friends at bar where he works or sits and watches TV by himself or with his girlfriend in the evening. When not feeling well, he stays at girlfriend's apartment mostly sleeping or watching TV. Gets about, dresses, feeds, and bathes himself without assistance, but describes this as becoming increasingly difficult due to fatigue. Describes increasing weakness, in legs especially. Present self-care abilities are decreased from 2 months ago.

***Self-Care Ability***

| | |
|---|---|
| Feeding—0 | Grooming—II |
| Bathing—II | General mobility—II |
| Toileting—I | Cooking—IV |
| Bed mobility—0 | Home maintenance—IV |
| Dressing—II | Shopping—IV |

## *Activity/Exercise — Continued*

> ### *Functional Levels Code*
> 0 — Full self-care
> I — Requires use of equipment or device
> II — Requires assistance or supervision from another person
> III — Requires assistance or supervision from another person and equipment or device
> IV — Is dependent and does not participate

## *Oxygenation/Perfusion*

In last 6 weeks the patient has noted increasing exertional dyspnea; climbs stairs only with extreme difficulty. He has cough on awakening, which is usually productive. Does not remember dates of last chest x-ray or electrocardiogram prior to this admission nor whether any abnormalities were noted. "I guess they were normal; they didn't tell me otherwise, except that I should stop smoking."

### *Cardiac Risk Factors*

|  | Positive | Negative |
|---|---|---|
| Sedentary life-style | X | |
| Hyperlipidemia | | X |
| Cigarette smoking | X | |
| Diabetes | | X |
| Obesity | | X |
| Hypertension | | X |
| Hypervigilant personality | | X |
| Family history of heart disease | X | |

## Sleep/Rest Pattern

### *Sleep/Rest*

Usual pattern has been to stay up late at night (e.g., 2–3 AM) and sleep late in the morning. "I don't have to be to work until the afternoon, so no sense getting up early." In past 6 weeks or so, however, pattern has changed and Mr. Barr reports that he now falls asleep in the early evening in the lounge chair and sleeps fitfully, arising for the day in the early morning. He also now naps frequently throughout the day. He attributes his spontaneous waking periods during the night to difficulty in finding a comfortable position due to increasing ascites. States that he never has needed sleeping pills. Also reports that sleeping in the hospital has been difficult because of noise on the unit.

## Cognitive/Perceptual Pattern

### *Hearing*

Mr. Barr occasionally experiences ringing in the ears; denies any difficulty with hearing.

### *Vision*

Needs glasses for reading, but has not replaced his prescription since breaking a lens in a fall 2 weeks ago. Describes itching sensation in both eyes, associated with tearing and redness; has also noted slight yellowish color of sclera in past few weeks.

### *Sensory Perception*

Denies any unusual difficulty with sensory perception. Describes perception of time as being somewhat off since becoming ill. Denies auditory or visual hallucinations, but is concerned about DTs (delerium tremens). He is right-hand dominant.
*Pain Perception:* Relates experiences of abdominal pain with past "stomach troubles"; denies present abdominal pain of that same magnitude.

| | |
|---|---|
| *Learning Style* | Claims his memory is "as good as anyone else my age"; however, he reports that when drinking heavily he often may not remember large segments of time. Says he sometimes finds it difficult to learn new things. Could not identify a "best" learning style. |

## SELF-PERCEPTION/SELF-CONCEPT PATTERN

| | |
|---|---|
| *Self-Perception/Self-Concept* | Mr. Barr has always considered himself a good and agreeable person who is willing to help others when asked. States he doesn't believe that anymore. "Just look at what I've done to my life. I sure haven't been a good father to my kids. They say I'm no damn good and they're probably right. They're grown up now and I hardly know them. What kind of a father is that? I guess I'm a real loser." He says he gets along well with his closest friends, although he tends to become argumentative when drinking and has lost friends in the past because of this. His drinking has also caused trouble for him with his girlfriend and was an important factor in the breakup of his first marriage. |

## ROLE/RELATIONSHIP PATTERN

| | |
|---|---|
| *Role/Relationship* | Mr. Barr lives alone in a rooming house, but often eats an evening meal at his girlfriend's house if not working. Has only occasional contact with his ex-wife and the 2 of his grown children who still live at home. Has not contributed to his children's support for many years and this is an issue in his relationship with both his ex-wife and children. Another son is married and lives out of state; the patient does not know where. His brother talks with him frequently and is able to help him out financially for serious problems, but he has family responsibilities of his own. Leisure time is spent with his girlfriend and longtime friends, and these are the people he would ask for help. He enjoys the contact he has with his girlfriend's grandson, who visits frequently. "I think I have a grandson, but I've never seen him. My own fault. . . . " |

## SEXUALITY/REPRODUCTIVE PATTERN

| | |
|---|---|
| *Sexuality/Reproductive* | Patient is heterosexual; infrequent sexual activity with girlfriend for past couple of years due to his decreased libido. Says girlfriend "doesn't nag about it," for which he is glad. Denies problems with prostate, hernias, discharge, or lesions of penis. |

## COPING/STRESS TOLERANCE PATTERN

| | |
|---|---|
| *Coping/Stress Tolerance* | When people "get on his case," Mr. Barr leaves the situation. When forced to associate with people he doesn't like or who make him feel uncomfortable, he avoids arguments by "just not talking." Admits to the use of alcohol to deal with stress; says this was a pattern begun in adolescence, that is, when he felt uncomfortable or stressed, he took a drink and it made him feel better. Major stressor at present is concern for his health. He has seen acquaintances (including a brother) die from the effects of drinking and relates his symptoms to his longtime use of alcohol. He has been unsuccessful in attempts to quit the use of alcohol by spending time in a detoxification program or attending Alcoholics Anonymous and is convinced that he must accomplish it on his own, although he expresses doubts that this can happen. |

## VALUE/BELIEF PATTERN

*Value/Belief*

Mr. Barr was raised as Catholic but hasn't gone to church for about 30 years. He expresses regret that he is "out of the church." Says he sometimes thinks he would like to go back to church, but "it's too late now for me. I've really blown it, and I'm getting what I deserve. I don't think God could forgive all that I've done, and I couldn't even say that I wouldn't do the same things again, so there's no hope for me. What do you think, nurse?"

# Physical Examination

*General Survey*

A 53-year-old white male, who looks older than his stated age. Complexion is grayish in color with a yellowish cast. Abdomen is distended. Movement is slow. Affect is pleasant but somewhat sad. Cooperates with interviewer.

*Vital Signs*

**Temperature:** 99.0°F (37.2°C) (oral)
**Pulse:** 104 regular (apical)
**Respirations:** 22 shallow
**BP:** 136/76 (right arm, Fowler's position).

*Integument*

**Skin.** Slightly icteric, warm and dry; overall intact, but with scratches on extremities. Prominent venules on nose, telangiectasias on cheeks; palms of hands are deep-red color. Body hair is sparsely distributed; spider angiomas on upper torso, and several ecchymotic areas on arms.
**Mucous Membranes.** Pale pink, slightly moist, and intact.
**Nails.** No lesions, deformity, or clubbing noted.

*HEENT*

**Head.** Symmetrical, normocephalic, no tenderness. No tenderness or lesions of scalp; hair is gray and balding. Face is symmetrical; no areas of tenderness. Temporomandibular joint has no tenderness; no crepitation or pain with movement.
**Eyes.** Sclera slightly icteric; palpebral conjunctiva reddened. Peripheral vision equal to examiner's; full range of extraocular movements (EOMs); no nystagmus noted. Pupils are equal, round, reactive to light and accommodation (PERRLA).
**Ears.** Auricles intact; no tenderness. Able to hear whispered word at 18 in. (45.7 cm).
**Nose.** No septal deviation; identifies smells accurately. No discharge, no inflammation.
**Mouth/Throat.** Edentulous. No lesions noted; mucous membrane intact; tongue somewhat dry; uvula is midline. Tonsils are evident; no evidence of infection or inflammation.

*Neck*

Full range of motion; cervical nodes palpable. No carotid bruits, jugular venous distention 8–10 cm (3.1–3.9 in).

*Pulmonary*

Somewhat barrel-shaped chest, with anteroposterior (AP)/lateral diameter 1:1. Crackles heard in right and left lower lobes.

*Breast*

Gynecomastia noted. No masses or tenderness.

*Cardiovascular*

Tachycardia, regular rhythm; no murmurs, rubs, or extra sounds.

**Peripheral Vascular**

Two-plus edema of both legs; capillary refill slow.

***Peripheral Pulses***
Temporal—4 bilaterally
Carotid—4 bilaterally
Brachial—4 bilaterally
Radial—4 bilaterally
Femoral—3 bilaterally
Popliteal—3 bilaterally
Posterior tibial—3 bilaterally
Dorsalis pedis—3 bilaterally

***Peripheral Pulse Scale***

0—Absent
1—Markedly diminished
2—Moderately diminished
3—Slightly diminished
4—Normal

**Abdomen**

Protuberant, symmetrical. Venous pattern prominent around umbilicus. Liver margin felt at 2 cm below right costal border. Positive fluid wave. Abdominal girth at umbilicus is 51 in. (129.5 cm).

**Musculoskeletal**

No joint tenderness or swelling, full range of motion of all joints without difficulty. Muscle wasting noted in both upper and lower extremities; muscle strength somewhat diminished bilaterally.

**Neurological**

***Mental Status.*** Alert, oriented, answers questions appropriately; affect somewhat flat.
***Cranial Nerves.*** I–XII intact.
***Motor.*** Negative Romberg sign, some difficulty with balance during heel-to-toe walking; otherwise gross motor evaluation normal.
***Sensory.*** Can identify soft touch and pinprick in all areas.

***Deep Tendon Reflexes***

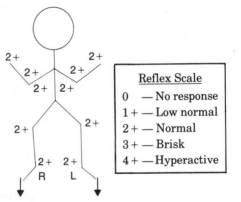

Reflex Scale

0 — No response
1+ — Low normal
2+ — Normal
3+ — Brisk
4+ — Hyperactive

**Rectal**

External hemorrhoids; stool guaiac slightly positive; prostate normal-sized, firm, smooth.

**Genitalia**

Adult male, some testicular atrophy.

## Laboratory Data/Diagnostic Studies

**Laboratory Data**

***Hgb:*** 10.2 g/100 ml
***Hct:*** 48%
***Na:*** 142 mEq/L
***K:*** 3.5 mEq/L
***Cl:*** 103 mEq/L
***BUN:*** 10 mg/dl
***Serum Cholesterol:*** 130 mg/dl

***Alk Phos:*** 78 Bodansky units/ml
***Serum Globulin:*** 5.5 g/100 ml
***Serum Albumin:*** 3.2 g/100 ml
***Serum Ammonia:*** 118 mg/dl
***Prothrombin Time:*** 16.2/12.8
***SGOT:*** 158 U/L

*Serum Triglycerides:* 40 mg/dl       *SGPT:* 160 U/L

*Total Bilirubin:* 3.1

*Direct Bilirubin:* 2.3 mg/dl

**Diagnostic Studies**

*Chest X-Ray.* Evidence of chronic obstructive pulmonary disease; no areas of consolidation noted.

*ECG.* Rate 108, normal sinus rhythm, right axis deviation; otherwise within normal limits.

*Radioisotope Liver Scan.* Diffuse areas of nonfunction, consistent with cirrhosis.

*Barium Contrast Esophagography.* Esophageal varices noted.

# COLLABORATIVE PLAN OF CARE

**Diet**

High calorie, moderate protein, low-salt diet.

**Medications**

Chlordiazepoxide hydrochloride (Librium) 50 mg PO q4h.

Multivitamins 1 tab PO bid.

Folic acid 0.5 mg PO once daily.

Docusate sodium (Colace) 100 mg PO bid.

Menadiol sodium diphosphate (Synkayvite) 5 mg PO once daily for prothrombin time of 16 seconds.

Spironolactone (Aldactone) 50 mg PO bid.

**Intravenous Therapy**

1000 ml of 5% D/W with 1 ampule of a vitamin preparation (Berocca-C) and 20 mEq KCl IV at 50 ml/hr today.

Salt-poor albumin 25 g/day for 3 days.

**Therapeutic Measures**

Vital signs q4h while awake.

Bed-to-chair ambulation as tolerated.

Commode at bedside.

Egg-crate foam on bed.

Elastic stockings.

Special skin care including cleansing, lotion, and massage, especially over bony prominences qid.

Test each stool for guaiac.

Accurate intake and output.

Daily weights and abdominal girth.

Daily BUN, serum ammonia level, and prothrombin times.

Observe closely for signs of impending DTs.

Report any change in mental status to physician.

**Consults**

Nutrition consultation.

Alcohol services consultation.

**Preoperative Plan**

Does not apply.

# NURSING DIAGNOSES DEVELOPED IN CARE PLAN

Self-Esteem Disturbance, p. 209

Altered Nutrition: Less Than Body Requirements, p. 210

Spiritual Distress (Distress of the Human Spirit), p. 211

# ADDITIONAL NURSING DIAGNOSES TO BE CONSIDERED

## I (At Present):

Activity Intolerance
Altered Thought Processes
Anticipatory Grieving
Bathing/Hygiene Self-Care Deficit
Body Image Disturbance
Decreased Cardiac Output
Diarrhea
Dressing/Grooming Self-Care Deficit
Fatigue
Fear
Hopelessness
Impaired Physical Mobility
Impaired Tissue Integrity
Ineffective Airway Clearance
Ineffective Breathing Pattern
Ineffective Individual Coping
Potential Fluid Volume Deficit
Potential for Infection
Potential for Trauma
Powerlessness
Sleep Pattern Disturbance

## II (Prior to Discharge):

Altered Health Maintenance
Altered Sexuality
Diversional Activity Deficit
Impaired Home Maintenance Management
Impaired Social Interaction
Noncompliance (Alcohol Abstinence)

# NURSING CARE PLAN BASED ON IDENTIFIED NURSING DIAGNOSES

| | |
|---|---|
| ***Self-Esteem Disturbance*** | ***Related to:*** Deteriorating physical condition; perceived role failure; and inability to control alcohol intake.<br>***Evidenced by:*** Self-negating verbalizations; expressions of shame and guilt, for example, "I'm a real loser"; agreement with his children that he's "no good." |
| ***Desired Patient Outcome*** | Patient will view himself as a worthwhile and capable person. |
| ***Evaluation Criteria*** | ***Prior to the Time of Discharge, the Patient Will:***<br>• Verbalize acceptance of himself in the present situation.<br>• Recognize and verbalize his strengths.<br>• Demonstrate willingness to participate in his own health care by creating a written plan to address his health care needs. |

| Interventions | Rationale |
|---|---|
| Encourage communication, especially with significant others. | Elicits support and relieves tension (Doenges, Moorhouse, and Geissler, 1989, pp. 698, 779). |
| Provide opportunities for listening to the patient's concerns and questions; provide information as needed. | Lessens feelings of rejection; conveys interest and concern; and can offer encouragement and support as well as give the patient a sense of value and self-worth (Doenges, Moorhouse, and Geissler, 1989, pp. 666, 779). |
| Assist patient to cope with changes in appearance. | Patient's appearance due to ascites, jaundice, and ecchymoses is unattractive, and he or she may need help to adjust to this image (Doenges, Moorhouse, and Geissler, 1989, pp. 489, 779). |
| Establish therapeutic nurse-patient relationship. | The patient will be freer to verbalize fears and other feelings about himself or herself in such a relationship (Doenges, Moorhouse, and Geissler, 1989, p. 344). |
| Avoid making moral judgments, and be aware of your own reaction to the patient. | The nurse needs to deal with own feelings so they do not interfere with the care of the patient or contribute to his or her feeling of low self-esteem (Doenges, Moorhouse, and Geissler, 1989, pp. 368, 378). |
| Help the patient to focus on strengths and past accomplishments. | Helps to diminish feelings of low self-worth, and allows the patient to feel good about himself or herself (Doenges, Moorhouse, and Geissler, 1989, pp. 666, 699). |
| Encourage maximum participation in self-care within limits of activity restriction. | Increasing independence can help in the redevelopment of the patient's self-esteem (Ulrich, Canale, and Wendell, 1986, p. 586). |
| Discuss and refer the patient to support groups upon discharge. | Provides a place for the patient to exchange concerns and feelings with others with similar experiences (Doenges, Moorhouse, and Geissler, 1989, pp. 369, 378, 427, 678). |
| Refer to professional counseling as necessary. | The patient may need additional help to resolve feelings of low self-esteem (Doenges, Moorhouse, and Geissler, 1989, pp. 378, 759, 780). |

| | |
|---|---|
| ***Altered Nutrition: Less Than Body Requirements*** | ***Related to:*** Poor eating habits, decreased appetite, and high alcohol intake. <br> ***Evidenced by:*** Weight loss of 19 lb (8.6 kg), fatigue, muscle wasting, anemia, reported inadequate food intake relative to minimum daily requirements. |
| ***Desired Patient Outcomes*** | The patient will have a daily caloric intake greater than 2500 calories, an improved appetite, increased strength, and decreased fatigue. |
| ***Evaluation Criteria*** | • By tomorrow and each day thereafter, the patient will have a daily calorie count above 2500 calories. <br> • Before the time of discharge, the patient will report improved appetite. <br> • By the time of discharge, the patient will report increased strength, and will be able to participate in activities of daily living with less fatigue than he is presently experiencing. |

| Interventions | Rationale |
|---|---|
| Identify patient's food likes and dislikes. | He is more likely to eat preferred food (Dudek, 1987, p. 398). |
| Offer small, frequent feedings. | There may be difficulty in consuming a large meal (Dudek, 1987, p. 398). Small meals are easier to tolerate (Brunner and Suddarth, 1988, p. 878). |
| Offer high-calorie, high-carbohydrate liquids. | The patient may tolerate liquids better than traditional meals (Dudek, 1987, p. 399). |
| Provide oral care before meals. | Improved oral hygiene can enhance appetite and improve oral intake (Ulrich, Canale, and Wendell, 1986, p. 570). Reduces unpleasant taste and stimulates appetite (Brunner and Suddarth, 1988, p. 878). |
| Increase patient's intake of foods high in vitamin $B_{12}$, folic acid, thiamine, and iron. | There is reduced metabolism and storage of nutrients by the liver due to a reduction of functional tissue (Ulrich, Canale, and Wendell, 1986, p. 570). |
| Limit sodium intake. | Ascites is present (Dudek, 1987, p. 400). |
| Do a daily calorie count with the patient. | The patient can assess his or her own progress; become an active participant in the process (Carrieri, Lindsey, and West, 1986, pp. 115,116). |
| Promote bed rest and/or rest periods. | Conserving energy reduces metabolic demands on the liver and promotes cellular regeneration (Doenges, Jeffries, and Moorhouse, 1984, p. 327). |
| Provide multivitamins and mineral supplements, especially iron, B vitamins, and vitamins C and K. | Liver damage profoundly affects the metabolism of almost all nutrients (Dudek, 1987, p. 400). |

| | |
|---|---|
| **Spiritual Distress (Distress of the Human Spirit)** | **Related to:** Separation from religious origins, guilt. **Evidenced by:** Ambiguity about church/religion; feelings of being punished; doubts about the possibility of God's forgiveness; hopelessness: "It's too late for me." |
| **Desired Patient Outcome** | The patient will believe he is worthy of forgiveness and experience spiritual peace. |
| **Evaluation Criteria** | • Throughout his hospital stay, the patient will be able to identify the mechanism(s) for contacting the chaplain/pastoral counselor. **By the Time of Discharge, the Patient Will:** • Verbalize positive feelings about his relationship with God. • Report spiritual peace. |

| Interventions | Rationale |
|---|---|
| Listen to the patient's concerns; offer him support and comfort. | Being present, available, and an empathetic listener can help a person who is spiritually distressed (Thompson, et al, 1986, p. 1851). |

## Interventions

Encourage the patient's expression of feelings in an atmosphere of acceptance.

Suggest, but do not insist, that the patient talk with a clergyperson.

Offer to contact pastoral care department or clergyperson if the patient would like to talk with a spiritual resource person. Be sure the patient does not interpret your offer of referral to mean that you do not want to discuss these issues with him.

## Rationale

Development of trust may decrease the patient's sense of alienation with God, self, and others (Thompson, et al, p. 1847).

Hospital chaplains are usually perceptive about the importance of resolving these psychological issues and can relieve the guilt that people may have been carrying (Barry, 1988, p. 245).

The patient may or may not be ready or willing to have this type of involvement, but should know of its availability if he or she wants to talk with clergypersons at any point since they are viewed as experts in spiritual care (Thompson, et al, 1986, p. 1851).

# QUESTIONS FOR DISCUSSION

1. Other than Laennec's cirrhosis, what other diseases of the liver might result in similar physiological problems as those of Mr. Barr?
2. Richard Barr is at risk for bleeding esophageal varices. Discuss the signs, symptoms, dangers, and treatments for this medical problem.
3. What surgical procedure(s) may be performed to assist in the management of portal hypertension? Would this surgery be a likely choice for Mr. Barr?
4. In the collaborative plan of care there is an order to administer salt-poor albumin. Why might Mr. Barr's physicians think this would help him? What are the advantages and disadvantages of this treatment modality?
5. What are your teaching priorities for Mr. Barr at present? When he is closer to discharge?
6. Why are patients with cirrhosis at high risk for bleeding and infection and, therefore, what are the implications for nursing care of these patients?

# REFERENCES

Barry, PD: Psychosocial Nursing Assessment and Intervention Care of the Physically Ill Person, ed 2. JB Lippincott, Philadelphia, 1988.

Brunner, LS and Suddarth, DS: Textbook of Medical-Surgical Nursing, ed 6. JB Lippincott, Philadelphia, 1988.

Carrieri, VK, Lindsey, AM, and West, CM: Pathophysiological Phenomena in Nursing: Human Responses to Illness. WB Saunders, Philadelphia, 1986.

Doenges, ME, Moorhouse, MF, and Geissler AC: Nursing Care Plans: Guidelines for Planning Patient Care, ed 2. FA Davis, Philadelphia, 1989.

Dudek, SG: Nutrition Handbook for Nursing Practice. JB Lippincott, Philadelphia, 1987.

Lieber, C: Medical Disorders of Alcoholism: Pathogenesis and Treatment. WB Saunders, Philadelphia, 1982.

Matheny, NM: Fluid and Electrolyte Balance: Nursing Considerations. JB Lippincott, New York, 1987.

Sherlock, S: Diseases of the Liver and Biliary System, ed 7. Blackwell Scientific Publications, Oxford, 1985.

Thompson, JM, et al: Clinical Nursing. CV Mosby, St. Louis, 1986.

Ulrich, SP, Canale, SW, and Wendell, SA: Nursing Care Planning. Guides: A Nursing Diagnosis Approach. WB Saunders, Philadelphia, 1986.

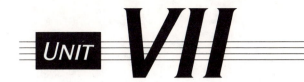

# UNIT VII

# THE PATIENT WITH ALTERATIONS IN METABOLISM RELATED TO THE ENDOCRINE SYSTEM

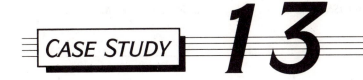

CASE STUDY **13**

# A PATIENT WITH DIABETES MELLITUS

Sharon P. Sullivan, M.S., R.N.

Diabetes mellitus is a chronic disorder of abnormal carbohydrate, fat, and protein metabolism resulting from an imbalance between insulin availability and insulin need (Porth, 1986, p. 632). It is not a single disease but rather a group of diseases of differing etiology that have common signs and symptoms. The classic profile seen in diabetes mellitus is a fluctuating blood glucose level.

## ANATOMY AND PHYSIOLOGY

Diabetes mellitus is a systemic disorder that involves the endocrine system, in particular the islets of Langerhans of the pancreas. The pancreas, located in the upper posterior abdominal region, and the hormones it secretes play an important role in the digestion and metabolism of food. The islets of Langerhans contain 4 types of cells, 2 of which, beta and alpha, secrete hormones that affect glucose levels by their opposing effects. Beta cells secrete insulin, lowering glucose levels, and alpha cells secrete glucagon, causing a hyperglycemic effect. Normal blood glucose levels are achieved by the opposing action of these 2 hormones and other counterregulatory hormones.

Insulin is essential for normal carbohydrate metabolism and is the only hormone known to reduce blood glucose levels. It has diverse metabolic effects that involve fat, carbohydrate, and protein metabolism. Functioning primarily as a storage hormone, insulin provides for glucose storage, prevents fat breakdown, and increases protein synthesis (Bullock and Rosendahl, 1984, p. 454). Its primary function is to promote cellular uptake of glucose for storage and aerobic glycolysis. Insulin acts by aiding in the transport of glucose across the cell membrane by combining with a receptor in the cell membrane. Defects or abnormalities that affect glucose uptake and utilization by cells make up the diabetic syndrome.

### Classification System

A classification system has been devised dividing diabetes mellitus into three groups: type I, type II, and other. Type I diabetes is insulin-dependent diabetes mellitus (IDDM) and is characterized by an absolute insulin-deficient state. Previously it had been referred to as juvenile-onset diabetes, but, since it may occur at any age, the term "juvenile" is misleading. Type II is noninsulin-dependent diabetes mellitus (NIDDM) and is associated with a relative lack of insulin availability or effectiveness. This form of diabetes has been called maturity-onset diabetes. The "other" classification refers to types that occur secondary to other disorders such as pancreatic diseases or endocrine disorders, or are drug related (Guthrie and Guthrie, 1983, p. 619).

# PATHOPHYSIOLOGY

Diabetes mellitus is characterized by an alteration in the mechanisms that regulate blood glucose resulting in impaired glucose tolerance and a hyperglycemic state. Blood glucose levels are difficult to regulate due to the absolute or relative lack of the metabolic effectiveness of insulin. In the absence of insulin due to beta-cell inability to secrete insulin, type I IDDM, glucose transport across the cell membrane is reduced to one fourth of normal. Type II NIDDM occurs when there is a deficiency or abnormality of the receptors, defects in the cell membrane, or intracellular abnormalities. Regardless of the etiology, the outcome is similar—defective use of glucose.

An insulin deficiency causes "(1) decreased glucose uptake and storage as glycogen and fat, (2) excess glucose breakdown from storage, (3) defective glucolysis, and (4) excess fat breakdown" (Guthrie and Guthrie, 1983, p. 622). The net results of these actions are elevated glucose levels, accumulation of free fatty acids and ketone bodies, and cellular starvation.

# RISK FACTORS

A number of factors have been implicated in the development of diabetes. Inheritance seems to play a greater role in those who develop NIDDM than in those with IDDM. A large percentage of persons with NIDDM are overweight, linking obesity as a significant risk factor. Exposure to beta-cell toxins and viruses has been associated with the development of IDDM. Gestational diabetes that develops during pregnancy indicates that a woman is at increased risk even though glucose tolerance returns to normal after childbirth. The risk of diabetes increases with age, with a higher incidence in the over-40 age-group and with more frequency in the older woman (Bullock and Rosendahl, 1983, p. 458).

# COMMON CLINICAL FINDINGS

The onset of diabetes mellitus can be either rapid or by slow progression. The most common signs and symptoms are polyuria, polyphagia, and polydipsia. These symptoms are related to the elevated glucose levels in both the urine and blood. Weight loss is a common manifestation in those with uncontrolled IDDM, whereas the NIDDM patient has problems with obesity. Other indicators include visual disturbances, fatigue, and an increased incidence of yeast infections.

The complications of diabetes include both short-term acute complications and long-term chronic complications. The short-term complications are a result of an acute change in glucose levels and include diabetic ketoacidosis, hypoglycemia, and, in the NIDDM patient, hyperosmolar coma. The long-term chronic complications develop in the setting of the chronic abnormality in metabolism caused by insufficient insulin secretion (Price and Wilson, 1986, p. 893). These include atherosclerosis, retinopathy, nephropathy, and peripheral and autonomic neuropathy.

# TREATMENT MODALITIES

The treatment plan for diabetes includes diet therapy, exercise, and, in some cases, the use of a hypoglycemic agent. The goal of diet therapy is to provide a diet that is nutritionally adequate and allows for maintenance of recommended body weight. Improving glucose tolerance has been shown to occur with a planned program of regular exercise. Oral hypoglycemic agents, for example, sulfonylurea, are used in NIDDM, in which some residual beta-cell function remains. They act by causing the release of insulin from the pancreas. The IDDM diabetic requires daily administration of an insulin preparation to control the illness (Lewis, 1986, p. 344). Recent advances have made available the use of a continuous subcutaneous insulin infusion pump providing controlled doses of insulin. Other more experimental therapies include the artificial pancreas and islet cell transplantation (Porth, 1986, p. 645).

# PATIENT ASSESSMENT DATA BASE

## Health History

> *Client:*
> Mrs. Lillian Fontaine
>
> *Address:* 10 Blossom Ln, Dallas, TX 75227
> *Telephone:* 214-555-1122
> *Contact:* Harold (husband)
> *Address of contact:* Same
> *Telephone of contact:* Same
> *Age:* 55    *Sex:* Female    *Race:* White
> *Educational background:* High school    *Religion:* Catholic
> *Marital status:* Married
> *Usual occupation:* Secretary (disabled)
> *Present occupation:* Housewife
> *Source of income:* Husband (works full-time)
> *Insurance:* Dallas Mutual
> *Source of referral:* Diabetes Clinic
> *Source of history:* Patient
> *Reliability of historian:* Reliable
> *Date of interview:* 2/21/90
> *Reason for visit/Chief compliant:* Ulcer of the right foot

### HEALTH PERCEPTION/HEALTH MANAGEMENT PATTERN

*Present Health Status*

One of many hospitalizations for this diabetic woman, present admission is for treatment of new right-foot ulcer. This ulcer developed from wearing ill-fitting shoes, and treatments done at home over the past 2 months have been unsuccessful in healing the wound. She denies any pain in the foot.

*Past Health Status*

**General Health.** Mrs. Fontaine describes a poor health state over the past 2 years. She has had several hospitalizations for regulation of insulin and treatment of leg ulcers. She was diagnosed with diabetes at age 11 and has been insulin dependent for 44 years. During her adolescence, she was athletic and had insulin reactions about once a month that she self-treated with food and never needed hospitalization.

She has had 2 episodes of diabetic coma: at ages 20 and 24, both of which occurred shortly after 2 of her 5 miscarriages. She describes herself as a brittle diabetic throughout most of her adult life with blood sugars fluctuating to both extremes, despite following prescribed diet as much as possible. She has a history of repeated infections, including cystitis, vaginitis, and upper respiratory tract infections.

**Prophylactic Medical/Dental Care.** Three-month medical checkup. Nine months ago Mrs. Fontaine began being seen in the diabetes clinic after her primary physician retired. She canceled her last visit. Wears a Medic-Alert bracelet. Podiatrist last seen 1 year ago. Has yearly dental care.

**Childhood Illnesses.** Measles, mumps, chickenpox.

**Immunizations.** Flu vaccine, yearly.

**Past Health
Status—Continued**

### Major Illnesses/Hospitalizations

*Age 11:* Diagnosed with diabetes.
*Ages 20, 24:* Hospitalized for diabetic coma.
*1984:* Pneumonia.
*1985:* Cellulitis of left leg; right-wrist fracture.
*1987–1989:* Several hospitalizations for control of diabetes.
*1987:* Left-foot ulcer debridements.

### Current Medications

*Prescription:* NPH insulin 42 units q AM, CZI insulin 8 units q AM, ascorbic acid 500 mg PO bid.
*Nonprescription:* Acetaminophen (Tylenol) prn.
**Allergies.** Sulfa drugs: "gets a rash."

### Habits

*Alcohol:* Rare glass of wine.
*Caffeine:* Four cups of tea per day; 24–32 oz of diet cola per day.
*Drugs:* See Current Medications.
*Tobacco:* None.

### Family Health History

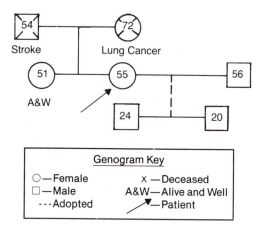

```
Genogram Key
○—Female          x —Deceased
□—Male            A&W—Alive and Well
---Adopted        ↗—Patient
```

## NUTRITIONAL/METABOLIC PATTERN

**Nutritional**

Mrs. Fontaine eats 3 meals a day; her diet reflects poor compliance with 1800-calorie American Diabetes Association (ADA) diet. Poor appetite noted over the past year: 1 on a scale of 1–5 (1 = poor, 5 = excellent). "Food doesn't have much appeal to me. I eat because I have to keep my blood sugar under control." She avoids concentrated sweets and uses low-calorie items. Carries candy bar in purse.

She is able to draw up and inject her own insulin. Generally she rotates sites for injection. Performs urine testing sporadically, 2–3 times a week. In the past, has refused to consider doing self-monitoring of blood glucose. Over the past 2 weeks, she has had several hypoglycemic reactions after omitting meals, manifested as feelings of light-headedness, weakness, and trembling. Treated with a glass of orange juice or candy bar.

### Usual Daily Menu

*Breakfast:* Orange juice (6 oz), 1 slice of toast with butter and diet jelly, and 1 cup of tea with milk and sugar substitute (Sweet and Low).

*Lunch:* Tossed salad with low-calorie dressing, 1 slice of bread and butter, 12-oz diet cola.

*Afternoon snack:* Crackers (1–2) with peanut butter, 12-oz diet cola.

*Dinner:* One small serving of fish, 1 small baked potato with butter, low-calorie jello, 2 cups of tea with milk and Sweet and Low.

*Daily fluid intake:* Six 8-oz glasses.

## Metabolic

*Height:* 5 ft 1 in. (154.94 cm). *Weight:* 85 lb (38.6 kg). Weight loss of 15 lb (6.8 kg) in the last year "without really trying." Poorly healing ulcer on right leg. Skin has patchy areas of dryness, especially on the legs. Routine skin care includes use of bath oils and emollients, 1–2 times per week. Special foot care was routinely done in the past, but at present she no longer feels this is necessary. "It's not going to make a difference. I'll still get these leg ulcers no matter what I do."

# ELIMINATION PATTERN

## Bowel

Normal bowel pattern is 1 soft-formed, brown stool daily. Denies history of constipation. Last bowel movement was the day prior to admission.

## Bladder

Urinates 6–8 times a day. Patient reports several bouts of cystitis in the past and was told to increase her daily fluid intake. At present, she denies burning, urgency, or difficulty. Urine is clear and yellow and tested positive for glucose.

# ACTIVITY/EXERCISE PATTERN

## Activity/Exercise

Mrs. Fontaine has a sedentary lifestyle. Performs no regular exercise program. Does light housework and cooking. Employs a homemaker for heavier chores. Complains of fatigue if she does too much work. Visits with friends occasionally, but most of her time is spent at home. Enjoys crafts, reading, and watching TV. Naps every day before dinner.

### Self-Care Ability

| | |
|---|---|
| Feeding—0 | Grooming—0 |
| Bathing—0 | General mobility—0 |
| Toileting—0 | Cooking—0 |
| Bed mobility—0 | Home maintenance—II |
| Dressing—0 | Shopping—II |

---

**Functional Levels Code**
0—Full self-care
I—Requires use of equipment or device
II—Requires assistance or supervision from another person
III—Requires assistance or supervision from another person and equipment or device
IV—Is dependent and does not participate

---

## Oxygenation/Perfusion

Had a chest x-ray this admission. Denies having dyspnea at rest or upon exertion, wheezing, cough, or sputum production. Does report experiencing frequent colds and flus during winter months. Denies complaints of palpitations, irregular heartbeat, or chest pain.

*Oxygenation/Perfusion—*
*Continued*

*Cardiac Risk Factors*

|  | Positive | Negative |
|---|---|---|
| Sedentary life-style | X |  |
| Hyperlipidemia |  | X |
| Cigarette smoking |  | X |
| Diabetes | X |  |
| Obesity |  | X |
| Hypertension |  | X |
| Hypervigilant personality | X |  |
| Family history of heart disease |  | X |

## SLEEP/REST PATTERN

*Sleep/Rest*

Usually sleeps 6–8 hours at night. Mrs. Fontaine falls asleep easily at home but has difficulty when she is hospitalized. Requested a sedative at bedtime while hospitalized. Awakes feeling well rested. At present, sleep is disturbed by the need to urinate. She is able to sleep flat, with 1 pillow. Daily routine includes rest periods following mealtimes, especially after dinner.

## COGNITIVE/PERCEPTUAL PATTERN

*Hearing*

Has no hearing problems. No earaches, vertigo, or ringing in ears.

*Vision*

Wears glasses, prescription changed $2\frac{1}{2}$ years ago.

*Sensory Perception*

Mrs. Fontaine has poor tolerance to pain. Requires pain relief medication for any pain. She is right-hand dominant.

*Learning Style*

Learns best by use of visual aids.

## SELF-PERCEPTION/SELF-CONCEPT PATTERN

*Self-Perception/Self-Concept*

Mrs. Fontaine describes herself as someone who relies on others for support. She wants to be more independent and care for her family but is hindered by her health state. Feels others see her as a person who tries hard to do her best. She describes herself as an outgoing and friendly person who enjoys being with other people. Has no difficulty with expressing thoughts and feelings, especially to those close to her.

## ROLE/RELATIONSHIP PATTERN

*Role/Relationship*

Mrs. Fontaine has been happily married for 35 years and has 2 adopted sons, ages 20 and 24. The older son lives and works out of state; the younger son lives at and attends a state college. The family is close, and the sons call and visit on a regular basis. Family problems are discussed openly and resolved.

For the last 30 years, her home has been a ranch-style house in a suburban community with shopping and recreational facilities nearby. The family owns a car, but Mrs. Fontaine no longer drives because of loss of sensation in her feet. She has been employed as a secretary in a construction firm for the last 10 years, but has been disabled for the past 10 months.

## SEXUALITY/REPRODUCTIVE PATTERN

*Sexuality/Reproductive*

Mrs. Fontaine describes her sex life as unsatisfactory. Her recent illnesses and ongoing problems related to her diabetes have affected her relationship with her husband.

Menstrual history: menarch, age 12; menopause, age 48. Last Pap smear — 2 years ago. Self – breast examination — does every 3–4 months. Obstetrical history: gravida 5; para 0. Repeated miscarriages were a cause of sadness earlier in her life but feels that this has been satisfactorily resolved.

## COPING/STRESS TOLERANCE PATTERN

*Coping/Stress Tolerance*

In the past year, because of problems with her legs and feet, Mrs. Fontaine has been forced to give up her job, which she had enjoyed doing. The loss of the job affected her greatly, but she has adjusted and now does various projects around the house. Her usual way of handling stress is by "being active and doing things." Her husband and sons are very supportive and have helped her "get through the bad times." "The death of my mother, 5 years ago from cancer, was especially trying for me. I got through it because I had my husband and my sons to support me."

She describes feelings of being depressed, especially when she is not feeling well or during the times she has been hospitalized.

## VALUE/BELIEF PATTERN

*Value/Belief*

Mrs. Fontaine was raised as a Roman Catholic, but no longer belongs to any church or attends religious services. Recently, she has been giving some thought to joining a community church. Raised in a Polish-speaking family, she feels it is important to pass on one's heritage to one's own children.

# Physical Examination

*General Survey*

A 55-year-old thin woman, appearing stated age; cooperative; in no distress.

*Vital Signs*

**Temperature:** 98.2°F (36.7°C) (oral)
**Pulse:** 92 regular (apical)
**Respirations:** 20
**BP:** 140/76 (seated, left arm).

*Integument*

**Skin.** Fair complexion; skin is warm and dry. Lower legs have no hair; skin is smooth, shiny, and has a cellophanelike appearance. No edema present. Left foot has scars from healed ulcers. Right foot has a 5 × 3 cm ulcer on medial aspect. Small amount of yellow drainage.
**Mucous Membranes.** Pink, moist, intact.
**Nails.** Beds smooth, no clubbing; toenails ragged.

*HEENT*

**Head.** Hair is dull, dry, and brittle; color is light brown and gray; scalp — no tenderness; face is symmetrical. Temporomandibular joint (TMJ) without pain.
**Eyes.** Vision (not tested) is corrected with glasses; conjunctivae are clear. Pupils equal, round, reactive to light and accommodation (PERRLA).
**Ears.** Auricles intact; canals clear; able to hear whispered word at 1 ft (30 cm) and 2 ft (60 cm).

*Nose.* Septum deviated to the left.
*Mouth/Throat.* Membranes and pharynx pink and moist; teeth are intact.

**Neck**

Full range of motion (ROM); no jugular venous distention (JVD); carotids full; no enlarged nodes.

**Pulmonary**

Thorax oval; anteroposterior (AP) diameter 2:1; bilateral chest excursion; lungs resonant and clear.

**Breasts**

Symmetrical; no lumps, pain, or discharge.

**Cardiovascular**

Normal $S_1$, $S_2$; point of maximal impulse (PMI) at fifth intercostal space at left midclavicular line.

**Peripheral Vascular**

*Peripheral Pulses*
Temporal — 4 bilaterally
Carotid — 4 bilaterally
Brachial — 4 bilaterally
Radial — 4 bilaterally
Femoral — 3 bilaterally
Popliteal — 2 bilaterally
Posterior tibial — 1 bilaterally
Dorsalis pedis — 1 bilaterally

*Peripheral Pulse Scale*

| |
| --- |
| 0 — Absent |
| 1 — Markedly impaired |
| 2 — Moderately impaired |
| 3 — Slightly impaired |
| 4 — Normal |

**Abdomen**

Flat abdomen, no tenderness, masses. Liver, spleen, and kidney not palpated. Active bowel sounds in all 4 quadrants.

**Musculoskeletal**

Full range of motion in all extremities; muscle strength normal for age; gait not tested.

**Neurological**

*Mental Status.* Alert; oriented to time, place, and person.
*Cranial Nerves.* II–XII intact.
*Sensory.* Diminished sensation to pain and light touch below both knees; loss of sensation in toes.

*Deep Tendon Reflexes*

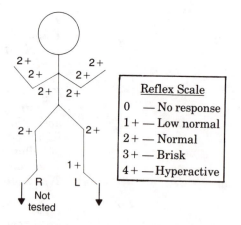

| Reflex Scale | |
| --- | --- |
| 0 | — No response |
| 1+ | — Low normal |
| 2+ | — Normal |
| 3+ | — Brisk |
| 4+ | — Hyperactive |

**Rectal**

External hemorrhoids; negative findings on stool guaiac test.

**Genitalia**

Normal female. Vaginal examination deferred.

## Laboratory Data/Diagnostic Studies

**Laboratory Data**

*Na:* 142 mEq/L
*K:* 3.4 mEq/L
*Cl:* 101 mEq/L
$CO_2$: 24 mEq/L
*BUN:* 32 mg/dl
*Creatinine:* 1.2 mg/dl

$HbA_{1C}$: 10.2%
*Blood Sugar:*
8 AM (fasting) 189
3 PM 348
8 PM 329

**Diagnostic Studies**

*Vascular Lab.* Bilateral popliteal and tibial artery disease and bilateral small vessel disease. Some progression of disease since 2/88 in right leg; no change in left leg. Marginally compensated on right leg; well compensated on left leg.

# COLLABORATIVE PLAN OF CARE

**Diet**

1800-calorie ADA diet.

**Medications**

Insulin NPH 42 units q AM, CZI 8 units q AM.
Docusate sodium (Colace 100 mg PO tid.
Vitamin C 500 mg PO bid.
Methenamine mandelate (Mandelamine) 1 g PO bid.
Heparin 5000 units SC bid.
Multivitamins 1 tab PO qd.
Milk of magnesia 30 ml PO qd prn.
Tylenol 650 mg PO q4–6h prn.

**Intravenous Therapy**

Does not apply.

**Therapeutic Measures**

Bed-to-chair activity with legs elevated.
No weight bearing on right foot.
Vital signs every 4 hours.
Weight every other day.
Foot cradle.
Egg-crate foam on bed, 3-in. (7.5-cm) thick.
Minimum fluid intake of 1500 ml per day.
Wound care: Normal saline wet-to-dry dressings tid.
Wound culture.
Finger sticks for glucose at 7 AM, 3 PM, 8 PM.

**Consults**

Nutritionist.
Diabetes Unit Clinical Specialist.

# NURSING DIAGNOSES DEVELOPED IN CARE PLAN

Altered Nutrition: Less than Body Requirements, p. 224
Impaired Tissue Integrity, p. 225
Noncompliance, p. 226

# ADDITIONAL NURSING DIAGNOSES TO BE CONSIDERED

Altered Sexuality Patterns
Knowledge Deficit
Potential for Activity Intolerance

Potential for Infection
Potential for Injury
Sleep Pattern Disturbance

# NURSING CARE PLAN BASED ON IDENTIFIED NURSING DIAGNOSES

| | |
|---|---|
| ***Altered Nutrition: Less than Body Requirements*** | ***Related to:*** Poor appetite.<br>***Evidenced by:*** Body weight 20% below ideal body weight; reported lack of interest in food; reported food intake below recommended daily allowance. |
| ***Desired Patient Outcomes*** | • The patient's weight progresses toward ideal body weight.<br>• The patient will be knowledgeable about diet prescription, meal planning, and exercise and its role in the management of diabetes. |
| ***Evaluation Criteria*** | ***By Discharge, the Patient Will:***<br>• Choose and consume foods that are consistent with her diet prescription.<br>• Express enjoyment of meal times.<br>• Verbalize information that reflects an understanding of her diet prescription, and knowledge of meal planning and food preparation. |

## Interventions

Monitor serum glucose levels.

Monitor urine ketones.

Weigh the patient.

Monitor food intake.

Promote a pleasant, relaxing environment at meals.

Encourage the patient to choose foods that are appealing.

Limit fiber/bulk food to dietary allowances and discourage excessive fluids at mealtimes.

## Rationale

Achieving and maintaining near-normal blood glucose values is the focus of the diabetic diet (Heins, 1983, p. 633).

"Ketones are found in the urine when the body's fat stores are metabolized for energy thus producing an excess of metabolic end products. This occurs in uncontrolled diabetes" (Luckmann and Sorensen, 1987, p. 1163).

Weighing the patient helps to assess the patient's needs and response to diet therapy (Kneisl and Ames, 1986, p. 205).

Careful measurement of intake should be kept and used as guidelines in determining nutritional needs (Kneisl and Ames, 1986, p. 460).

Emotional stressors may lead to a decrease in food intake (Lewis, 1986, p. 331).

A diet that allows many choices usually results in more success (Guthrie and Guthrie, 1982, p. 105).

Foods high in fiber and increased fluid levels with meals give temporary satiety and decrease the appetite for the more substantial part of the meal (Lewis, 1986, p. 332).

## Interventions

Review with the patient diet prescription, meal planning, and food preparation. Discuss their rationale and the role of diet and exercise in diabetes management.

Consult the nutritionist.

## Rationale

The successful diabetic diet contains "the necessary elements for good nutrition, maintains near normal glucose ranges" (Heins, 1983, p. 642), and mealtimes that are planned to match activities and the kind and dosage of insulin (Guthrie and Guthrie, 1982, p. 102). Exercise is important in the management of diabetes. Exercise lowers blood glucose levels by increasing the glucose uptake of exercising muscles (Lewis, 1986, p. 347).

The nutritionist is responsible for setting up the diet plan for the diabetic patient (Lewis, 1986, p. 351).

---

**Impaired Tissue Integrity**

*Related to:* Altered circulation to lower extremities, history of tissue trauma.
*Evidenced by:* Presence of right-foot ulcer; diminished peripheral pulses; diminished sensitivity to pressure, temperature, and pain in the lower extremities.

**Desired Patient Outcomes**

• Ulcer on right foot will be healed and/or complications will be minimized or prevented.
• The patient will be knowledgeable about practices and measures to prevent tissue trauma and injury.
• The patient will be knowledgeable about signs and symptoms that require medical attention.

**Evaluation Criteria**

*During the Hospital Stay:*
• The skin remains intact and further skin breakdown is prevented.

*After Instruction, the Patient Will:*
• Verbalize and demonstrate proper skin and foot care techniques.
• Discuss the rationale for skin and foot care.
• Identify the signs and symptoms that require follow-up care.
• Identify factors that promote wound healing.

---

## Interventions

Monitor leg ulcer, noting size, color, drainage, and odor.

Perform dressing changes.

Employ the use of egg-crate mattress, sheepskin, and bed cradle.

Institute skin and foot care program.

Instruct and demonstrate proper skin and foot care measures. Discuss their purpose, the consequences of improper care, and the importance of early detection of skin changes.

## Rationale

Wounds must be observed closely during therapy because subsequent response may require prompt changes in therapeutic modalities (Kneisl and Ames, 1986, p. 2171).

Open wounds require dressings that not only protect but also maintain their physiological integrity (Sieggren, 1987, p. 445).

Use of pressure-relieving devices aids in the prevention of tissue trauma (Gosnell, 1987, p. 412).

For diabetics, meticulous skin care and foot care are key factors in the prevention of infections (Donahue-Porter, 1985, p. 196).

Demonstration is the best method for teaching routine foot hygiene and treatment of problem areas (Resler, 1983). Diabetics who are taught to practice proper foot care as well as how to recognize early signs of trouble, may prevent further complications (Graham and Morley, 1984, p. 889).

## Interventions

Discuss the role of nutrition in wound healing.

## Rationale

An adequate supply of nutrients aids healing and tissue repair (Bobel, 1987, p. 379).

---

| | |
|---|---|
| ***Noncompliance*** | ***Related to:*** Burnout. <br> ***Evidenced by:*** Lack of adherence to ADA diet, frequent hypoglycemic reactions, and inadequate skin and foot care. |
| ***Desired Patient Outcome*** | Patient verbalizes intent to practice and participate in planning self-care activities. |
| ***Evaluation Criteria*** | ***By Discharge, The Patient Will:*** <br> • Verbalize reasons for noncompliance with treatment regimens. <br> • Express a more positive approach to self-care activities. <br> • Make appropriate choices based on accurate information. <br> • Be willing to negotiate and work toward meeting treatment goals. <br> • Have family involvement in the treatment program. |

---

## Interventions

Encourage the patient to discuss concerns and feelings about diabetes and how it affects her life.

Explore reasons or experiences that promote noncompliance.

Emphasize the person's choices as much as possible in planning interventions.

Counsel and assist the patient in determining what constitutes compliant behavior.

Set reasonable goals for the treatment program.

Provide encouragement through positive reinforcement of any progress made with therapy.

Encourage the use of self-reward.

Involve the patient's family as much as possible in the treatment program.

Encourage participation in discussion groups, that is, self-help groups.

## Rationale

An individual's failure to follow a treatment regimen usually stems from a complicated array of reasons (Trekas, 1984, p. 58; Padrick, 1986, p. 19).

The nurse can assist the patient in identifying barriers to adherence (Brunner and Suddarth, 1988, p. 936).

A treatment program that has flexibility and is tailored to the person's lifestyle and circumstances and is described in relevant terms fosters better adherence (Thompson, et al., 1986, p. 1883).

Continuing education reinforces learning and is necessary for self-management of diabetes. The more in control the person feels, the more likely he or she is to accept and adhere to treatment regimens (Lewis and Collier, 1987, p. 1280).

Goals should be formulated so that success is achievable (Squyres, 1980, p. 233).

Positive consequences following an action lead to an increase in the desired behavior (Young, 1986, p. 35).

A consistent and reliable source of reward and positive feedback is oneself. Planning positive thoughts or rewarding oneself following a specific behavior can help to maintain the desired behavior (Squyres, 1980, p. 241).

Family involvement in the treatment program can foster cooperation and understanding (Kneisl and Ames, 1986).

"Discussion groups facilitate learning from the experience of others, foster a feeling of belongingness, and reinforce previous learning" (Rankin and Duffy, 1983, p. 170). Self-help groups are important sources of support for patients and family (Rankin and Duffy, 1983, p. 170).

| Interventions | Rationale |
|---|---|
| Consult the diabetes unit clinical specialist. | The diabetic nurse specialist can provide consultation and collaborate with the nursing staff in the management of the patient with diabetes (Lewis and Collier, 1987, p. 1284). |

## QUESTIONS FOR DISCUSSION

1. Review the sequelae that occur in persons with advanced diabetes.
2. Why are patients with diabetes more highly susceptible to infection?
3. Review the different types of insulin used to treat diabetes—names, action, onset, peak, and duration.
4. If Mrs. Fontaine had been a newly diagnosed diabetic, what topics would be covered when teaching her about self-care?
5. Compare and contrast the signs and symptoms of hypoglycemia and diabetic ketoacidosis. What is the treatment for each?
6. Explain why IDDM predisposes to the development of ketoacidosis and NIDDM does not.
7. What types of discharge planning needs does Mrs. Fontaine have? Identify nursing interventions for those you identify.

## REFERENCES

Bobel, L: Nutritional implications in the patient with pressure sores. Nurs Clin North Am 22:379, 1987.

Brunner, LS and Suddarth, DS: Textbook of Medical-Surgical Nursing. JB Lippincott, Philadelphia, 1988.

Bullock, B and Rosendahl, P: Pathophysiology. Little, Brown & Co, Boston, 1984.

Donahue-Porter, P: Insulin-dependent diabetes mellitus. Nurs Clin North Am 20:191, 1985.

Gosnell, D: Assessment and evaluation of pressure sores. Nurs Clin North Am 22:399, 1987.

Graham, S and Morley, M: What "foot care" really means. Am J Nurs 84:889, 1984.

Guthrie, D and Guthrie, R: Nursing Management of Diabetes Mellitus. CV Mosby, St. Louis, 1982

Guthrie, D and Guthrie, R: The disease process of diabetes mellitus. Nurs Clin North Am 18:617, 1983.

Heins, J: Dietary management in diabetes mellitus. Nurs Clin North Am 18:631, 1983.

Kneisl, C and Ames, S: Adult Health Nursing. Addison-Wesley, Menlo Park, Calif, 1986.

Lewis, CM: Nutrition and Nutritional Therapy in Nursing. Appleton-Century-Crofts, Norwalk, Conn, 1986.

Lewis, SM and Collier, IC: Medical-Surgical Nursing Assessment and Management of Clinical Problems. McGraw-Hill, New York, 1987.

Luckmann, J and Sorensen, KC: Medical-Surgical Nursing: A Psychophysiologic Approach. WB Saunders, Philadelphia, 1987.

Padrick, K: Compliance: Myths and motivators. Topics Clin Nurs 7:17, 1986.

Porth, C: Pathophysiology. JB Lippincott, Philadelphia, 1986.

Price, SA and Wilson, LM: Pathophysiology: Clinical Concepts of Disease Processes. McGraw-Hill, New York, 1986.

Rankin, SH and Duffy, KL: Patient Education: Issues, Principles and Guidelines. JB Lippincott, Philadelphia, 1983.

Resler, M: Teaching strategies that promote adherence. Nurs Clin North Am 18:799, 1983.

Sieggren, M: Healing of physical wounds. Nurs Clin North Am 22:439, 1987.

Squyres, WD (ed): Patient Education: An Inquiry into the State of the Art. Springer Publishing, New York, 1980.

Thompson, JM, et al: Clinical Nursing. CV Mosby, St. Louis, 1986.

Trekas, J: It takes 2 to achieve compliance. Nursing '84 14:58, 1984.

Young, M: Teaching strategies that promote adherence. Topics Clin Nurs 7:31, 1986.

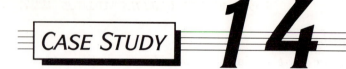

# CASE STUDY 14

# A PATIENT WITH HYPERTHYROIDISM

Dorothy Bagnell Kelliher, M.S., R.N.

## ANATOMY AND PHYSIOLOGY OF THE THYROID GLAND

The thyroid gland is located in the anterior portion of the neck just below the thyroid cartilage. It consists of 2 lateral lobes about the size and shape of a plum cut vertically. The normal estimated weight in an adult is between 10 and 50 g. The normal gland is smooth and firm on palpation. These lobes lie to the right and left of midline on either side of the trachea. The lateral lobes are joined by an isthmus that transverses the second to the fourth tracheal rings, just below the thyroid cartilage.

The thyroid gland has a blood flow about 5 times its weight each minute. This flow rate exceeds every other area of the body with perhaps the exception of the adrenal cortex. This reflects the high metabolic activity of this gland.

The thyroid gland produces 3 different hormones: thyroxine ($T_4$), which contains 4 iodine molecules; triiodothyronine ($T_3$), which contains 3 iodine molecules; and calcitonin. $T_4$ and $T_3$, referred to collectively as thyroid hormone, are involved with iodine metabolism and the regulation of basal metabolic rates. Calcitonin is a hormone involved with calcium metabolism that promotes the deposition of calcium in the bones and thus decreases calcium concentration in the extracellular fluid. When compared on a milligram for milligram basis, $T_3$ is about 4 times as potent as $T_4$ in stimulating metabolism and causing other intracellular effects. However, $T_4$ has at least a duration of action that is 4 times as long as the action of $T_3$. Thus it is felt that the integrated effect of each of the hormones is about equal.

One of the principal functions of the thyroid gland is the regulation of iodine metabolism. The thyroid gland takes up between 10% and 40% of circulating iodine. The remainder of iodide is excreted in the urine. The thyroid gland stores the converted iodide loosely coupled with a protein in the form of thyroglobulin. The rate at which iodine is absorbed from the bloodstream is regulated by the thyroid-stimulating hormone (TSH), which is secreted by the pituitary gland. TSH also controls the rate at which $T_4$ and $T_3$, stored as thyroglobulin in the thyroid cells, are released from storage and secreted into the bloodstream. This is an example of feedback control.

The pituitary gland is also stimulated by the thyrotropin-releasing hormone (TRH) of the hypothalamus. Environmental factors, such as a fall in temperature, may lead to an increased secretion of TRH and thereby result in elevated secretion of thyroid hormones. An example of this reaction to cold is that people moving to arctic regions have been known to develop basal metabolic rates 15%–20% above normal.

The important actions of $T_4$ and $T_3$ are stimulation of calorigenesis, enhancement of epinephrine, lowering of serum cholesterol, and stimulation of growth. In addition, they may stimulate oxidative processes within the mitochondria of the cells on which they act. The thyroid hormones are also involved in the normal development of the central nervous system. In the absence of $T_4$ and $T_3$, mental retardation may be present at birth and in infancy.

# PATHOPHYSIOLOGY OF HYPERTHYROIDISM (THYROTOXICOSIS)

Hyperthyroidism may be defined as the body tissue's response to excessive thyroid hormone. Graves' disease is the most common form of hyperthyroidism, most commonly seen in females under 40 years. In this type of hyperthyroidism there may be 2 major groups of features, thyroidal and extrathyroidal. The thyroidal features of hyperthyroidism are the result of the excessive secretion of thyroid hormone and possibly a goiter, caused by diffuse hyperplasia of the thyroid gland. It is felt that the antibodies that cause hyperthyroidism are almost certainly a result of an autoimmunity that develops against thyroid tissue. It is presumed that earlier an excess of thyroid cell antigens was released from the thyroid cells, which resulted in the formation of antibodies against the thyroid gland itself. One of these antibodies found in over 50% of patients with hyperthyroidism is called long-acting thyroid stimulator (LATS). In this event, the high level of thyroid hormone secretion caused by LATS in turn suppresses the anterior pituitary formation of TSH.

Hyperthyroidism may also result from the development of a localized adenoma that develops in the thyroid tissue and secretes a large amount of thyroid hormone. This is not associated with autoimmune disease.

## RISK FACTORS

Women are 7–10 times more commonly affected than men, and there is a higher incidence between 20 and 40 years of age. Hyperthyroidism often appears after increased stress, emotional upheaval, or infection, and it seems to occur frequently in people who have had other endocrine disorders. Populations living in geographical regions where the natural supply of iodine is deficient are prone to develop simple goiters. Some goiters are associated with hyperthyroidism and are termed "toxic."

## COMMON CLINICAL FINDINGS

Findings may be insidious and nonspecific but they are all related to an increase in the basal metabolic rate, increased cardiac and respiratory stimulation, and increased neurological activity.

Most frequently signs of nervousness predominate. Patients are often hyperemotional, apprehensive, and irritable. They experience palpitations, and tachycardia with rates ranging from 90–160 beats per minute. They are intolerant to heat, perspire freely, and have flushed skin. They experience increased weakness and fatigue as well as an increased appetite that is accompanied by weight loss and dyspnea. Some patients complain of an increased frequency of bowel movements and diarrhea. Fine tremors of the hands are frequently present. Exophthalmia may be present if the cause of hyperthyroidism is Graves' disease (toxic diffuse goiter). Women may experience decreased menstruation or amenorrhea. In men there may be a decrease in libido. Patients with underlying cardiac conditions may be seriously threatened due to the increases in blood volume, cardiac output, and blood pressure.

Metabolic abnormalities such as glucose intolerance may develop due to decreased insulin release. Increased serum calcium may be seen because of increased bone breakdown and increased plasma volume.

## TREATMENT MODALITIES

Treatment is aimed at relief of symptoms and reducing thyroid hormone. As yet no treatment for the basic cause of hyperthyroidism has been discovered. The most common modalities for treating hyperthyroidism are the administration of antithyroid medication, radioiodine therapy, and surgery. Antithyroid drugs, such as propylthiouracil and methimazole, are used to block thyroid hormone synthesis. Iodine drugs such as saturated solution of potassium iodide (SSKI) and Lugol's solution are given to reduce the vascularity of the thyroid gland and to treat "thyroid storm." Other drugs such as adrenergic blocking agents are used to control the activity of the sympathetic nervous system; an example is propranolol. Radioiodine therapy is used mainly in the middle-aged and elderly population and is contraindicated for pregnant women, and seldom used for children. Its advantage is that it is safe, economical, and can be used on an outpatient basis. However, because it destroys thyroid cells, its major complication is hypothyroidism.

The third modality is surgical removal of a part of the thyroid gland (Fig. 14–1). Approximately five

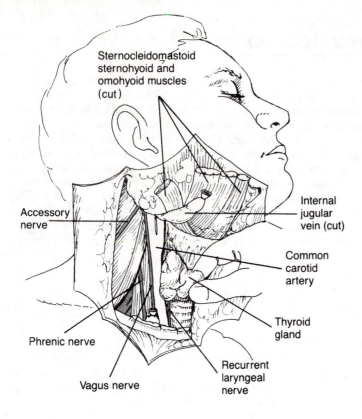

Sternocleidomastoid
sternohyoid and
omohyoid muscles
(cut)

Accessory
nerve

Internal
jugular
vein (cut)

Common
carotid
artery

Thyroid
gland

Phrenic nerve

Vagus nerve

Recurrent
laryngeal
nerve

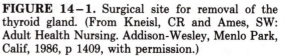

**FIGURE 14–1.** Surgical site for removal of the thyroid gland. (From Kneisl, CR and Ames, SW: Adult Health Nursing. Addison-Wesley, Menlo Park, Calif, 1986, p 1409, with permission.)

sixths of the gland is removed and thus hormonal replacement may not be necessary. If surgery is the treatment of choice, a euthyroid state must be achieved by use of appropriate medication before surgery is attempted. A euthyroid state is having the thyroid gland return to normal functioning. Thus by achieving a euthyroid state, the operative mortality is reduced to 1 in 1000, whereas, prior to giving propylthiouracil and iodine preparations, the operative mortality was as high as 1 in 25 due to occurrence of hemorrhage or thyroid storm. Other treatment interventions are aimed at providing adequate rest, good nutrition, and prevention of damage to the eyes in the case of exophthalmos.

# PATIENT ASSESSMENT DATA BASE

## Health History

*Client:*
Lynn Swartz

*Address:* 4 Lake View Drive, Apt. 49, Chicago, IL 60611
*Telephone:* 312-555-6398
*Contact:* Mrs. Emma Swartz (mother)
*Address of contact:* 1623 Buena Vista Blvd., Dallas, Texas 54204
*Telephone of contact:* 909-555-5507
*Age:* 35    *Sex:* Female    *Race:* White
*Educational background:* Master's degree, University of Texas
*Religion:* Jewish    *Marital status:* Single
*Uusal occupation:* Buyer of apparel
*Present occupation:* Same
*Source of income:* Employment
*Insurance:* Health Maintenance Organization of Chicago
*Source of referral:* Clinic M.D.
*Source of history:* Patient
*Reliability of source:* Reliable
*Date of interview:* 2/1/90
*Reason for visit/Chief complaint:* Sensitivity to heat, bouts of tachycardia, weight loss, tremor of hands, and diarrhea.

## HEALTH PERCEPTION/HEALTH MANAGEMENT PATTERN

### Present Health Status

Since moving to Chicago 6 months ago to assume the position of buyer for the Neiman-Marcus Cruisewear Department, Lynn has noticed that she has become exceptionally tense and irritable. She attributed this at first to the stress of her new job and change in location. She has also noticed that she has become very sensitive to heat and has been perspiring excessively. She states that she is concerned about a recent 10-lb (4.5-kg) weight loss and also with bouts of diarrhea. Lynn has noticed that she seems to have a fine tremor in both hands. Although normally used to jogging 3–5 miles a day, she has had to stop this due to increasing fatigue and dyspnea. She says that sometimes, unexpectedly, her heart will start pounding so hard that she is sure it can be heard. During these episodes, she has taken her pulse and found it to be 110–140, which frightened her. These particular symptoms finally caused her to seek medical advice.

### Past Health Status

*General Health.* Excellent. She had been jogging 3–5 miles per day. Denies any health problems, physical or psychological, until this present upset.
*Prophylactic Medical/Dental Care.* Had a complete physical after arriving for her new job. Dental checkup every 6 months; has not contacted a dentist in Chicago yet.
*Childhood Illnesses.* Chickenpox—age 3. Appendectomy—age 12.
*Immunizations.* Vaccination—age 5. Diphtheria-pertussis-tetanus (DPT) vaccine—on entering kindergarten. Tetanus vaccine—1980. Measles-mumps-rubella (MMR) vaccine—1963?

**Past Health
Status—Continued**

*Major Illnesses/Hospitalizations.* Other than appendectomy in 1965, she has had no illnesses.

*Current Medications*
*Prescription:* Saturated solution of potassium iodide (SSKI) 5 gtt PO tid; propylthiouracil (PTU) 300 mg PO q8h; propranolol hydrochloride (Inderal) 10 mg PO tid.
*Nonprescription:* An analgesic (Bufferin) for occasional headache; daily multivitamin capsule; diphenoxylate hydrochloride/ atropine (Lomotil) for diarrhea.

*Allergies.* None.

*Habits*
*Alcohol:* Social drinker only (wine mainly).
*Caffeine:* 4–5 cups coffee (black) a day.
*Drugs:* None. See Current Medications.
*Tobacco:* Nonsmoker.

*Family Health History*

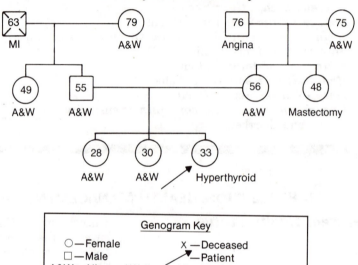

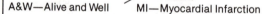

# NUTRITIONAL/METABOLIC PATTERN

*Nutritional*

Patient is a vegetarian but does eat fish and dairy products. She has maintained the same weight for the past 15 years. Over the last several months, she has been losing weight although she has been eating a lot more food. She claims, even though she has been upset over her "condition," she has been ravenously hungry. She has no problems with dentition at this time.

*Usual Daily Menu**
*Breakfast:* One large glass of orange juice, 2 cups of coffee, no sugar, 1 bran muffin with margarine.
*Lunch:* Tofu sandwich on whole wheat bread; 2 cups of coffee; yogurt, ice cream, or fruit.
*Dinner:* Medium portion of fish, 1 cup green beans, large mixed salad with creamy Italian dressing, whole wheat roll, margarine, 3 cookies or other dessert, 1 large glass of milk.
*Night snack:* Tea with milk, cookies.

*Feels she has recently increased these amounts and is also snacking more between meals.

| | |
|---|---|
| *Metabolic* | *Height:* 5 ft 8 in. (172.7 cm). *Weight:* 115 lb (52.3 kg). She has lost approximately 10 lb (4.5 kg) over the last 2 months. Skin has become very smooth feeling and moist. Has noted nails are splitting. Hair is also very fine and hard to manage. |

## ELIMINATION PATTERN

| | |
|---|---|
| *Bowel* | Bowel movement is always regular, 1 stool a day, soft-formed, medium brown in color. Over the last 3–4 months, she has been experiencing frequent episodes of diarrhea. |
| *Bladder* | Voids 7–8 times during waking hours. Urine is pale yellow in color, clear, with no odor noted; seldom wakes at night to void. |

## ACTIVITY/EXERCISE PATTERN

*Activity/Exercise*

Lynn has always been very active; she enjoys swimming, tennis, and racquetball. Jogged 3–5 miles per day rain or shine until these past few months when she has become very tired and experienced episodes of a "pounding heart."

*Self-Care Ability*

| | |
|---|---|
| Feeding—0 | Grooming—0 |
| Bathing—0 | General mobility—0 |
| Toileting—0 | Cooking—0 |
| Bed mobility—0 | Home maintenance—0 |
| Dressing—0 | Shopping—0 |

---

*Functional Levels Code*
  0—Full self-care
  I—Requires use of equipment or device
 II—Requires assistance or support from another person
III—Requires assistance or support from another person and equipment or device
 IV—Is dependent and does not participate

---

*Oxygenation/Perfusion*

Developed dyspnea while jogging—this is a recent happening. No other problems.

*Cardiac Risk Factors*

| | Positive | Negative |
|---|---|---|
| Sedentary life-style | | X |
| Hyperlipidemia | | X |
| Cigarette smoking | | X |
| Diabetes | | X |
| Obesity | | X |
| Hypertension | | X |
| Hypervigilant personality | X | |
| Family history of heart disease | X | |

## SLEEP/REST PATTERN

*Sleep/Rest*

Usually sleeps 5–6 hours, falling asleep easily and waking up refreshed. Last vacation was just prior to coming to Chicago (2 weeks in Cancún, Mexico). Recently she has been having some periods of wakefulness. Will wake suddenly and be unable to fall back to sleep for 1–2 hours. This is causing her to feel tired and not well rested.

## Cognitive/Perceptual Pattern

**Hearing**

Normal.

**Vision**

Wears contact lenses; has had 1 or 2 episodes of double vision recently.

**Sensory Perception**

Is very sensitive to heat; perspires freely; prefers a cold environment. States again that these are unusual for her. Has developed a fine tremor in her hands.

**Learning Style**

Feels she learns best by verbal explanation and visual demonstration. Now feels it is difficult to concentrate on things.

## Self-Perception/Self-Concept Pattern

**Self-Perception/Self-Concept**

Normally Lynn is a very self-reliant, happy, confident person. Lately she has been tense and irritable. This has caused her to feel quite insecure and anxious: "I just don't know what is happening to me; I'm not the nervous type but I'm frightened by all these changes. I hope the doctor can find out what's wrong with me." Sees herself as a warm, friendly person but not "gushy." Also very concerned about her appearance. "I'm afraid the surgical scar will be so ugly that I'll have to wear high-necked clothing from now on. I really hate that thought—in the fashion world, I'm noted for my classic V-neck style of dress." Her physical appearance is very important to her and in essence her self-concept.

## Role/Relationship Pattern

**Role/Relationship**

Pattern lives alone in a very comfortable apartment. She has made 2 or 3 good friends since arriving in Chicago. Feels she can contact them anytime but does not want to bore them with health problems. She is close to her family—talks with her parents once a week; also in close contact with her 2 sisters (1 in Iowa, 1 in Indiana). Younger sister lives in Terra Haute, Indiana. She has seen her once a month since coming to Chicago. Is not currently dating but looks forward to meeting a person she could form a permanent relationship with.

## Sexuality/Reproductive Pattern

**Sexuality/Reproductive**

Menarch, age 11; no problem with dysmenorrhea. Since age 32 has had regular 33-day cycle; period lasts 4–5 days. Has had a yearly gynecological examination and Pap smear since age 28. Is not currently sexually active—has used birth control pills in the past. Has recently experienced two 2-day periods with scanty flow; this is unusual for her.

## Coping/Stress Tolerance Pattern

**Coping/Stress Tolerance**

Lynn has no problem with stress—if something is bothering her she is able to talk it out. Jogging also helps her straighten a difficult problem out. She is usually quite calm and not given to outbursts (this is why she is so upset about her current behavior). Feels that all her positive coping strategies have "disappeared." She now feels very anxious and upset about her short temper at work and is afraid she will alienate her new co-workers. She cries "at the drop of a hat." When she wakes at night all these fears seem overwhelming and have caused her to lose sleep or have difficulty falling back to sleep.

## VALUE/BELIEF PATTERN

*Value/Belief*

Feels very strongly about good health practices. Is a religious person but mainly attends temple on holidays. She is planning to join a congregation near her apartment in the very near future. She treats others as she would like to be treated. Has a strong work ethic.

# Physical Examination

*General Survey*

Very attractive, tall, slim, white female who looks slightly younger than her stated age. Pleasant and cooperative; appears somewhat anxious.

*Vital Signs*

*Temperature:* 101.0°F (38.3°C) (oral)
*Pulse:* 98 regular (apical) (increased to 140–150 at times)
*Respirations:* 18 regular
*BP:* 132/56 (left arm, sitting).

*Integument*

*Skin.* Skin is smooth, moist, and slightly flushed.
*Mucous Membranes.* Smooth, moist, and pink.
*Nails.* Nails have been splitting and they are hard to keep clean.

*HEENT*

*Head.* Well-shaped head, no areas of tenderness; scalp clean, no scaling. Hair is very fine and friable, dark brown in color. Facial features are even and symmetrical. Expression is appropriate.
*Eyes.* No exophthalmia. Pupils equal, round, reactive to light and accommodation (PERRLA). Extraocular movements (EOMs) are normal. Conjunctiva are quite pink but not inflamed; sclerae are clear. Acuity is 20/20, corrected with contact lenses bilaterally.
*Ears.* Within normal limits.
*Nose.* Midline; mucous membranes are moist and pink.
*Mouth/Throat.* Mucous membranes are pink and moist; teeth in good condition. Tonsils are present; pharynx pink, no inflammation noted. Does have a feeling of fullness in the throat.

*Neck*

No nodes. Trachea is midline. Slightly firm and enlarged thyroid; bruit and palpable thrill over thyroid gland. Venous hum present.

*Pulmonary*

Lungs are clear; no rales; expansion equal bilaterally.

*Breast*

Moderate size, round, and symmetrical breasts. Skin is smooth and supple, nipple light pink with light brown areola; no discharge expressed. No axillary or clavicular nodes palpable; no masses present. Does self-breast examination (SBE) monthly.

*Cardiovascular*

Systolic murmur over the pulmonic and aortic area; systolic click; prominent third heart sound. Point of maximal impulse (PMI) palpable and visible at fifth intercostal space in midclavicular line.

*Peripheral Vascular*

All pulses are strong, bounding, and regular. Extremities are warm; no mottling. Good capillary refill.

**Peripheral Vascular — Continued**

*Peripheral Pulses*
Temporal — 4 bilaterally
Carotid — 4 bilaterally
Radial — 4 bilaterally
Femoral — 4 bilaterally
Popliteal — 4 bilaterally
Posterior tibialis — 4 bilateral
Dorsalis pedis — 4 bilaterally
Brachial — 4 bilaterally

*Peripheral Pulse Scale*

| 0 — Absent |
| 1 — Markedly diminished |
| 2 — Moderately diminished |
| 3 — Slightly diminished |
| 4 — Normal |

**Abdomen**

Flat; no bruits; bowel sounds present in all quadrants. Hyperactive on auscultation; no tenderness.

**Musculoskeletal**

Within normal limits (WNL) bilaterally. Total range of motion (ROM) in all extremities. Complains of recent muscle fatigue and weakness and questions some loss of muscle mass. Has difficulty maintaining legs in extended position for more than count of 20. Total ROM of spine, no limitation, no pain or tenderness; vertebrae straight, no deviations.

**Neurological**

*Mental Status.* Clear, intelligent, and logical responses to questions. Mood is slightly anxious. Pleasant attitude.
*Cranial Nerves.* I–XII intact.
*Sensory.* Response to light touch and pinprick is within normal limits (WNL). Negative Romberg sign; Babinski reflex is normal. Fine tremor of upper extremities noted.
*Deep Tendon Reflexes.* All points register 3+ on a scale of 0–4+.

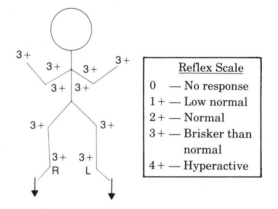

Reflex Scale

| 0 — No response |
| 1+ — Low normal |
| 2+ — Normal |
| 3+ — Brisker than normal |
| 4+ — Hyperactive |

**Rectal**

Deferred.

**Genitalia**

Deferred (last examination 10/88).

## Laboratory Data/Diagnostic Studies

**Laboratory Data**

*WBC:* 5200/mm³
*RBC:* 5.3 million/mm³
*Ca:* 8.5 mg/dl
*Type and Cross Match:* 0+

*K:* 3.5 mEq/L
*Na:* 135 mEq/L
*T₃ RIA:* 240 mg/dl
*T₄ RIA:* 15 mg/dl

**Additional Data**

Lynn was diagnosed as having a hyperthyroid condition and a medical/surgical approach was decided on. Surgery is now scheduled for 2/5/90.

# COLLABORATIVE PLAN OF CARE

| | |
|---|---|
| *Diet* | Diet as tolerated—high calorie, high protein. |
| *Medications* | SSKI 5 gtt PO in water tid. |
| | Propylthiouracil 30 mg PO tid. |
| | Propranolol 10 mg PO tid. |
| | Multivitamin 1 capsule PO qd. |
| | Acetaminophen (Tylenol) 2 tabs PO prn for fever $> 100°F$ (37.7°C) |
| | Sodium pentobarbital (Nembutal) 60 mg PO prn for sleep. |
| | Lomotil 5 mg PO prn q6h for diarrhea. |
| *Intravenous Therapy* | Does not apply. |
| *Therapeutic Measures* | Weigh daily. |
| | Maintain cool environment. |
| | Provide quiet atmosphere. |
| | Preoperative teaching for surgery on 2/5/90. |
| *Consults* | Cardiology. |
| *Preoperative Plan* | NPO after midnight. |
| | Diazepam (Valium) 10 mg PO with sip of water on call. |

# NURSING DIAGNOSES DEVELOPED IN CARE PLAN

Ineffective Individual Coping, p. 237
Diarrhea, p. 239
Hyperthermia, p. 240

# ADDITIONAL NURSING DIAGNOSES TO BE CONSIDERED

Activity Intolerance
Altered Nutrition: Less than Body Requirements
Anxiety
Body Image Disturbance
Fatigue
Sleep Pattern Disturbance

# NURSING CARE PLAN BASED ON IDENTIFIED NURSING DIAGNOSES

| | |
|---|---|
| *Ineffective Individual Coping* | **Related to:** Physiological changes, increased anxiety, and irritability. |
| | **Evidenced by:** Emotional tension, verbalization of inability to cope, diarrhea, sleep disturbance, and fatigue. |

| *Desired Patient Outcomes* | *Patient Will:*<br>• State awareness of her own positive coping abilities.<br>• Understand underlying conditions causing physical and emotional stress. |
|---|---|
| *Evaluation Criteria* | *Before Surgery, the Patient Will:*<br>• Discuss positive coping strategies.<br>• Verbalize feelings of being in control.<br>• Recognize the importance of a support group.<br>• Verbalize understanding of diagnosis and its implication.<br>• Demonstrate stress management techniques that she finds useful. |

## *Interventions*

## *Rationale*

Provide emotional reassurance to patient.

The patient with hyperthyroidism needs assurance that the emotional reactions that he or she is experiencing are a result of the disorder and that with effective treatment these symptoms will be controlled (Brunner and Suddarth, 1988, p. 956).

Investigate the patient's usual methods of coping.

Exploring past coping patterns, as well as perceptions of current stressors and anticipated outcomes, assists the nurse in identifying the person's overall ability to handle stress (Brunner and Suddarth, 1988, p. 59).

Assist the patient to verbalize a positive self-concept.

Health concerns may threaten how a person perceives himself or herself. Body image is vulnerable as a result of certain medical and surgical interventions (Brunner and Suddarth, 1988, p. 58).

Assist the patient to understand the cognitive appraisal and coping activity she utilizes in stress response.

In Lazarus's theory, appraisal is a cognitive process through which an event is evaluated with respect to what is at stake and what coping resources and options are available (Brunner and Suddarth, 1988, p. 90).

Assist the patient to evaluate her support system.

The ability to cope effectively is utilized by a person's resources (Brunner and Suddarth, 1988, p. 90). Social support facilitates coping behaviors of a person . . . but the necessary support comes only when there is a deep level of involvement and concern (Brunner and Suddarth, 1988, p. 93). Using the support of others helps the person to maintain mastery of a situation and to keep self-esteem intact (Brunner and Suddarth, 1988, p. 98).

Assist the patient's family to understand the present situation.

Family and close friends should be made aware that this behavior is a result of the disease and not to be taken personally. Voiced anger or retaliatory remarks may only aggravate the patient's condition (Patrick, et al, 1986, p. 1025).

Provide information regarding diagnosis and medical-surgical treatment.

Nursing research by Leventhal and Johnson has indicated that people acquire a sense of control over events when they are given information that makes it possible for them to form a mental image of them. If people were provided with a description of sensations, if the routine of the procedure was described, and if they were given instructions in coping behaviors, they would experience less distress and have better outcomes (Brunner and Suddarth, 1988, p. 96).

Teach the patient methods of stress management.

Stress management embraces a self-management orientation, emphasizing personal responsibility and participation in treatment. The goal of treatment is to provide the behavioral, cogni-

## Interventions

## Rationale

tive, and psychophysiological skills necessary for persons to manage their own responses. It is designed to enhance the person's ability to take charge of his or her own wellness-illness behaviors (Phipps, Long, and Woods, 1987, p. 137).

---

| | |
|---|---|
| **Diarrhea** | ***Related to:*** Hypermetabolism.<br>***Evidenced by:*** Increased episodes of watery stools. |
| **Desired Patient Outcomes** | The patient will understand how to correct bowel problem by proper dietary intake and will experience a return to normal bowel functioning. |
| **Evaluation Criteria** | ***By the Time of Discharge, the Patient Will:***<br>• Have soft and formed bowel movements approximately once per day.<br>• Be taking 2500 ml of fluids daily.<br>• Be selecting a high-calorie, high-protein, low-fiber diet.<br>• Have gained a small amount of weight (1–2 lb [0.45–0.9] kg). |

---

## Interventions

Weigh the patient daily.

Increase fluid intake to 2500–3000 ml over 24 hours. Offer cola, bouillon, juices, Gatorade.

Evaluate present dietary intake and modify the diet as necessary.

Teach the patient the relationship of the diagnosis to diarrhea.

Administer medications to decrease gastrointestinal motility.

## Rationale

Inability to meet metabolic requirements results in weight loss (Patrick, et al, 1986, p. 1060).

Diarrhea causes fluid and electrolyte losses. These losses must be replaced. Fluids such as colas, bouillon, and juices should be encouraged (Patrick, et al, 1986, p. 1025). Rapid transit of feces through the large intestine results in less water absorption, which increases the risk of dehydration (Patrick, et al, p. 1061). Correction of fluid and electrolyte imbalances is of primary importance in the treatment of diarrhea (Spenser, et al, 1986, p. 650).

Omit milk products because diarrhea temporarily depletes gastrointestinal disaccharidase required for digestion of lactose (Spenser, et al, 1986, p. 53). Provide a well-balanced diet. Six full meals a day may be needed to satisfy appetite. Encourage foods that are high in protein, carbohydrates, fats, and minerals. Avoid foods that cause increased peristalsis, that is, highly seasoned, bulky, or fibrous foods (Luckmann and Sorensen, 1987, p. 1449).

Effective patient teaching not only minimizes the patient's stress and increases his or her coping abilities, but also dramatically affects the course and management of most endocrine problems (Patrick, et al, 1986, p. 1026). The hypermetabolic effects of disease cause gastrointestinal hypermotility, leading to increased bowel tone and diarrhea (Patrick, et al, 1986, p. 1055).

Anticholinergic drugs that reduce parasympathetic nerve activity alleviate intestinal hypermotility and hypersecretion and are used in the treatment of diarrhea. They usually are used as adjuncts in combination with absorbent agents. Opiates are also used as antidiarrheal agents (Spenser, et al, 1986, pp. 650–651).

| Interventions | Rationale |
|---|---|
| Evaluate anal mucosa for irritation. | When irritation to the anal mucosa is severe, apply a thin coat of mineral oil, petroleum jelly, or A and D ointment (a petrolatum-lanolin preparation) to help relieve discomfort (Luckmann and Sorensen, 1987, p. 1260). |

---

| | |
|---|---|
| **Hyperthermia** | **Related to:** Increased metabolic rate.<br>**Evidenced by:** Temperature of 101°F (38.3°C), skin flushed and warm to the touch, and episodes of tachycardia. |
| **Desired Patient Outcomes** | **The Patient Will:**<br>• Experience a return of temperature to normal range.<br>• Understand factors contributing to elevated temperature.<br>• Identify methods of preventing hyperthermia. |
| **Evaluation Criteria** | **By the Time of Discharge, the Patient's:**<br>• Temperature will have returned to normal range— 98.4F°–98.6°F (36.8°C–37°C).<br>• Fluid intake will be between 2000–3000 ml/day.<br><br>**By the Time of Discharge, the Patient Will:**<br>• Verbalize factors that can reduce temperature.<br>• Be able to monitor her own temperature. |

---

| Interventions | Rationale |
|---|---|
| Administer antipyretics to lower body temperature. | Antipyretic drugs are used to moderate temperatures in febrile illnesses. The therapeutic goal is not to restore temperature to normal levels but to reduce discomfort and physiological depletion characteristic of prolonged or marked fever (Spenser, et al, 1986, p. 339). |
| Provide a cool environment. | Patients with hyperthyroidism experience increased body temperature and intolerance to heat (Phipps, Long, and Woods, 1987, p. 560). |
| Increase fluid intake to 2500–3000 ml spaced over 24 hours. | Severe diaphoresis can cause a loss of up to 2500 ml/day. Continued loss without replacement results in dehydration (Patrick, et al, 1986, p. 1060). All patients with fever need replacement of fluids since insensible water loss is increased (Patrick, et al, 1986, p. 212). Increased sweat gland activity promotes heat loss through evaporation. In order to increase sweat production, the person must be well hydrated (Atkinson and Murray, 1985, p. 490). |
| Provide lightweight bed linen and cool clothing. | A response to circulating catecholamines in hyperthyroidism results in exaggerated increase in metabolic rate with vasodilation and heat intolerance (Patrick, et al, 1986, p. 1060). Light covering and loose garments enhance natural heat loss during the course of a fever (Luckmann and Sorenson, p. 1987, p. 130). |
| Tepid sponge bath for temperature over 102°F (38.8°C). | Cool baths accelerate heat loss through conduction and evaporation (Atkinson and Murray, 1985, p. 516). |

| *Interventions* | *Rationale* |
|---|---|
| Bedrest or low level of activity. | Muscle tone is decreased, which means less activity within the muscle cells and thus less heat production (Atkinson and Murray, 1985, p. 488). |
| Monitor temperature q4h. | When the thyroid gland releases increased amounts of $T_4$, it accelerates the cellular metabolic rate, thus increasing heat production (Atkinson and Murray, 1985, p. 492). Frequent temperature checks are important in all activities causing accelerated heat loss in order to determine the effectiveness of the treatment and the need for additional measures or cessation of efforts (Atkinson and Murray, 1985, p. 516). |

## QUESTIONS FOR DISCUSSION

1. Identify the clinical manifestations of hyperthyroidism.
2. Discuss the tests used to diagnose thyroid dysfunction.
3. What are the modes of treating hyperthyroidism?
4. What are the antithyroid drugs used to bring about a euthyroid state?
5. Develop a nursing care plan for a patient experiencing hyperthyroidism.
6. Surgery is being planned—what preoperative teaching is needed for patients undergoing a thyroidectomy?
7. What are the major postoperative complications? What nursing assessments should be done in the immediate postoperative phase?
8. What are the long-term implications for a patient who has had a thyroidectomy?

## REFERENCES

Atkinson, L and Murray, M: Fundamentals of Nursing. Macmillan, New York, 1985.

Brunner, L and Suddarth, D: Medical-Surgical Nursing. JB Lippincott, Philadelphia, 1988.

Luckmann, J and Sorensen, K: Medical-Surgical Nursing. WB Saunders, Philadelphia, 1987.

Patrick, M, et al: Medical-Surgical Nursing. JB Lippincott, Philadelphia, 1986.

Phipps, WJ, Long, B, and Woods, N: Medical-Surgical Nursing. CV Mosby, St. Louis, 1987.

Spenser, R, et al: Clinical Pharmacology and Nursing Management. JB Lippincott, Philadelphia, 1986.

## BIBLIOGRAPHY

Bayliss, RJS: Thyroid Disease. Oxford University Press, New York, 1982.

Blonde, L, et al: Answer to questions on hyperthyroidism. Hosp Med, December 1984, pp 131–132, 142–143.

Carpenito, L: Nursing Diagnosis. JB Lippincott, Philadelphia, 1983.

Doenges, M and Moorhouse, M: Nursing Diagnoses With Interventions. FA Davis, Philadelphia, 1988.

Gettrust, K, Ryan, S, and Engleman, D: Applied Nursing Diagnosis. John Wiley & Sons, New York, 1985.

Gorall, A, et al: Primary Care Medicine. JB Lippincott, Philadelphia, 1981.

Gordon, M: Manual of Nursing Diagnosis 1986–1987. McGraw-Hill, New York, 1987.

Guyton, A: Textbook of Medical Physiology. WB Saunders, Philadelphia, 1986.

Johnson, D: Pathophysiology of thyroid storm: Nursing implications. Crit Care Nurse, November–December 1983, pp 80–86.

Mathewson, MK: Thyroid disorder. Crit Care Nurse, January–February, 1987, pp 74–85.

McConnell, EA: Assessing the thyroid. Nursing, May 1985, pp 60–62.

Wood, L, et al: Your Thyroid. Houghton Mifflin, Boston, 1982.

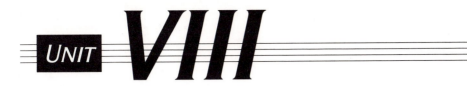

# UNIT VIII

# THE PATIENT WITH ALTERATIONS IN THE MUSCULOSKELETAL SYSTEM

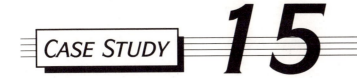
# A PATIENT WITH RHEUMATOID ARTHRITIS

Meg Doherty, M.S., R.N.

Rheumatoid arthritis is a chronic, inflammatory disease that is systemic in nature but characterized by inflammation of the synovial membrane of the joints. Although primarily thought of in terms of joint involvement, it can involve all connective tissues of the body and cause multisystem disease and complications. Many misconceptions about rheumatoid arthritis have led to a general lack of awareness of the seriousness of this disease.

## ANATOMICAL ALTERATIONS

Rheumatoid arthritis begins as an inflammation of the synovium, producing edema, vascular congestion, fibrin exudate, and infiltration of leukocytes. There is an increase in synovial fluid as well as alterations in its character, such as increased turbidity and decreased viscosity. The synovium thickens and grows out and over the articular cartilage, eventually destroying the cartilage and the bone beneath it. As the cartilage is destroyed, the bony surfaces articulate and adhere resulting in a permanently fused, rigid, immobile joint. Tendons, ligaments, and muscles become weakened causing instability and/or partial subluxation of the joint. The common deformities of rheumatoid arthritis occur because of joint destruction, soft-tissue weakness, and tendon rupture. Initially, small joints such as those of the hands and feet are most commonly involved progressing to the larger joints. Classically arthritis appears to be symmetrical, although the identical bilateral joints of the hands and fingers may not always be involved.

Involvement of hands and wrists is characteristic of rheumatoid arthritis. Deformities of different types develop depending on the site of the rheumatoid lesions, such as ulnar deviation and swan-neck and boutonnière deformities. Loss of grasp and pinch, functional limitations of the wrist, evidenced by the inability to remove a lid from a jar, and inability to extend the fingers are commonly encountered.

Synovitis of the elbow joint and inflammation and nodules in the olecranon bursa are common in established rheumatoid arthritis.

Pain in 1 or both shoulders with or without swelling is common in rheumatoid arthritis of the glenohumeral joint.

The end-stage pathology of rheumatoid disease with its typical cartilage loss produces a similar functional abnormality as osteoarthritis of the hip joint. However, isolated involvement of the hips is uncommon in contrast to frequent isolated involvement of the knee of the rheumatoid patient.

Not only is the knee the most common single joint initially involved in rheumatoid arthritis, but it often remains the site of significant disease. Persistent synovitis eventually produces limitation in walking as a result of cartilage destruction, ligament weakness, joint instability, and contractures.

Inflammation of the small joints of the feet and of the ankle joints is common. The metatarsophalangeal joints are the site of early synovitis that results in pain in the ball of the foot on weight bearing. Occasionally, patients may be unaware of arthritis until the foot is squeezed to produce localized metatarsophalangeal pain. Hallux valgus occurs as a typical foot deformity.

Cervical spine disease is frequent and may result in neurological complications. Besides neurological symptoms and pain, cervical arthritis may produce bizzare head and neck sensations. Joints of the thoracic, lumbar, and sacral spine are relatively unaffected.

Synovitis of the temporomandibular joint may produce pain on chewing and may lead to limitation of jaw motion.

# SYSTEMIC ALTERATIONS

The most frequent ocular disturbance of rheumatoid arthritis is Sjögren's syndrome, manifested by sensations of grittiness, an accumulation of dried mucoid material, and decreased tear formation. Other features of Sjögren's syndrome may include dryness of the mouth, nose, rectum, and vagina as well as enlargement of the lacrimal and salivary glands. Other ocular pathologies include episcleritis, scleritis, and corneal and conjunctival lesions.

Pleurisy with or without effusion, pulmonary fibrosis, and pulmonary rheumatoid nodules are examples of pulmonary involvement. Rheumatoid nodules occur in the pulmonary parenchyma as well as on the pleural surface.

The frequency of cardiac involvement in rheumatoid arthritis is high and includes pericarditis, myocarditis, endocarditis, and valvular fibrosis. Cardiac involvement may also be associated with the presence of rheumatoid nodules in structures such as the valves and the conduction system.

Vasculitis of the coronary, cranial, and mesenteric vessels may be seen in patients with advanced disease and can include visceral ischemia such as perforated bowel, and myocardial and cerebral infarctions. In many patients with rheumatoid arthritis, some degree of vasculitis is present at some time or another but it is usually limited to synovial vessels.

Rheumatoid nodules are usually subcutaneous and often are found over the extensor surface of the elbows, Achilles tendons, and the toes. They are firm and freely movable but can be uncomfortable since they are found over bony pressure points. Nodules, as previously mentioned, are also found in viscera such as the heart, lungs, and intestinal tract and in the dura.

# PATHOPHYSIOLOGY

The most popular causative theory is that the rheumatoid disease process is the result of an autoimmune response. A specific antibody, rheumatoid factor (RF), has been found in the serum of 80% of adult patients; however, it is nonspecific for rheumatoid arthritis since it has also been found in high titers in a number of other diseases. Current theory suggests that RF plays a role in perpetuating disease activity as it reacts to the patient's own IgG, but the disease process is triggered by some other agent or mechanism. Whether this is a metabolic reaction or a specific virus continues to be a mystery.

There are 2 areas of intense study of the rheumatoid disease process. In the first area, the genetic basis of the disease and specifically the immunogenetic basis for the generation of RF is being examined. It has been firmly established that the host response to the initiating agent determines the outcome, rheumatoid arthritis. Most humans probably have the ability to make RF, given stimulation with immune complexes. Research is presently focusing on the genetic basis of human leukocyte antigen (HLA) associations.

The second area of investigation focuses on the lymphocytic abnormalities that cause persistence of the disease and chronic inflammation. The evidence to date indicates that helper lymphocytes in rheumatoid arthritis make deficient amounts of interleukin-2. Whether this is because of a primary abnormality or is induced by excessive macrophage stimulation is not known.

Immunoregulation, interleukins, and the various cell types involved in the immune response in rheumatoid inflammation are also current areas of investigation.

# RISK FACTORS

What is known about the incidence of definite rheumatoid arthritis is that the average annual age-adjusted incidence rates are 21.6 per 100,000 for males and 48 per 100,000 for females. The incidence rate increases with age in both sexes, with an overall sex ratio of 2.3 : 1 (female to male). Of particular interest is a finding identified by the disease registry of Rochester, Minnesota, conducted by the Mayo Clinic; a marked decrease in the incidence rate (by almost 50%) for women was noted between 1960–1964 and between

1970–1974. The data suggested that this finding may be related to the introduction and widespread acceptance of oral contraceptives in the 1960s.

The prevalence of definite rheumatoid arthritis for North American whites and blacks is 1%. Studies of 2 American Indian tribes indicate that prevalence rates are 3–7 times higher than in whites. The prevalence rate is 2–3 times greater in females than in males and, as is true for incidence, the prevalence of definite rheumatoid arthritis increases with increasing age. The rate approaches 2% in males and 5% in females over 55 years. Climate, geography, latitude, and altitude do not appear to influence prevalence.

Increasing age, female sex, certain ethnic groups (North American Indians), relatives of those with rheumatoid arthritis, lower income and education, and the presence of HLA-DR4, HLA-Dw4, and HLA-DR1 (Asian Indian and Jewish populations) are the currently identified risk factors. A reduction in risk postulated by exposure to oral contraceptives has been noted.

## COMMON CLINICAL FINDINGS

Rheumatoid arthritis is most commonly insidious in onset with some degree of polyarticular involvement, usually the small joints of the hands and feet, followed by the wrists and knees in a symmetrical pattern. Rheumatoid arthritis is characterized by joint swelling and pain that may be present for years or even a lifetime. It has been suggested that stress, for example, emotional or physical trauma, plays some role in inducing, exacerbating, and affecting the ultimate outcome in the disease. How such events related to pathogenesis has yet to be identified in a scientifically acceptable fashion. Anorexia, malaise, weight loss, fatigue, and low-grade fever may be present because of the systemic effect of the inflammatory process. The rheumatoid patient may complain of morning stiffness or "gelling" in affected joints that only begins to disappear after a considerable length of time (30 minutes to many hours). This is a characteristic feature and may give a clue to the diagnosis even when joint swelling is uncertain. The course of the disease is difficult to predict. Lengthy and complete remissions have been reported but generally it tends to become a chronic, progressive situation. The course of events (progression, remissions, and exacerbations) is frequently associated with type of onset, age at onset, and initial high titers of RF.

Diagnosis can often be made clinically; however, the presence of RF (present in 80% of patients) lends credibility to the diagnosis. An elevated erythrocyte sedimentation rate (ESR) is usually found and serves as a gross guide to the level of clinical activity. Other laboratory abnormalities may include a slight increase in white blood cell (WBC) count, increased C-reactive protein, and abnormal synovial fluids. X-ray examination early in the disease shows soft-tissue swelling and periarticular osteoporosis. As the disease progresses, narrowing of the joint space and bony erosions can be visualized. Late x-ray findings demonstrate malalignment and ankylosis.

## TREATMENT MODALITIES

Since there is no cure, treatment is aimed at controlling the disease and preventing deformities. A full treatment program must be individualized for each patient's situation, the purpose of which is to relieve pain, reduce inflammation, prevent joint damage, prevent or correct existing deformities, and keep joints movable and functioning. Components of the treatment program may include medications, rest, exercise, splints, assistive devices, heat, surgery, rehabilitation, and education of the patient and family members.

The aim of medication is to reduce pain and decrease inflammation. Salicylates remain the mainstay of pharmacological therapy. Analgesia is usually achieved with smaller doses of aspirin. When a full anti-inflammatory effect is needed, aspirin is taken in large doses regularly, even during periods when pain and swelling have subsided and the patient is feeling better. Nonsteroidal anti-inflammatory drugs (NSAIDs) such as ibuprofen, fenoprofen, indomethacin, and naproxen may be used as an alternative to aspirin when aspirin is ineffective or not tolerated. Other remissive agents helpful in the treatment of rheumatoid arthritis include gold, penicillamine, and the antimalarials, such as hydroxychloroquine sulfate (Plaquenil). Adrenocorticosteroids are seldom used except in a severe exacerbation or for intra-articular injections. Intra-articular injections of corticosteroids are helpful to temporarily relieve acute inflammation of specific joints. Methotrexate is one immunosuppresive agent that has been found to be effective in approximately 70% of patients tested. Its use is reserved for patients who have been refractory to conventional therapy.

Surgical procedures are used to relieve symptoms, improve function, and prevent or correct deformities. In the past, surgery was only considered late in the course of arthritis after severe joint destruction or deformity had developed. Preventive surgery is now being performed during the early, active phases of the disease and includes tendon transfer, osteotomy, synovectomy, specific joint replacement, and hip arthroplasty.

# PATIENT ASSESSMENT DATA BASE

## Health History

*Client:*
Martha Thompson

*Address:* 1112 Forest St., Jacksonville, FL 32209
*Telephone:* 904-934-0275
*Contact:* Thomas (husband)
*Address of contact:* Same as above
*Telephone of contact:* Same as above
*Age:* 42   *Sex:* Female   *Race:* White
*Educational background:* 2 years of college
*Religion:* Roman Catholic   *Marital status:* Married
*Usual occupation:* Homemaker
*Present occupation:* Same
*Source of income:* Husband's salary
*Insurance:* Blue Cross/Blue Shield
*Source of referral:* Self
*Source of history:* Patient and current chart
*Reliability of Historian:* Reliable
*Date of interview:* 5/20/89
*Reason for visit/Chief complaint:* Monthly follow-up, Rheumatology Clinic, University Hospital.
"These pills aren't helping me." "I am so stiff in the morning I can't seem to get myself going for hours."

## HEALTH PERCEPTION/HEALTH MANAGEMENT PATTERN

*Present Health Status*

Martha states that she was in excellent health until 5 months ago when she wore a pair of shoes that were "too tight." Her feet began to bother her to the point that she could barely walk. She saw a podiatrist who referred her to her family doctor. Within 2 weeks she experienced generalized exhaustion and "stiffness" on getting up in the morning. She states, "even my fingers hurt." The family doctor "did some blood tests and told me he thought I had rheumatoid arthritis and I should see Dr. Mills at the clinic here." "I started coming here 2 months ago; I took more tests that indicated I do have rheumatoid arthritis, and I'm here for a monthly visit to check on how I am doing.

This is the third clinic visit for Martha since her definitive diagnosis 2/21/89. The purpose of this visit is to monitor disease activity and to provide education and counseling for the patient and her husband about the disease and the therapeutic program. A home evaluation visit is scheduled for early June 1989.

During the last visit, Martha discussed her "devastation" about having an "incurable" disease. She was provided with medication instructions and was able to demonstrate comprehension of the rationale for dosage and schedule and the side effects to watch for. Her emotional response to her diagnosis somewhat limits her comprehension of physical activity instructions. "I can't let my poor husband have all the responsibility for the kids." It was suggested that her husband accompany her for this visit.

*Past Health Status*

**General Health.** General health has been good. No recent illnesses or health complaints until now.

***Prophylactic Medical/Dental Care.*** The patient has a physical examination every few years. Last gynecological exam (Pap smear) with postpartum visit of last child, 5 years ago. Last dental visit was 1 year ago. At age 18, all her upper teeth were extracted because of "infected gums." She wears a well-fitting upper appliance. Bottom teeth are in good repair. Has no problem with chewing.

***Childhood Illnesses.*** "I think I've had them all—chickenpox, measles, mumps, scarlet fever—All before age 10."

***Immunizations.*** All childhood immunizations and 1 tetanus shot when "I cut myself 5 years ago. I was vaccinated at age 25 to travel to Europe."

***Major Illnesses/Hospitalizations.*** "I've been pretty healthy; I've only been in the hospital to have my children in 1976, 1982, and 1983 and to have my teeth extracted in 1970."

### Current Medications

*Prescription:* Ascriptin (an analgesic preparation)—"16 tablets daily."

*Nonprescription:* None. "Once in a while I may take pseudoephedrine hydrochloride (Sudafed) when I have a cold or the flu.

***Allergies.*** No known allergies to food or medications.

### Habits

*Alcohol:* "Socially."

*Caffeine:* 2–3 cups of caffeinated coffee in the morning "to get me going and 1 cup in the late afternoon."

*Drugs:* See Current Medications.

*Tobacco:* "I tried it once at a party and didn't like it."

### *Family Health History*

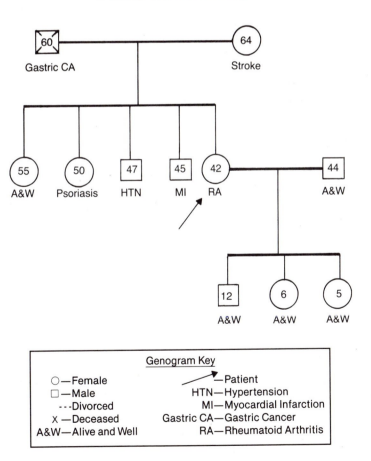

**Past Health Status — Continued**

No significant past family history for rheumatoid arthritis except that patient reports a maternal aunt as having "rheumatism."

## NUTRITIONAL/METABOLIC PATTERN

### Nutritional

Usually eats 3 well-balanced meals per day and a late afternoon snack "with the kids when they get home from school." States that she and her husband have a snack during the evening while watching television.

**Usual Daily Menu**
*Breakfast:* Orange juice, cottage cheese, toast with jelly, coffee.
*Lunch:* Sandwich, usually lunch meat or tuna fish, 1 glass of milk.
*Snack:* Cookies, peanut butter crackers or cake, 1 cup of coffee.
*Dinner:* Meat or fish, potato, vegetable, salad, and dessert.
Patient reports an evening snack of popcorn, ice cream, coffee, or a glass of wine.

### Metabolic

*Height:* 5 ft 2 in. (157 cm). *Weight:* 135 lb (61.3 kg). "I'm about 15 lb (6.8 kg) overweight. I've been on Weight Watchers' diets in the past and have lost the weight but right now I'm not able to concentrate on that."

## ELIMINATION PATTERN

### Bowel

Has 1 formed bowel movement every day, usually in the morning. Has never had problems with bowel movements or relied on laxatives.

### Bladder

Urinates about 5–6 times per day. Patient denies any problems or need to get up during the night to void. No history of urinary tract infections.

## ACTIVITY/EXERCISE PATTERN

### Activity/Exercise

"For the past several months, I have been just exhausted. I was never one for much physical exercise, maybe to trim down, but I figure I've always gotten enough exercise with the kids and keeping house." Patient describes leisure activities as sedentary and creative, "working with my hands." "I design and make pierced and cut lamp shades; I needlepoint, knit, and sew handmade pillows, usually after the kids go to bed; things I can do while watching TV. I also enjoy reading."

"When you ask me these questions I become afraid that maybe someday I will need to be in a wheelchair and have people waiting on me. So far I have been able to do things for myself, except for the shopping. My husband does that now. I keep pushing myself to do the things I ordinarily do."

**Self-Care Ability**

| | |
|---|---|
| Feeding—0 | Grooming—0 |
| Bathing—0 | General mobility—0 |
| Toileting—0 | Cooking—0 |
| Bed mobility—0 | Home maintenance—0 |
| Dressing—0 | Shopping—0 |

> ### *Functional Levels Code*
> 0—Full self-care
> I—Requires use of equipment or device
> II—Requires assistance or support
> III—Requires assistance or support from another person and equipment or device
> IV—Is dependent and does not participate

**Oxygenation/Perfusion**

*Last Chest X-Ray:* "Can't remember; I think it was normal."
*Last ECG:* 2/21/89—Within normal limits (WNL).
*Sinus Rhythm:* Rate 84.

*Cardiac Risk Factors*

|  | Positive | Negative |
|---|---|---|
| Sedentary life-style | X | |
| Hyperlipidemia | | X |
| Cigarette smoking | | X |
| Diabetes | | X |
| Obesity | X | |
| Hypertension | | X |
| Hypervigilant personality | | X |
| Family history of heart disease | X | |

## SLEEP/REST PATTERN

**Sleep/Rest**

Patient reports no problems with sleep, once in bed. "I've always been a night owl, watching the late show till 1 o'clock in the morning." States she usually awakens at 7 AM "to see the kids off to school." "Since this started I'm having a hard time getting up because I am so stiff. It's getting more difficult to get going in the morning." Denies the use of sleep aids and is not in the practice of resting during the day.

## COGNITIVE/PERCEPTUAL PATTERN

**Hearing**

Patient denies hearing problems; no report of "ringing" in ears.

**Vision**

Excellent vision; she does not wear glasses or contacts.

**Sensory Perception**

Martha is right-hand dominant. She describes past experiences with pain management as "ignoring it as best I can. I have never liked taking pills and usually use them as the last resort." The sensations of taste, touch, and smell are intact.

**Learning Style**

Learns best by explanation and demonstration. Patient describes herself as someone who is interested in learning new skills, and that she frequently takes evening courses with friends to learn crafts. Does not anticipate difficulty with learning "all she can about the disease or with following instructions." "I like to try new things."

## SELF-PERCEPTION/SELF-CONCEPT PATTERN

**Self-Perception/Self-Concept**

Martha describes herself as a strong person. "I basically feel good about myself, although I tend to be insecure and intimidated with new people." "I wish I looked a little better. I feel much more positive about myself when I am thinner." Martha states

*Self-Perception/Self-Concept—Continued*

that she hopes her body won't change because of the disease. "When I am in the waiting room and see some of the other patients with deformities or in wheelchairs I pray that won't happen to me. I don't think I could take it. I don't like the idea that maybe someday I will be dependent on others. I don't want to be a burden on anyone." She also states, "It makes me angry and depressed that I am feeling tired and that I am pushing myself to do just ordinary household chores. I frequently get annoyed and frustrated with small things when I am in a situation I can't seem to control. I feel so helpless about not being able to do the things I normally do. I am afraid of the outcome of this and sometimes it helps to pretend it is not happening. Lately I have become somewhat depressed with my situation. I have done what I have been told and I don't feel any better. All this aspirin, and they don't seem to be working. Sometimes I forget to take them, and then I think, what's the sense of this since they don't seem to help anyway. There is no cure! In the past when I have been upset about something, I usually get angry or hurt and then I seem to pull myself together and work through it somehow on my own."

## ROLE/RELATIONSHIP PATTERN

*Role/Relationship*

Martha lives in a small cape-style home with her 3 children and her husband. "Usually I make the major decisions about handling money, the general operation of the home, and enforcing the rules." Her husband works 2 jobs and is off 2 or 3 evenings a week and on weekends. "My husband is very supportive; he will do anything to help out the situation, but I guess sometimes I wish he would be more understanding of how I feel without me having to tell him or ask him to do things. He has no idea how frustrating this is for me. I don't like having to ask him to assume more responsibility for the children or for the maintenance of our home."

In handling family problems she stated, "I usually handle things myself and my husband goes along with it. He is good like that. My family is very dependent on me right now; my children are small (ages 12, 6, and 5); they need me to do everything for them. I don't like having to depend on other mothers for rides to lessons or games when I'm not sure I can reciprocate. I don't want the children to know I am not feeling well; they wouldn't understand anyway."

The patient describes many old and "good" friends who are supportive but "I can't ask them for help; they have their own lives and families. What is the sense in telling them you don't feel well—no one likes to listen to that all the time. I just try to make the best of it." In general she describes herself as "not a joiner"; she does participate in social activities with old friends or with parents of children's friends. "I am beginning to feel somewhat isolated when I see my friends going on with their lives, and I am so concerned with what will happen to me. Sometimes you just can't explain that to people. I feel no one understands how I really feel."

Income is described as sufficient to meet the family needs with her husband working a second job. "My immediate neighbors are good neighbors although I do not socialize with them. We are friendly and I could call on any one of them for an emergency, but my friends are mostly those from the past who do not live in the immediate area, although we visit often."

## SEXUALITY/REPRODUCTIVE PATTERN

*Sexuality/Reproductive*

The patient reports regular monthly periods, "heavier now that I am in my forties," with age of menarche at 13 years. Last menstrual period was "2 weeks ago." When asked about birth control, the patient states, "I am Catholic, which means we must rely on the rhythm method of birth control." The patient is para 3, gravida 3, normal vaginal deliveries. She describes the birthing experiences as not problematic and states that during her pregnancies, she "never felt better in her life."

When questioned about her sexual relationship she hesitated, and replied, "I am somewhat uncomfortable discussing this. I've really never discussed sexual intercourse with anyone. My husband and I have not had relations for the past couple of months since all this started. I am just so tired, and I think he feels afraid he will hurt or bother me but we haven't talked about it." Does not routinely perform self–breast examinations.

## COPING/STRESS TOLERANCE PATTERN

*Coping/Stress Tolerance*

"I feel that in general I have been able to handle stress fairly well. Usually when I get annoyed or am under stress I may yell at the kids and let it out, although I try not to let things bother me. I have noticed that sometimes rather than say how I really feel I just keep my mouth shut; then later I am angry with myself and, it seems, everyone around me. In terms of coping with the pain, the feeling tired, and the morning stiffness, I tend to keep it to myself; even the fears of what is to come I keep to myself. I know this is not good but my husband does so much already, I don't want to worry him, and the children wouldn't understand. Sometimes I find it very difficult since I have good days and other days it is so hard to get going and keep going."

"When I am not there to supervise things, like in the morning when the kids are getting dressed for school, I feel I am losing control of things. I have always been particularly concerned about how they are dressed and it seems they don't look as good when I'm not right there to organize the situation."

"I am feeling overwhelmed right now about some of these things; I can talk to my sister and a few friends who sometimes provide me with ideas on how to cope, but for the most part it is up to me to handle this myself." When questioned about coping with major problems in the past the patient stated that she learned to "handle things herself." She stated that "there are things I would do differently in retrospect, but in general things usually work themselves out for the best."

Denies use of medications to help with stressful situations in the past. Denies use of pain medications since "I've never really had any pain in the past to speak of."

## VALUE/BELIEF PATTERN

*Value/Belief*

"I believe if you are a good person the things you want in life will be attained. My family and home are the most important things to me. I feel I will let my family down if I cannot be there for them. Until all this happened, we have had a fairly good life; we've worked hard but we are happy. I am a fairly religious person, attending Mass every Sunday, and I do have faith that God will help us all with this." Religion is described as important to the patient and her family although she states that "religion is a private experience; I get comfort from the peace in attending

*Value/Belief—Continued*

church." When asked specifically what the major concerns for this visit are she stated, "The pain. Isn't there something besides aspirin that will help me? What can I do about the stiffness in the morning, and how can I feel better about myself and my situation?"

## Physical Examination

*General Survey*

A 42-year-old female, slightly overweight, appearing stated age and moderately anxious; neatly groomed, well-dressed, alert, and cooperative. The patient is accompanied by her husband.

*Vital Signs*

**Temperature:** 99°F (37.7°C) (oral)
**Pulse:** 80 regular (apical)
**Respirations:** 16 regular
**BP:** 130/76 left arm, 124/78 right arm, seated.

*Integument*

**Skin.** Skin on head, arms, torso, lower extremities is warm, slightly moist, and supple; no bruising, scarring, or lesions noted.
**Mucous Membranes.** Pink, slightly dry, and intact.
**Nails.** Neatly trimmed, deeply ridged, brittle, normal in color.

*HEENT*

**Head.** Scalp is normocephalic; no palpable masses. Hair is thick, shiny, and well groomed. Face is symmetrical, without drooping or swelling; without tenderness or crepitus on palpation; no bruising or scarring. Temporomandibular joint (TMJ) fully movable without pain or crepitation.
**Eyes.** Pupils equal, round, reactive to light and accommodation (PERRLA). Extraocular movements (EOMs) intact. Fundi are without edema, hemorrhage, or exudate. Gross visual acuity is intact.
**Ears.** Able to hear whisper at 2 ft (61 cm). Ears are bilaterally symmetrical and equal in size and shape. Left and right canals contain small amount of cerumen. Tympanic membranes are intact; no scarring or infection. Weber-Rinne test: air conduction greater than bone conduction.
**Nose.** Nostrils are pink, patent, and without septal deviation.
**Mouth/Throat.** Uvula is midline. Tonsils are nonvisual. Edentulous; upper appliance in good repair. Lower teeth are in excellent condition. No reported problems with dentition.

*Neck*

Trachea is midline; thyroid is palpable; nonenlarged; no palpable nodes. No limitation or pain on range of motion (ROM).

*Pulmonary*

Bilaterally symmetrical chest expansion; no pain or abnormalities noted on palpation. Breath sounds clear throughout on auscultation, anterior and posterior.

*Breast*

Well-developed normal female breasts, symmetrical in shape; skin is smooth and soft, without palpable masses, swelling, or tenderness; nipples are pink and prominent, without discharge.

*Cardiovascular*

Apical pulse 80 and regular. $S_1$ and $S_2$ of good quality; no murmurs or rub. Point of maximal impulse (PMI) at fifth intercostal space, midclavicular line. No audible carotid bruits.

**Peripheral Vascular**

All arterial pulses are palpable and within normal limits (WNL). No edema noted in lower extremities.

**Peripheral Pulses**
Temporal — 4 bilaterally
Carotid — 4 bilaterally
Brachial — 4 bilaterally
Radial — 4 bilaterally
Femoral — 4 bilaterally
Popliteal — 4 bilaterally
Posterior tibial — 4 bilaterally
Dorsalis pedis — 4 bilaterally

**Peripheral Pulse Scale**

0 — Absent
1 — Markedly diminished
2 — Moderately diminished
3 — Slightly diminished
4 — Normal

**Abdomen**

Active bowel sounds in all 4 quadrants; nontender, nondistended, soft, depressible abdomen; nonpalpable liver, spleen, and kidneys; no masses or bruits; no scarring or rashes noted.

**Musculoskeletal**

Upper extremities are bilaterally equal with normal muscle tone, mass, and strength. Joint inflammation and limited mobility are noted bilaterally in the metacarpophalangeal and proximal interphalangeal joints. The patient is unable to make a complete fist, and grip strength is weak. Bilateral wrists are swollen and painful on ROM. All other upper extremity joints are benign for pain and swelling. In the lower extremities, the hip joints are benign for pain on ROM and swelling. There is mild suprapatellar swelling, and the knees are painful with movement bilaterally; bilateral bulge sign is negative. Ankle joints are benign. The feet are painful with applied pressure to the metatarsophalangeal joints.

**Neurological**

***Mental Status.*** Alert and oriented to time, place, and person.
***Cranial Nerves.*** I through XII intact.
***Motor.*** As described above under Musculoskeletal.
***Sensory.*** Normal sensation to light touch bilaterally in upper and lower extremities.

***Deep Tendon Reflexes***

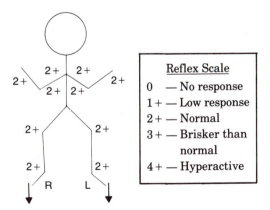

Reflex Scale

0 — No response
1+ — Low response
2+ — Normal
3+ — Brisker than normal
4+ — Hyperactive

| | |
|---|---|
| *Rectal* | Normal sphincter tone; no tenderness, nodules, or irregularities noted. Stool for occult blood is negative. |
| *Genitalia* | Normal female external genitalia. No bulging, ulcerations, nodules, bleeding, or discharge noted in vagina or cervix. Pap smear of 2/21/89 — negative. |

## Laboratory Data/Diagnostic Studies

*Laboratory Data*

*2/21/89*
*Rheumatoid Factor:* 1:250   *WBC:* 9.6/mm$^3$
(latex fixation)           *Hgb:* 12.4 g/100 ml
*Erythrocyte*              *Hct:* 37%
*Sedimentation Rate (ESR):*
60 mm/hr

*2/21/89: Synovial Fluid Analysis*
*Color:* Yellow          *Mucin Clot:* Poor
*Quantity:* 3 ml         *Clarity:* Cloudy
*WBC:* 20,000/70%        *Viscosity:* 4.0
*Bacteria:* No growth    *RA cells:* Positive

*4/18/89*
*Blood Salicylate Level:* 22
mg/dl
*ESR:* 52 mm/hr

*Diagnostic Studies*

*2/21/89*
*Bilateral Hand/Wrist Films:* Moderate soft-tissue thickening surrounding the metacarpophalangeal and interphalangeal joints, bilaterally. Minimal soft-tissue thickening surrounding bilateral wrists; question of old healed fracture in distal right radius.

## COLLABORATIVE PLAN OF CARE

*Diet*

1800 calorie, weight reduction diet.

*Medications*

*5/20/89:* Increase Ascriptin dose to 20 300-mg tablets/day.
Reinforce medication teaching: dosage increase, side effects, and administration schedule.

*Activity*

Continue with therapeutic exercise program as prescribed on 4/18/89, and rest/activity as outlined 4/18/89.

*Therapeutic Measures*

ESR next clinic visit — 6/17/89.
Home evaluation by skilled nursing and occupational therapist (OT) on 6/10/89.
Continue with patient/family education program as outlined on 2/21/89.
Continue with relaxation techniques as contracted with patient on 4/18/89.

## NURSING DIAGNOSES DEVELOPED IN CARE PLAN

Knowledge Deficit: Pain and Pain Control, p. 257
Disturbance in Self-Concept, p. 259
Alteration in Comfort, Stiffness, p. 261

## ADDITIONAL NURSING DIAGNOSES TO BE CONSIDERED

Anxiety
Fatigue
Fear
Impaired Physical Mobility
Ineffective Family Coping: Compromised
Knowledge Deficit: Disease Process
Knowledge Deficit: Physical Activity
Noncompliance, Potential for
Pain, Acute and Chronic
Self-Care Deficit, Dressing/Grooming, Potential for
Sexual Dysfunction, Potential

## NURSING CARE PLAN BASED ON IDENTIFIED NURSING DIAGNOSES

| | |
|---|---|
| **Knowledge Deficit: Pain and Pain Control** | **Related to:** Acute and chronic pain caused by rheumatoid arthritis and pain management techniques.<br>**Evidenced by:** The patient's description of inconsistent use of anti-inflammatory/analgesic agents. Complaints of pain and activity intolerance. |
| **Desired Patient Outcomes** | **The Patient Will:**<br>• Develop an understanding of pain and pain management in relation to the disease process.<br>• Incorporate appropriate pain management techniques into her daily life. |
| **Evaluation Criteria** | **During the Clinic Visit, the Patient Will:**<br>• Verbalize pain as characteristic of rheumatoid arthritis.<br>• Identify factors that exacerbate or influence the pain response.<br>• Reestablish realistic pain control goals.<br>• Verbalize an understanding of aspirin therapy and its side effects.<br>• Verbalize an understanding of daily activity log and pain rating scale.<br>• Verbalize plan for daily activity/rest schedule.<br>• Reestablish commitment to utilize relaxation techniques daily.<br>• Verbalize an understanding of and demonstrate the ability to actively participate in relaxation techniques.<br>• Report the use of appropriate pain management strategies on the next clinic visit. |

### Interventions

Assess and evaluate the patient's understanding of pain as a common problem of rheumatoid arthritis.

### Rationale

Total pain response is in part determined by patient expectations and perceptions (Thompson, et al, 1986, p. 1971). As patients learn that their sensations are typical and do not necessarily indicate the severity of disease, they may be less anxious when experiencing discomfort (Johnson and Repp, 1984, p. 585).

## Interventions

Reinforce previously taught disease concepts in relation to pain and physical expectations.

Assess and evaluate the patient's pain experience since the last visit utilizing the pain assessment tool with a subjective pain rating scale completed by the patient.

Assess the patient's expectations of pain control.

Teach/reinforce pain management strategies:

• Pharmacological

## Rationale

Instruction about arthritis should include information on the physical sensations experienced by persons who have the disease. Use of the word "discomfort" may decrease the patient's fear of coping with a long-term, physically and emotionally crippling disease (Johnson and Repp, 1984, p. 585). The degree of pain may fluctuate during the disease process and may vary in different areas of the body. Pain may be chronic due to structural joint changes or may be acute during disease exacerbation. Acute and chronic pain may be simultaneous (Smith-Pigg and Schroeder, 1984, p. 700).

The nurse must be able to assess the subjective and objective characteristics of both acute and chronic pain (Thompson, et al, 1986, p. 1978). In the assessment of chronic pain, the patient's description of the pain sensation is a more reliable indicator than objective measurements (American Nurses Association, 1986, p. 3). Physical assessment may yield some measure on the status of the disease process, but the only reliable measure of pain is the patient's description, satisfaction with present comfort level, and use of a pain rating scale. This prevents the assumption that acute pain is more severe than chronic pain (Smith-Pigg and Schroeder, 1984, p. 700). The person may not offer information about pain because of a desire to be a "good patient" or the person may assume that the nurse is already aware of how he or she is experiencing pain (Thompson, et al, 1986, p. 1976). The pain assessment tool should provide a holistic approach to pain assessment including physiological, psychological, and social components. On an outpatient basis, a daily activity log, identifying when pain occurs, intensifies, and subsides, and its precipitating factors and changes (using the pain rating scale) is most helpful. In addition, for analgesia administration, a graphic or flowsheet display documents the effectiveness of the analgesic. Trends need to be identified in order to evaluate nursing interventions in relation to expected patient outcomes (Thompson, et al, 1986, pp. 1978–1979). Pain response is influenced by a number of factors including disease activity, fatigue, depression, anxiety, tension, physical activity, and past experience with pain (American Nurses Association, 1986, p. 3).

Unrealistic expectations promote noncompliance. The patient who expects too much too soon will be disappointed with treatment and reach the unjustified conclusion that it has failed (Johnson and Repp, 1984, p. 585). Since the pain is not usually controlled as rapidly as the person would desire, or is never completely eliminated, it is not uncommon for the patient to seek nontraditional or unproved treatment methods (Smith-Pigg and Schroeder, 1984, p. 700). The impact of pain on an individual's life often leads to the use of non-traditional and unproven self-treatment methods (American Nurses Association: Outcome Standards or Rheumatology Nursing Practice, 1986, p. 3).

Rheumatoid arthritis does respond to aspirin. It is one of the safest and most effective drugs available for its treatment. In addition to relieving pain, it reduces inflammation. It is given in repeated doses and must be continued daily even when arthritic symptoms are absent. Many patients underestimate the value of aspirin and believe the physician is not doing enough when

| *Interventions* | *Rationale* |

prescribing "only aspirin." Taking aspirin is the medication program, which is only part of the total program for managing arthritis (Arthritis Foundation, Publication 4100/9-82, 1982, p. 7).

Frequent doses of aspirin are required to keep blood salicylate levels high. Aspirin is usually prescribed in doses sufficient to produce mild symptoms of drug intoxication. Once symptoms are produced, the dose is reduced slightly. To reduce gastric irritation, aspirin should be taken with food, and the patient instructed to watch for signs of bleeding, dark stools, and bruising (Luckmann and Sorensen, 1987, p. 1547).

• Nonpharmacological (positioning, activity and rest, relaxation)

Nonpharmacological pain management focuses on increasing the patient's tolerance to pain and decreasing the suffering in situations in which it may not be possible to eliminate or even alleviate the pain sensation (Johnson and Repp, 1984, p. 584). Interventions such as physical and emotional rest, pacing of activities, heat and cold, and positioning and relaxation techniques should be incorporated as basic pain control measures (Smith-Pigg and Schroeder, 1984, p. 701).

Positioning is one of the simplest pain-reducing techniques employed by the nurse. Posture is important; poor posture puts a strain on joints and increases pain. The nurse should assist the patient in understanding and performing ROM exercises and in identifying those positions that promote contracture development. Joints should be maintained in a functional position (Johnson and Repp, 1984, p. 586). Assisting the patient to develop a plan for balancing activity and rest is an important strategy in controlling fatigue and inflammation. At home, the patient needs to establish a balance. The nurse will need to consider helping the patient plan home and work routines and assist with developing a daily rehabilitation program for joint protection, strengthening, and posture building (Johnson and Repp, 1984, p. 586; Luckmann and Sorensen, 1987, p. 1547).

Relaxation is becoming well recognized as a method of controlling stress and pain. Relaxation techniques begin with an explanation of the procedure and a discussion of the usefulness of the technique. The relaxation response can be explained to the patient as a new way of responding to pain or stress, and teaching the physiological changes occurring with this response can help the patient understand the rationale behind this strategy. A contract may be developed to clarify the nurse and patient responsibilities. The patient must learn a sequence of steps to promote relaxation and must practice twice a day for several weeks until the relaxed feeling can be obtained through recall. The patient must be an active planner and participant (Johnson and Repp, 1984, pp. 586–588).

**Disturbance in Self-Concept**

*Related to:* Role changes in the family structure.
*Evidenced by:* Patient's reports: "I feel so helpless about not being able to do the things I normally do." "I don't like having to rely on my family for help with even the simplest things." "Sometimes I get so angry and depressed. I feel no one understands how I really feel."

### Desired Patient and Family Outcomes

**The Patient Will:**
- Understand that changes in self-concept are normal responses to rheumatoid arthritis.
- Be able to openly express feelings and concerns with nurse and family members.
- Utilize coping strategies that enhance self-concept.

**The Husband Will:**
- Understand the need for role changes.
- Identify role changes.
- Identify strategies to cope with role changes.

### Evaluation Criteria

**The Patient Will:**
- Verbalize that alterations of self-concept are normal responses to rheumatoid arthritis.
- Be able to discuss/describe feelings in relation to the impact of the disease.
- Identify realistic, attainable goals for herself.
- Recognize and articulate her own strengths and abilities.
- Recognize controllable situations and those that are beyond her capabilities.
- Be able to identify and articulate needs.
- Report feeling less "helpless" by her next clinic visit.
- Report contacting and/or participating in a local support group within the next month.
- Verbalize how to access community resources.

**The Husband Will:**
- Verbalize understanding of the disease process and the physical, psychological, and social impact on his spouse.
- Identify necessary role changes.
- Articulate a willingness to accept role changes.
- Identify and/or access community resources.

## Interventions

Explain the role of rheumatoid arthritis in relation to altered self-concept to the patient and spouse.

Reinforce the need for and assist with identification of role changes with the patient and spouse (e.g., the husband may assume responsibility for early morning activities of family members).

Assist the patient and spouse with identification of strategies to cope with role changes:

- Provide and promote discussion of alternatives and options.
- Provide educational materials.
- Identify and refer to community resources and supports.
- Suggest local arthritis support groups.
- Acquaint with local chapter of Arthritis Foundation.

## Rationale

Rheumatoid diseases may present with remissions and exacerbations or follow a declining trajectory. This places the person's self-concept in constant jeopardy. During exacerbations, the person may not be able to maintain previous roles, responsibilities, and leisure activities. Self-care abilities are also compromised. A disturbed self-concept creates feelings of reduced self-worth and helplessness (Smith-Pigg and Schroeder, 1984, p. 706).

The family must also adjust to changes in the individual's self-concept. The family may need to carry out roles previously accomplished by the person (Smith-Pigg and Schroeder, 1984, p. 707).

Education and client/family involvement in decision making and care requirements are important to the impact of arthritis on the patient's self-esteem and the quality of life (Kneisl and Ames, 1986, p. 1733). Experiences increase the person's knowledge and ability to cope. In addition, observing others making successful plans and actions as well as using other forms of social support contributes to coping responses (Thompson, et al, 1986, p. 1896). Written materials provide useful information. Health care providers must remember that "telling is not teaching." Family education is needed concerning the disease process, impact, and treatment to enlist support.

## Interventions

Assess and evaluate:

- Patient perception and appraisal of physical, psychological, and social self.
- Patient's ability to set realistic goals.
- Patient's strengths.

Establish open, accepting, and empathetic communication.

Reinforce the patient's assets and strengths whenever possible. Verbalize and reinforce past and present successes.

Assist the patient with realistic goal setting and identification of coping strategies.

Assist with planning activities that promote the patient's self-concept in relation to the physical, psychological and social self.

## Rationale

Nurses encounter numerous situations of role change and are in the most opportune position to assess the patient's psychosocial needs during role transitional periods and provide the necessary interventions based on the persons' needs and deprivations created by role transitions. Health/illness transitions denote a change in role relationships, expectations, and abilities (Thompson, et al, 1986, pp. 1817–1818). In forming appropriate intervention strategies for disturbance in self-concept, the nurse should employ major interventions (requiring skill in assessment, communication, and counseling techniques) (Thompson, et al, 1986, p. 1823).

The patient needs to feel valued, worthwhile, and trusted.

Positive values of self-worth help persons seek and deal with their environmental experiences constructively. Success experiences can help with feeling less powerless. As the patient increases self-help skills, there will be a concurrent decrease in feelings of helplessness, a renewed feeling of wellness, and a decrease in suffering (Johnson and Repp, 1984, p. 585).

In order to adjust successfully to role transitions a person must be able to incorporate new knowledge, alter expressive and instrumentive behaviors, and change the concept of self. Patients need to recognize and control those aspects of experience that are within their control (Thompson, et al, 1986, p. 1818).

Effective coping strategies must be preserved, augmented, and developed; effective coping strategies result in a decrease in uncomfortable feelings, generation of hope, enhancement of self-esteem, maintenance of positive interpersonal relationships, and maintenance of or improvement in the state of coping (Thompson, et al, 1986, p. 1827).

---

| **Alteration in Comfort, Stiffness** | *Related to:* Joint inflammation, rheumatoid arthritis. *Evidenced by:* Patient reports of inability to "move in the morning. I just can't seem to get my joints to move." |
| --- | --- |
| **Desired Patient Outcomes** | **The Patient Will:**<br>• Understand the relationship between morning stiffness, disease activity, medications, and activities of daily living.<br>• Identify measures to manage morning stiffness.<br>• Incorporate measures to manage morning stiffness as part of daily activities.<br>• Experience decreased morning stiffness. |
| **Evaluation Criteria** | **The Patient Will:**<br>• Explain "morning stiffness," its relationship to disease activity, medication, and activities of daily living.<br>• Describe appropriate methods of decreasing morning stiffness.<br>• Describe a schedule of daily activities that take into account the intensity and duration of stiffness.<br>• Use appropriate measures for decreasing morning stiffness.<br>• Verbalize a decrease in the intensity and duration of morning stiffness. |

## Interventions

The patient recognizes "morning stiffness" as a problem that needs to be assessed separately from pain, addressed at each clinic visit.

## Rationale

Stiffness is not identified on the National Conference List of Accepted Nursing Diagnoses but presents a problem that can be diagnosed by nurses and influenced by nursing interventions. Stiffness can range from a temporary localized condition occurring after a period of inactivity and relieved by easy exercise movements to a profound, generalized immobilization lasting for several hours. The duration of morning stiffness and the accompanying fatigue time are more accurate indicators of the control of the inflammatory rheumatic disease than pain (Smith-Pigg and Schroeder, 1984, pp. 701–702).

---

Assess and evaluate:

- Patient's understanding of morning stiffness and its implications.
- Morning stiffness with the patient using a daily activity log and including its intensity and duration.

Morning stiffness is measured by the amount of time elapsed from awakening until movement is at its optimum for the rest of the day. The nurse and the patient use this assessment as an indicator of improvement or lack of adequate disease control (Smith-Pigg and Schroeder, 1984, p. 702). Supervision of a patient's progress with self-management techniques can be by reviewing records that the person may keep. Supervision also may help the person build self-assurance. With response to therapy, morning stiffness should decrease. If the time is decreased to 30 minutes, it is 1 indication that the patient is improved and the treatment is effective (Jarvis, 1985, p. 603).

---

Identify measures to relieve morning stiffness:

- Ascriptin taken on awakening, while still in bed; the patient remains in bed at least 60 minutes.
- Use of an electric blanket, flannel sheets, down comforter, or other light-weight sleeping materials.
- Other heat-providing measures; early morning hot showers/tub soaks, hot packs, heating pad, or paraffin baths for fingers and feet.

The earlier the intervention, the sooner the results are secured and the stiffness relieved. Medication and water can be kept at the bedside for early-morning administration. Warmth may be effective in providing a comfortable sleeping environment and relief. Cold usually increases stiffness. Heat is an old and effective means of relaxing muscles and relieving pain. Most people with rheumatoid arthritis feel their pain and stiffness the most in the morning. A hot shower or bath just after getting up may help with this. (Arthritis Foundation, 1983, p. 6).

---

Assist the patient with identification of role change needs in relation to morning stiffness.

Daily living skills such as personal care and mobility are greatly affected by morning stiffness. The ability to carry out activities may fluctuate and challenge the individual's and family's ability to adapt. Helping the family examine realistic approaches to and expectations of the situation provides structure and support in spite of the disequilibrium being experienced. Giving choices helps the family feel the important need of control over what is happening (Thompson, et al, 1986, p. 1933).

---

Teach the patient that increased time may be necessary to complete activities of daily living (ADLs). Capitalize on individual strengths.

More time may be needed to complete ADLs independently. Accomplishment of *realistic* tasks provides an opportunity for a greater sense of self-confidence and self-worth (Doenges and Jeffries, 1989, p. 760).

## QUESTIONS FOR DISCUSSION

1. What are the common signs and symptoms of rheumatoid arthritis? Identify the risk factors.
2. The patient develops "tinnitus." Explain the significance of this finding in relation to the continuance of Ascriptin therapy.
3. Outline the therapeutic plan of care for the patient with rheumatoid arthritis.

4. What is the significance of the erythrocyte sedimentation rate (ESR) in relation to the disease process?
5. Identify the nursing actions following a synovial fluid tap.
6. What assessment parameters are used to distinguish between pain and stiffness in evaluating the disease activity of the rheumatoid arthritis patient?
7. What role does stress play in the onset and exacerbation of rheumatoid arthritis?

# REFERENCES

American Nurses Association: Outcome Standards for Rheumatology Nursing Practice, MS-121.5 M 86 R. ANA, Kansas City, MO, 1986.

Arthritis Foundation: Arthritis Medical Information Series, Publication 4030/5-83. Arthritis Foundation, Atlanta, GA, 1983.

Arthritis Foundation: Arthritis Practical Information, Publication 4100/9-82, Atlanta, GA, 1982.

Doenges, M and Jeffries, M: Nursing Care Plans: Nursing Diagnoses in Planning Patient Care, ed 2. FA Davis, Philadelphia, 1989.

Jarvis, L: Community Health Nursing: Keeping the public healthy. FA Davis, Philadelphia, 1985.

Johnson, J and Repp, E: Nonpharmacologic pain management in arthritis. Nurs Clin North Am 19:583, 1984.

Kneisl, C and Ames S: Adult Health Nursing: A Biopsychosocial Approach. Addison-Wesley, Reading, Mass, 1986.

Luckmann, J and Sorensen, K: Medical-Surgical Nursing: A Psychophysiologic Approach. WB Saunders, Philadelphia, 1987.

Smith-Pigg, J and Schroeder, P: Frequently occurring problems with rheumatic diseases. Nurs Clin North Am 19:699, 1984.

Thompson, J, et al: Clinical Nursing. CV Mosby, St. Louis, 1986.

# BIBLIOGRAPHY

Bacon, P and Salmon, M: Modes of action of second line agents. Scand J Rheumatol 64:17, 1987.

Banwell, B: Exercise and mobility in arthritis. Nurs Clin North Am 19:605, 1984.

Bates, B: A Guide to Physical Examination, ed 3. JB Lippincott, Philadelphia, 1986.

Doenges, M and Moorhouse, M: Nurse's Pocket Guide: Nursing Diagnoses with Interventions. FA Davis, Philadelphia, 1988.

Hart, F: Current concepts in the rheumatic diseases: Etiology and treatment. Semin Arthritis Rheum 15:4, 1985.

Koener, M and Dickenson, G: Adult arthritis: A look at some of its forms. Am J Nursing, February 1983, p 253.

Neuberger, J and Neuberger, G: Epidemiology of the rheumatic diseases. Nurs Clin North Am 19:597, 1984.

Maskowitz, R: Clinical Rheumatology, ed 2. Lea & Febriger, Philadelphia, 1982.

Meinhart, N and McCaffrey, M: Pain: A Nursing Approach to Assessment and Analysis. Appleton-Century-Crofts, Norwalk, Conn, 1983.

Price, S and Wilson, L: Pathophysiology: Clinical Concepts of Disease Processes, ed 3. McGraw-Hill, New York, 1986.

Rodman, G and Schumacher, H: Primer on Rheumatic Diseases. Atlanta, Ga, Arthritis Foundation, 1983.

Scherman, S: Community Health Nursing Care Plans, John Wiley & Sons, New York, 1985.

Spiegel, J, et al: Are rehabilitation programs for rheumatoid arthritis patients effective? Semin Arthritis Rheum 16:260, 1987.

Spitz, P: The medical, personal and social costs of rheumatoid arthritis. Nurs Clin North Am 19:575, 1984.

Wallace, D: The role of stress and trauma in rheumatoid arthritis and systemic lupus erythematosus. Semin Arthritis Rheum 16:575, 1987.

Wolf, F: Arthritis and musculoskeletal pain. Nurs Clin North Am 19:565, 1984.

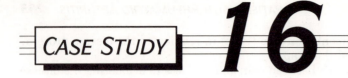

# A PATIENT WITH A HIP FRACTURE

Jean D'Meza Leuner, M.S., R.N.

## ANATOMY AND PHYSIOLOGY OF THE MUSCULOSKELETAL SYSTEM

The musculoskeletal system comprises the bones, the joints that connect the bones, and the muscles that move the bones. The 206 bones of the body are either long, short, flat, irregular, or round. The shape of the bone reflects the function the bone will serve. The bones of the body produce red blood cells within the red bone marrow. In addition, calcium and phosphorus are stored in the bone. Approximately 99% of the body's calcium and 90% of its phosphate is within bone. Bones give the body the rigidity it requires as well as protection from injury to internal structures. The skeleton of the body works with the muscles to produce coordinated movements.

Upon examination of a long bone within the body (Fig. 16–1), the diaphysis or long shaft of the bone can be observed with an epiphysis at either end of the bone. The bone is covered with periosteum except where an articulating surface is found. At these areas, a thin hyaline cartilage is present. The periosteum acts to protect the bone, and the blood vessels in the periosteum bring nutrients to the bone and remove wastes.

Dense compact bone is found in the diaphysis of long bones and to a much lesser extent in the epiphysis of these bones. Cancellous bone that is soft and spongy with red bone marrow for hematopoiesis is found at the end of long bones and at the ridges and crests of the ileum and the tibia. In the center of the shaft of the long bones, fat cells, called yellow marrow, replace red bone marrow with the aging process. Bones that are not long bones contain no marrow cavity but have cancellous bone internally and a thin layer of compact bone on the exterior surface of the bone.

The microscopic unit found within compact bone is the haversian system. A haversian system comprises concentric layers of compact bone cells called lamellae, and a central canal with blood vessels and a nerve. Lacunae, small cavities with bone cells and tissue fluid, communicate with the haversian canal through smaller canals, the canaliculi. The purpose of the haversian canal is to provide nutrients to osteocytes and bone-forming cells and to remove the wastes from bone growth.

New bone formation occurs continuously along with the process of reabsorption. A balance is struck whereby bones do not become excessively thick with new bone formation or too thin from reabsorption. This balance is related to the calcium and phosphate levels as well as the process of metabolism in the body.

Muscles move the body parts as a result of the tightening and shortening of the fibers that comprise each motor unit. A muscle gains its strength in response to the number of motor units contracting within the muscle and the frequency with which the motor unit is stimulated. Muscle fibers can arise from a bone and be considered fleshy, or they can be fibrous attachments called tendons. Skeletal muscles are responsible for approximately 40%–45% of the body's total weight.

Two bone surfaces that come together and articulate form a joint. Joints are classified according to their degree of movement. Most joints are diarthrotic, or freely movable.

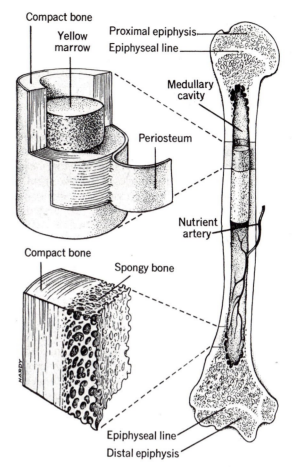

**FIGURE 16–1.** Diagram of a long bone shown in longitudinal section. (From Patrick, ML, et al: Medical-Surgical Nursing: Pathophysiological Concepts. JB Lippincott, Philadelphia, 1986, p 1274, with permission.)

On the inner surface of a diarthrotic joint is a membrane, the synovial membrane. This membrane consists of villous folds that contain blood and lymph vessels. Synovial fluid is stored in the villous folds for the purpose of lubricating the articular surface to facilitate movement and adequate functioning of the joint. A joint capsule formed by ligaments and tendons houses the bones, articular cartilage, synovial fluid, nerves, and blood as well as the lymph vessels found in a diarthrotic joint.

The hip joint (Fig. 16–2) comprises the head of the femur and the concave acetabulum of the pelvic bone. The pelvic bones unite anteriorly at the symphysis pubis and posteriorly at the sacrum. On the margin of the

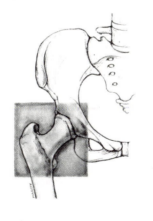

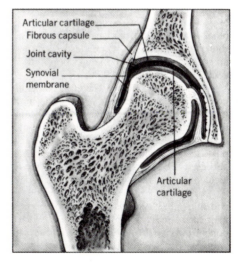

**FIGURE 16–2.** Hip joint, showing structure of synovial joints. Joint cavities have been enlarged. (From Patrick, ML, et al: Medical-Surgical Nursing: Pathophysiologic Concepts. JB Lippincott, Philadelphia, 1986, p 1276, with permission.)

acetabulum, a fibrocartilaginous labrum can be observed. The head of the femur sits deeply into the acetabulum, thus preventing the removal of the femoral head without damage to the labrum. The labrum extends across the acetabular notch and is referred to as the transverse acetabular ligament. The synovial membrane, the membrane that contains the joint-lubricating fluid lining the capsule of the hip, arises from the labrum and continues toward the articular cartilage. The synovial membrane passes across the notch of the acetabulum covering the fat and connective tissue of the acetabular fossa.

The fibrous membrane of the hip contains three prominent ligaments and an area of circular fibers called the zona orbicularis, which forms a collar around the neck of the femur. The ligaments (iliofemoral, ischiofemoral, and pubofemoral) extend from the pelvis to the femur. In addition, the ligament of the head (capitate ligament) lies within the cavity of the hip joint. Surrounded by the synovial membrane, it originates at the acetabular fossa and transverse ligament and extends to the fovea of the head. An unusually long ligament of the head is presumed to be the reason why dislocation of the hip is sometimes present in the neonate.

Nerves that supply the hip joint include the femoral nerve supplying the anterior portion of the joint, the obturator nerve, and occasionally the accessory obturator supplying the anteroinferior part of the joint. The posterior aspect is supplied by a small branch of the nerve to the quadratus femoris. A branch of the superior gluteal may innervate the upper lateral portion of the joint as well.

The ligaments in the hip area are primarily avascular. The small vessels that supply the joint include both femoral circumflex, both gluteals, the obturator, and the upper perforating branch of the profunda femoris. While the femoral circumflex vessels are prominent in size, they primarily supply the femur and to a much lesser extent supply the capsule.

Movements at the hip occur with coordination from the knee and the ankle. The specific movements that occur at the hip include flexion, extension, adduction, abduction, and medial as well as lateral rotation.

# PATHOPHYSIOLOGY: FRACTURE OF THE HIP

A fracture of the upper end of the femur, also known as the proximal end, can be classified as either intracapsular or extracapsular (Fig. 16–3). An intracapsular fracture is any break through the head of the femur, just below the head of the femur, or through the neck of the femur. An extracapsular fracture occurs in a point distal to the neck of the femur and may extend about 2 in. (5 cm) below the lesser trochanter. Extracapsular fractures are also known as intertrochanteric or subtrochanteric fractures.

A fracture that occurs as a result of a fall is often preceded by a rotational force that fractures the fragile femur and ends with the patient on the ground. This type of fracture causes the patient to be immobile. An impacted femoral neck fracture allows the afflicted person to continue weight bearing on the affected leg.

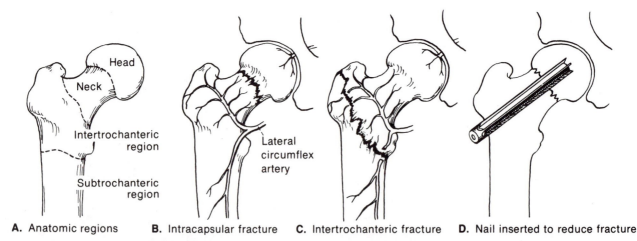

**A.** Anatomic regions      **B.** Intracapsular fracture      **C.** Intertrochanteric fracture      **D.** Nail inserted to reduce fracture

**FIGURE 16–3.** (*A*) Normal proximal end of femur. (*B*) Intracapsular fracture of proximal end of femur. Note blood supply. (*C*) Extracapsular intertrochanteric fracture. Note effect of fracture on blood supply. (*D*) Intracapsular fracture with nail inserted for reduction. (From Luckmann, J and Sorensen, KC: Medical-Surgical Nursing: A Psychophysiologic Approach, ed 3. WB Saunders, Philadelphia, 1987, p. 1536, with permission.)

# RISK FACTORS

Within the community, 30% of the population that is older than the age of 65 fall annually. In the group of individuals older than the age of 80, the rate increases to 40%. Falls are considered the sixth most common cause of death for the elderly (Tinetti, et al, 1988, p. 1701). A fracture in the neck of the femur is most often seen in debilitated elderly patients. Intertrochanteric fractures are often observed in older, more active persons. The elderly population is more prone to fractures of the hip due to osteoporosis and a lack of stability on their feet as well as other factors.

Hip fractures are more common in whites and Orientals than in blacks. This is directly proportional to the increased prevalence of osteoporosis in the first two groups.

Age-related changes that contribute to the prevalence of hip fractures in the elderly include a decrease in visual acuity, a change in the perception of spatial relationships, a decrease in muscle mass and strength, orthostatic hypotension, hearing loss, caloric malnutrition, and vitamin deficiencies. In addition, elderly patients tend to be ingesting several medications at one time without a thorough evaluation of possible adverse drug interactions. Drug effects or interactions could impair a person's cognitive abilities as well as physical state.

Osteoporosis can be caused by specific disease processes; however, it is also related to postmenopausal bone loss in women and age-related bone loss in men.

A diet poor in calcium has been associated with the presence of osteoporosis in the elderly. Other factors that have been noted to contribute to osteoporosis include a sedentary lifestyle, alcohol abuse, cigarette smoking, and the excessive use of corticosteroids.

Risk factors in the environment that might predispose one to a fall include the presence of obstacles, slippery floors, poor lighting, poorly defined floors and stairs, and improperly fitting clothing.

# COMMON CLINICAL FINDINGS

The patient who has suffered a fracture at the hip presents with the affected leg shortened, adducted, and externally rotated. A femoral fracture in the extracapsular area (outside of the joint and capsule, through the greater and lesser trochanter or the intertrochanteric area) demonstrates a more pronounced external rotation and shortness of the extremity as compared with an intracapsular fracture. In addition, in the presence of an extracapsular fracture the patient exhibits spasms of the muscle with intractable pain, and ecchymosis may be visible at the fracture site. Positioning the leg in external rotation with flexion may relieve some of the discomfort for the patient.

When an impacted femoral neck fracture is present, the patient may have weight bearing on the affected extremity, and shortening of the extremity may not be visible. Pain is present with movement.

The most frequently seen complications include shock and hemorrhage at the time of the injury and immediately postoperatively. Avascular necrosis of the head of the femur and delayed healing are most often seen with fractures. Fat emboli syndrome can occur with fractures of the lower extremities, particularly the long bones, and also when multiple fractures occur.

Complications may arise as a result of immobility. Dislocation of the femur may be evident postoperatively and devices used for the internal fixation of the hip may become dislodged, weaken, or break causing damage to the adjacent soft tissue.

# TREATMENT MODALITIES

The treatment plan for a person with a fractured hip depends on the type of fracture sustained and the person's mental and physical condition. Fractures of the femur are usually treated with an open reduction. Through this surgical opening into the hip joint, the fracture can be assessed and stabilized with the use of internal fixation devices.

Internal fixation allows the patient to resume activity soon after the accident has occurred. Fractures of the head or proximal femoral neck may be treated with the use of a femoral prosthesis. A prosthesis is the treatment of choice when a concern for nonunion or avascular necrosis exists or if the fracture is difficult to reduce. Distal neck fractures are often nailed or pinned. Also screws, wires, or rods can be used. Plates may be used as well, which are secured to the shaft of the femur.

# PATIENT ASSESSMENT DATA BASE

## Health History

*Client:*
Mrs. Grace Carr

*Address:* 18 Lansdowne Street, Baltimore, Maryland 21205
*Telephone:* 301-555-5019
*Contact:* Mr. Barbara Bondreau (daughter)
*Address of contact:* 112 Great Pond Road, Towson, Maryland 21204
*Telephone of contact:* 301-555-0218
*Age:* 83     *Sex:* Female     *Race:* White
*Educational background:* High school graduate
*Religion:* Methodist     *Marital status:* Widowed
*Former occupation:* Secretary
*Present occupation:* Retired
*Source of income:* Social Security
*Insurance:* SSI
*Source of referral:* Self
*Source of history:* Self
*Reliability of historian:* Reliable
*Date of interview:* 1/7/90
*Reason for visit/Chief complaint:* "Pain in my left hip and I am unable to walk."

### HEALTH PERCEPTION/HEALTH MANAGEMENT PATTERN

*Present Health Status*

Patient slipped on some water on the kitchen floor (melted snow after retrieving mail). She arrived in the emergency department by ambulance. Was in excruciating pain when she arrived at the hospital. The affected leg was externally rotated and appeared to be shortened. Any motion of the stretcher caused the patient pain. She was examined by Dr. Blevins in the emergency department and admitted to the orthopedic unit with the diagnosis of left intertrochanteric fracture.

*Past Health Status*

*General Health.* Mrs. Carr stated that her health has been generally "good." She does suffer from degenerative joint disease. After long periods of sitting, she experiences marked stiffness and discomfort. Her left knee has been quite stiff and daily activities are somewhat limited because of the knee problem. Has had varicosities of both legs, and a vein stripping in the left leg in 1948. No phlebitis or related problems since 1948.
*Prophylactic Medical/Dental Care.* Sees her local doctor when the need arises. "If I saw the doctor for every ache and pain I have, I would be at the doctor's office all the time." Last visit to the dentist was approximately 3 years ago when her denture did not fit well.
*Childhood Illnesses.* Cannot recall.
*Immunizations.* Unknown.
*Major Illnesses/Hospitalizations. 1948:* Left-leg vein stripping and ligation. In 1968 she developed pneumonia, which subsided after a lengthy course of medication.

*Current Medications*
*Prescription:* Takes chloral hydrate pills to help her sleep at night.

*Nonprescription:* Takes an analgesic (Excedrin) for joint pain; may take 2 every 3 hours with severe pain and stiffness; occasionally takes a laxative (Ex-Lax) for constipation.
**Allergies.** No known food or drug allergies.

### Habits
*Alcohol:* Enjoys a drink in the evening, usually a scotch before dinner.
*Caffeine:* Three cups of tea daily, maybe a cup of coffee in the morning.
*Drugs:* None. See Current Medications.
*Tobacco:* Denies use of tobacco.

### Family Health History

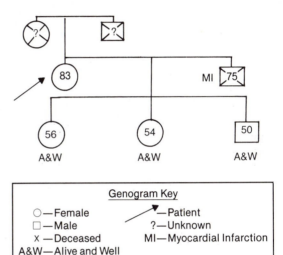

Genogram Key
○—Female          ➤—Patient
□—Male            ?—Unknown
x —Deceased       MI—Myocardial Infarction
A&W—Alive and Well

## NUTRITIONAL/METABOLIC PATTERN

### Nutritional

Mrs. Carr states, "I enjoy eating, although being alone for meals is not pleasant." She shops for her own food and prepares her own meals. She does note that at times it is difficult to get to the store and bring home the bundles. Neighbors are helpful, and a small local convenience store is not far away.

**Usual Daily Menu**
*Breakfast:*   Juice or fruit, toast or cereal, coffee or maybe tea, prunes once or twice a week.
*Lunch:*   Half a sandwich, tea, and a cookie.
*Dinner:*   Meat, potatoes, vegetable (pork chop, chicken breast, hamburger). Prefers cauliflower and peas as vegetables. Patient states that she keeps frozen dinners in the freezer because she usually does not feel like making dinner for herself. For dessert has ice cream or cookies (occasionally makes pudding) and tea.

### Metabolic

Mrs. Carr states that she thinks her weight is about 110 lb (50 kg) and she is 5 ft 3 in. (160 cm) tall. When asked about any skin problems she states, "My skin is very dry. I try to use cream and take fewer baths because at times it cracks and bleeds. Also, if I bump my leg or arm, I bruise easily and it doesn't go away." Patient has a full set of dentures that she knows how to care for. They fit well. Denies any difficulty with swallowing.

## ELIMINATION PATTERN

### Bowel

States she occasionally has a "problem with constipation, but I eat bran cereal and prunes on occasion and it really helps." Ex-Lax is helpful also when she cannot move her bowels. Bowel movements are usually very firm and dark brown. Her usual pattern is once every 3–4 days.

### Bladder

States she has "occasional burning with urination." She urinates infrequently, maybe 3 times a day but she regularly has to get up at night to urinate. Urine is yellow and not a large amount.

## ACTIVITY/EXERCISE PATTERN

### Activity/Exercise

Enjoys keeping the house "clean and tidy" and doing light gardening. Enjoys reading very much. States she doesn't have the energy she did when she was younger, but frequent rest breaks "keep me going." Occasional knee discomfort also "slows me down a bit."

#### Self-Care Ability

| | |
|---|---|
| Feeding—0 | Grooming—0 |
| Bathing—0 | General mobility—0 |
| Toileting—0 | Cooking—0 |
| Bed mobility—0 | Home maintenance—0 |
| Dressing—0 | Shopping—0 |

> ### Functional Levels Code
> 0—Full self-care
> I—Requires use of equipment or device
> II—Requires assistance or support from another person
> III—Requires assistance or support from another person and equipment or device
> IV—Is dependent and does not participate

### Oxygenation/Perfusion

**Last Chest X-Ray:** Unsure. Denies dyspnea, chest pain, wheezing, cough, sputum production, night sweats, bronchitis, thoracic trauma, or surgery.

#### Cardiac Risk Factors

| | Positive | Negative |
|---|:---:|:---:|
| Sedentary life-style | X | |
| Hyperlipidemia | | X |
| Cigarette smoking | | X |
| Diabetes | | X |
| Obesity | | X |
| Hypertension | | X |
| Hypervigilant personality | | X |
| Family history of heart disease | X | |

## SLEEP/REST PATTERN

### Sleep/Rest

Sleeps 5–6 hours a night. Wakes up 1–2 times a night for the past 10 years or so. Urinates once in the night time. Varies as to whether she falls back to sleep easily or stays awake. Does not feel rested in the morning. Has a big glass of warm milk prior to bed and takes a sleeping pill to help her fall asleep. During the day, she may take 3–4 rest breaks. "Sleeping on my back hurts;

my tail bone is always sore." Can't remember when she took a "real vacation" but she is content where she lives and her schedule is comfortable at home.

## COGNITIVE/PERCEPTUAL PATTERN

### Hearing

Mrs. Carr states, "I'm slightly hard of hearing." Denies use of hearing aid, tinnitus, vertigo, earaches, infection, or discharge.

### Vision

Wears bifocal glasses. Last seen by optometrist 8/81. Denies redness, double vision, glaucoma. The optometrist told Mrs. Carr she had "the beginnings of cataracts."

### Sensory Perception

"I don't like spicy foods, my taste buds seem to work fine." Denies any difficulty with smell. "I try to keep my aches and pains under control. If I complain all day long, I'll have no friends. I always have an ache somewhere. This leg pain is the worst I've had."
Patient is left-handed.

### Learning Style

Patient states that she likes to be shown things. "I can read about anything and then try. If someone demonstrates for me, I can remember pretty well. That's how I learned to do some new needlework, and I took a pottery course not long ago with friends."

## SELF-PERCEPTION/SELF-CONCEPT PATTERN

### Self-Perception/Self-Concept

"I am a determined woman; I'm not going to let this hip slow me down! I usually speak my mind and take care of myself." Patient states that she has had a good life and loves Maryland. "Maryland has always been my home, and it gives me the strength I need to go on."

## ROLE/RELATIONSHIP PATTERN

### Role/Relationship

Mrs. Carr lives alone in a 1-floor home that she has had since her husband retired. It is small, with 2 bedrooms and a small garden in the backyard. She has 2 daughters and 1 son. They are all very helpful. One daughter lives in Towson, Maryland; the other is in Baltimore. Her son lives in Concord, Massachusetts. All are close-by, except her son in Concord. "I don't know what will happen to me now with this fracture. I don't want to go to a nursing home. I expect to resume my activities as soon as I am able."

## SEXUALITY/REPRODUCTIVE PATTERN

### Sexuality/Reproductive

Menarche at age 13; menopause at age 50. No recollection of postmenopausal bleeding. Denies performing self–breast examination and cannot recall ever having a Pap smear. Gravida—4, para—3. One spontaneous abortion. Three children were delivered vaginally without any difficulties.

## COPING/STRESS TOLERANCE PATTERN

### Coping/Stress Tolerance

"The most difficult thing I've had to face was the death of my husband. We were very close. We loved to walk and talk and just be together. With time I learned to cope with being alone. I have learned to enjoy my friends' companionship because it's lonely all alone."

**Coping/Stress Tolerance—Continued**

The patient's family offers assistance. Her children invite her for holidays and special events. The patient notes that her family is available when she needs them, but she doesn't want to be dependent on them for too much.

## VALUE/BELIEF PATTERN

**Value/Belief**

Patient states she is content with her relationship with God. Enjoys reading the Bible. Goes to church each Sunday and enjoys the special gatherings at church. States her health is important because without it a big part of her life would be closed off. "My ability to be with friends, keep my home, and remain independent are the pearls I treasure."

# Physical Examination

**General Survey**

Mrs. Carr is an elderly white female, appearing younger than stated age. In moderate distress at this time. Patient is alert, cooperative, and oriented to time, place, and person.

**Vital Signs**

*Temperature:* 99.8°F (37.6 C)
*Pulse:* 90 regular (apical)
*Respirations:* 18 regular
*BP:* 136/82 right arm, 134/78 left arm, lying down.

**Integument**

*Skin.* Her skin appears very dry, with poor skin turgor and several ecchymotic areas noted on her extremities. Seborrheic keratosis can be seen on the neck and hands. Circumscribed reddened area noted at sacrum with an approximately 1-inch (2.54 cm) wide break in the skin with a small amount serous drainage present.
*Mucous Membranes.* Smooth, slightly dry; no inflammation or lesions noted.
*Nails.* Nails are rough, but well kept. No clubbing or ridges noted.

**HEENT**

*Head.* Hair is clean and well kept. Scalp appears dry with some flaking. Face is symmetrical; no areas of tenderness noted. Temporomandibular joint (TMJ) is fully mobile without crepitation or pain.
*Eyes.* Evidence of cataracts noted bilaterally. With corrective lenses in place, vision is 20/30 in right eye and 20/20 in left eye with the use of the Rosenbaum eye chart. Conjunctiva and sclera are clear. pupils equal, round, reactive to light and accommodation (PERRLA). Upon visual field testing diminished peripheral vision noted bilaterally. No evidence of extraocular movements (EOMs).
*Ears.* Unsure if she heard the watch tick at 1 in. (2.5 cm) with right ear and 2 in. (5 cm) with left ear. Weber test: Lateralization to right ear predominantly (poorest hearing noted in right ear). Rinne test: Bone conduction greater than air conduction (normal conduction through right ear is blocked).
*Nose.* No discharge noted; no deviations. Nasal mucosa is pink. No sinus tenderness noted.
*Mouth/Throat.* Mucous membranes in mouth are pink and slightly dry. No pain noted upon tapping of teeth. Soft and hard palate are without lesions. Trachea appears midline; thyroid not palpable.

**Neck**

Moderate range of motion of neck without venous distention or pulsation. Carotid pulses are equal and without bruits.

**Pulmonary**

Slight barrel chest seen with symmetrical thorax. Slight hyper-resonance on percussion with diminished breath sounds. No adventitious sounds heard.

**Breast**

Breasts were examined with patient lying down. No masses or lesions noted. No dimpling or nipple discharge.

**Cardiovascular**

$S_1$ and $S_2$ heard; no extra sounds or murmurs noted. Point of maximal intensity (PMI) noted at fifth intercostal space at the left midclavicular line.

**Peripheral Vascular**

Extremities are warm to the touch with minimal hair distribution. Bilateral lower limb varicosities noted.

*Peripheral Pulses*
Temporal—4 bilaterally
Carotid—4 bilaterally
Brachial—4 bilaterally
Radial—4 bilaterally
Femoral—4 right; unable to palpate left
Popliteal—4 right; unable to palpate left
Posterior tibialis—4 bilaterally
Dorsalis pedis—4 bilaterally

*Peripheral Pulse Scale*

| |
|---|
| 0—Absent |
| 1—Markedly diminished |
| 2—Moderately diminished |
| 3—Slightly diminished |
| 4—Normal |

**Abdomen**

Bowel sounds are present but diminished in all 4 quadrants. No scars or deformities present.

**Musculoskeletal**

Limited range of motion in upper extremities; lower extremities were not evaluated due to patient discomfort. Left hip area red, edematous, and painful to the touch.

**Neurological**

*Mental Status.* Alert, oriented to time, place, and person. Mrs. Carr is cooperative given the degree of discomfort she is experiencing.
*Cranial Nerves.* CN I deferred and CN VII and IX for taste deferred; otherwise, CN II–XII intact. CN VIII impaired.
*Sensory.* Responds appropriately to light touch and pinprick bilaterally in upper extremities and lower right extremity. Did not test left lower extremity. Unable to test gait, balance, and coordination.

### *Deep Tendon Reflexes*

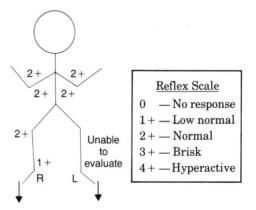

| Reflex Scale | |
|---|---|
| 0 | — No response |
| 1+ | — Low normal |
| 2+ | — Normal |
| 3+ | — Brisk |
| 4+ | — Hyperactive |

**Rectal**

Deferred at this time.

**Genitalia**

Deferred at this time.

# Laboratory Data/Diagnostic Studies

**Laboratory Data**

*Hgb:* 12.4 g/100 ml
*Hct:* 36%
*WBC:* 12,300/mm³
*Blood Sugar:* 113 mg/dl
*BUN:* 12 mg/dl
*Creatinine:* 0.9 mg/dl
*Na:* 138 mEq/L
*K:* 4.2 mEq/L
*Cl:* 98 mEq/L
*Co₂:* 22 mM
*Ca:* 8.0 mg/dl

*P:* 2.7 mg/dl
*Prothrombin Time:* 9.8/10.5 seconds
*Partial Thromboplastin Time:* 40 seconds
*Bleeding Time:* 4 minutes

*Urinalysis*
Clear yellow
pH 5.7
Specific gravity 1.015
Trace bacteria
Glucose — negative
Acetone — negative

**Diagnostic Studies**

*Left Hip X-Ray.* Findings reveal a comminuted intertrochanteric fracture.
*Chest x-ray.* Normal findings.
*ECG.* No specific ST-T changes.
*Normal Sinus Rhythm.* Rate 80.

**Additional Data**

*Medical Diagnosis.* Comminuted intertrochanteric fracture of the left hip.

# COLLABORATIVE PLAN OF CARE

**Diet**

Full liquid diet on admission.

**Medications**

Meperidine (Demerol) 50–75 mg q3h for 24 hr, then q3h prn.
Acetaminophen 650 mg q4h PO prn for temperature above 101°F (38.3°C).
Lorazepam (Ativan) 1 mg PO qhs prn.

**Intravenous Therapy**

Begin IV 1000 ml 5% dextrose and 0.5 Normal saline at 100 ml/hr. Add 20 mEq KCl to each liter.

**Therapeutic Measures**

Place patient in Buck's extension — 5 lb (2.25 kg).
Complete bed rest.

**Consults**

Does not apply.

## Preoperative Plan of Care

**Diet**

NPO after midnight.

**Medications**

Cefazolin (Ancef) 3 g in 250 ml 5% D/W. Give 83 ml q8h for 4 doses, then discontinue. Give first dose on call to OR.

**Intravenous Therapy**

Continue IV with 1000 ml of 5% dextrose and 0.5 Normal saline at 100 ml/hr.

**Therapeutic Measures**

Insert indwelling Foley catheter before surgery.
Wash left hip with PhisoHex preoperatively.
To OR in bed.
Type and cross match for 2 units of blood on call to OR.

**Consults**

Does not apply.

*Additional Information*    On 1/9/90 Mrs. Carr was taken to surgery at 8:00 AM for an uneventful open reduction and internal fixation (ORIF) and hip pinning of the left hip. Spinal anesthesia was used for the procedure. The patient returned to her room at 3:00 PM after an uneventful stay in the recovery room.

# Postoperative Plan of Care

*Diet*    Clear liquids after surgery and advance to regular diet once nausea subsides.

*Medications*    Heparin 5000 units subcutaneously q12h.
Ancef 3 g in 250 ml 5% D/W. Give 83 ml q8h for 4 doses, then discontinue. First dose should have been given on call to OR.
Prochlorperazine maleate (Compazine) 10 mg IM prn for nausea.
Morphine sulfate 5 mg or 8 mg or 10 mg SC q3h prn for pain.
Milk of magnesia (MOM) 30 ml PO q12h prn.
Bisacodyl (Dulcolax) suppository 1 per rectum once a day (OD) prn.
Triazolam (Halcion) 0.125–0.25 mg PO qhs prn for sleep.

*Intravenous Therapy*    IV 5% dextrose and 0.5 Normal saline at 80 ml/hr. May use heparin lock (intermittent venous access) when taking PO greater than 1000 ml in 24 hours.

*Therapeutic Measures*    Bed rest with operative leg in neutral position.
Turn to unoperative side and back, supporting operative side q2h.
Reinforce dressing as needed.
Maintain intake and output.
Empty Jackson-Pratt drainage prn.
Bed rest.
Up in chair 2 times on second postoperative day with no weight bearing. Keep affected leg elevated and supported.
Complete blood count (CBC), electrolytes in AM and daily for 4 days.
Discontinue indwellng urinary catheter on first postoperative evening.

*Consults*    Physical therapy consult to assist patient out of bed with walker third postoperative day without weight bearing.

# NURSING DIAGNOSES DEVELOPED IN CARE PLAN

# ADDITIONAL NURSING DIAGNOSES TO BE CONSIDERED

Anxiety
Bathing/Hygiene Self-Care Deficit
Body Image Disturbance
Chronic Pain
Dressing/Hygiene Self-Care Deficit
Hopelessness
Potential for Injury
Sleep Pattern Disturbance
Social Isolation

# NURSING CARE PLAN BASED ON IDENTIFIED NURSING DIAGNOSES

| | |
|---|---|
| ***Impaired Skin Integrity*** | ***Related to:*** Immobility, alteration in skin turgor.<br>***Evidenced by:*** Patient verbalization of pain in sacral area, small open area at sacral bony prominence circumscribed by redness. |
| ***Desired Patient Outcomes*** | • The wound will progressively decrease in size and depth.<br>• Patient participation in the treatment plan to promote wound healing.<br>• Skin will remain intact. |
| ***Evaluation Criteria*** | ***During this Hospitalization:***<br>• The wound will remain clean with an increase in granulation tissue and epithelialization complete by discharge.<br>• There will be no evidence of additional impairment in skin integrity at the time of discharge.<br>• The patient will verbalize measures to maintain skin integrity by the time of discharge.<br>• The patient will demonstrate body movements without friction or shearing motions. |

## Interventions

Provide local wound care every 8 hours. Wound care will consist of:

• Cleansing with an antimicrobial agent.
• Drying the intact skin area thoroughly.
• Application of a protective dressing that minimizes disruption to wound and protects newly formed granulation tissue.

Apply a lubricating spray to affected area with each dressing change.

Apply a covering to the wound that will facilitate healing.

Provide the patient with a trapeze bar over the bed.

Provide the patient with pressure-relieving device when lying in bed or sitting up in chair, for example, a solid foam surface or alternating pressure pads.

Utilize a pressure-sore flow sheet to document patient progress.

## Rationale

Wound management requires vigilant nursing care to enhance healing. A nonirritating liquid preparation can be used. Antimicrobial agents act to destroy microorganisms or suppress their growth. Monitoring and dressing the wound site should be done at least every 8 hours (Fowler, 1987, pp. 450, 457).

A lubricating spray acts to promote healing by means of capillary stimulant action (Fowler, 1987, p. 467).

According to recent research, wound healing occurs best when the wound surface is slightly moist and the dressing does not adhere to the wound site. Adherence of a dressing to the wound site causes a disruption in the healing process with damage to granulation tissue (Fowler, 1987, p. 453).

A trapeze will enable the patient who can assist with movement to do so (Fowler, 1987, p. 459).

A pressure-relieving device redistributes pressure and provides more even weight distribution when the patient is lying or sitting (Fowler, 1987, p. 458).

A flow sheet enhances the individualization for patient care and provides a means of communication concerning patient progress (Maklebust, 1987, p. 374).

## Interventions

Plan with the patient to maintain a turning schedule that may consist of modified movements based on her level of mobility.

Provide the patient with protective heel pads and elbow pads.

Explain to the patient the need to keep body skin dry and apply minimal lubricants. Use a bland (mild) lotion or thin layer of silicone cream on the skin.

Plan to perform active and passive range of motion to the extremities every 8 hours without compromising the surgical site.

Discuss with the patient the importance of a diet that is high in protein, including additional iron supplements and vitamin C to assist with wound healing. In addition, a daily diet should include a balance of carbohydrates, fats, vitamins, and minerals.

Discuss with the patient the importance of not wearing clothing or encountering a situation that increases the temperature on the surface of the skin. An example of this would be the use of an electric blanket or excessively warm clothes that trap body heat.

Teach the patient to mobilize with avoidance of shearing forces, for example, lifting her body into a position rather than pulling it into position.

## Rationale

The obstruction of capillary blood flow due to pressure in a localized area results in tissue ischemia and hypoxia (Maklebust, 1987, p. 362).

Prevention of friction between skin and other surfaces decreases the chance of depleting the outer stratum corneum of the dermis, thus making skin susceptible to pressure necrosis (Maklebust, 1987, p. 366).

Moisture on the skin reduces the skin's resistance to infection and ulceration. It has been shown to increase the risk of decubitus ulcer formation fivefold (Maklebust, 1987, p. 369).

Exercise assists in stimulating circulation and maintains joint function and strength (Brunner and Suddarth, 1988, p. 1591).

Protein depletion contributes to altered cellular exchange and the quality of the tissue is decreased, thus weakening body resistance to skin breakdown (Bobel, 1987, p. 380). Iron is an essential mineral in the healing process. It is needed for collagen formation (Carrieri, Lindsey, and West, 1986, p. 349). Vitamin C is required for angiogenesis and hydroxylation of proline and lysine for the formation of collagen (Carrieri, Lindsey, and West, 1986, p. 349). Carbohydrates provide the energy needed for metabolic processes, while fats supply a concentrated form of energy. Vitamins assist with all metabolic processes. Vitamin A aids in epithelialization and vitamin K aids in tissue repair. Minerals are necessary for normal cellular function (Bobel, 1987, pp. 380–381).

A rise in temperature of $1°C$ ($33.8°F$) will cause a 10% increase in tissue metabolism along with oxygen demand, thus increasing the susceptibility of the tissue to necrosis (Maklebust, 1987, p. 370).

Shearing forces have been noted to be responsible for the presence of sacral decubiti (Maklebust, 1987, p. 365). The aging process results in a change in collagen synthesis, and the integument has a decrease in mechanical strength and is less pliable (Maklebust, 1987, p. 369).

---

| **Constipation** | *Related to:* Immobility.<br>*Evidenced by:* Patient demonstrating difficulty moving the bowels. |
| --- | --- |
| **Desired Patient Outcomes** | *The Patient Will:*<br>• Demonstrate an improvement in bowel elimination.<br>• Describe factors that contribute to a change in bowel pattern and effective interventions. |

*Evaluation Criteria*

**The Patient Will:**
- Demonstrate a change in her diet and activity level consistent with an improvement in her elimination pattern.
- Verbalize factors that contribute to a change in her bowel pattern by the time of discharge.
- Experience a change in her elimination pattern once she has advanced her diet postoperatively.

## Interventions

Discuss with the patient her food preferences to plan a diet to aid in bowel elimination. Characteristics of a diet should include:

- Foods high in fiber.
- Unprocessed bran.
- At least 4 servings of fruit and vegetables daily (offer them fresh or raw if available).
- Drink 6–8 glasses of water daily.
- Offer prunes, figs, dates.
- May add fat to the diet.
- Offer hot tea, coffee, and warm lemon water in the morning.

Develop a schedule for fluid intake offering fluids the patient likes. Plan with the patient a regular time for a bowel movement and provide privacy for the patient.

Place the patient in a sitting position for elimination.

Discuss with the patient the need to increase mobility and exercise within acceptable limits.

Discuss with the patient the importance of planning her care so that there is time to defecate based on a schedule that is best for the patient.

## Rationale

High fiber foods increase gastrointestinal motility, increase fecal weight, and stimulate peristalsis. Offer foods with laxative effects to stimulate peristalsis (Dudek, 1987, p. 372).

Planning for bowel movements within a daily schedule is necessary to avoid constipation (Luckmann and Sorensen, 1987, p. 1261).

A sitting position provides a more natural position for defecation and enhances elimination (Luckmann and Sorensen, 1987, p. 1260).

A decrease in mobility and exercise is responsible for a decrease in gastric motility and weak abdominal and perineal muscles (Luckmann and Sorensen, 1987, p. 1261).

Not responding to the urge to defecate and not allowing time to defecate are common causes of constipation (Potter and Perry, 1985, p. 1145).

*Impaired Physical Mobility*

*Related to:* Weakness, decreased level of energy.
*Evidenced by:* Inability to get out of bed or make transfers without assistance, and decreased motor agility.

*Desired Patient Outcomes*

**The Patient Will:**
- Increase mobility using assistive devices.
- Demonstrate an awareness of safety factors to minimize the potential for injury.
- Verbalize an increase in strength in the upper extremities.

*Evaluation Criteria*

*By the Time of Hospital Discharge, the Patient Will:*
- Acknowledge increasing strength in her upper and lower extremities.

- Verbalize an understanding of a plan for her daily activities that she can initiate.
- Describe safety factors that would affect ambulation.
- Demonstrate an ability to independently tend to self-care needs.

## Interventions

Discuss with the patient her prefracture level of mobility.

Discuss with the patient the need to think positively about recovery and rehabilitation.

Provide passive range of motion (ROM) in the affected limb within guidelines at least once a shift. Encourage active ROM of all joints at least once a shift.

In collaboration with physical therapy, increase mobility with the use of safe and effective techniques. Instruct the patient to have a supportive pair of shoes with a nonskid sole or a pair of sneakers in the hospital for safe ambulation.

Encourage the use of an overbed trapeze hourly for upper extremity exercise. Instruct the patient in lower extremity exercise (quadriceps and gluteal setting exercises).

Encourage the patient to invite a family member or significant other to become involved in her care and plan for discharge.

Discuss with the patient the use of a walker and home considerations concerning the use of assistive devices. Have the patient describe the steps to take to achieve daily ambulation and encourage her to initiate the activities.

Include the patient in the decisions that must be made daily. All activities that affect the patient should be discussed with her. The patient should understand that she is viewed as a significant contributor in planning her own care. For example: plan with the patient the time for the daily bath, getting out of bed, and when and how additional activities will be accomplished.

## Rationale

An awareness of the prefracture level of mobility serves as a goal for postfracture activities (Lukens, 1986, p. 206).

Research has demonstrated that a positive attitude toward personnel, emotions, and motivation can positively influence progress in a rehabilitation program (Lukens, 1986, p. 203).

With an impairment in joint mobility, the aim is to preserve full ROM, prevent contractures, and to foster self-help activities. Active ROM activities and strength-building activities prepare the person for postfracture ambulation (Lukens, 1986, p. 205).

Explain transfer maneuvers to the patient. Have the patient verbalize to the nurse how the transfer maneuver will occur. A transfer should not occur if the patient cannot comprehend and assist with the movement (Potter and Perry, 1985, p. 736).

Encourage movement of all joints and muscles to improve the level of strength needed for walking with ambulatory aids (Brunner and Suddarth, 1988, p. 1589).

In planning for a patient's discharge, it is useful to call upon resources that will help the patient return to the home environment (Lukens, 1986, p. 206).

Assisting a patient with walking requires preparation. Determine distance, evaluate the environment, and plan a slow, steady program of ambulation (Potter and Perry, 1985, p. 778).

A sudden traumatic experience for an older person can result in the loss of his or her control of the environment. This is a stressor that can be minimized by including the person in decisions that need to be made (Lukens, 1986, p. 205).

## Interventions

Allow time daily to discuss the patient's concerns with regard to mobility and self-care once she is discharged.

Discuss with the patient external factors in the environment that could be hazardous. Review the importance of watching for slippery floors, wires, rugs, inadequate lighting, and furniture that is low and/or unstable.

## Rationale

Discharge planning should occur at admission. It promotes continuity of care, recognizes patient independence, and considers comfort and the economics of health care needs (Bulechek and McCloskey, 1985, pp. 385–386).

Most elderly people fall due to an environmental hazard in their home (Peck, 1986, p. 72).

# QUESTIONS FOR DISCUSSION

1. Discuss why Buck's extension was ordered for Mrs. Carr after she was admitted to the orthopedic unit.
2. Why is avascular necrosis seen more frequently with a fracture of the neck of the femur (intracapsular fractures)?
3. Discuss age-related needs to be considered when caring for Mrs. Carr.
4. Confusion is often seen in the elderly patient who has a fracture of the hip. Discuss possible etiologies for this confusion and nursing interventions to aid in eliminating this problem.
5. Mrs. Carr tells you that she is disgusted with her progress on day 4 and believes she will "never recover." What can you do to raise her hope and belief in her ability to recover and gain independence.
6. Mrs. Carr does have osteoporosis. Develop a teaching plan that will aid her in managing this condition.
7. Mrs. Carr is at high risk for complications related to immobility. Discuss these complications and associated interventions (independent and collaborative) to alleviate the complications.
8. Mrs. Carr tells you that she wants to return to her own home at the time of discharge, but she is afraid of another fall. What can you suggest to this patient that might help her at home?

# REFERENCES

Bobel, LM: Nutritional implications in the patient with pressure sores. Nurs Clin North Am 22:379, 1987.

Brunner, LS and Suddarth, DS: Textbook of Medical-Surgical Nursing, ed 6. JB Lippincott, Philadelphia, 1988.

Bulechek, GM and McCloskey, JC: Nursing Interventions: Treatments for Nursing Diagnoses. WB Saunders, Philadelphia, 1985.

Carrieri, VK, Lindsey, AM, and West, CM: Pathophysiological Phenomena in Nursing: Human Responses to Illness. WB Saunders, Philadelphia, 1986.

Dudek, SG: Nutrition Handbook for Nursing Practice. JB Lippincott, Philadelphia, 1987.

Fowler, EM: Equipment and products used in management and treatment of pressure ulcers. Nurs Clin North Am 22:449, 1987.

Luckmann, J and Sorensen, KC: Medical-Surgical Nursing: A Psychophysiologic Approach. WB Saunders, Philadelphia, 1987.

Lukens, L: Six months after hip fracture. Geriatr Nurs, July/August 1986, p 202.

Maklebust, J: Pressure ulcers: Etiology and prevention. Nurs Clin North Am 22:359, 1987.

Peck, WA: Falls and hip fracture in the elderly. Hosp Pract, Dec 15, 1986, p 72.

Potter, PA and Perry, AG: Fundamentals of Nursing Concepts: Process and Practice. CV Mosby, St. Louis, 1985.

Tinetti, ME, Speechley, M, and Ginter, SF: Risk factors for falls among elderly persons living in the community. N Engl J Med 319:1701, 1988.

# BIBLIOGRAPHY

Aisenbrey, JA: Exercise in the prevention and management of osteoporosis. Physical Therapy 67:1100, 1987.

Beil, AV: Osteoporosis: How to avoid its crippling effects. RN, August 1986, p 14.

Billig N, et al: Assessment of depression and cognitive impairment after hip fracture. J Am Geriatr Soc 34:7, 1986.

Campbell, EB, Williams, MA, and Mlynarczyk, SM: After the fall—Confusion. Am J Nurs, February 1986, p 151.

Clarke, M and Kadhom, HM: The Nursing prevention of pressure sores in hospital and community patients. J Adv Nurs 13:365, 1988.

Fowler, E: Nursing diagnosis: Actual impairment of skin integrity. J Gerontol Nurs 12:10, 1986.

Furstenberg, AL: Expectations about outcome following hip fracture among older people. Social Work in Health Care 11:4, 1986.

Jones, PL and Millman, A: A three-part system to combat pressure sores. Geriatr Nurs, March/April 1986, p 78.

Osteoporosis: JAMA 252:6, 1984.

White, L, Farmer, M, and Brody, J: Who is at risk? Hip fracture epidemiology report. J Gerontol Nurs 10:10, 1986.

Williams, MA, et al: Reducing acute confusional states in elderly patients with hip fractures. Res Nurs Health 8:329, 1985.

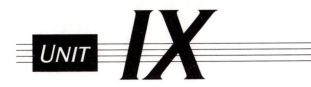

# THE PATIENT WITH ALTERATIONS RELATED TO SEXUALITY AND REPRODUCTION

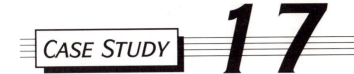

# A PATIENT WITH CANCER OF THE BREAST

Jean D'Meza Leuner, M.S., R.N.

## ANATOMY AND PHYSIOLOGY OF THE BREAST

The breasts, also called mammary glands, are accessory organs of reproduction. Located on the anterior chest, the breast extends from the second rib to the sixth rib vertically and horizontally from the sternum to the midaxillary line. The mammary glands are anterior to the pectoralis major muscle and consist of lobular epithelium and a system of ducts embedded within adipose and interstitial tissue.

Cooper's ligaments are fibrous bands that serve to maintain the position of the breast on the chest wall. These ligaments are found between the skin and the deep fascia and can readily stretch to accommodate a change in breast size.

A breast (Fig. 17–1) consists of 15–20 lobes surrounded by fatty tissue. The lobes, which subdivide into lobules, form a circular pattern with the nipple at the center. Each of the lobes is drained by a duct that opens into the nipple. The ducts extend distally toward the chest wall and in doing so unite the lobules, which contain the milk-secreting cells, also known as alveoli or acini. A lobule can contain 10–100 alveoli, while 20–40 lobules can be found in each of the 15–20 lobes in each breast.

The circular, darker pigmented area around the nipple is the areola. Within the areolar epithelium, small hairs can be seen. The small sebaceous glands (Montgomery's glands) located under the areola give it a rough appearance.

The tail of Spence is the area of breast tissue that extends from the upper lateral quadrant to the axilla. The significance of this area of the breast rests with the fact that greater than 50% of the lobes of the breast extend laterally in the tail of Spence and under the pectoralis muscle group. Thus, an asymmetrical distribution of lobes can be seen throughout the breast. Fewer than 20% of the ducts are located in the medial region of the breast and approximately 30% are below the area of the areola and the central portion of the breast.

The breast receives its blood supply from the lateral mammary artery and the lateral thoracic artery. The lymphatic drainage of the breast is mainly to the axilla and medially near the axillary vein. The medial portion of the breast has lymphatic drainage directed toward the sternum and into the internal mammary chain inside the thoracic cavity. Additional lymph nodes drain into the epigastric, supraclavicular, and anterior cervical lymphatics. Lymph nodes are frequently a site of breast cancer metastases. Disease spread to the nodes causes them to become enlarged and firm. Nervous innervation to the breast is by way of the anterior and lateral branches of the fourth and sixth intercostal nerves.

The primary function of the mammary glands is milk secretion and ejection. Lactation occurs in response to the release of the hormone prolactin from the anterior pituitary gland. During pregnancy, hypothalamic prolactin-releasing factor stimulates the release of prolactin; however, no milk is secreted at this time because the blood levels of estrogen and progesterone cause the hypothalamus to release prolactin-inhibiting factor. After the baby is born, a decrease in the blood levels of estrogen and progesterone occurs, and the inhibition of prolactin is lifted.

Prolactin secretion is maintained as long as the infant sucks at the breast. Sucking stimulates impulses

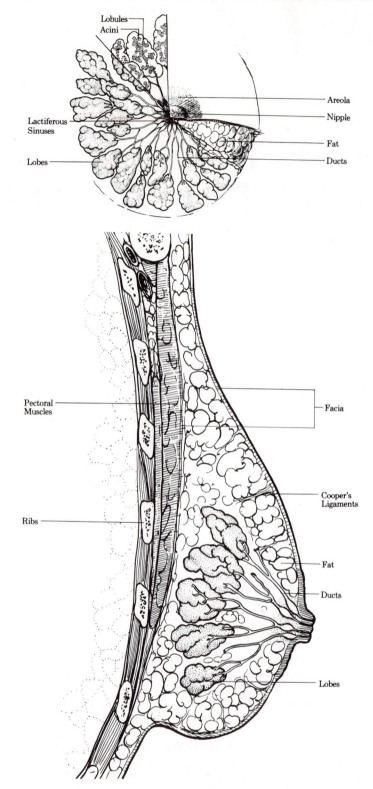

**FIGURE 17–1.** Diagram of the breast. (From The Breast Cancer Digest, ed 2. National Cancer Institute, Bethesda, Md, US Department of Health and Human Services, April 1984, NIH Publication No. 84-1691, p. 5.)

from the receptors present in the nipples to the hypothalamus. The impulses stimulate the release of the hormone oxytocin. This hormone affects the cells surrounding the alveoli and causes contractions, thus causing alveolar compression. Milk is projected from the alveoli into the ducts and sucked by the infant, who has latched onto the areola surrounding the nipple.

# PATHOPHYSIOLOGY RELATED TO CANCER OF THE BREAST

Cancer of the breast can be categorized generally as either originating within the ductal system or arising from the glandular tissue of the mammary lobules. Ductal or intraductal carcinoma constitutes approximately 70% of all breast cancers, whereas lobular carcinoma, or adenocarcinoma, accounts for 25%–30%. Paget's disease is an additional form of breast cancer, as is a small group of highly undifferentiated carcinomas that do not fit into the previous 3 categories.

Breast cancer can be invasive or in situ. Most breast tumors arise from the ducts and are invasive (invasive ductal, infiltrating ductal), while the in situ tumors are self-contained growths. The upper outer quadrant of the breast is often the site for tumorous growth.

Invasive ductal tumors that are not otherwise specified (NOS) are characterized by their hardness to the touch and ability to cause connective tissue to proliferate. The tumor may be fixed to the skin, chest wall, or nipple. This type of cancer often spreads to the axillary lymph nodes and has a poor prognosis. Invasive lobular tumors are similar in appearance and behave like invasive ductal tumors. The prognosis for the patient tends to be unfavorable as well.

Medullary carcinoma, comedocarcinomas, and mucinous and tubular carcinoma are all forms of invasive ductal cancer. Each of these tumors exhibits a characteristic cell growth and has a prognosis that is more favorable than the NOS invasive ductal tumors.

Inflammatory breast cancer carries a poor prognosis. It is often characterized by skin induration and redness. The lymphatics are consumed with tumor, and the overwhelming appearance of a breast infection can be seen.

Paget's disease of the nipple is a form of breast cancer infrequently seen in women and constitutes approximately 3% of all breast cancers. In this particular form of cancer, the tumor extends through the ducts and onto the surface of the nipple. The prognosis associated with this cancer depends on whether the tumor is invasive or noninvasive.

Lobular and ductal carcinoma in situ are tumorous growths that have not extended beyond the boundaries of the lobules of the ducts. These lesions are recognized microscopically and are therefore often first detected on a mammogram or when the tissue is being examined for other purposes. In situ cancers may progress to an invasive state.

Fibrocystic disorders of the breast are commonly seen in many women. Breast changes that occur as a result of monthly fluctuating hormone levels result in nodular or lumpy breasts. The fibrocystic changes involve excessive cell growth in the ducts of the breast as well as within the lobules and the connective tissue. The fibrocystic changes within the breast can take 1 of 2 paths. The first is clinically nonsignificant and results in the presence of a simple cyst and sclerosing adenosis. The second results in ductal hyperplasia in the ducts of the breast and is thus seen as a precursor to breast cancer. The hyperplastic lesions may develop into dysplasia and can eventually result in the evolution of carcinoma in situ. Although not a true cancer, carcinoma in situ requires early recognition and intervention to prevent further tumor growth.

# RISK FACTORS

The careful evaluation of women at risk for the development of breast cancer will aid in the early recognition and treatment of this disease. Women who are at high risk for the development of breast cancer include women who have a family history of breast cancer, particularly a mother or sister. Women who became pregnant and delivered their first child after the age of 30 are in the high-risk category, as are women who are nulliparous. Natural menopause occurring after the age of 50 is an additional risk factor. Women who have had a history of ductal or lobular hyperplasia are in the high-risk group. Women who have had cancer in one breast are at an increased risk for the development of cancer in the other breast.

Additional, less critical risk factors have been identified. They include obesity with and without the presence of diabetes mellitus, diets high in fat content and animal protein, women who have had a large exposure to radiation, and women who have been exposed to environmental carcinogens.

# COMMON CLINICAL FINDINGS

A patient with breast cancer usually presents with a lump in the breast. The typical breast cancer tumor is characteristically solitary and unilateral with an irregular shape. In addition, it is hard, nonmobile, and nontender to the touch. Skin changes such as dimpling or axillary lymphadenopathy may be evident. The presence of a discharge from the nipple that is serosanguineous, bloody, or watery is usually indicative of a malignancy. Once a diagnosis of breast cancer is suspected, a breast biopsy is performed at which time estrogen receptor status may be evaluated. If a positive biopsy report is obtained, the patient is presented with treatment options.

The complications that may arise following surgical intervention include edema of the arm with or without paresthesia. The disease may recur due to the incomplete removal of the tumor or the involved nodes. The rate of recurrence has been closely associated with the size and type of the cancerous mass as well as with the extent of metastases. A recurrence of breast cancer most likely occurs within the first 2 years, with a peak incidence during the second year after surgery. Approximately one third of the population at risk develop a recurrence within 3 years following a mastectomy (Hassey, 1988, p. 441). The importance of emotional support during this critical time cannot be overlooked.

Data are inconclusive concerning the effects of pregnancy on a woman with breast cancer. Women who are pregnant when a diagnosis of breast cancer is made should be counseled individually concerning the duration of pregnancy and the effects of the disease and treatment options on the fetus as well as on the mother.

Women who have had treatment for breast cancer and are of childbearing age should be counseled by a health care provider. It has been suggested that childbearing be postponed for at least 2 years after treatment with surgical intervention or radiation. Waiting for this period of time would respect the critical 2-year period following initial treatment. The concerns regarding pregnancy following treatment with adjuvant chemotherapy are still being debated. These patients need to be counseled concerning the degree of nodal involvement and long-term survival. The increased risk of disease recurrence or metastases when nodal involvement is identified at the time of diagnosis should be evaluated in relation to a desire for pregnancy. Infertility, ovarian dysfunction, and the possibility of germ cell mutations that are cytotoxically induced are a few of the concerns that have been raised with regard to adjuvant chemotherapy (Hassey, 1988, p. 441).

# TREATMENT MODALITIES

Treatment options include a modified radical mastectomy for Stages I and II carcinoma of the breast. This procedure consists of the removal of the entire breast along with the pectoralis minor muscle. Additionally, some or most of the axillary lymph nodes are removed. The evaluation and resection of lymph nodes at the time of surgery assist in the planning for adjuvant therapy. A simple mastectomy, also called a total mastectomy, consists of the removal of the entire breast without the removal of the axillary nodes.

Limited surgical procedures are also viable options for the woman with Stage I and possibly Stage II disease. A segmental mastectomy (lumpectomy, quadrectomy, partial mastectomy) is a procedure to remove the tumor. This is usually done in conjunction with radiation therapy. It has been determined that the survival and recurrence rates with this regimen are similar to those for a modified radical mastectomy. Studies

## TNM CLINICAL STAGING OF BREAST CARCINOMA

### STAGE I
Tumor—Less than 2 cm in diameter
Nodes—Negative
Metastases—No distant metastases

### STAGE II
Tumor—Greater than 2 cm but less than 5 cm in diameter
Nodes—Positive or negative; if positive they are not fixed to one another or to other structures
Metastases—No distant metastases

### STAGE III
Tumor—Greater than 5 cm, or tumor of any size with direct extension to the chest wall
Nodes—Supraclavicular or infraclavicular involvement
Metastases—No distant metastases

### STAGE IV
Tumor—Tumor of any size
Nodes—Positive or negative
Metastases—Distant metastases present

with regard to this combination treatment are still being performed, and a long-term evaluation of treatment plans will demonstrate more definitive guidelines.

The treatment options for women with Stage III or Stage IV disease are less clear. These patients are viewed individually, and a combination of surgery, radiation therapy, and systemic chemotherapy may be employed. Oral endocrine agents such as tamoxifen, aminoglutethimide, diethylstilbestrol, and megestrol acetate may be prescribed.

Breast cancer is viewed by most clinicians as a systemic disease. This is due to the fact that approximately two thirds of these patients demonstrate signs of distant metastasis regardless of the treatment plan utilized. This belief has led practitioners to recommend chemotherapy as adjunctive treatment for patients with curable disease and positive axillary node involvement. The goal of this form of therapy is to eliminate occult metastases.

# PATIENT ASSESSMENT OF DATA BASE

## Health History

*Client:*
Mrs. Elizabeth Heller

*Address:* 150 W. Main St., Washington, D.C. 20205
*Telephone:* 202-555-8034
*Contact:* Mr. Wellesley Heller (husband)
*Address of contact:* Same
*Telephone of contact:* Same
*Age:* 64   *Sex:* Female   *Race:* White
*Educational background:* BA from George Washington University
*Religion:* Episcopalian   *Marital status:* Married
*Former occupation:* Office manager for government agency office for 14 years (age 23–37)
*Present occupation:* Housewife
*Source of income:* Husband (works full time)
*Insurance:* Health Maintenance Organization
*Source of referral:* Dr. Ronald Bartholin (gynecologist)
*Source of history:* Self
*Reliability of historian:* Reliable
*Date of interview:* 10/15/89
*Reason for visit/Chief complaint:* In June 1985 Mrs. Heller first noted pain in the right breast. Mammogram at that time was negative with some obvious fibrous changes. In July 1988, she noted a lump in the right breast while taking a shower and realized that the breast was noticeably enlarged and "different." She delayed seeking medical advice for 3 months. The right breast had an obvious "dimpled" look and Mrs. Heller knew she needed to seek assistance from a physician. "I felt a hard mass; I couldn't believe it was there because I had no pain. I guess I wanted it to go away but I knew it wouldn't."

### Health Perception/Health Management Pattern

*Present Health Status*

Mrs. Elizabeth Heller, having discovered a lump in her right breast, saw a clinical nurse specialist and a physician at a breast evaluation clinic. At the clinic, she had an extensive examination that included a breast biopsy to confirm the diagnosis. The physician and clinical nurse specialist spoke with Mrs. Heller confirming the fact that the tumor was malignant. She could consider conservative surgery or a modified radical mastectomy. Each of these procedures might be followed with additional treatments if necessary. The physician discussed the plans for her admission to the hospital, and Mrs. Heller decided to have the modified radical mastectomy.

**Past Health Status**

**General Health.** "I knew what was wrong with me the day I went to see the doctor (October 1988). It was very obvious because in July [1988] while I was taking a shower I was sure that I felt a lump. As I was dressing, I looked closely at myself in the mirror and I was quite surprised at what I saw. I knew then, but I tried to suppress my concerns, because I didn't want to make our world come to a stop because of me. My husband, my daughter, and I had been planning a trip to Hong Kong. I thought to myself, 'We're going to have a great time and when I get back I'll see the doctor.' I didn't say anything to my husband to worry him." The patient states that she is generally in good health and revealing this new discovery would have upset their lives too much.

**Prophylactic Medical/Dental Care.** Doesn't see a doctor unless there's a problem. Last doctor visit was 2 years ago for a persistent chest cold and fever lasting 3 days. She was treated with antibiotics and cough medicine with codeine. Sees a dental hygienist every 6 months.

**Childhood Illnesses.** Had measles, mumps, rubella, and chickenpox, but she is unsure of the dates.

**Immunizations.** Polio, diphtheria, tetanus; negative tuberculosis test.

**Major Illnesses/Hospitalizations.** Uterine fibroidectomy, January 1956; total abdominal hysterectomy, 1963. History of repeated infections (systemic or localized): None known.

**Current Medications**

*Prescription:* None at this time; took diethylstilbestrol throughout pregnancy. Premarin (estrogen combination) posthysterectomy until 1975 when patient voluntarily stopped because of pain in both breasts and weight gain.

*Nonprescription:* Aspirin for tension headaches.

**Allergies.** No known allergies.

**Habits**

*Alcohol:* Occasional social drink.

*Caffeine:* 3–4 cups of coffee a day (in the morning), 1–2 glasses of iced tea in the afternoon, 1 cup of coffee after dinner.

*Drugs:* None.

*Tobacco:* Never smoked.

## Family Health History

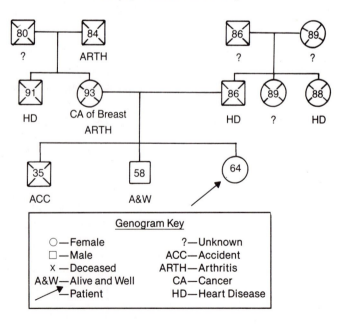

## Nutritional/Metabolic Pattern

*Nutritional*

Mrs. Heller has 3 meals a day; tries to limit fat and carbohydrates in diet. She is aware that salt isn't good but has difficulty staying away from the salt shaker. Her appetite continues to be good. Likes all foods; no particular likes or dislikes. Reports no changes in appetite since onset of illness. Patient is responsible for buying the food and preparing the meals. No religious dietary restrictions.

*Usual Daily Menu*

| | |
|---|---|
| *Breakfast:* | Juice (if in season, melon or grapefruit), toast or a bagel with cream cheese, and coffee (several cups). |
| *Lunch:* | Sandwich (tuna, bologna, or turkey on wheat bread), iced tea or a glass of milk. |
| *Afternoon snack:* | Cookies and iced tea or hot tea. |
| *Dinner:* | Hamburger, chicken, chops, or steak; potato, rice, occasionally pasta; vegetable (broccoli, cauliflower, or green beans); ice cream or cake; coffee. |

*Metabolic*

Patient reports no apparent weight loss or gain. No changes in skin; denies dryness or lesions. No difficulty with healing or intolerance to heat or cold. Has own teeth, all intact. Reports no difficulty with swallowing. *Weight:* 154 lb (70 kg). *Height:* 5 ft 4 in. (163 cm).

## Elimination Pattern

*Bowel*

One daily bowel movement (usually midmorning), moderate in size, soft-brown consistency. Denies use of aids to assist with elimination.

*Bladder*

Urinates probably 5–6 times a day; clear amber color. No associated pain or discomfort. Denies nocturia or ever having a urinary tract infection.

## Activity/Exercise Pattern

*Activity/Exercise*

Mrs. Heller considers herself "too old" for vigorous exercise. Has noticed an increase in fatigue the last 3 weeks. States she realized she had very little energy 1 month prior to admission. She likes to read; walks approximately ½ mile (0.8 km) a day mostly in her own yard and neighborhood. No associated difficulty with activities.

*Self-Care Ability*

| | |
|---|---|
| Feeding — 0 | Grooming — 0 |
| Bathing — 0 | General mobility — 0 |
| Toileting — 0 | Cooking — 0 |
| Bed mobility — 0 | Home maintenance — 0 |
| Dressing — 0 | Shopping — 0 |

---

*Functional Levels Code*
  0 — Full self-care
  I — Requires use of equipment or device
  II — Requires assistance or support from another person
  III — Requires assistance or support from another person and equipment or device
  IV — Is dependent and does not participate

*Oxygenation/Perfusion*

**Chest X-Ray.** Multiple chest x-rays throughout teen and early adult years. Chest x-ray done during this admission. Results not available at this time. Denies pulmonary problems, shortness of breath, dyspnea. Denies palpitations, pain in the chest, rapid heartbeat, or irregular rhythm.

**Cardiac Risk Factors**

|                            | Positive | Negative |
|----------------------------|----------|----------|
| Sedentary life-style       |          | X        |
| Hyperlipidemia             |          | X        |
| Cigarette smoking          |          | X        |
| Diabetes                   |          | X        |
| Obesity                    | X        |          |
| Hypertension               |          | X        |
| Hypervigilant personality  |          | X        |
| Family history of heart disease | X   |          |

## SLEEP/REST PATTERN

*Sleep/Rest*

Averages 6–7 hours of sleep each night. Since she found the lump, sleep has been interrupted; has dreams and can't seem to relax. Denies waking feeling rested. "My lack of sleep may be contributing to my fatigue. I never used to nap during the day, but lately I have been resting off and on all day. I never really sleep, I just close my eyes."

## COGNITIVE/PERCEPTUAL PATTERN

*Hearing*

Denies difficulty with hearing.

*Vision*

Denies visual difficulties.

*Sensory Perception*

Has not noticed any changes in sensation. No difficulty with taste or smell. Patient denies having pain at this time. She states that she "hates pain, has a low tolerance for pain, and has no difficulty requesting medications." Mrs. Heller is right-hand dominant.

*Learning Style*

Patient states that she learns best with audiovisual aids and a return demonstration. She has no difficulty learning something new, but she wants to be sure that she has mastered the task properly.

## SELF-PERCEPTION/SELF-CONCEPT PATTERN

*Self-Perception/Self-Concept*

"I have always felt independent and strong." When asked how she feels about her body image, she states, "I want to look appealing to my husband, and I want to look good for myself. My breasts are an important part of my sexuality and feeling good about myself. I would be kidding myself if I said I wasn't scared about how I'll look. What will happen to my life? I will look strange and disfigured, and everyone will know I have cancer." Rates herself as a good listener, 3 on a scale of 1–5 (1 = poor, 5 = good). Doesn't mind being touched by others, but prefers to know the person before being touched. Denies difficulty with direct contact with others.

## ROLE/RELATIONSHIP PATTERN

*Role/Relationship*

Patient lives with her husband in a 2-story home in a suburban neighborhood. Daughter, Brittany, lives in Georgetown. Brittany is 29 years old, fully independent, and works as a junior law partner in a law firm. The patient's brother lives in Dallas, Texas, and therefore they seldom get together.

Patient states that she is a content housewife with several volunteer activities. She is a volunteer for the local chapter for abused children; she participates in church activities and is a volunteer in the hospital. Reports an active social life with dinner parties and activities related to her husband's job. "We're lucky to have many good friends and we have fun together."

## SEXUALITY/REPRODUCTIVE PATTERN

*Sexuality/Reproductive*

Could not identify problems with sexuality prior to this current health problem. "My husband and I are very close. Yes, we are sexually active and enjoy being together." Expresses great concern over future sexual encounters. Worried that her husband won't want to touch her or be near her. "My breasts are a very important part of our sex life."

Menarche at age 13, periods lasting 4–7 days with a moderate flow. Denies dysmenorrhea; however, experienced menorrhagia (heavy menses) and metrorrhagia (intermenstrual bleeding) prior to fibroidectomy in 1956. The symptoms recurred with dyspareunia present and patient underwent a total abdominal hysterectomy in 1963. Surgically induced menopause at age 38 (Premarin was prescribed). Denies postmenopausal bleeding.

She is gravida 4, para 1. "Three miscarriages prior to one and only one full-term delivery in 1960." Denies vaginal discharge. Does have vaginal dryness that seems itchy at times. The dryness does cause discomfort with intercourse. Denies ever having practiced self–breast examinations (SBE). Patient states, "I have never been taught how, and I guess I was afraid if I did it, I'd find something."

## COPING/STRESS TOLERANCE PATTERN

*Coping/Stress Tolerance*

Patient defines stress for herself as "having no appetite and feeling nervous. Unable to sleep or attend to any activity for a period of time." Two stressful moments patient could recall were when her brother died in a car accident, and when her mother died. When her brother died the family was in shock. As the oldest in the family, Mrs. Heller had to help the members of the family "keep from falling apart." She stated that she's not sure where she got the strength, but she had to look ahead and not stay locked in her grief. Mrs. Heller states that she was in total shock at first and then took hold of the situation and got all the information necessary to make plans for the funeral. She could recall speaking with the church priest for guidance and relying on her friends. After the funeral, Mrs. Heller recalls trying to remember all the good things that her brother did and that was when she began volunteering in the local hospital 1 day a week.

Mrs. Heller's mother had breast cancer that resulted in a mastectomy. The disease continued to spread and her mother eventually died in a great deal of pain. "Watching my mother die was very painful. I know I was unfit to live with at that time because I was so upset that nothing could be done to help her through her suffering." Mrs. Heller continued to talk about her fear of cancer, "because it never goes away."

## Value/Belief Pattern

*Value/Belief*

Could not relate to any specific cultural traditions or practices. Mrs. Heller notes that she is a practicing Episcopalian. She attends church each Sunday and holy days. She has always had a special place for religion in her life. When their daughter was young, Mrs. Heller taught religious education classes. When asked what Mrs. Heller finds most meaningful in her life she replied, "My family, my health, and my values." She continued to say that honesty and love have been the driving force in her family.

# Physical Examination

*General Survey*

Slightly obese, alert, white female who looks older than stated age of 64 years old. Moves without difficulty; no gross abnormalities apparent. Is neatly groomed, responsive, and cooperative. Responds appropriately and smiles frequently.

*Vital Signs*

*Temperature:* 98.8°F (37.1°C) (oral)
*Pulse:* 80 beats/minute, strong and regular (apical)
*Respirations:* 18 regular
*BP:* 112/70 (left arm, sitting); 118/74 (right arm, sitting).

*Integument*

*Skin.* Skin uniformly light tan in color; soft, warm, moist, elastic, of normal thickness.
*Mucous Membranes.* Smooth, pink, moist, intact. No inflammation or lesions noted.
*Nails.* Nailbeds pink, smooth; no clubbing or ridges noted.

*HEENT*

*Head.* Head is normocephalic, without tenderness. Hair is evenly distributed, thick, and light brunette in color. Face is symmetrical at rest and with movement. Temporomandibular joint (TMJ) is fully mobile without crepitation or pain.
*Eyes.* Vision with Rosenbaum hand-held chart, right eye 20/20, left eye 20/30. Extraocular movements (EOMs) intact bilaterally. Conjunctiva is clear; sclera white; lacrimal glands palpated and without tenderness or discharge. Pupils equal, round, reactive to light and accommodation (PERRLA).
*Ears.* External auricles are without lesions. Whisper test: Distinguished soft whisper at 2 in. (5 cm) bilaterally. Rinne test: Air conduction (AC) greater than bone conduction (BC) 2:1. Weber test: Noted equal lateralization.
*Nose.* Nostrils are patent; odors identified; no obvious septal deviations. Nasal membranes are pink, moist, with no discharge.
*Mouth/Throat.* Membranes are pink, moist, and intact. Buccal mucosa and gingiva are pink and moist, without lesions. Soft and hard palate are intact. Teeth in good repair with many fillings. Uvula rises midline. Tonsil tags are intact without redness.

*Neck*

Full range of motion (ROM), strong symmetrically. Trachea is midline. No enlargement of head and neck regional nodes. Carotid pulse is strong, regular bilaterally, and without bruits.

*Pulmonary*

Thorax is symmetrical at rest and with movement. Anteroposterior (AP) diameter greater than lateral. Fremitus equal bilaterally; resonance in lung fields. Vesicular breath sounds bilaterally; no adventitious sounds.

**Breast**

Breasts were evaluated with arms elevated, hands on hips, hands stretched out in front of patient, and with patient lying down. No nodes palpable, axillary or supraclavicular. Approximately 1.5–2 in. (3.7–5 cm) × 2 in. (5 cm) firm mass palpated in right upper outer quadrant of the right breast. Mass was nontender to the touch, irregular in shape. Dimpling noted in area of the mass. No discharge was evident from the nipple. Left breast round and pendulous, without lumps or changes in the skin texture; no nipple discharge.

**Cardiovascular**

No lifts or heaves. Apical pulse noted at fifth intercostal space, midclavicular line. Apical rate 80, regular. $S_1$ greater than $S_2$ at the apex; no additional sounds, murmurs, or rubs.

**Peripheral Vascular**

Patient denies leg pain; extremities are warm to the touch, pink in color. Slight evidence of varicosities on both legs.

***Peripheral Pulses***
Temporal — 4 bilaterally
Carotid — 4 bilaterally
Brachial — 4 bilaterally
Radial — 4 bilaterally
Femoral — 4 bilaterally
Popliteal — 4 bilaterally
Posterior tibial — 4 bilaterally
Dorsalis pedis — 4 bilaterally

***Peripheral Pulse Scale***

| |
|---|
| 0 — Absent |
| 1 — Markedly diminished |
| 2 — Moderately diminished |
| 3 — Slightly diminished |
| 4 — Normal |

**Abdomen**

Slightly obese, protuberant, symmetrical abdomen. Bowel sounds present in all quadrants; no bruits, no visible pulsations; no lesions or tenderness.

Liver edge at the costal margin is smooth; liver height 9 cm (3⅝ in.) at the midclavicular line (MCL). Tympany noted in left upper quadrant.

**Musculoskeletal**

Full ROM of hands, wrists, elbows, shoulders, spine, hips, knees, and ankles. No crepitation or swelling noted. No pain on palpation over bony prominences.

**Neurological**

***Mental Status.*** Alert, oriented to person, place, and time. Remote and recent memory intact. Coordinated movements, gait, and balance are normal. Sensory system is intact for light touch, superficial pain, and vibrations.
***Cranial Nerves.*** I–XII intact.

***Deep Tendon Reflexes***

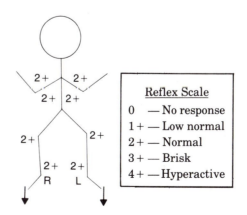

Reflex Scale
0  — No response
1+ — Low normal
2+ — Normal
3+ — Brisk
4+ — Hyperactive

| | |
|---|---|
| *Rectal* | Deferred. |
| *Genitalia* | Deferred. |

## Laboratory Data/Diagnostic Studies

*Laboratory Data*

*Na:* 136 mEq/L
*K:* 3.3 mEq/L
*Cl:* 96 mEq/L
*$CO_2$:* 29 mEq/L
*BUN:* 20 mg/dl
*Glucose (Fasting):* 92 mg/dl
*Hct:* 42.8%
*Hgb:* 13.8%

*Differential Leukocyte Count*
  Polymorphonuclear leukocytes, 52%
  Lymphocytes, 38%
  Monocytes, 10%
  Eosinophils, 2.6%
  Basophils, 0.3%

*Erythrocyte Sedimentation Rate:* 26 mm/hr
*Alk Phos:* 38 U/L
*Ca:* 9.2 mg/dl
*Bleeding Time:* 4.5 minutes
*Prothrombin Time:* 9.7/11.3 seconds
*Carcinoembryonic Antigen:* 2.9 ng/ml

*Urinalysis*
*Ph:* 6; yellow, clear
*Protein:* Negative
*Bile:* Negative
*Specific gravity:* 1.012
*Ketones:* Negative
*Sediment:* 2 WBC; 0–2 RBC; rare WBC casts; 0–5 hyaline casts

*Diagnostic Studies*

**ECG.** Sinus rhythm without ectopic activity. Ventricular rate 88 beats/minute.
**Chest X-Ray.** Clear lung fields.
**Bone Scan.** Negative for metastases.

## COLLABORATIVE PLAN OF CARE

| | |
|---|---|
| *Diet* | House diet. |
| *Medications* | Flurazepam hydrochloride (Dalmane) 30 mg PO qhs prn. |
| *Intravenous Therapy* | Does not apply. |
| *Therapeutic Measures* | Out of bed ad lib. Type and cross match 2 units of blood for OR in AM. |
| *Consults* | Does not apply. |

## Preoperative Plan

| | |
|---|---|
| *Diet* | NPO after midnight. |
| *Medications* | Diazepam (Valium) 7 mg with a sip of water on call for OR. (Ancef) 1 g IM on call for OR. |
| *Intravenous Therapy* | In the AM begin an intravenous (IV) infusion with dextrose 5% and 0.45% NaCl solution to run at 80 ml/hr. |
| *Therapeutic Measures* | Shave the right axillary area the morning before surgery. |
| *Consults* | Does not apply. |

# Postoperative Orders

| | |
|---|---|
| *Diet* | NPO until fully awake and alert; advance diet as tolerated. |

*Medications*

Morphine sulfate 4 mg or 6 mg or 8 mg IM q3h prn for pain.
Percocet 1–2 tabs PO q4h prn for pain.
Prochlorperazine maleate (Compazine) 10 mg IM q6h prn for nausea.
Triazolam (Halcion) 0.125 mg PO hs prn for sleep.
Cefazolin (Ancef) 3 g/250 ml of 5% D/W to run at 83 ml q8h × 48 hours.

*Intravenous Therapy*

Dextrose 5% and 0.45 NaCl solution to run at 80 ml/hr. Can convert IV to a heparin lock (intermittent venous access) when taking greater than 1000 ml PO in 24 hours.

*Therapeutic Measures*

Out of bed on the evening of surgery. Out of bed at least tid on the first postoperative day.
Elevate right arm on 3 pillows at all times.
Cough, turn, deep-breathe at least q2h.
Measure and record Hemovac drainage each shift.
Call physician for output greater than 50 ml q2h.
Notify physician if temperature is greater than 101.6°F (38.6°C).
Insert a straight urinary catheter if unable to void by 6 PM.

*Consults*

Call Reach to Recovery representative to visit patient.

*Additional Data*

*Postoperative physician's note:* Right modified radical mastectomy was performed, with removal of 4 involved axillary nodes. Estimated blood loss of 250 ml. One Hemovac drainage tube is in place. Surgery without complications; condition is stable. *Stage:* T2–N1–M0.

# NURSING DIAGNOSES DEVELOPED IN CARE PLAN

Body Image Disturbance, p. 298
Fear of Recurrence of Cancer, p. 300
Potential for Infection, p. 301

# ADDITIONAL NURSING DIAGNOSES TO BE CONSIDERED

Altered Sexuality Patterns
Dysfunctional Grieving
Family Coping: Potential for Growth
Hopelessness
Impaired Physical Mobility
Pain
Powerlessness
Sexual Dysfunction
Sleep Pattern Disturbance

# NURSING CARE PLAN BASED ON IDENTIFIED NURSING DIAGNOSES

| | |
|---|---|
| ***Body Image Disturbance*** | ***Related to:*** Removal of breast. <br> ***Evidenced by:*** Verbalized negative feelings about the change in her body; fear of rejection by husband; not looking at her incision site. |
| ***Desired Patient Outcomes*** | ***The Patient Will:*** <br> • Demonstrate a positive approach toward her altered body image. <br> • Use past coping strategies and personal strengths to gain control over her current health status. <br> • Reestablish presurgical social activities. <br> • View her incision site before discharge. <br> • Interact with a support system that she has identified to help her adjustment process. |
| ***Evaluation Criteria*** | ***By the Time of Discharge, the Patient Will:*** <br> • Identify coping mechanisms and strengths that have been successful in the past and apply them to the present. <br> • Develop and participate in a plan to view her surgical incision site. <br> • Discuss initiating a conversation with her husband concerning his reactions to the surgery and their combined need to share feelings with one another. <br> • Identify support systems to assist her in the rehabilitation process. <br> • Describe the presurgical activities that will be reinstated after her discharge. <br> • Describe ways to enhance her appearance and self-concept after surgery. |

## Interventions

Plan a time each day with the patient when the nurse will be with her to engage in conversation with regard to the patient's feelings.

Demonstrate support and concern for the patient.

Validate with the patient that her feelings are real and acceptable and should be discussed.

Allow adequate time for the patient to grieve the loss of her breast.

Be accepting of the patient's need to discuss the loss of her breast. Discussion

## Rationale

Presence on the part of the nurse is demonstrated by (1) verbal communication of empathy or understanding in regard to the patient's experience; (2) trust and genuineness, a positive regard for the patient; and (3) being physically available (Bulechek and McCloskey, 1985, p. 317).

Allowing the patient to have time to mourn the loss of a breast will help her progress toward an improved body image (Glasgow, Halfin, and Althausen, 1987, p. 326).

By deemphasizing the breast as a sexual organ and by referring to it as a diseased organ that threatened her life, the incision site

## Interventions

of the surgery should focus on the fact that a diseased organ was removed and the fact that it should not affect her sexual functioning and femininity.

Encourage discussion of the patient's strengths and coping strategies that were effective in the past.

Invite the patient to discuss contacting other sources of support that could be beneficial at this time, for example, a woman who has had a mastectomy, a priest, a psychiatric clinical nurse specialist, or an oncology clinical nurse specialist.

Encourage discussion of the patient's sexual self-concept to include her role as wife, lover, mother, and friend. Focus on the positive aspects of the roles and relationships that have existed for her.

Discuss ways to enhance appearance after the mastectomy. Wide shoulder straps, armholes without constrictions, opaque night gowns, and shopping in specialty shops for women who have experienced mastectomies are a few examples. Plan to have the patient fitted for a bra before her discharge. Invite a consultant to discuss the use of an external prosthetic device to enhance the patient's appearance in preparation for discharge.

Provide the patient with the opportunity to discuss the option of breast reconstruction.

Discuss with the patient the need to include her husband in a discussion concerning the recent changes in her body structure. Encourage her to discuss her feelings about resuming an intimate relationship with her husband.

## Rationale

for a woman who has had a mastectomy can be given a positive value (Glasgow, Halfin, and Althausen, 1987, p. 325).

The ability of a person to cope with a crisis depends in part on the coping skills she can use to adapt to a crisis (Barry, 1984, p. 84). Assessing the patient's strengths and previous coping skills provides the health care professional with a data base to help the patient reinforce her sense of self-worth (Bulechek and McCloskey, 1985, p. 284).

Patients are more comfortable expressing emotion to a person not directly responsible for the delivery of care. This additional supportive person may be viewed as a source of information, confidant, advocate, and facilitator (Youssef, 1984, p. 310).

Positive self-esteem is a result of the interactions with people close to oneself. Self-esteem can suffer during an illness due to the fact that the patient may perceive that negative appraisals will be forthcoming from significant others (Meisenhelder, 1985, pp. 127–135). A marital relationship that was supportive with good sexual adjustment preoperatively will have less adjustment difficulties postoperatively than a nonsupportive marital relationship (Woods, 1984, p. 346).

The reintegration of body image includes restoring feelings of attractiveness as well as being able to participate in discussions about breast reconstruction (Scott, 1983, p. 32).

Physiological adaptation to the effects of losing a breast may be improved when reconstruction is presented as an option (Woods, 1984, p. 349).

Offering a time to explore her husband's concerns and express his feelings regarding cancer can serve to decrease guilt over uncontrollable emotions. Husband and wife should discuss resumption of sexual relations. This will facilitate adaptation and increase the level of comfort between man and wife concerning issues surrounding sexual matters (Carroll, 1981, p. 31). Recent research suggests that when a patient and her husband have a high degree of social support from each other, family members, friends, nurses, and physicians they experience fewer adjustment problems (Northouse, 1988, p. 94).

## Interventions

Develop a plan with the patient to view the incision site. This includes assessing the patient's readiness to look at the incision. A sample plan might be this: On day 3 after surgery, the nurse removes the dressing and discusses what the scar looks like. On day 4, the patient looks at the incision site in the presence of the nurse. At that time, the patient agrees to discuss her feelings about the surgical site.

Discuss with the patient the need to maintain social contacts and continue with presurgical activities as a means of maintaining a positive self-concept.

## Rationale

The ability to look at what has happened to one's body is one step in the ability to cope with a body change. This should be encouraged throughout the patient's stay (Carroll, 1981, p. 31).

Patients have reported an improvement in the quality of their lives when they could gain control over their lives (Lindsay, 1985, p. 33). One of the goals in the reintegration of body image is the ability to participate in normal pleasurable activities (Scott, 1983, pp. 32–33).

---

**Fear of Recurrence of Cancer**

**Related to:** Perceived inability to control the spread of cancer.
**Evidenced by:** Verbalization of fear concerning a recurrence of cancer; recounting her mother's experience with cancer.

**Desired Patient Outcomes**

**The Patient Will:**
• Discuss her concerns about the recurrence of cancer.
• Develop an awareness of positive health habits.

**Evaluation Criteria**

**By the Time of Discharge, the Patient Will:**
• Understand that it is helpful to verbalize one's fears and concerns about cancer.
• Know that being an informed patient promotes hopefulness and aids in decreasing fears.
• Be knowledgeable about specific health care practices aimed at early detection and prevention of cancer recurrence.

---

## Interventions

Encourage discussion with the patient concerning her fear of cancer recurrence. Acknowledge her concerns and be available for future discussions about mastectomy-related fears.

Discuss with the patient her feelings about and knowledge of self–breast examination (SBE). Discuss the usefulness of this technique in order to have more control over her own body.

Teach the technique of SBE and emphasize the importance of assessing the

## Rationale

While it has been noted that most women worry about the spread of cancer, women who had a greater number of people with whom they could discuss their fears had a decreased fear of recurrence as compared with women who had few people to talk to and discuss their fears (Scott, 1983, p. 28).

Breast cancer is considered one of the leading causes of cancer death in women, and the teaching of breast self-examination has been considered a major strategy in an effort to achieve early detection (Lindsay, 1985, p. 29). The knowledge of the benefits from this preventive behavior is helpful in overcoming barriers against using this technique. Women with prior experience of this disease are more likely to practice SBE on a monthly basis or more frequently (Hirschfield-Bartek, 1982, p. 80).

Interventions aimed at early recognition of breast cancer result in a decreased mortality rate (Howard, 1987, p. 33; Wertheimer

operative chest wall as well as the unaffected breast. Provide the patient with relevant literature to read and discuss. Teach the patient to evaluate her breasts with the use of soapy water.

Discuss the importance of frequent mammograms. Encourage the patient to continue to have regular follow-up visits with a health care provider.

Encourage frequent self-examination of the surgical incision site.

Discuss with the patient the importance of being hopeful and maintaining a positive outlook concerning her prognosis and long-term survival with cancer.

et al, 1986, p. 1314). Examination done with soapy fingers assists the fingers in sliding with ease over the entire breast and axilla (Pfeiffer and Mulliken, 1984, p. 9). Women who master the SBE technique do feel a greater sense of control over their bodies (O'Malley and Fletcher, 1987, p. 2202).

A reduction in breast cancer mortality in women 50 years of age and older has been associated with mammography (O'Malley and Fletcher, 1987, p. 2197).

Local recurrence occurs at 2 principle sites: either at the adjacent skin flap or at the scar/grafted site (Mueller, 1987, p. 189).

Patients who exhibit a high degree of hope can be observed as persons who are more actively involved in their own care. It has been suggested that being well informed fosters hope by diminishing fear and anxiety (Brandt, 1987, p. 36).

---

| | |
|---|---|
| ***Potential for Infection*** | ***Related to:*** Surgical procedure to remove lymph nodes and vessels in the right axillary area in conjunction with the removal of the right breast.<br>***Evidenced by:*** Risk Factors—Suppressed inflammatory response, invasive surgical procedure, insufficient knowledge concerning exposure to pathogenic organisms; and tissue destruction. |
| ***Desired Patient Outcomes Evaluation Criteria*** | ***The Patient Will:***<br>• Be free from infection postmastectomy.<br>• Have minimal edema in the affected arm and hand.<br><br>***During this Hospitalization, the Patient Will:***<br>• Discuss ways to prevent trauma from occurring to the affected extremity.<br>• Describe the signs and symptoms associated with an infection and acknowledge what to do if they are present.<br>• Keep the affected arm elevated on pillows after surgery.<br>• Perform the prescribed exercise regimen at predetermined intervals and discuss continuance of the exercises once discharged. |

---

## Interventions

Discuss with the patient the need to avoid trauma to the affected arm and hand. The teaching plan would include the following points of emphasis:

• Avoid cuts or abrasions.
• Prevent burns by the use of padded pot holders in the kitchen and the use of water faucets that blend hot and cold water rather than individual hot and cold water faucets.
• Avoid sunburns.
• Do not have blood drawn, receive injections, or have blood pressures taken on the affected arm.

## Rationale

The axillary node dissection places the patient at an increased risk for the development of an infection and lymphedema (Pfeiffer and Mulliken, 1984, p. 55). The severity of an injury can affect the person's ability to heal without a wound impairment. A severe injury increases the risk of wound impairment. Healing can be disrupted when substrates for repair or regeneration are unavailable, when biochemical processes are disrupted, or when stressors alter the tissue response to the injury (Carrieri, Lindsey, and West, 1986, p. 344).

- Avoid constrictive clothing or jewelry.
- Avoid carrying heavy objects on the affected side.
- Use gloves when gardening.
- Use rubber gloves in hot water.
- Do not cut cuticles or pick hangnails.

Teach the patient to observe for the signs of infection in the affected arm or hand. She should watch for redness, swelling, or drainage at the site of the alteration in skin integrity. She may also experience pain. The physician should be contacted if these problems arise.

Postoperative teaching should include an emphasis on recognizing signs of infection since the patient is at an increased risk of developing an infection as a result of impaired lymph flow (Nail et al, 1984, p. 1123).

Teach the patient to keep the affected arm elevated on pillows immediately after surgery.

In the immediate postoperative period it is important to promote lymph drainage by elevating the affected arm (Luckmann and Sorensen, 1987, p. 1824).

Teach the patient to perform the prescribed arm exercises and develop a plan to continue them on a regular basis.

In order to regain strength and mobility in the affected arm, an exercise regimen is usually established after surgery (Pfeiffer and Mulliken, 1984, p. 193).

## QUESTIONS FOR DISCUSSION

1. Specimens of a breast cancer tumor are evaluated for estrogen receptor status. Discuss the significance of this test and its implications for both premenopausal and postmenopausal women.
2. The TNM system of classification is used for the clinical staging of the tumor. Explain what the T, N, and M refer to and discuss the patient's findings. When a woman is told she has a Stage I, II, or III tumor, what does this mean?
3. Chemotherapy is used as an adjuvant treatment for the patient with breast cancer. (a) Discuss what you would include in a teaching plan for the patient who will receive chemotherapy. (b) Discuss the following side effects associated with chemotherapeutic drugs: bone marrow suppression, alopecia, nausea and vomiting, stomatitis, and renal effects.
4. An alternative treatment to a mastectomy is local excision of the tumor followed by radiation therapy. Discuss the nursing care for the woman who is about to undergo her first radiation treatment.
5. Breast cancer is diagnosed with the use of a tissue biopsy. Discuss this procedure and explain the 2-step approach for the diagnosis and treatment of breast cancer.
6. Mrs. Heller asks about breast reconstruction. Discuss the procedures for breast reconstruction. What should be included in a patient teaching plan with regard to reconstructive surgery?

## REFERENCES

Barry, P: Psychological Nursing Assessment and Intervention. JB Lippincott, Philadelphia, 1984.

Brandt, BT: The relationship between hopelessness and selected variables in women receiving chemotherapy for breast cancer. Oncol Nurs Forum 14:35, 1987.

Bulechek, GM and McCloskey, JC: Nursing Interventions: Treatments for Nursing Diagnoses. WB Saunders, Philadelphia, 1985.

Carrieri, VK, Lindsey, AM, and West, CM: Pathophysiological Phenomena in Nursing: Human Responses to Illness. WB Saunders, Philadelphia, 1986.

Carroll, RM: The impact of mastectomy on body image. Oncol Nurs Forum 8:29, 1981.

Glasgow, M, Halfin, V, and Althausen, A: Sexual response

and cancer. CA—A Cancer Journal for Clinicians 37:322, 1987.

Hassey, KM: Pregnancy and parenthood after treatment for breast cancer. Oncol Nurs Forum 15:439, 1988.

Hirschfield-Bartek, J: Health beliefs and their influence on breast self-examination practices in women with breast cancer. Oncol Nurs Forum 9:77, 1982.

Howard, J: Using mammography for cancer control: An unrealized potential. CA—A Cancer Journal for Clinicians 37:33, 1987.

Lindsay, AM: Building the knowledge base for practice. II. Alopecia, breast self-exam and other human responses. Oncol Nurs Forum 12:27, 1985.

Luckmann, J and Sorensen, KC: Medical-Surgical Nursing: A Psychophysiologic Approach, ed 3. WB Saunders, Philadelphia, 1987.

Meisenhelder, JB: Self-esteem: A closer look at clinical interventions. Int J Nurs Stud 22:127, 1985.

Mueller, CB: Valid alternatives in the management of early breast cancer. Adv Surg 20:183, 1987.

Nail, L, et al: Sensations after mastectomy. Am J Nurs 84:1121, 1984.

Northouse, L: Social support in patients' and husbands' adjustment to breast cancer. Nurs Res 37:91, 1988.

O'Malley, MS and Fletcher, SW: Screening for breast cancer with breast self-examination. JAMA 257:2197, 1987.

Pfeiffer, CH and Mulliken, JB: Caring for the Patient with Breast Cancer: An Interdisciplinary/Multidisciplinary Approach. Reston Publishing, Reston, Va, 1984.

Scott, DW: Quality of life following the diagnosis of breast cancer. Topics Clin Nurs, January 1983, p 20.

Wertheimer, MD, et al: Increasing the effort toward breast cancer detection. JAMA 255:1311, 1986.

Woods, NF: Human Sexuality, ed 3. CV Mosby, St. Louis, 1984.

Youssef, FA: Crisis interventions: A group therapy approach for hospitalized breast cancer patients. J Adv Nurs 9:307, 1984.

# BIBLIOGRAPHY

Knobf, MT: Physical and psychologic distress associated with adjuvant chemotherapy in women with breast cancer. J Clin Oncol 4:678, 1986.

Oberst, M and James, R: Going home: Patient and spouse adjustment following cancer surgery. Topics Clin Nurs 7:46, 1985.

Schwarz-Appelbaum, J, et al: Nursing Care Plans: Sexuality and treatment of breast cancer. Oncol Nurs Forum 11:16, 1984.

Valanis, BG and Rumpler, CH: Helping women to choose breast cancer treatment alternatives. Cancer Nurs 8:167, 1985.

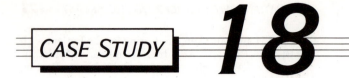

# A PATIENT WITH PREGNANCY-INDUCED HYPERTENSION

Maria N. Bueche, Ph.D., RNC

## ANATOMY AND PHYSIOLOGY OF THE FEMALE REPRODUCTIVE SYSTEM AND ASSOCIATED SYSTEMS AFFECTED BY PREGNANCY AND PREGNANCY-INDUCED HYPERTENSION

The female reproductive system consists of the external genitalia and the internal reproductive organs. The body surface containing the external female reproductive organs is called the vulva. The vulva consists of the vagina, labia minora and majora, clitoris, urethral orifice, Bartholin's ducts, Skene's ducts, the hymen, and the perineum.

The internal female reproductive organs consist of the uterus, the 2 ovaries, and the 2 fallopian tubes. The uterus is a pear-shaped, thick-walled muscular organ located between the bladder and the rectum and is supported by ligaments and the muscles of the pelvic floor. It consists of 3 parts: the upper portion known as the fundus, the middle portion known as the corpus, and the lower portion called the cervix. The cervix extends into the vagina and has an internal and external os or opening.

The wall of the uterus consists of the outer serosal, the middle myometrial, and the inner endometrial layers. The endometrial layer undergoes characteristic changes during the menstrual cycle and also serves as the attachment site for the developing embryo. During pregnancy, the myometrium thickens primarily through hypertrophy of pre-existing muscle cells. The main blood supply to the uterus comes from the ovarian and uterine arteries. The main nerve supply comes from the sympathetic and parasympathetic nervous systems. The endocervical glands, under hormonal influence, increase cervical mucous production throughout pregnancy.

The ovaries are 2 oval-shaped structures located in the upper part of the pelvic cavity. They are held in place near the uterus by several ligaments (Reeder and Martin, 1987, pp. 104–110). They ripen and expel the ovum. Each ovary has a lifetime supply of germ cells present at birth. From puberty to menopause, a follicle ruptures each month and releases an ovum. The corpus luteum, formed at the site of the follicular rupture, secretes progesterone and estrogen. If fertilization takes place, the corpus luteum continues to secrete these hormones until this function is taken over by the placenta (Reeder and Martin, 1987, pp. 107–110; Thompson et al, 1986, pp. 943–966).

The fallopian tubes are two flexible, trumpet-shaped, muscular tubes extending from the upper portion of the uterus. One end opens into the uterus and the other fimbriated end opens into the abdominal area and lies near the ovary.

The fimbriated ends of the fallopian tube convey the ovum into the tube itself. The ovum is propelled by cilia and the peristaltic contractions of smooth muscles of the tube. The major blood supply comes from the ovarian and uterine arteries. The tubes are innervated by the same nerves as the uterus. Fertilization takes place in the distal and middle segment of the tube. The oocyte takes 3–4 days to reach the uterus.

In addition to the female reproductive system, the cardiovascular, renal, and placental systems play a critical role in a normal pregnancy. These are also the systems most affected by the development of pregnancy-induced hypertension (PIH), a syndrome characterized by edema, hypertension, and proteinuria.

During a normal pregnancy, the total blood volume increases by as much as 30%–50%. This increase gradually reaches its peak between 20–24 weeks. The number of red blood cells also increases dramatically but not as rapidly as the plasma fluid expansion. The hematocrit and hemoglobin values decrease slightly (but still remain within normal limits) due to this diluting effect. During the third trimester, the plasma fluid level stabilizes, the body continues its red blood cell production, and the "physiological anemia of pregnancy" disappears.

Cardiac output is increased by 25%–50% and reaches its peak around the 28th–32nd week. It is reflected in an average increase of the heart rate by 10 beats per minute. During the third trimester, cardiac output gradually decreases. This is thought to be partially due to the pressure exerted on the vena cava by the enlarging uterus.

Blood pressure essentially remains unchanged. In some women, a slight decrease may be noted during the first half of pregnancy. During the latter half, it rises to its prepregnant level (Neeson and May, 1986, pp. 265–266).

During labor, delivery, and the early postpartum period, dramatic changes again occur in cardiac output. Factors affecting cardiac output include position of the mother, use of anesthesia, and method of delivery (Pillitteri, 1985, p. 308; Pauerstein, 1987, pp. 627–628).

The renal system adapts in a number of ways to the presence of the growing fetus. Because of an increase in the load of excretory products, the amount of urine produced is slightly increased. Due to the production of steroid hormones by the placenta and the adrenal cortex, there is a greater absorption of sodium, chloride, and water by the renal tubules. At the same time, there is a noticeable increase in the glomerular filtration rate (GFR) resulting in an increased loss of water and electrolytes in the urine. However, a balance between absorption and loss is maintained between the two mechanisms resulting in minimal retention of water and salt by the mother (Guyton, 1981, p. 1030).

The ureters become dilated during pregnancy due to the pressure of the enlarging uterus and the elaboration of hormones that contribute to the softening of the ureteral walls (Reeder and Martin, 1987, p. 295).

The placenta is involved in the transfer of gases and heat, in the transport of nutrients, in the excretion of wastes, and in the production of hormones. The maternal side of the placenta contains approximately 20 cotyledons or lobes. These lobes are further subdivided into approximately 200 lobules, each of which contains a single spiral artery. The mother's blood flows from the uterine arteries, through the maternal spiral arteries, and into the large maternal blood sinuses. These blood sinuses surround the placental villi, bringing oxygen-rich blood to the fetus; the oxygen-depleted blood then leaves by way of the uterine veins of the mother. The fetus's blood flows through 2 umbilical arteries to the capillaries of the placental villi and returns through the one umbilical vein. It is clear that there is normally no direct connection between the circulations of the mother and fetus. Diffusion of gases, nutrients, and wastes takes place at the level of the placental villi and maternal blood sinuses.

During normal labor, uterine contractions compress the spiral arteries in the myometrium. The healthy fetus readily tolerates this temporary decrease in oxygen supply (Reeder and Martin, 1987, pp. 162–164).

# PATHOPHYSIOLOGY OF PREGNANCY-INDUCED HYPERTENSION

PIH is a syndrome characterized by hypertension, proteinuria, and edema. It generally occurs after the 20th week and may be progressive in nature. The condition may be mild, affecting only a few organ systems, to severe, affecting many organ systems. Indications that PIH is increasing in severity are the presence of epigastric pain, hyperreflexia, headache, visual disturbances, oliguria, drowsiness, nausea, and vomiting. The onset of convulsions indicates a significant increase in severity.

The following classification system is now generally accepted (Ouimette, 1986, p. 117):

    I. PIH

        A. Pre-eclampsia—a term used to describe the occurrence of hypertension, proteinuria, and edema after the 20th week of gestation.

        B. Eclampsia—a term used to describe the symptoms of pre-eclampsia plus seizures.

    II. Hypertension (chronic) existing prior to the pregnancy (any etiology).

    III. Chronic hypertension with superimposed PIH.

IV. Late or transient or gestational hypertension—during pregnancy or within 10 days postpartum.

In PIH, significant pathological changes occur in the circulatory, renal, and placental systems. Generalized vasospasm is a major alteration found in the circulatory system. It is postulated that the vasculature of the woman with PIH is extremely sensitive to vasopressors, such as renin synthesized by the kidney. Prostaglandins of the E series are also present and act as vasodilators. It is thought that an imbalance in the action between the vasoconstrictors and the vasodilators is responsible for the resultant hypertension (Braunwald, et al, 1987, p. 1204).

Hemoconcentration also occurs in the presence of severe PIH. The expected increase in plasma fluid volume that occurs in normal pregnancy does not appear to take place. The heart responds to this decreased plasma fluid volume by increasing the pulse rate. Despite the tachycardia, there is decreased cardiac return and cardiac decompensation may occur. Hemoconcentration and the fact that red blood cell production is unaffected both contribute to an increased hematocrit level (Thompson, et al, 1986, p. 1011).

Generalized vasospasm also contributes to a decrease in renal perfusion and the glomerular filtration rate. A characteristic change in the kidney is the development of glomeruloendotheliosis. This renal lesion shows a number of changes including edema of the glomerular tuft and thickening of the glomerular basement membrane (Thompson, et al, 1986, p. 1011). These changes are partially reflected in the retention of fluid and the decrease in urinary output. Evidence of retention is seen in edema of the extremities, hands, and face. With worsening of the condition, edema of the brain may occur resulting in convulsions; fluid may collect in the lungs leading to pulmonary edema; and urine output may decrease leading to oliguria.

In addition, constriction of the maternal distal spiral arteries in the placenta takes place. Because of the constriction, the blood supply to the lobules is decreased, resulting in a decrease in gas, nutrient, and waste transport. The extent of constriction, the size of the area involved, and the timing and duration of the pathology all will influence the well-being of the fetus. Labor imposes an additional stressor on this compromised blood supply. Uterine contractions result in further compression of the spiral arteries in the myometrium, which may be evidenced as fetal distress. Cumulative effects on the fetus during pregnancy may be evidenced by IUGR (intrauterine growth retardation). During labor, the effects of a decreased oxygen supply may range from mild hypoxia to stillbirth (Reeder and Martin, 1987, pp. 162–163; Pauerstein, 1987, p. 648).

Although the major organs involved in PIH are the cardiovascular, renal, and uteroplacental systems, other organs may be involved when the condition is severe. The liver may show damage from edema, coagulation defects, and thrombi formation; the brain may be affected by edema, thrombi, rupture, and infarction of blood vessels; and the retina may show the effects of edema and constriction of arterioles.

## RISK FACTORS

Risk factors frequently associated with the development of PIH are a maternal age of under 18 years or over 35 years; primigravidity; chronic hypertension; previous obstetrical history of PIH; family history of hypertension, PIH, or vascular disease; and conditions such as diabetes mellitus, multiple gestation, and hydatidiform mole. Dietary deficiencies, especially decreased protein intake, and being underweight or obese are also significant factors. PIH is also more commonly found in women of a lower socioeconomic level and in women who do not receive prenatal care.

## COMMON CLINICAL FINDINGS

Common clinical findings are excessive edema, weight gain, proteinuria, and an increase in blood pressure. Almost every woman experiences some edema during pregnancy, particularly of the feet and ankles in the third trimester. However, edema of the hands and face may be pathological. Weight gain is vital but a sudden gain of more than 2 lb (0.9 kg) per week is reason for concern. Proteinuria may range from 1+ on a dipstick reading to a loss of 0.5 g/L or more in a 24-hour specimen. In terms of blood pressure, an increase of 30 mmHg in systolic and an increase of 15 mmHg diastolic over the baseline is significant, as are readings above 140/90.

A progression of signs and symptoms may occur despite prompt diagnosis and early treatment. The common clinical findings, previously discussed, may increase in severity. In addition, pathophysiological changes will occur in a number of other systems throughout the body. Early central nervous system effects may be experienced by the woman as hyperreflexia and headache, and later effects, as convulsions. Liver edema may be reflected as epigastric pain; renal changes as oliguria; retinal changes as blurring of vision; and respiratory changes as dyspnea.

Maternal complications of PIH include placenta abruptio, disseminated intravascular coagulopathy (DIC) with or without hypofibrinogenemia, and maternal cerebrovascular accident (Pauerstein, 1987, p. 656). Recent reports indicate that another outcome of severe PIH is the HELLP syndrome. The incidence of this syndrome is not yet known, but it is characterized by hemolysis (H), elevated liver enzymes (EL), and low platelets (LP) (Shannon, 1987, pp. 395–396).

Fetal and newborn complications relate primarily to the fact that many of these infants are born or delivered prematurely. Because of placental insufficiency, the fetus may be small for gestational age (SGA). However, the stress of the intrauterine environment appears to increase fetal lung maturation and therefore these infants tend to do better than others of equal weight and/or gestational age (Bobak and Jensen, 1987, p. 780).

The woman who has coped with PIH during her first pregnancy will be concerned about its recurrence rate. Pauerstein found that "there is one category of patients who may be predisposed to recurrent severe pre-eclampsia/eclampsia (i.e., PIH): those who have a maternal genetic component for the disease as characterized by previous obstetric history, positive maternal history, or siblings who have had similar problems" (1987, p. 656).

PIH remains one of the 3 major causes of maternal morbidity and mortality. Fortunately, only a small percentage of women develop convulsions. Once a woman develops convulsions, she and the fetus are at an increased risk of mortality.

## TREATMENT MODALITIES

Treatment modalities for PIH consist of preventive measures, bed rest, dietary modifications, monitoring of maternal and fetal well-being, and use of medications to prevent convulsions and treat the hypertension.

The best treatment for PIH is its prevention through early, regular prenatal care. Patient/family and lifestyle risk factors may be identified and possibly modified. An increase in blood pressure, proteinuria, and hyperreflexia are not usually apparent to the woman but may be readily identified by the nurse or physician. PIH often responds to home management of bed rest, dietary modification, assessment of fetal well-being, and assessment for signs and symptoms of increasing severity of PIH. Should hospitalization become necessary, additional assessments of maternal and fetal well-being and administration of medications to prevent convulsions and treat hypertension are utilized. If the severity of PIH continues to increase, the fetus may be assessed for fetal lung maturity. If necessary and time permits, fetal lung maturity may be hastened through the administration of steroids to the mother. Delivery of the fetus usually resolves the maternal signs and symptoms of PIH within 8–48 hours.

## PATIENT ASSESSMENT DATA BASE

## Health History

*Client:*
Susan D. Brown

*Address:* 24 Long St., Iowa City, IA 52240
*Telephone:* 319-555-9352
*Contact:* Mary (mother)
*Address of contact:* Same
*Telephone of contact:* Same
*Age:* 17    *Sex:* Female    *Race:* White
*Educational background:* A junior in high school
*Religion:* Catholic    *Marital status:* Single
*Usual occupation:* Student
*Source of income:* Family. Father works as a janitor in local elementary school; mother is at home.
*Insurance:* Covered by father's Blue Cross/Blue Shield
*Source of referral:* Self
*Source of history:* Patient and current chart
*Reliability of historian:* Reliable
*Date of interview:* 3/1/90
*Reason for visit/Chief complaint:* "Last time I was here they told me I had to come back in to be checked in a week. They thought I was gaining too much weight or something, but honest, I haven't been eating too much lately. Something about my blood pressure being up a little, too. I might even have to be hospitalized. I don't know what they're so worried about; I feel OK."

## Health Perception/Health Management Pattern

*Present Health Status*

Susan states that she was in "pretty good" health prior to her pregnancy. At this time, her pregnancy is interfering with her ability to achieve the following developmental tasks of adolescence.

***Achievement of New and More Mature Relationships with Age Mates of Both Sexes.*** She no longer has her boyfriend, an 18-year-old high school senior, nor is she able to maintain a number of peer relationships. The latter has occurred because she has left school.

***Achievement of a Feminine Social Role.*** Pregnancy is the taking on of a feminine role but it has limited her opportunity to grow and develop other aspects of her role.

***Acceptance of Her Physique and Effective Use of Her Body.*** As an adolescent, she experienced very rapid and dramatic growth throughout her body and was concerned about the normalcy of these changes. Because body image is still in the formative stage, she is finding the many changes associated with pregnancy difficult to accept.

***Achievement of Independence From Parents and Other Adults.*** At a time when she is attempting to distance herself and become more autonomous, pregnancy forces her to again become more dependent on her parents. Not only does she require their financial assistance but the pregnant state itself causes her to be more dependent and vulnerable.

***Establishment of a Life-style that Is Personally and Socially Satisfying.*** This pregnancy was unplanned. She had not used contraception. She feels that she was not making conscious choices regarding sexual relationships, parenthood, and career. At this time, she has interrupted her high school education. Because of this, she thinks she may be considerably older before she completes this task. She also states that her career plans are "up in the air" and have to be changed because of her new responsibilities.

***Acquisition of an Ethical System that Will Serve as a Guide to Socially Responsible Behavior.*** Her ethical system is sufficiently developed for her to feel guilty about this pregnancy. She recognizes that this is not socially responsible behavior and is now attempting to make a decision as to what would be best for the baby, for her family, and herself (Bobak and Jensen, 1987, pp. 950–952).

She came to the Prenatal Clinic for the first time about 8 weeks ago. Assessment of uterine size, fetal heart sounds, and fetal movement by ultrasound confirmed a pregnancy of 20 weeks. She had not sought prenatal care earlier because she felt that "I just couldn't be pregnant. My father would kill me."

She was encouraged to continue to come for prenatal care and was seen at 24 and 28 weeks, respectively. At her 28th-week visit, a slight increase in blood pressure and an 11-lb (5-kg) weight gain was noted. Susan received instructions regarding diet, bed rest, and the potential complications of PIH and was asked to return today, 1 week later.

## Past Health Status

***General Health.*** Susan's health has been good. She states that she experiences dysmenorrhea with every cycle. Has not sought medical help for these cramps but takes a variety of over-the-counter medications for them.

***Prophylactic Medical/Dental Care.*** Does not have her own physician. Went to a "Health Stop" clinic 8 months ago when she had a sore throat. Last visit to a dentist was 2 years ago; had several dental caries filled.

***Childhood Illnesses.*** Chickenpox—age 9 years; does not recall any other childhood illnesses. Rubella titer is 1:10.

***Immunizations.*** None since entry into first grade.

***Major Illnesses/Hospitalizations.*** None.

### Current Medications

*Prescription:* None.

*Nonprescription:* Aspirin—"One or 2 when I have a headache;" Ibuprofen (Advil)—"One 200-mg tablet for my cramps"; Ibuprofen (Motrin)—"Sometimes I take Motrin instead of Advil."

***Allergies.*** No known allergies to medications or foods.

### Habits

*Alcohol:* Does not drink.

*Caffeine:* Drinks 3–4 glasses of Coke every day; does not drink coffee.

*Drugs:* None. See Current Medications.

*Tobacco:* One pack a day for the past 2 years. Does not want to quit. "All my friends smoke. It doesn't hurt the baby, does it?"

### *Family Health History*

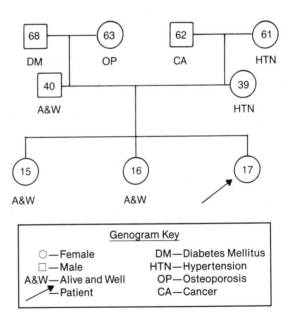

Family history is significant in that the maternal grandmother and mother are being treated for chronic hypertension and the paternal grandfather is being treated for diabetes mellitus.

## NUTRITIONAL/METABOLIC PATTERN

### Nutritional

Usually eats 2 meals per day and 2–3 snacks. States that she likes to eat, especially "junk" food such as potato chips, Coke, sweets.

***Usual Daily Menu***
*Breakfast:* Does not eat breakfast.
*Lunch:* One–2 bagels with cream cheese, potato chips, Coke, chocolate chip cookies.
*Snack:* Coke, vanilla ice cream topped with small package of plain M&M's.
*Dinner:* Double cheeseburger, large french fries, 1 apple snack pie.
*Snack:* Coke, and some Oreo cookies.

**Metabolic**

At 29 weeks, Susan has gained a total of 30 lb (13.6 kg). Pattern of weight gain is as follows: 14 lb (6.3 kg) by 24 weeks; 11 lb (5 kg) from 24–28 weeks; and 5 lb (2.3 kg) this past week.
*Current weight:* 180 lb (82 kg).
*Prepregnant weight:* 150 lb (68 kg).
*Height:* 5 ft 3 in. (160 cm).

## Elimination Pattern

**Bowel**

Has 1 formed bowel movement every other day. States that flatus has increased since her pregnancy.

**Bladder**

Urinates about 8 times per day. Gets up once during the night to void. Denies dysuria, frequency, or urgency.

## Activity/Exercise Pattern

**Activity/Exercise**

Susan dropped out of school a couple of weeks ago. She usually sleeps until noon, eats, goes shopping or "hangs out" at the mall, calls her girlfriend, and watches TV. States, "I feel tired most of the time." Has no self-care deficits related to bathing, feeding, dressing, toileting, or ambulation. Is dependent on her mother for cooking, shopping, and home maintenance.

***Self-Care Ability***

| | |
|---|---|
| Feeding — 0 | Grooming — 0 |
| Bathing — 0 | General mobility — 0 |
| Toileting — 0 | Cooking — II |
| Bed mobility — 0 | Home maintenance — II |
| Dressing — 0 | Shopping — II |

***Functional Levels Code***

  0 — Full self-care
  I — Requires use of equipment or device
 II — Requires assistance or supervision from another person
III — Requires assistance or supervision from another person and equipment or device
IV — Is dependent and does not participate

**Oxygenation/Perfusion**

Has not had a chest x-ray. Has no history of chest pain or palpitations.

**Cardiac Risk Factors**

|  | Positive | Negative |
|---|---|---|
| Sedentary life-style | X |  |
| Hyperlipidemia |  | X |
| Cigarette smoking | X |  |
| Diabetes |  | X |
| Obesity | X |  |
| Hypertension | X |  |
| Hypervigilant personality |  | X |
| Family history of heart disease |  | X |

## SLEEP/REST PATTERN

### Sleep/Rest

Stays up late; often watches TV movies. Sleeps 11 hours a night but often does not feel rested. Occasionally wakes up with leg cramps but readily falls asleep again.

## COGNITIVE/PERCEPTUAL PATTERN

### Hearing

Reports no difficulties with hearing.

### Vision

Susan has worn glasses since third grade for nearsightedness; changed to soft contact lenses upon entry into junior high school.

### Sensory Perception

Notices a tightness in both feet and ankles by the end of the day. Occasionally gets a sudden cramping in the calf of one or the other leg during the night.

### Learning Style

States she has been an average student in high school. Likes to learn by doing. Is able to learn when she is interested in a topic. Likes music and typing.

## SELF-PERCEPTION/SELF-CONCEPT PATTERN

### Self-Perception/Self-Concept

Susan has experienced difficulty in achieving the developmental tasks of pregnancy, that is, accepting the pregnancy, adjusting to changes in self, adjusting to changes in the couple relationship, and in preparing for birth and early motherhood. Initially she ignored the signs and symptoms of pregnancy using denial until she began to show. When she shared the news with the father of the baby (FOB) he responded with anger and left. States she is very upset about losing her boyfriend. Now feels that he did not love her enough to go through this pregnancy with her. Wishes she had someone to pay attention to her and take care of her.

Her parents were very upset, especially her father. He did not like her boyfriend and always tried to keep her from going out with him. He was always very strict with her and insisted that she was too young to be dating. Both parents "screamed and yelled," and threatened to throw her out of the house. She says she fantasizes that her baby will look like the brother she always wishes she had.

States she hates getting "fatter and fatter." "I've always felt too fat and now being pregnant has made me feel even worse. I don't even look at myself in the mirror. A lot of times I really feel down on myself but I hide it. My family thinks I'm cheerful and outgoing most of the time. Sometimes when I'm really moody, I

*Self-Perception/Self-Concept—
Continued*

shut the door to my bedroom, flop on the bed, and put on my music real loud."

Susan is undecided as to whether she will attend childbirth education classes. States that her mother will probably help her get things ready for the baby when the time comes. (Neeson and May, 1986, pp. 343–347). Also relates that she is very "bossy" with her two younger sisters and argues a lot with her mother. Says her mother "just won't let me grow up."

## ROLE/RELATIONSHIP PATTERN

*Role/Relationship*

Susan lives at home with her parents and sisters. States that since she has dropped out of school, her friends do not seem to care about her anymore and are calling her less and less on the phone. Lots of times she feels lonely and does not know what to do with herself.

States that although her family is close, they are pretending that nothing has changed. Her sisters do not mention that she is pregnant, and they do not ask her how she feels.

States she resents the fact that she is now more dependent on her parents for their support and financial assistance. They are trying to persuade her to give the baby up for adoption. She hasn't decided yet but thinks that someday she would like to finish high school and be happily married.

## SEXUALITY/REPRODUCTIVE PATTERN

*Sexuality/Reproductive*

Patient is a gravida 1, para 0; has had 1 boyfriend, the father of the baby; engaged in unprotected sexual intercourse. States she does not know much about the menstrual cycle, that is, when one can or cannot become pregnant. Age of menarche was 12½ years; thinks periods have become more regular during the past year but does not keep track; flow lasts 5 days, is moderate in amount, with the second day being the heaviest.

## COPING/STRESS TOLERANCE PATTERN

*Coping/Stress Tolerance*

Susan states she has been under a lot of stress lately. She had to decide how to tell her parents about the pregnancy but before she could do so, her mother confronted her about it. Usually copes with stress by making jokes, eating, and smoking. Since leaving school, she has also been sleeping more. States that she has 1 aunt, who lives nearby, whom she can talk with. She feels that this aunt has always liked her and is very accepting of her as a person.

When asked what she would like to change in her life, she said "I wish I had never given in to him, but he was my first boyfriend, and I was afraid of losing him. I wish I could be with my friends, back in school."

## VALUE/BELIEF PATTERN

*Value/Belief*

Susan relates that she feels very guilty about being pregnant without being married. She is upset that she even thought about having an abortion at one time. States that she feels that it would have been morally wrong. Identifies herself as a strong Catholic. Usually goes to church once a week with her family. Believes in God.

# Physical Examination

## General Survey

A 17-year-old, G1P0, 29th week of pregnancy, single, female, estimated date of confinement (EDC) May 17th, cooperative.
*Height:* 5'3" (160 cm).
*Prepregnant Weight:* 150 lb (68 kg).
*Current weight:* 180 lb (82 kg).

## Vital Signs

*Temperature:* 98.6°F (37°C) (oral)
*Pulse:* 88 regular
*Respirations:* 22 regular
*BP:* 150/100 (right arm with patient in left lateral position).
*Pattern of BP Increase:* At 20 weeks, 120/70, at 24 weeks, 130/80, at 28 weeks, 140/90, all taken on right arm and same position, as above.

## Integument

*Skin.* Oiliness of skin on nose and cheeks; striae gravidarum on abdomen, thighs, and breasts; linea nigra from symphysis pubis to top of fundus. Skin on torso, arms, and legs is warm and adequately hydrated with no evidence of lesions or scarring.
*Mucous Membranes.* Moist, pink; no lesions noted.
*Nails.* Nails on hands and toes are smooth.

## HEENT

*Head.* Symmetrical and smooth; brown hair is oily, symmetrically distributed; no evidence of nits. Face is symmetrical with some puffiness of eyes. Temporomandibular Joint (TMJ) is fully mobile without crepitation or pain.
*Eyes.* Irises are blue in color; ophthalmoscopic examination of the retina reveals no arteriospasm or edema. Pupils equal, round, reactive to light and accommodation (PERRLA). Visual acuity in left eye is 20/30 and in right eye is 20/40 with soft contact lenses in place, using the Rosenbaum chart for testing near vision (Seidel et al, 1987, pp. 32–33).
*Ears.* Cerumen in left and right external auditory canal. Left and right tympanic membranes show increased vascularity; no evidence of scarring or infection.
*Nose.* Slight congestion of mucous membranes; deep pink in color, increased vascularity.
*Mouth/Throat.* Lips are dry and chapped; buccal mucosa is pink and moist; teeth are present and in good repair; gums slightly swollen, reddened, and spongy; tonsils are present; not enlarged. Trachea is midline; slight enlargement of thyroid gland consistent with pregnancy; no palpable masses.

## Pulmonary

Anteriorposterior chest diameter and circumference slightly enlarged due to enlarging uterus; respirations 22 per minute; breath sounds, anterior and posterior chest, within normal limits; no rales or adventitious sounds heard.

## Breast

Convex and symmetrical in shape; skin texture is smooth and soft; bilateral venous pattern visible; areolae are dark brown in color with increased diameters; nipples are prominent, dark, and erect; Montgomery's tubercles are prominent; able to express colostrum; Tanner stage V breast development.

## Cardiovascular

Apical pulse 88 per minute; normal $S_1$ and $S_2$ sounds at each of the cardiac areas; no $S_3$ or $S_4$ sounds heard.

## Peripheral Vascular

Arterial pulses are palpable and normal in both upper and lower extremities; negative Homans' sign; no evidence of superficial

**Peripheral Vascular—Continued**

varicosities in lower extremities; dependent pitting edema (+2) in both feet and ankles; some puffiness of fingers.

**Peripheral Pulses**
Temporal—4 bilaterally
Carotid—4 bilaterally
Brachial—4 bilaterally
Radial—4 bilaterally
Femoral—4 bilaterally
Popliteal—4 bilaterally
Posterior tibial—4 bilaterally
Dorsalis pedis—4 bilaterally

**Peripheral Pulse Scale**

0—Absent
1—Markedly diminished
2—Moderately diminished
3—Slightly diminished
4—Normal

**Abdomen**

No scars, rashes, lesions; no liver enlargement or tenderness. Striae gravidarum and linea nigra are present; umbilicus is flat; fetal movement observed; Leopold's maneuvers reveal cephalic presentation; fundal height measurement 29 cm (11.4 in.); no diastasis of abdominal recti muscles; bowel sounds decreased; fetal heart rate is 160 beats per minute, with point of maximum intensity slightly left of the umbilicus.

**Musculoskeletal**

Full range of motion of upper and lower extremities. No pain on movement. Lordosis of lower spine; increased mobility of sacroiliac, sacrococcygeal, and pubic joints.

**Neurological**

**Mental Status.** Oriented; responds appropriately to questions; makes eye contact.
**Cranial Nerves.** Cranial nerves I–XII intact.
**Sensory.** Response to light touch on upper and lower extremities is within normal limits.

**Deep Tendon Reflexes**

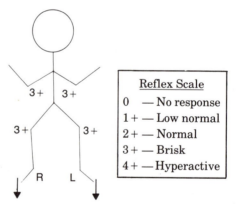

Reflex Scale

0  — No response
1+ — Low normal
2+ — Normal
3+ — Brisk
4+ — Hyperactive

Brisk deep tendon reflexes, 3+; no ankle clonus.

**Rectovaginal Examination**

Rectal tone is adequate; rectovaginal septum is intact; sacral shape, ischial spines, and sacrospinous ligaments are within normal limits; no evidence of rectal masses or hemorrhoids.

**Vaginal Examination**

Inspection and palpation of external genitalia—within normal limits; speculum examination reveals a small, round nulliparous cervical os. Presence of white vaginal discharge; vagina bluish in color with rugae present. Bimanual examination reveals soft cervical os; ovoid-shaped uterus—nontender; ovaries not palpable; gynecoid pelvis; irregular Braxton-Hicks contractions.

## Laboratory Data/Diagnostic Studies

**Laboratory Data**

### Blood Tests
**WBC:** 16,000/mm$^3$
**RBC:** 3.6 million/mm$^3$
**Hgb:** 10.5 g/100 ml
**Hct:** 32%
**Platelets:** 200,000/mm$^3$
**Antithrombin III:** Less than 80% of normal
**Fibrinogen:** 450 mg/dl
**Serum Iron:** 48 mg/dl
**Serum Folate:** 1.9 mg/ml
**Blood Sugar Level:**
Fasting: 65 mg/dl
2-hour postprandial: 130 mg/dl
**Blood Group and Rh Factor:** A, Rh+
**Serology or VDRL Test:** Negative
**Serum Creatinine:** 2.4 mg/dl
**BUN:** 12 mg/dl

### Electrolytes
**Na:** 148 mEq/L
**K:** 5.0 mEq/dl
**Cl:** 108 mEq/L

### Urine Tests
**Urinalysis:**
pH: 6.0
Color: Yellow
Specific gravity: 1.026
**Protein:** 2+
**Glucose:** 1+
**Ketones:** Negative
**Urine Culture and Sensitivity:** Negative
**Uric Acid — 24-Hour Urine Specimen:** 500 mg/24 hr — normal diet

### Cultures
**Gonorrhea:** Negative
**Herpes:** Negative
**Chlamydia:** Negative

**Diagnostic Studies**

*Nonstress Test (NST).* Reactive. Fetus responded with 3 heart rate accelerations associated with fetal movement during a 20-minute testing period (ACOG Technical Bulletin No. #107, 1987).

*Daily Fetal Movement Count.* Eight episodes of fetal activity noted during a 2-hour maternal rest period. Fetus demonstrated more than the minimum 6 episodes per 2-hour period (Pauerstein, 1987, p. 264).

*Biophysical Profile (BPP).* Score: 6/8. A score of 6 out of 8 indicates that the fetus is doing well. However, fetus received a score of 0 for fetal breathing because respiratory movement was not observed during the 30-minute testing period (Pauerstein, 1987, pp. 261–264).

*Ultrasound.* Initial measurement of biparietal diameter (BPD) of fetal head at first prenatal visit indicated a pregnancy of 20 weeks. No evidence of intrauterine growth retardation (IUGR). Another BPD measurement will be obtained at 33 weeks to evaluate dates more precisely (Pauerstein, 1987, p. 269) and reassess for IUGR.

# COLLABORATIVE PLAN OF CARE FOR MILD TO MODERATE PIH

**Diet**

Eighty-gram protein diet; no salt restriction.

**Medications**

Prenatal vitamin preparation with 1 mg of folic acid 1 tablet PO qd.
Ferrous sulfate 325 mg PO tid.

**Intravenous Therapy**

Does not apply.

| | |
|---|---|
| ***Therapeutic Measures*** | BP and pulse qid. |
| | Assess deep tendon reflexes qid with vital signs. |
| | Weigh qd. |
| | Measure intake and output. |
| | Urine protein qd; if greater than 1+, obtain 24-hour urine for a total protein level. |
| | Complete bed rest on left side with bathroom privileges. |
| | Fetal surveillance: Fetal heart rate (FHR) qid; fetal movement chart qd; NST twice weekly. |
| | Obtain baseline laboratory values: Complete blood count (CBC), BUN, serum creatinine, antithrombin III, serum free iron, platelet count, fibrinogen level, liver profile studies, and electrolytes. |
| | Hct qd × 4 days. |
| ***Consults*** | Nutrition and social service consult. |
| ***Preoperative Plan*** | Does not apply. |

# COLLABORATIVE PLAN OF CARE FOR SEVERE PIH

| | |
|---|---|
| ***Diet*** | Clear liquid diet. |
| ***Medications*** | Prenatal vitamin preparation with 1 mg of folic acid 1 tablet PO qd. |
| | Ferrous sulfate 325 mg PO tid. |
| | Magnesium sulfate ($MgSO_4$) 4 g in 250 ml of 5% D/W over 20 minutes as a loading dose, followed by a continuous infusion of 1–2 g/hr. |
| | Calcium gluconate 1 g intravenous (IV) push—antidote for magnesium sulfate toxicity, that is, hypotension, urine <25 ml/hr, respirations <12/minute, absence of deep tendon reflexes, serum levels above 10 mg/dl, and decrease in fetal heart rate. |
| | Hydralazine (Apresoline) 5–10 mg IV push or 6–12 mg/hr by IV infusion to maintain diastolic pressure at 90–100 mmHg. |
| | Administer betamethasone (steroid) 12 mg intramuscularly (IM) if indicated, that is, for fetal lung maturity. Give at least 24–48 hours prior to delivery. |
| ***Intravenous Therapy*** | IV fluids—1000 ml of Ringer's lactate at 125 ml/hr. |
| ***Therapeutic Measures*** | BP, pulse, and respirations q1h. |
| | Assess deep tendon reflexes q1h. |
| | Weigh qd. |
| | Measure intake and output. |
| | Insert Foley catheter—check urine output q1h; check urine for protein q4h; check specific gravity q4h; collect 24-hour urine for protein. |
| | Complete bed rest on left side. |
| | Continuous external electronic fetal monitoring. |
| | Amniocentesis—Lecithin/sphingomyelin (L/S) ratio, phosphatidylglycerol, saturated phosphatidylcholine—to determine fetal lung maturity. |
| | Repeat previously obtained baseline laboratory values including Hct. |
| | Perform fundoscopic examination of the eyes daily. |
| ***Consults*** | Does not apply. |

| | |
|---|---|
| *Preoperative Plan* | Deliver by vaginal or cesarean birth, depending on fetal and maternal conditions.<br>Begin preoperative teaching for possible cesarean section. |
| *Additional Data* | Since Susan responded well to the collaborative plan of care for mild to moderate PIH, the collaborative plan of care for severe PIH did not need to be instituted. She was sent home with discharge instructions. |

# COLLABORATIVE PLAN OF CARE FOR PATIENT DISCHARGE

| | |
|---|---|
| *Diet* | Eat a high (80-g) protein diet, drink 6–8 glasses of fluid, and include roughage in diet. |
| *Medications* | Take 1 prenatal vitamin preparation with 1 mg of folic acid PO qd.<br>Take ferrous sulfate 325 mg PO tid. |
| *Intravenous Therapy* | Does not apply. |
| *Therapeutic Measures* | Take blood pressure and record qid; maintain left lateral position and take recording on right arm.<br>Weigh and record qd.<br>Check and record urine for protein qd using dipstick.<br>Maintain bed rest on left side qd; may get up for bathroom, meals, and visits to the prenatal clinic.<br>Keep a 2-hour fetal movement chart while on bed rest.<br>Report immediately decreased urine output, headaches, "feeling jittery," vision problems, nausea and vomiting, epigastric pain.<br>Report immediately if any of the maternal/fetal assessments are not within normal limits (WNL).<br>Return for visit to prenatal clinic in 3 days. |
| *Consults* | Does not apply. |
| *Preoperative Plan* | Does not apply. |

# NURSING DIAGNOSES DEVELOPED IN CARE PLAN

Altered Family Processes, p. 318
Social Isolation, p. 319
Knowledge Deficit, p. 320

# ADDITIONAL NURSING DIAGNOSES TO BE CONSIDERED

Altered Growth and Development
Altered Health Maintenance
Altered Nutrition: More than Body Requirements
Fluid Volume Excess, Edema

# NURSING CARE PLAN BASED ON IDENTIFIED NURSING DIAGNOSES

| | |
|---|---|
| ***Altered Family Processes*** | ***Related to:*** Pregnancy and hospitalization of teenage daughter (sibling). |
| | ***Evidenced by:*** Family members not talking with one another about the impact of the pregnancy on the family unit; siblings ignoring the fact that their sister is pregnant; family members not meeting one another's emotional needs. |
| ***Desired Patient/Family Outcomes*** | ***The Family Will:*** |
| | • Utilize support systems to help them cope with the crisis of pregnancy. |
| | • Increase the level of support and communication among family members. |
| ***Evaluation Criteria*** | ***By the Time of Hospital Discharge, the Patient/ Family Will:*** |
| | • Meet with the social worker and nutritionist. |
| | • Begin to share their concerns and feelings with one another. |
| | ***Prior to Labor and Delivery, the Patient/Family Will:*** |
| | • Watch prenatal classes on videocassettes. |
| | • Reach agreement regarding keeping/adoption of the infant. |

## Interventions

Refer family for a social service evaluation.

Refer appropriate family member and patient to nutritionist.

Meet with the family and patient to discuss their concerns and feelings regarding this pregnancy and the development of PIH.

Ask a family member to watch prepared childbirth education classes on videocassettes with the patient.

## Rationale

An initial evaluation of available family resources provides pertinent data to the nurse. Assessment of such factors as family support, health insurance, current use of community services, school attendance, and employment experience often reveals that patients need assistance in coping with current stressors (Bobak and Jensen, 1987, p. 895).

The appropriate family member is the one who does the meal planning and cooking. The nutritionist will explore knowledge of basic nutrition and the diet needed for this high-risk pregnancy. He or she will also assess the patient's eligibility for the Special Supplemental Food Program for Women, Infants and Children (WIC) (Goldberg, et al, 1986, pp. 265–266).

Provides an opportunity for the family to communicate their concerns with one another in a supportive, safe environment with the nurse present. Family members will gain insight into factors such as personality and developmental stage, as well as cultural and religious beliefs that influence how each of them reacts to the pregnancy. The family may also feel guilty about the PIH complication and feel that they contributed toward its development (Kemp and Page, 1986, p. 234).

Involvement of a family member will increase the patient's sense of support and may contribute to a sense of closeness (Bobak and Jensen, 1987, pp. 3–4). Classes geared to the special interests of adolescents, such as bodily changes, will hold their attention (Olds, et al, 1984, p. 305).

## Interventions

Involve the entire family in the decision-making process regarding keeping the infant or adoption.

## Rationale

Family input is critically important to the adolescent who needs help in the decision-making process. Family support for a particular course of action will influence whether the patient keeps the baby or gives it up for adoption (Olds, et al, 1984, p. 302).

| | |
|---|---|
| *Social Isolation* | ***Related to:*** Pregnancy, dropping out of school, 5-day hospitalization, and enforced bed rest after discharge.<br>***Evidenced by:*** Verbalization of losing boyfriend, losing contact with girlfriends, and changes in sleeping, physical activity, and mood behavior. |
| *Desired Patient Outcomes* | ***The Patient Will:***<br>• Discuss with the nurse ways of increasing social contact with others.<br>• Participate in diversional activity within the home.<br>• Report positive behavior changes in sleeping and mood.<br>• Maintain decreased physical activity, that is, bed rest with bathroom privileges. |
| *Evaluation Criteria* | ***Throughout the Remainder of this Pregnancy, the Patient Will:***<br>• Establish social relationships and participate in activities with her peers, tutor, extended family, and church group.<br>• Express decreased feelings of guilt over the pregnancy.<br>• State that she is sleeping less, is maintaining bed rest, and is less irritable with her siblings and parents. |

## Interventions

Have the patient invite a friend to her home once a week for a visit.

Encourage the patient to telephone her favorite aunt once a day.

Encourage the family to tape the weekly church service for the patient.

Encourage the patient to listen to music on the radio or to her records.

## Rationale

The need for social support during pregnancy is so strong that lack of it has been shown to result in an increased rate of complications during pregnancy. The social support may come from family, friends, and health care providers (Kemp and Page, 1986, p. 234).

The patient is working on the developmental task of achieving emotional independence from her parents. Thus it is often another adult, such as the favorite aunt identified by the client, who is taken as a role model (Bobak and Jensen, 1987, p. 124; Jensen and Bobak, 1985, p. 1155). This aunt can also help her meet her love and belonging needs, which is a basic human need (Potter and Perry, 1985, p. 91).

The patient is working on the developmental task of acquiring a set of values and an ethical system (Bobak and Jensen, 1987, p. 123; Jensen and Bobak, 1985, p. 1156). Church participation, by listening to the tapes, may help the patient to continue growth in this dimension (Potter and Perry, 1985, pp. 404–409).

Due to enforced bed rest, the patient has time to build on her previous interest in rock music, which contributes to the developmental task of establishing a lifestyle that is personally and socially satisfying (Bobak and Jensen, 1987, p. 123; Jensen and Bobak, 1985, p. 1156).

## Interventions

Have the patient work with a tutor (obtained through the public school system) to help her complete some of her junior year course work.

## Rationale

The patient is in the formal operations stage in terms of cognitive functioning. Thus she is able to plan and reason and come up with solutions to problems. She is able to recognize that further education may ultimately assist her in finding a job (Bobak and Jensen, 1987, pp. 119–120).

---

### Knowledge Deficit

*Related to:* PIH, smoking and its effects on the mother and baby, diet required in PIH, meaning of bed rest and assessment of blood pressure, edema, and proteinuria.

*Evidenced by:* Patient's comments indicating lack of understanding about diet, smoking, and blood pressure; patient's comments indicating lack of knowledge regarding role of hospitalization in controlling PIH; and objective data showing an increase in blood pressure and presence of edema and proteinuria.

### Desired Patient/Family Outcomes

*The Patient Will Participate in the Following Self-Care Activities:*
- Discuss the signs and symptoms of PIH.
- Describe the diet in terms of protein, sodium, fluid, and roughage needs.
- Maintain bed rest except for meals, use of bathroom, and visits to the prenatal clinic.
- Maintain blood pressure within normal limits (WNL).
- Maintain a normal pattern of weight gain, no evidence of edema, and no protein in urine.
- Report normal fetal movement.

### Evaluation Criteria

*Throughout the Remainder of this Pregnancy, the Patient Will:*
- Assess for signs and symptoms of increasing severity of PIH on a daily basis.
- Eat a high 80-g protein diet.
- Remain on bed rest on left side except for use of bathroom, meals, and visits to the prenatal clinic.
- Monitor blood pressure, weight gain, edema, proteinuria, and fetal movement.
- Verbalize the understanding that despite compliance with treatment regimen, the condition may worsen.
- Perceive increased self-esteem through mastery of self-care activities.

---

## Interventions

Teach the patient the signs and symptoms of PIH that she needs to report immediately, during hospitalization, and after discharge.

Teach the patient and family member the necessity for a high-protein and adequate sodium, fluid, and roughage diet.

## Rationale

The patient needs to know that one or more of the following, that is, an increase in blood pressure, rapid weight gain, edema, proteinuria, epigastric pain, hyperreflexia, severe headaches, visual disturbances, oliguria, drowsiness, or nausea and vomiting, indicate a worsening of her condition that needs immediate intervention to lessen the danger of eclampsia (seizures) to herself and the baby (Bobak and Jensen, 1987, p. 780).

Because this patient is an adolescent and has PIH, she needs 1.5 g/kg/day of protein above the nonpregnant state. This provides sufficient protein to meet her own growth needs, those of the fetus, and the loss experienced through proteinuria. To combat the slight anemia already present, iron and folic acid supplements are given. Recommended daily sodium intake is 2–3 g/day. It has been found that sodium is needed in the fluid that is normally retained during pregnancy. Constipation is prevented by drinking 6–8 glasses of fluid per day plus including high-fiber foods in the diet (Neeson, 1987, pp. 132–133).

| | |
|---|---|
| Discuss the meaning of bed rest with the patient. | After hospital discharge, bed rest is prescribed for a minimum of 6 hours per day in the left lateral recumbent position. In this position, pressure on the aorta, renal arteries, and iliac veins is minimized. Thus cardiac output, and blood flow to the uterus, renal arteries, and extremities are optimized. Bed rest results in an increased glomerular filtration rate, with subsequent dramatic fluid loss and a decrease in blood pressure (Ouimette, 1986, p. 121). |
| Teach the patient and family member to assess her own blood pressure at home. | A slowly increasing blood pressure usually goes undetected unless measured. Self-assessment gives the patient immediate feedback on her condition. An increase of 30 mmHg in the systolic and 15 mmHg in the diastolic over the prepregnant baseline is one of the triad of symptoms of PIH (Neeson and May, 1986, p. 536). |
| Teach the patient to weigh herself daily. | Recording of daily weight will give the patient immediate feedback on whether she is gaining at an acceptable rate, that is, less than 2 lb (0.9 kg) per week (Neeson and May, 1986, p. 536). |
| Teach the patient to assess for the presence of edema. | The patient should inspect and palpate her feet and ankles, check for tightness of her rings, and look at her face for puffiness around the eyes (Neeson and May, 1986, p. 536). |
| Teach the patient to check her urine for protein qd. | The use of the dipstick is readily learned by the patient. She records readings and brings the results with her to the prenatal clinic. Participation in self-care activities raises her self-esteem (Potter and Perry, 1985, p. 92). |
| Teach the patient to record episodes of fetal movement. | The normally developing fetus demonstrates a minimum of 6 episodes of fetal movement during a 2-hour period. The patient should choose the same time of day, each day, for her assessment (Jensen and Bobak, 1985, p. 533). |

## QUESTIONS FOR DISCUSSION

1. Susan experienced PIH. What risk factors are you able to identify from her history?
2. What nursing interventions would be necessary if Susan were to be rehospitalized with severe PIH including convulsions?
3. Using the data base provided in the case study and the accepted list of nursing diagnoses from North American Nursing Diagnosis Association (NANDA), identify other potential nursing diagnoses that Susan is at risk for.
4. What major organs undergo pathophysiological changes in PIH? Specifically, what is the impact of the placental changes on the fetus?
5. The collaborative plan of care for moderate to severe PIH indicates that Susan would receive magnesium sulfate 1–2 g/hr IV. What are the nursing implications when a patient receives this medication?
6. Susan's fetus received a score of 8 on the Biophysical Profile (BPP), an antepartum test. In addition to the nonstress test (NST), 4 other parameters are assessed. Describe the parameters, method of scoring, and interpretation of the score.
7. What is the significance of the laboratory tests presented for uric acid, serum free iron, antithrombin III, and platelets?
8. Susan has been smoking a pack of cigarettes per day for the past 2 years. Explain to her why it would be helpful if she smoked less or quit.

# REFERENCES

American College of Obstetricians and Gynecologists Technical Bulletin: Antepartum Fetal Surveillance. No. 197. Washington, DC, August 1987.

American College of Obstetricians and Gynecologists Technical Bulletin: Management of Pre-eclampsia. No. 91. Washington, DC, February 1986.

Auvenshine, MA and Enriquez, MG: Maternity Nursing: Dimensions of Change. Wadsworth Health Sciences, Monterey, Calif, 1985.

Bobak, IM and Jensen, MD: Essentials of Maternity Nursing: The Nurse and the Childbearing Family, ed 2. CV Mosby, St. Louis, 1987.

Braunwald, E, et al: Harrison's Principles of Internal Medicine. McGraw-Hill, New York, 1987.

Carpenito, LJ: Nursing Diagnosis: Application to Clinical Practice, ed 2. JB Lippincott, Philadelphia, 1987.

Fischbach, F: A Manual of Laboratory Diagnostic Tests, ed 3. JB Lippincott, Philadelphia, 1988.

Goldberg, BD, et al: Teen pregnancy service: An interdisciplinary health care delivery system utilizing certified nurse–midwives. J Nurse–Midwifery 31:6, November/December 1986.

Guyton, AC: Textbook of Medical Physiology, ed 7. WB Saunders, Philadelphia, 1981.

Jensen, MD and Bobak, IM: Maternity and Gynecologic Care: The Nurse and the Family. CV Mosby, St. Louis, 1985.

Kemp, VH and Page, CA: The psychosocial impact of a high-risk pregnancy on the family. J Obstet Gynecol Neonatal Nurs 15:3, May/June 1986.

Neeson, JD: Clinical Manual of Maternity Nursing. JB Lippincott, Philadelphia, 1987.

Neeson, JD and May, KA: Comprehensive Maternity Nursing: Nursing Process and the Childbearing Family. JB Lippincott, Philadelphia, 1986.

Olds, SB, et al: Maternal–Newborn Nursing: A Family-Centered Approach, ed 2. Addison-Wesley, Reading, Mass, 1984.

Ouimette, J: Perinatal Nursing: Care of the High Risk Mother and Infant. Jones & Bartlett, Boston, Mass, 1986.

Pauerstein, CJ: Clinical Obstetrics. John Wiley & Sons, New York, 1987.

Pillitteri, A: Maternal–Newborn Nursing: Care of the Growing Family, ed 3. Little, Brown & Co, Boston, Mass, 1985.

Potter, PA and Perry, AG: Fundamentals of Nursing. CV Mosby, St. Louis, 1985.

Reeder, SJ and Martin, LL: Maternity Nursing: Family, Newborn and Women's Health Care, ed 16. JB Lippincott, Philadelphia, 1987.

Seidel, HM, et al: Mosby's Guide to Physical Examination. CV Mosby, St. Louis, 1987.

Shannon, DM: HELLP syndrome: A severe consequence of pregnancy induced hypertension. J Obstet Gynecol Neonatal Nurs 16:6, November/December 1987.

Thompson, JM, et al: Clinical Nursing. CV Mosby, St. Louis, 1986.

# BIBLIOGRAPHY

Bobak, IM and Jensen, MD: Essentials of Maternity Nursing: The Nurse and the Childbearing Family, ed 2. CV Mosby, St. Louis, 1987.

Brengman, SL, et al: Hypertensive crisis in L & D. Am J Nurs 88:325A, 1988.

Carpenito, LJ: Nursing Diagnosis: Application to Clinical Practice, ed 2. JB Lippincott, Philadelphia, 1987.

Fischbach, F: A Manual of Laboratory Diagnostic Tests, ed 3. JB Lippincott, Philadelphia, 1988.

Koniak-Griffin, D, et al: Severe pregnancy-induced hypertension: Postpartum care of the critically ill patient. Heart Lung 16:661, 1987.

Minakami, H, et al: Preeclampsia: A microvesicular fat disease of the liver? Am J Obstet Gynecol 159:1043, 1988.

Poole, JH: Getting perspective on HELLP syndrome. Am J Maternal Child Nurs 13:432, 1988.

Remich, MC and Youngkin, EQ: Factors associated with pregnancy-induced hypertension. Nurse Practitioner 14:20, 1989.

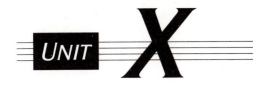

# THE PATIENT WITH ALTERATIONS IN THE HEMATOPOIETIC SYSTEM

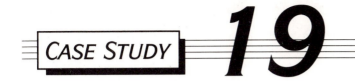

# A PATIENT WITH LEUKEMIA

Sharon P. Sullivan, M.S., R.N.

## ANATOMY AND PHYSIOLOGY

### Formation of White Blood Cells

The process by which white blood cells (leukocytes), red blood cells (erythrocytes), and platelets are formed is called hematopoiesis. In the adult, hematopoiesis takes place in the bone marrow of the ribs and sternum, the ends of long bones, and in the lymphoid tissue of the lymph nodes, spleen, thymus, and intestinal mucosa. Hematopoiesis is a continuous, ongoing process since blood cells have a limited life span and lost cells need to be replaced. It is in the bone marrow with its precursors that all blood cells will be produced (Porth, 1986, p. 158).

The stem cell theory explains the various stages of cell differentiation that result in mature leukocytes erythrocytes, and platelets (Fig. 19–1). The primordial, or uncommitted, stem cell differentiates into committed stem cells, which are the precursor cells for the blood cell lines. The committed stem cells differentiate and are transformed into more specialized cell types, such as the myeloblasts from which mature granulocytes develop. It should be noted that the immature or blast forms of blood cells do not normally appear in the peripheral circulation. As cell lines develop, cell function becomes specialized and the mature cells are no longer capable of further division (Bullock and Rosendahl, 1984, p. 185).

### Differential White Cell Count

Normal adult blood contains between 5000/mm³ and 10,000/mm³ leukocytes. Leukocytes are composed of neutrophils, lymphocytes, monocytes, eosinophils, and basophils. The proportion of these various types of leukocytes found in a smear of peripheral blood is referred to as the differential count.

Leukocytes are divided into 2 categories: granulocytes and nongranulocytes. Granulocytes, so called because of the large granules in their cytoplasm, include the neutrophils, eosinophils, and basophils. Neutrophils are the most numerous of all leukocytes, making up between 50%–70% of all leukocytes. The nongranulocytes are the lymphocytes and monocytes, and they make up the remaining cell types in the differential count.

### Function of White Blood Cells

The function of leukocytes is to defend the body against invasion by foreign substances and to provide the defensive elements necessary for the immune response. Leukocytes are divided, according to their primary function, into 2 major groups, phagocytes and lymphocytes (immune cells). Each type has its own unique function in the body's defense mechanism.

Phagocytes include the granulocytes and monocytes, both of which are derived from a common commit-

**325**

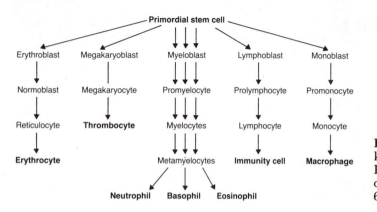

**FIGURE 19–1.** Illustrates development of leukocytes, erthyrocytes, and thrombocytes. (From Patrick ML, et al: Medical-Surgical Nursing: Pathophysiological Concepts. JB Lippincott, 1986, p. 667, with permission.)

ted stem cell and have phagocytic properties. They are effective against microbial invaders but, in order to accomplish their defensive purpose, there must be sufficient numbers to attack and engulf the foreign substance and then dispose of the debris (Bullock and Rosendahl, 1984, p. 189).

Lymphocytes are not capable of phagocytosis but function by protecting the body against specific antigens. They begin as lymphoblasts in the bone marrow and are processed elsewhere in the lymphoid system. Two types, T lymphocytes and B lymphocytes, emerge that are capable of immunological specificity, or the ability to recognize and respond to a specific antigen. The immune system response takes 2 forms: cellular immunity mediated by T lymphocytes and humoral immunity mediated by B lymphocytes (Griffin, 1986b, p. 47; Kottra, 1983, p. 11).

## PATHOPHYSIOLOGY

The leukemias are malignant disorders involving the leukocytes and the precursor cells. A malignant transformation of the stem cells takes place, producing a new group of leukocytes that are often immature, poorly differentiated, and dysfunctional, especially in the acute forms. These leukemic cells are unable to perform the functions of the mature leukocytes and thus are ineffective as phagocytes or immune cells. There is a rapid proliferation of leukemic cells, with increasing numbers of cells capable of proliferating along with a life span that is prolonged. Because of the mobile nature of all blood cells, leukemic cells disseminate throughout the body. This results in replacement of normal bone marrow cells with leukemic cells, the presence of immature or blast cells in peripheral blood, and infiltration of liver, spleen, and lymph nodes along with other tissues.

### Classification

The leukemias are classified according to the predominant cell type and tissue involved. The use of the terms acute and chronic describes the different clinical course. The acute leukemias are commonly divided into 2 groups, myelogenous (AML) or lymphoblastic (ALL). Onset is usually abrupt, and the therapy is intensive. It is important to distinguish between these 2 types because the prognosis in AML is generally poorer and survival, even with treatment, is limited.

Chronic leukemias, lymphocytic (CLL) and granulocytic (CGL), have a gradual onset, and the affected cells are more mature. The course of the disease is much slower and treatment protocols are less intense.

## RISK FACTORS

Certain factors have been identified as possible links in the development of leukemia. These are grouped into 3 categories: (1) congenital and hereditary conditions, (2) chemical and physical agents, and (3) preexisting hematological disorders. A number of congenital conditions, including Down's and Bloom's syndromes, are associated with an increased incidence of leukemia, and it has been seen in a significant number of twins. Leukemia can follow an exposure to radiation, benzene, and cytotoxic drugs. Acquired diseases also represent an increased risk. These include Hodgkin's disease, multiple myeloma, aplastic anemia, and preleukemic syndromes (Ersek, 1984, p. 185).

## COMMON CLINICAL FINDINGS

Symptoms seen in the leukemias are similar, despite the difference in cell type. The characteristic signs and symptoms are a result of the growth and infiltration of the leukemic cells into bone marrow and other organs and tissues.

Leukemic infiltration and the replacement of normal bone marrow cells result in a decrease in the number and functioning of red blood cells and platelets. Anemia occurs along with fatigue, malaise, and pallor. Thrombocytopenia and bleeding tendencies result in petechiae, ecchymoses, and gingival and visceral bleeding. Fever and increased vulnerability to infections reflect the immune deficiencies and ineffective leukocytes. Anorexia and weight loss are also seen due to a hypermetabolic state. Leukemic cells can invade bone causing bone pain, tenderness, and swelling. If there is infiltration of the central nervous system, there are complaints of visual disturbances, headache, dizziness, nausea, and vomiting.

## TREATMENT MODALITIES

Chemotherapy is most often the treatment of choice for leukemia. The goal of treatment is to induce a remission by selectively killing leukemic cells and allowing the bone marrow to repopulate with normal cells. A remission is defined as "the existence of fewer than 5% blast cells in the bone marrow with normal bone marrow functioning, no clinical signs of leukemia, and a normal peripheral blood cell count" (Ersek, 1984, p. 185). Administration of a combination of chemotherapeutic agents is used for the initial or induction therapy to achieve a remission. A protocol of multidrugs increases the effectiveness of therapy by combining their antitumor effects, and decreases the toxicity of individual agents on normal tissue. To prevent a relapse or reappearance of leukemic cells, consolidation therapy (readministration of the same or similar drug protocol) is begun after bone marrow recovery at the end of induction therapy. Maintenance therapy is administered after consolidation therapy. Its goal is to maintain remission (Jones, Dunbar, and Jirovec, 1984, p. 288).

Other treatment modalities used in leukemia therapy include radiation, immunotherapy, surgery, and bone marrow transplantation.

## PATIENT ASSESSMENT DATA BASE

### Health History

*Client:*
Richard Palazzo

*Address:* 12 Lincoln Road, Cleveland, OH 44114
*Telephone:* 216-555-8657
*Contact:* Maria or Frank Palazzo (parents)
*Address of contact:* Same
*Telephone of contact:* Same
*Age:* 23     *Sex:* M     *Race:* White
*Educational background:* Vocational-technical school
*Religion:* Catholic     *Marital status:* Single
*Usual occupation:* Auto mechanic
*Present occupation:* Same
*Source of income:* Job (full-time)
*Insurance:* Regional Health Plan
*Source of referral:* Community Hospital
*Source of history:* Patient, hospital records
*Reliability of historian:* Reliable
*Date of interview:* 10/21/89
*Reason for visit/Chief complaint:* Fevers, fatigue, and pain in leg and back; recent diagnosis of acute leukemia.

## Health Perception/Health Management Pattern

**Present Health Status**

About 2 months ago, Richard began experiencing right-leg pain. Seen by local physician, and, despite rest and medication, pain has spread to neck and back. He also has had intermittent fevers and complaints of fatigue and malaise. He was admitted on 10/5/89 to Bates Medical Center for treatment of acute leukemia.

**Past Health Status**

*General Health.* Usual health is described as excellent.
*Prophylactic Medical/Dental Care.* Sees physician only when necessary. Eye examination—none recently. Dental visits yearly.
*Childhood Illnesses.* Mumps, measles, chickenpox.
*Immunizations.* Routine; tetanus shot 1 year ago.
*Major Illnesses/Hospitalizations.* None.

*Current Medications*
*Prescription:* Codeine 30 mg PO every 4–6 hours as needed.
*Nonprescription:* None.
*Allergies.* None.

*Habits*
*Alcohol:* 1–2 beers per day.
*Caffeine:* 2–3 cups of coffee per day.
*Drugs:* See Current Medications.
*Tobacco:* Marijuana on a rare occasion.

### *Family Health History*

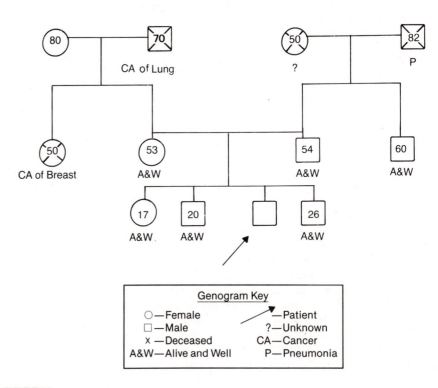

```
Genogram Key
○—Female            ↗—Patient
□—Male              ?—Unknown
x —Deceased         CA—Cancer
A&W—Alive and Well  P—Pneumonia
```

## Nutritional/Metabolic Pattern

**Nutritional**

*Usual Daily Menu*
Richard enjoys eating. Follows no special diet. Likes all foods, especially fried and Italian foods. Rates usual appetite as 5 (1 = poor, 5 = excellent). Gained 10 lb (4.5 kg) over the past years. "I

had been eating out a lot lately." During administration of chemotherapy, nausea was a big problem with a variable response to antiemetics. Oral intake and appetite were poor during this period. Currently, appetite remains poor (1 rating) due to mouth lesions that are causing difficulty with chewing and swallowing. Diet has been modified to a soft-solid, bland diet. Richard uses lidocaine (Xylocaine) as needed before meals and his oral intake has improved.

### *Usual Hospital Menu*
*Breakfast:* One serving of oatmeal with milk, 1 serving of scrambled eggs, 8 oz of milk.

*Lunch:* Macaroni and cheese (1 serving), 4 oz of custard, 8-oz milkshake.

*Dinner:* Cream soup (6 oz), 8 oz of yogurt, 1 ripe banana, 3 oz of ice cream, 8 oz of milk.

## Metabolic

Weight loss of 12 lb (5.4 kg) since admission. *Weight:* 237 lb (107.7 kg) on admission; current weight is 225 lb (102.3 kg). *Height:* 5 ft 10 in. (178 cm).

# ELIMINATION PATTERN

## Bowel

Usual bowel pattern is 1 soft, formed brown stool daily. Required no laxatives. At present, has experienced both diarrhea and, most recently, constipation requiring the daily use of laxatives.

## Bladder

Urinates 6–8 times per day. Denies burning, urgency, or any difficulty. Urine is clear, yellow, and in moderate to large amounts per void.

# ACTIVITY/EXERCISE PATTERN

## Activity/Exercise

Job-related activities include lifting, bending, and standing. Richard follows no regular exercise program. He enjoys woodworking and carpentry in his spare time. Participates in many social activities with his numerous friends. Reports that fatigue and pain have interfered with his usual activities. In the 3 weeks prior to admission, he was unable to work. Since admission, he reports feeling tired and listless, with activities limited to hygiene measures and moving from his bed to the chair. Pain is described as "a stiffness" in leg and back; rated 1–2 on a scale of 0–10 (0 = no pain, 10 = severe pain) and relieved with pain medications.

### *Self-Care Ability*

| | |
|---|---|
| Feeding—0 | Grooming—0 |
| Bathing—0 | General mobility—0 |
| Toileting—0 | Cooking—0 |
| Bed mobility—0 | Home maintenance—0 |
| Dressing—0 | Shopping—0 |

> *Functional Levels Code*
> 0—Full self-care
> I—Requires use of equipment or device
> II—Requires assistance or support from another person
> III—Requires assistance or support from another person and equipment or device
> IV—Is dependent and does not participate

**Oxygenation/Perfusion**

Denies any problems with wheezing, asthma, dyspnea, or colds. Routine chest x-ray during this admission was reported as normal. Denies history of chest pain or palpitations.

### Cardiac Risk Factors

|  | Positive | Negative |
|---|---|---|
| Sedentary life-style |  | X |
| Hyperlipidemia |  | X |
| Cigarette smoking |  | X |
| Diabetes |  | X |
| Obesity | X |  |
| Hypertension |  | X |
| Hypervigilant personality |  | X |
| Family history of heart disease |  | X |

## SLEEP/REST PATTERN

**Sleep/Rest**

Richard normally sleeps 5–7 hours per night. Prior to admission, back and neck pain had prevented him from getting to sleep at night. Taking codeine at bedtime helped to relieve pain, and he was able to fall asleep, but he awoke in the morning feeling tired and listless. While hospitalized, he requires a sedative at bedtime: "Otherwise, I lie there worrying about what is happening to me." Reports his sleep is frequently interrupted by nursing activities, that is, medications. States he experiences "bad dreams," and he is only able to sleep 3–4 hours at night. He awakes feeling tired. Attempts to nap in the midafternoon.

## COGNITIVE/PERCEPTUAL PATTERN

**Hearing**

Has no hearing problems; denies earaches, vertigo, or ringing in ears.

**Vision**

Normal.

**Sensory Perception**

Finds pain annoying and bothersome. "Pain medication helps a lot." He is right-hand dominant.

**Learning Style**

Learns best by demonstration and written material.

## SELF-PERCEPTION/SELF-CONCEPT PATTERN

**Self-Perception/Self-Concept**

Richard describes himself as outgoing, friendly, and a hardworking person. He has no problems in interactions with others. He is worried that his girlfriend will feel differently about him when he loses his hair.

## ROLE/RELATIONSHIP PATTERN

**Role/Relationship**

Lives at home with parents, 1 sister, and 2 brothers. He shares a room with his younger brother, with whom he is close. Has a special girlfriend whom he has considered marrying but says, "That's on hold until I feel better and I get back to work." Mother and father are very supportive, but he is closer to his mother. Father visits infrequently due to his working hours. Has 2 boyhood friends who visit regularly along with other close family members. Receives many cards and calls from other friends and relatives. For the last 2 years, he has worked as a mechanic in an auto repair shop. States "I really like my job and hope to own my own shop someday."

## SEXUALITY/REPRODUCTIVE PATTERN

*Sexuality/Reproductive*

Reports his sex life as satisfactory. Uses birth control and is aware of the need to employ safe sex practices.

## COPING/STRESS TOLERANCE PATTERN

*Coping/Stress Tolerance*

States he "finds it hard to believe he has leukemia. What did I do to deserve this? My life has been going along just the way I wanted. Now this. What's going to happen to me?" Tries to always look at the positive side, but he is having a difficult time coming to terms with his diagnosis. Usual method of dealing with stress is by talking with family and close friends and working on his woodworking projects.

## VALUE/BELIEF PATTERN

*Value/Belief*

Richard has a strong belief in God. Attends Mass sporadically. Feels God is testing him. Hospital chaplain visits regularly.

# Physical Examination

*General Survey*

Twenty-three-year-old overweight white male; lying in bed with eyes closed complaining of neck pain.

*Vital Signs*

**Temperature:** 99.8°F (37.6°C) (oral)
**Pulse:** 98 regular (apical)
**Respirations:** 20
**BP:** 110/68 (supine, right arm).

*Integument*

**Skin.** Tan color, warm, moist, and of normal thickness for age; petechiae noted over lower extremities; several small ecchymotic areas on both forearms and lower extremities.
**Mucous Membranes.** Pale pink (see additional findings under Mouth/Throat.
**Nails.** Nailbeds are smooth; no clubbing; edges ragged.

*HEENT*

**Head.** Black, short, thinning hair; loss of hair noted; scalp is clean and intact; face is symmetrical; temporomandibular joint (TMJ) without pain.
**Eyes.** Vision not tested; able to focus on objects and read newsprint. Conjunctivae are clear; extraocular movements (EOMs) are intact. Pupils equal, round, reactive to light and accommodation (PERRLA).
**Ears.** Auricles are intact; cerumen is present. Able to hear whispered word at 1 ft (30 cm) and 2 ft (60 cm).
**Nose.** Passages are patent.
**Mouth/Throat.** Mucous membranes are dry and red; several white lesions noted on buccal mucosa; gingiva is red, tender, and edematous; teeth are intact; oropharynx reddened; lips dry and cracked.

*Neck*

No enlarged nodes; no jugular venous distention (JVD). Carotids are full; pain with lateral movement.

*Pulmonary*

Thorax is oval; anteroposterior (AP) diameter 2:1; lungs are resonant and clear; Hickman catheter at right anterior chest.

*Breast*

No lumps, pain, or discharge.

**Cardiovascular**

Normal $S_1$, $S_2$; point of maximal impulse (PMI) at fifth intercostal space at midclavicular line.

**Peripheral Vascular**

**Peripheral Pulses**
Temporal — 4 bilaterally
Carotid — 4 bilaterally
Brachial — 4 bilaterally
Radial — 4 bilaterally
Femoral — 4 bilaterally
Popliteal — 4 bilaterally
Posterior tibial — 4 bilaterally
Dorsalis pedis — 4 bilaterally

**Peripheral Pulse Scale**

| |
|---|
| 0 — Absent |
| 1 — Markedly diminished |
| 2 — Moderately diminished |
| 3 — Slightly diminished |
| 4 — Normal |

**Abdomen**

Obese, protuberant, symmetrical abdomen, soft and nontender; liver, spleen, and kidney not palpable; bowel sounds present in all 4 quadrants.

**Musculoskeletal**

Full range of motion in all extremities; all movements coordinated.

**Neurological**

*Mental Status.* Alert, oriented to time, place, and person; memory intact.
*Cranial Nerves.* CN I–XII intact.
*Sensory.* Light touch, pain, and vibration to face, trunk, and extremities within normal limits.

***Deep Tendon Reflexes***

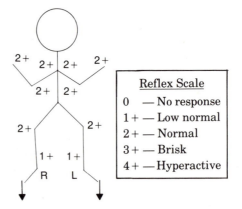

| Reflex Scale | |
|---|---|
| 0 | — No response |
| 1+ | — Low normal |
| 2+ | — Normal |
| 3+ | — Brisk |
| 4+ | — Hyperactive |

**Rectal**

Deferred.

**Genitalia**

Normal male.

## Laboratory Data/Diagnostic Studies

**Laboratory Data**

*Na:* 136 mEq/L
*K:* 3.5 mEq/L
*Cl:* 99 mEq/L
*$CO_2$:* 27 mM/L
*Urinalysis:* Specific gravity 1.024, protein 2+, blood 2+, glucose — negative.

*BUN:* 20 mg/100 ml
*Creatinine:* 1.2 mg/100 ml
*Uric Acid:* 7.5 mg/100 ml
*Cultures (mouth):* Candida albicans.
*Stool:* Positive guaiac test.

| DATE | Hct (%) | Hgb (g/dl) | WBC (no. $\times 10^3$/mm³) | PLATELETS (no. $\times 10^3$/mm³) |
|------|---------|------------|------------------------------|------------------------------------|
| 10/5* | 25.6 | 8.3 | 4.2 | 130 |
| 10/9 | 29.9 | 9.6 | 3.4 | 158 |
| 10/15 | 26.3 | 8.0 | 1.6 | 130 |
| 10/17 | 21.8 | — | 0.8 | 110 |
| 10/18 | 16.2 | 5.5 | 0.5 | 104 |
| 10/20 | 27.8 | — | 0.8† | 55 |
| 10/21 | 26.7 | 7.7 | 0.3 | 18 |
| 10/22 | 21.6 | — | 0.2 | 4 |
| 10/24 | 24.2 | — | 0.2 | 3 |
| 10/27 | 24.5 | 9.3 | 0.4‡ | 12 |

*Differential: 10% neutrophils, 70% myeloblasts.
†No polymorphonuclear leukocytes.
‡Blasts.

**Diagnostic Studies**

***Bone Marrow Biopsy.*** Hypercellular marrow packed with myeloblasts, Auer rods visualized. Diagnosis: acute myelogenous leukemia (AML).

# COLLABORATIVE PLAN OF CARE

**Diet**

Soft-solid, bland.

**Medications**

*Chemotherapy Protocol:* (administered beginning 10/9/89.
Cytarabine (ARA-C) 100 mg/m²/day by intravenous (IV) infusion × 7 days.
Daunorubicin 45 mg/m²/day by IV infusion × 3 days.
Allopurinol 300 mg PO qd.
Docusate sodium (Colace) 100 mg PO bid.
Prochlorperazine maleate (Compazine) 10 mg PO or 25 mg per rectum q4–6h prn.
Acetaminophen (Tylenol) 650 mg PO or per rectum q4h prn.
Triazolam (Halcion) 0.125 mg PO qhs prn.
Ceftazidime 1.5 g IV q6h.
Amikacin 160 mg IV q8h.
Milk of magnesia (MOM) 30 ml PO qd prn.
Metamucil (laxative preparation) 2 tsp PO q AM.
Codeine 30 mg PO q4h prn.
Nystatin 500,000 units orally qid.
Chlortrimazole troche orally qid.
2% Viscous Xylocaine 15 ml orally before meals prn.

**Intravenous Therapy**

Hickman catheter (placed on 10/7/89) flush with heparin solution every 8 hours.

**Therapeutic Measures**

Vital signs every 4 hours.
Weigh weekly.
Record intake and output.
Activity as tolerated.
Bleeding precautions.
Protective isolation/neutropenia precautions.
Daily laboratory studies: Complete blood count (CBC), platelet count, electrolytes, BUN, creatinine.
Test urine, stool, and vomitus for blood.

**Consults**

Nutritionist.

# NURSING DIAGNOSES DEVELOPED IN CARE PLAN

Alteration in Oral Mucous Membranes, p. 334
Potential for Infection, p. 335
Potential for Injury, p. 337

# ADDITIONAL NURSING DIAGNOSES TO BE CONSIDERED

Activity Intolerance
Alteration in Nutrition: Less Than Body Requirements
Anxiety
Constipation
Disturbance in Self-Concept
Fear
Knowledge Deficit
Pain
Powerlessness
Sleep Pattern Disturbance

# NURSING CARE PLAN BASED ON IDENTIFIED NURSING DIAGNOSES

| | |
|---|---|
| ***Alteration in Oral Mucous Membranes*** | ***Related to:*** Stomatitis, side effects of chemotherapy.<br>***Evidenced by:*** Buccal lesions, dry mucous membranes, and complaints of oral discomfort. |
| ***Desired Patient Outcomes*** | • Mucous membranes sustain no further increase in mucosal irritation and ulceration and complications are minimized or prevented.<br>• Oral pain/discomfort is relieved and oral intake improves.<br>• Patient is knowledgeable about oral care program and its rationale. |
| ***Evaluation Criteria*** | ***After Instruction, the Patient Will:***<br>• Perform prescribed oral care measures.<br>• Discuss the need for regular oral care.<br>• Inspect oral cavity daily and report any abnormalities.<br><br>***After Institution of Oral Care Program, the Patient Will:***<br>• Report increased comfort with chewing food and swallowing fluids.<br>• Have mucous membranes that appear pink, moist, and intact; teeth free of plaque; and lips soft, moist, and intact. |

| Interventions | Rationale |
|---|---|
| Assess oral status daily. Note patient's perception of changes in taste, voice, or comfort. Teach the patient to perform self-inspection. | Assessment of oral status aids in the early detection of problem areas and helps determine the needs and type of oral hygiene to be used (Daeffler, 1981, p. 29). |
| Monitor oral intake. | Oral lesions may interfere with nutritional and fluid intake causing decreased dietary intake and dehydration (Yasko, 1983, p. 213). |

## Interventions

Institute an oral care program done after meals and every 2–4 hours while awake:

- Clean teeth gently with a soft-bristle toothbrush, unless contraindicated by pain or bleeding. To increase softness soak in hot water before brushing).
- Gently floss teeth daily with unwaxed dental floss only if platelet levels are above 40,000/mm³ and the neutrophil count is above 1500/mm³.
- Rinse mouth thoroughly with hydrogen peroxide and saline (1:2 or 1:4); follow with rinse of saline.

Avoid use of commercial mouthwashes containing alcohol and agents that contribute to dryness, for example, lemon-glycerine swabs.

Moisten lips with lip balm/lubricant.

Modify diet avoiding hot food and beverages; coarse, spicy, and acidic foods; and any foods or fluids that cause discomfort.

Instruct the patient about oral care program and its rationale.

## Rationale

Frequent oral care "prevents accumulation of oral secretions which harbor pathogenic organisms" (Jones, Dunbar, and Jirovec, 1984, p. 285) and when performed before and after meals, freshens mouth and stimulates the appetite (Beck, 1979, p. 190).

Trauma to the mucous membranes can be minimized by avoiding agents that can cause irritation and drying of the oral mucosa (Simonson, 1988, p. 307).

Lubricants will maintain a moist surface and prevent cracking, which prevents access by bacteria (Doenges, Jeffries, and Moorhouse, 1984, p. 358).

Soft, bland foods served at room temperature and cool fluids may reduce irritation to sensitive tissues and increase the person's tolerance and willingness to eat and drink (Jones, Dunbar, and Jirovec, 1984, pp. 164, 285).

Patient education about oral complications of chemotherapy, oral care, and nutritional implications is an important part of the treatment protocol (Beck, 1979, p. 191). The informed patient is more attentive to oral care (Bersani and Carl, 1983, p. 586).

---

**Potential for Infection**

*Related to:* Disease process (leukemia), side effects of chemotherapy (bone marrow suppression).
*Evidenced by:* Neutropenia.

**Desired Patient/Family Outcomes**

- The patient is free of signs and symptoms of infection, or complications are minimized or prevented.
- The patient/family are knowledgeable about the signs and symptoms of infection and the factors that will reduce the risk of infection.

**Evaluation Criteria**

*During the Hospital Stay, the Patient Will:*
- Be free of signs and symptoms of infection.

*After Instruction, the Patient and/or Family Will:*
- State the signs and symptoms of infection.
- Discuss measures to be taken to prevent infection and the steps taken if infection is suspected/present.
- Perform prescribed daily hygiene.
- Consume a diet that is well balanced and has an adequate fluid intake.

| Interventions | Rationale |
|---|---|
| Observe and monitor for specific signs and symptoms of infection. | Neutropenia is associated with an increased frequency of infection. Some of the typical signs and symptoms of infection, such as inflammation, may be absent in the neutropenic patient (Carlson, 1985, p. 59). |
| Monitor potential sites of infection: skin, mouth, throat, respiratory tract, gastrointestinal tract, axilla, perineum, rectum, and Hickman catheter site. | In the neutropenic patient, careful inspection of all body sites with a high potential for infection should be made (Adams, 1985, p. 307). |
| Monitor temperature curve and vital signs. | Fever is an early and important sign of infection in the neutropenic patient since clinical signs of infection are frequently absent. Increased pulse rate may be indicative of infection (Jones, Dunbar, and Jirovec, 1984, p. 282). |
| Monitor white blood cell and neutrophil count. | White blood cells and neutrophils may continue to drift downward for a period of time after chemotherapy, and susceptibility to infection will increase inversely requiring an increased vigilance (Brandt, 1984, p. 25). The highest risk for infection occurs during the nadir about 1–2 weeks after the administration of chemotherapy (Brown et al, 1986, p. 75). |
| Maintain protective isolation. | The neutropenic patient should be protected from any obvious or potential source of infection (Reheis, 1985, p. 223). "Infection from external hospital borne organisms can frequently be avoided by careful assessment of the person's immediate environment and early control of any potential environmental sources" (Jones, Dunbar, and Jirovec, 1984, p. 286). |
| Prevent constipation and any injury to the rectal mucosa. | Constipation, enemas, and rectal medications and thermometers can cause trauma to intestinal and rectal mucosa already damaged by cytotoxic therapy, thus increasing the risk of infection (Fox, 1981, p. 463). |
| Initiate pulmonary hygiene measures. | Pulmonary hygiene "facilitates the removal of bronchial secretions which provide a reservoir to the growth of microorganisms" (Fox, 1981, p. 463). |
| Provide a restful environment and reduce the patient's anxieties. | Fear and anxiety precipitate the stress response, which may compromise the person's ability to resist infection (Kneisl and Ames, 1986, p. 275). |
| Encourage and instruct the patient to maintain a well-balanced diet and adequate fluid intake. | A well-balanced diet "promotes a general improvement of host resistance and provides nutrients necessary to meet energy demands" (Fox, 1981, p. 463). |
| Teach the patient to perform meticulous skin and hygiene care. | "Intact skin is the body's first line of defense." Infection of the skin or body may occur when the continuity of the skin is broken (Adams, 1985, p. 146). |
| Instruct patient/family about the factors that reduce the risk of infection, the signs and symptoms of infection, and steps to be taken if infection is suspected. | The patient and family need to be instructed in all aspects of infection prophylaxis. Infection is "the most frequently occurring serious complication" in the leukemic patient and requires a comprehensive approach for detection and prevention (Brandt, 1984, p. 28). |
| Consult the infection control nurse. | The infection control staff are responsible for monitoring the hospitalized patient for development of nosocomial infection, enforcing isolation procedures, and educating staff about infection control (Kneisl and Ames, 1986, p. 278). |

| | |
|---|---|
| ***Potential for Injury: Bleeding*** | ***Related to:*** Bone marrow depression.<br>***Evidenced by:*** Thrombocytopenia; presence of petechiae and ecchymoses; presence of occult bleeding. |
| ***Desired Patient/Family Outcomes*** | • Patient is free of signs and symptoms of bleeding, or complications are minimized or prevented.<br>• The patient/family are knowledgeable about bleeding precautions and safety measures, steps to be taken if bleeding occurs, and signs of bleeding to be reported. |
| ***Evaluation Criteria*** | ***During the Hospital Stay, the Patient Will:***<br>• Be free of bleeding due to trauma.<br><br>***Upon Instruction, the Patient and/or Family Will:***<br>• Comply with bleeding precautions and follow safety measures.<br>• Discuss the need for bleeding precautions and safety measures.<br>• State the steps taken if bleeding occurs. |

## Interventions

Assess skin for petechiae and ecchymoses.

Observe for signs of bleeding from nose, mouth, conjunctiva, and rectum. Monitor for occult bleeding.

Assess for changes in mental status.

Monitor vital signs.

Monitor CBC and platelet count.

Institute bleeding precautions:

• Avoid use of aspirin and aspirin-containing products.
• No rectal temperatures.
• No intramuscular injections.
• Apply pressure to puncture sites for 5 minutes.
• Use of electric razor for shaving.

Provide gentle nursing care. Avoid trauma to mucous membranes and tissues.

Instruct the patient/family on bleeding precautions and safety measures in activities of daily living (ADLs). Teach the early signs of bleeding and steps to be taken if bleeding occurs. Discuss rationale.

## Rationale

The presence of petechiae and ecchymoses on the skin are indicative of a low level of circulating platelets (Jones, Dunbar, and Jirovec, p. 282).

Thrombocytopenia can result in bleeding and hemorrhage, which, for the leukemic patient, can be life threatening (Kneisl and Ames, 1986, p. 934).

Neurological changes may be present when there is central nervous system (CNS) involvement, as a result of CNS hemorrhage secondary to thrombocytopenia (Kneisl and Ames, 1986, p. 883).

Vital signs are monitored for tachycardia and decreases in blood pressure, which may indicate serious bleeding (King, 1984, p. 26).

The hematological status can change daily. Knowledge of the most recent values can provide a base from which to plan care and identify priorities (Jones, Dunbar, and Jirovec, 1984, p. 287).

Bleeding precautions for the high-risk patient must be taken to prevent accidental bleeding and injuries (Griffin, 1986a, p. 39).

In the person with thrombocytopenia, especially if platelet counts are below 50,000/mm$^3$, trauma even in mild form may precipitate bleeding (Bullock and Rosendahl, 1984, p. 207).

The person with leukemia and his or her family need teaching with information provided about preventing injuries and the factors that can cause bleeding (Griffin, 1986a). Patient participation can decrease the complications associated with leukemia (Kneisl and Ames, 1986, p. 934).

# QUESTIONS FOR DISCUSSION

1. Discuss the rationale behind the chemotherapy prescribed for Richard Palazzo.
2. Compare the action of cell-cycle specific and cell-cycle nonspecific chemotherapeutic drugs.
3. What is "nadir"? Explain the nursing implications.
4. Identify some treatment modalities that are employed to treat nausea.
5. Explain why infection is a serious complication in leukemia.
6. Review the role platelets play in hemostasis.
7. Discuss some ways Richard's family can be involved in his care.

# REFERENCES

Adams, A: External barriers to infection. Nurs Clin North Am 20:145, 1985.

Beck, S: Impact of a systematic oral care protocol on stomatitis after chemotherapy. Cancer Nurs 2:185, 1979.

Bersani, G and Carl, W: Oral care for cancer patients. Am J Nurs 83:533, 1983.

Brandt, B: A nursing protocol for the client with neutropenia. Oncol Nurs Forum 11:24, 1984.

Brown, MH, et al: Standards of Oncology Nursing Practice. John Wiley & Sons, New York, 1986.

Bullock, BL and Rosendahl, PB: Pathophysiology. Little, Brown & Co, Boston, 1984.

Carlson, AC: Infection prophylaxis in the patient with cancer. Oncol Nurs Forum 12:56, 1985.

Daeffler, R: Oral hygiene measures for patients with cancer: III. Cancer Nurs 4:29, 1981.

Doenges, M, Jeffries, M, and Moorhouse, M: Nursing Care Plans. FA Davis, Philadelphia, 1984.

Ersek, MT: The acute leukemia patient in the intensive care unit. Heart Lung 13:183, 1984.

Fox, L: Granulocytopenia in the adult cancer patient. Cancer Nurs 4:459, 1981.

Griffin, JP: The bleeding patient. Nursing '86 86:34, 1986a.

Griffin, JP: Hematology and immunology. Appleton-Century-Crofts, Norwalk, Conn, 1986b.

Jones, D, Dunbar, C, and Jirovec, M: Medical-Surgical Nursing: A Conceptual Approach. McGraw-Hill, New York, 1984.

King, NH: Controlling bleeding when the platelet count drops. RN 47:25, 1984.

Kottra, C: Infection in the compromised host—An overview. Heart Lung 12:10, 1983.

Kneisl, C and Ames, S: Adult Health Nursing. Addison-Wesley, Reading, Mass, 1986.

Porth, C: Pathophysiology. JB Lippincott, Philadelphia, 1986.

Reheis, CE: Neutropenia causes, complications, treatment, and resulting nursing care. Nurs Clin North Am 20:219, 1985.

Simonson, G: Caring for patients with acute myelocytic leukemia. Am J Nurs 88:304, 1988.

Yasko, JM: Guidelines for Cancer Care: Symptom Management. Reston Publishing, Reston, Va, 1983.

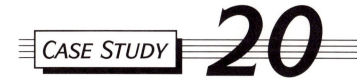

# A PATIENT WITH SICKLE CELL ANEMIA

Gloria F. Antall, M.S., R.N.

## ANATOMY AND PHYSIOLOGY OF THE HEMATOPOIETIC SYSTEM

Sickle cell anemia is a chronic, hereditary disease of abnormal hemoglobin production. It primarily affects the world's black population, although to a lesser extent sickle cell disease occurs in the populations of the Middle East, the Mediterranean area, Southern India, and the Caribbean. Sickle cell disease is the most-common genetic disorder in the United States (Phipps, Long, and Woods, 1987). In this disease, the abnormal Hb S replaces the normal Hb A in the erythrocyte, as a result of single amino acid substitution in the beta polypeptide chain. This polypeptide mutation results in abnormal cells that assume crescent or sickle shape when oxygen deprived. Once the cells sickle, they may obstruct capillary blood flow, resulting in more hypoxia and consequently more sickling.

The word *erythrocyte* is derived from two Greek words, *erythros* (red) and *kykos* (cell). The normal number of erythrocytes in a cubic millimeter of blood is approximately 5 million. The unique structure of an erythrocyte enables it to carry out its most important function, oxygen and carbon dioxide transport. The cell shape is that of a biconcave disc, which provides a large cell surface area on which absorption and release of oxygen and carbon dioxide are accomplished. It is also very flexible and elastic, which provides adaptability to blood vessel diameters.

Mature erythrocytes normally have a life span of approximately 120 days. As the aging cells become worn, they are replaced with new erythrocytes. Normally, the number of aged red blood cells and new red cells remains fairly constant, with new cells replacing old cells at a rate of approximately 180 million each minute (Luckmann and Sorenson, 1987, p. 1036).

## PATHOPHYSIOLOGY OF SICKLE CELL DISEASE

The basic anomaly in this disease state is contained in the globin fraction of the Hb. Hb S results when valine replaces glutamic acid on the beta chain of the hemoglobin molecule. When this abnormal substitution happens, an anomalous bonding occurs between Hb S molecules whenever blood oxygen content decreases (Luckmann and Sorenson, 1987, p. 1051). This sickling tendency is also related to hemoglobin concentration in the cell. Dehydration promotes sickling, due to the fact that hypertonicity of the blood plasma increases the intracellular concentration of hemoglobin (Whaley and Wong, 1987, p. 1526). This abnormal bonding results in contraction of the cell membrane and the characteristic "sickling" shape of the cell (Figure 20-1). In addition, the life span of these cells is shortened to 7–20 days.

The heavy preponderance of misshapen cells increases the blood viscosity, which in turn leads to sluggish

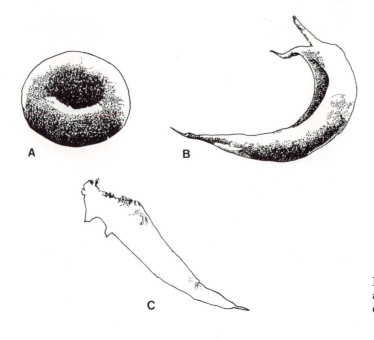

**FIGURE 20-1.** Unlike the normal cell (A), cells affected by sickle cell anemia (B and C) assume a crescent or sickle shape when deprived of oxygen.

circulation. Blood plasma hypertonicity increases the intracellular concentration of hemoglobin, which means that the sickling tendency is also related to the state of hydration, with dehydration promoting sickling of cells. Increased viscosity and cell shape irregularities cause cells to clump together within the smaller blood vessels. The resulting occlusion in the microcirculation causes hypoxia, which then causes more sickling of other erythrocytes and the vicious cycle repeats itself. The end result of repeated hypoxia with tissue ischemia is most evident as damage in the kidneys, brain, bone marrow, and spleen due to circulatory and oxygenation need.

There are several terminology variations of sickle cell disease. The critical and profound form of the disease is the homozygous condition Hb SS, which is the form inherited from both parents. The milder, usually asymptomatic form of the disease is Hb Sa, or sickle cell trait, which is inherited from 1 parent.

## Risk Factors

Sickle cell anemia is a potentially fatal disease, which occurs predominantly in the black race. It is a hereditary disease whereby an abnormal gene inherited from both parents is required to produce symptomatic sickle cell anemia. This is referred to as a homozygous state.

The heterozygous state is when a person inherits an abnormal gene from only 1 parent. This results in a condition referred to as sickle cell trait and is usually asymptomatic. Prevention of the disease through genetic counseling is the only avenue known to prevent its occurrence.

## COMMON CLINICAL FINDINGS

Sickle cell anemia commonly is diagnosed in childhood, usually in a toddler or preschooler during an acute crisis precipitated by an infection (Whaley and Wong, 1985, p. 1528). However, in rare cases symptoms do not appear until young adulthood. Symptoms that profoundly affect all organs and tissues are generally due to hemolytic anemia from sickle cell destruction and thrombosis with resultant infarction. Many organs including the spleen, liver, or penis may enlarge, and function may decrease or cease altogether. Circulation occlusion may affect all internal organs as well as extremities. Stasis ulcers occur in approximately 75% of older children and adults with the disease. Cerebral hemorrhage is also a common problem among sufferers of sickle cell anemia (Luckmann and Sorenson, 1987, p. 1052). Common clinical findings of sickle cell anemia include weakness, pallor, easy fatigability, and jaundice due to hemolysis and tissue hypoxia. Many children begin to show growth abnormalities around age 7. Both height and weight can be affected, and puberty can also be delayed (Foster, Hunsberger, and Anderson, 1989, p. 1354).

Episodes of pain are often severe and represent the most common symptom that causes victims to seek treatment. Pain is usually in the abdomen, back, chest, or extremities; it may be generalized, localized, or migratory.

Bone marrow changes can include compensatory proliferation that results in osteoporosis, osteosclerosis, and possibly osteomyelitis. Weakening of the bones can result in lordosis or kyphosis.

Bacterial infection is often a problem due to nonfunctioning of the spleen. Meningitis, sepsis, pneumonia, and urinary tract infection represent causes of increased morbidity and mortality, and can precipitate a crisis.

A sudden exacerbation of the symptoms of the disease due to either sickling or destruction of red blood cells can result in a situation known as a "sickle cell crisis." Common symptoms depend on the type of crisis, but can include pain, fever, vaso-occlusive crises, anemia, arthralgias, shock, hypoxia, extreme fatigue, and infection. There are four types of sickle cell crises: vaso-occlusive, splenic sequestration, aplastic, and hyperhemolytic. It is thought that several physical and emotional factors may precipitate a crisis. Physical factors include dehydration or other events that would change oxygen tension such as overexertion or smoking. Patients are cautioned to avoid high altitudes or air travel in unpressurized planes. Emotional factors include any highly stressful situation.

## TREATMENT MODALITIES

There is no specific treatment for sickle cell disease. Care is generally directed toward prevention of sickling and treatment of crises. In some cases, slow administration of packed cells or exchange transfusions may be used in an attempt to relieve severe symptoms of a sickle crisis. Other interventions include judicious use of pain management, enforced rest, use of IV replacement of fluids and electrolytes, sedation, and the use of oxygen. Folic acid is given to replace depletion of folic acid stores in the bone marrow. There is a great need for education in this population of clients for both successful disease management and genetic counseling about sickle cell disease and trait. Some researchers are currently investigating the use of antisickling agents and the induction of hyponatremia to induce hydration (Whaley and Wong, 1985, p. 1528).

## PATIENT ASSESSMENT DATA BASE

### Health History

*Client:*
Mr. Lonnie Campbell

*Address:* 12 Carlisle St, Salt Lake City, Utah
*Telephone:* (801) 555-4567
*Contact*: Mother—Dorothy Campbell
*Address of contact:* Same as client
*Telephone of contact:* Same as client
*Age:* 18    *Sex:* Male    *Race:* Black
*Education:* Currently student at John Hay High School
*Religion:* Baptist    *Marital status:* Single
*Usual occupation:* Burger King employee, 12 hours/week
*Source of income:* Mother—works full-time
*Insurance:* Allied Insurance
*Source of referral:* Hematology clinic
*Source of history:* Patient and his mother
*Reliability of historian:* Reliable
*Date of interview:* 5-9-89
*Reason for visit/Chief complaint:* Severe abdominal pain

## HEALTH PERCEPTION/HEALTH MANAGEMENT PATTERN

### Present Health Status

Lonnie describes his health as "pretty good." His mother relates that he is frequently ill from upper respiratory illnesses, refuses to "take care of himself," often runs with his gang until late at night, and refuses to get adequate rest or meals. Average hospitalizations are 2/yr, and, in addition, Lonnie has had an appendectomy and repair of trauma to head and chest from an automobile accident.

This is Lonnie's second hospital admission this year for sickle cell crises and related symptoms; the first admission was in January 1989. Lonnie is admitted with severe abdominal pain; temperature of 101° F; left ankle ulcer, and painful, swollen joints. Things done to keep healthy include "hanging out with friends and keeping myself happy." Finds it "hard" to follow the advice of the doctors and nurses; they "don't know how I feel." States the hospital can be most helpful in "getting rid of this pain."

### Past Health Status

**General Health.** Diagnosed with sickle cell disease at age 4 and has been hospitalized multiple times since. Has 1 sibling with sickle cell trait. Has a history of the usual childhood diseases, influenza, colds, croup, and frequent URIs. Has been hospitalized for pneumonia 3 times in addition to his usual sickle crisis admissions.

**Prophylactic Medical/Dental Care.** Sees private physician once yearly, last check up 2-6-89. Sees physician or nurse practitioner in the Hematology Clinic. Has not kept up dental appointments; last seen in 1980.

**Childhood Illnesses.** See above.

**Immunizations.** All usual childhood immunizations given. Pneumococcal and Haemophilus type B and meningococcal vaccine.

**Major Illnesses/Hospitalizations**
See above under past health status.

**Current Medications**
*Prescription:* Folic acid qd whenever patient feels like taking it.
*Nonprescription:* Ibuprophen tablets 1–2 q4h, PO prn
**Allergies.** Penicillin

**Habits**
*Alcohol:* Patient states he drinks once in a while. Mother states he drinks with the other boys every weekend; she thinks mostly beer but isn't sure.
*Caffeine:* Two cups of coffee qam. 3–4 cans of soda pop/d.
*Drugs:* Client denies any usage.
*Tobacco:* Smokes 1 pack of cigarettes per day.

**Family Health History**

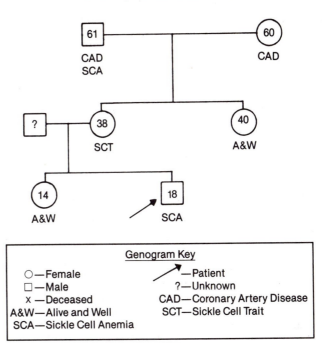

## NUTRITIONAL/METABOLIC PATTERN

**Nutritional**

Lonnie states he has a "good appetite." Denies weight loss in the last year. Denies difficulty in chewing, swallowing, nausea, or vomiting. His mother states he has nausea and vomiting when he is hospitalized for sickle cell crisis.

**Usual Daily Menu**
*Breakfast:* Cereal or doughnut and coffee.
*Lunch:* At school, hamburger or macaroni, ice cream, potato chips, soda.
*Snack:* Usually at the fast food restaurant, milkshake and french fries.
*Dinner:* Meat, potatoes and vegetable, although he admits to hating vegetables.

**Skin**

Lonnie says he generally "heals well, but slowly." Currently, he has an ulcer on his left ankle; it began 2 weeks pta. The ulcer is 1½" dia, and covered with a dressing. There is scant, serosanguinous drainage.

**Metabolic**

*Height:* 5 ft. 5 in. (165 cm); *Weight:* 118 lb (53.6 kg)

## ELIMINATION PATTERN

**Bowel**

Lonnie states he has no problem with bowel elimination. States he moves bowels qd or qod. Refuses to discuss further. His mother states he has had problems in the past with constipation, usually after coming home from a hospitalization. Treatment is with over-the-counter laxatives and is usually successful.

**Bladder**

Describes urinary elimination as "no problem," denies frequency and pain. Lonnie's mother states that he has had difficulty with urinary elimination when hospitalized with sickle cell crises;

### Bladder—Continued

episodes of hematuria predominate, with some pain on urination. She states that this is embarrassing to Lonnie, and he won't talk about it. She cannot remember what the doctor told her about the hematuria, except that it is connected to the sickle cell disease in some way.

## ACTIVITY/EXERCISE PATTERN

### Activity/Exercise

Usual pattern of activity includes attending school, part-time work at a fast food restaurant, and occasional basketball games with friends. Lonnie tries to help his mother with household chores but most often leaves that "to my sister." Lonnie feels that he has sufficient energy to accomplish tasks; has no special exercise regimen. Leisure activities usually consist of "hanging out with friends." Likes sports, both to participate and to observe, but doesn't get to attend sporting events much due to cost. Perceived ability for self care is level 0 at home and level II in the hospital. Since admission, has been essentially bedridden, complaining of joint and abdominal pain, and febrile.

#### Self-Care Ability

Feeding—0                Grooming—0
Bathing—0                General mobility—II
Toileting—II             Cooking—IV
Bed mobility—II          Home maintenance—IV
Dressing—II              Shopping—IV

> #### Functional Levels Code
> 0—Full self-care
> I—Requires use of equipment or device
> II—Requires assistance or supervision from another person
> III—Requires assistance or supervision from another person or device
> IV—Is dependent and does not participate

### Oxygenation/Perfusion

Chest x-ray this admission. Moderate cardiomegaly. Mild to moderate dyspnea related to low hemoglobin and hematocrit levels.

#### Cardiac Risk Factors

|                              | Positive | Negative |
|------------------------------|----------|----------|
| Sedentary life-style         |          | X        |
| Hyperlipidemia               |          | X        |
| Cigarette smoking            | X        |          |
| Diabetes                     |          | X        |
| Obesity                      |          | X        |
| Hypertension                 |          | X        |
| Hypervigilant personality    |          | X        |
| Family history of heart disease | X     |          |

## SLEEP/REST PATTERN

### Sleep/Rest

Lonnie generally feels well rested, usually sleeps 7–8 hr/night on weekdays and 9 hr/night on weekends. He denies insomnia, wakefulness, or nightmares. His mother states that infrequently he has difficulty sleeping due to joint pain, and other symptoms related to his sickle cell disease. He denies taking any naps during the day.

## Cognitive/Perceptual Pattern

**Hearing**

He is alert and oriented to person, place, and time; has intact memory and is able to recall events appropriately from recent past and distant past. Denies hearing difficulty; can hear whispered voice.

**Vision**

Wears corrective lenses for near-sightedness since age 13. Has not had vision exam for 2 years.

**Sensory Perception**

No problem. Right hand is dominant.

**Pain**

Lonnie describes himself as a person who "cannot take pain too much." On a scale of 1–10, with 1 being scant and 10 the most he can imagine, he describes current pain as an 8. Describes pain in abdomen as sharp and jabbing, joint pain as constant dull ache. Usual management of pain is by taking medicine, applying heat, and watching TV. Has never tried relaxation techniques.

**Learning Style**

States he cannot describe decision-making abilities, guesses he "makes decisions okay." Easiest learning method is a combination of visual and auditory styles. Describes self as "below average student."

## Self-Perception/Self-Concept Pattern

**Self Perception/Self Concept**

Lonnie describes himself as a "cool guy who can take care of himself." States he feels pretty good about himself most of the time. Feels like his body "lets me down a lot;" he wants to do more things than he is sometimes able to do. Sometimes feels very angry, jumpy; at these times, goes out with friends and drinks beer. Denies feelings of depression, sadness; does admit to feeling sometimes hopeless about his disease; wonders if he will "live a long time." Lonnie's mother states he is a generally moody person, with "ups and downs;" sometimes is very tense and will not talk to family members.

## Role/Relationship Pattern

**Role/Relationship**

Lonnie lives in an apartment, which he shares with his mother and 14-year-old sister. His mother works full-time as a maintenance worker in a museum. His father has never been involved in his life; father's whereabouts unknown. Extended family includes grandparents, aunt, uncle, 2 cousins, described as "fairly close" family. In terms of family problems, Lonnie describes his family as "okay," appears embarrassed in talking about these issues. He states his mother and sister are helpful about his illness but he doesn't want others to know much about it. The family handles problems by talking sometimes, arguing at other times. His mother states that income is not really adequate for needs; she is in debt to family members. His mother states that the neighborhood is not particularly desirable, that they have good friends there, but there is a moderate amount of crime.

## Sexuality/Reproductive Pattern

**Sexuality/Reproductive**

Lonnie is very uncomfortable with this topic, denies doing testicular self-exam, does not desire to talk about it; will admit that he has a girlfriend.

## Coping/Stress Tolerance Pattern

### Coping/Stress Tolerance

Lonnie denies any life changes in the previous year. Describes his mother as person he would talk things over with. States he is tense "a lot." Things done to relieve stress include basketball, spending time with friends, drinking beer, and watching television. When problems occur in his life, usual coping style is to "get mad, yell, and get what I need." Finds this method works for him. His mother states that he sometimes is "more than I can handle," describes angry outbursts as Lonnie's usual coping style.

## Value/Belief Pattern

### Value/Belief

Feels he generally gets what he wants out of life except for "money." He has no particular plans for the future. He is Baptist, an irregular church goer, and doesn't find religion very important in his life. Denies need to see minister while hospitalized.

# Physical Examination

### General Survey

17-year-old black male, appearing as stated age, slight of build, appears in acute distress due to abdominal and joint pain.

### Vital Signs

**Temperature.** 101°F oral
**Pulse.** 110 regular (apical)
**Respirations.** 30/min
**Blood pressure.** 118/76, right arm, sitting
**Height.** 5 ft. 5 in. (165 cm)
**Weight.** 118 lb (53.6 kg)

### Integument

**Skin.** Light-brown; face pale and dry; only breakdown is small left ankle ulcer with pink, regular smooth skin edges, scant serosanguinous drainage. Joints enlarged, skin over joints stretched and shiny.
**Mucous Membranes.** Pink, slightly dry, intact.
**Nails.** Beds smooth, no clubbing.

### HEENT

**Head.** Well-shaped, size appropriate for age. Scalp clean, smooth, no areas of tenderness. Hair is black, curly, and shiny.
**Eyes.** Vision corrected with lenses (not tested). Pupils equal, round, reactive to light and accommodation (PERRLA).
**Ears.** Canals clear, able to hear whispered word from 3'.
**Nose.** Nares open, light pink.
**Mouth/Throat.** Oral membranes slightly dry, pink, teeth intact. Uvula midline. Tonsils and adenoids are present.

### Neck

Range of motion (ROM) full, carotids full. No enlarged nodes.

### Pulmonary

Thorax oval. AP diameter 2:1. Bilateral chest excursion. Rales in bilateral lung bases.

### Breast

Normal male—no breast enlargement.

### Cardiovascular

$S_1$ $S_2$ point of maximal impulse at fifth intercostal space at midclavicular line—no murmurs. Apical rate 110, regular.

### Peripheral Vascular

All pulses regular and strong. No bruits heard. Extremities warm, slightly slow capillary refill.

| **Peripheral Vascular — Continued** | **Peripheral Pulses**<br>Temporal—4 bilaterally<br>Carotid—4 bilaterally<br>Brachial—4 bilaterally<br>Radial—4 bilaterally<br>Femoral—4 bilaterally<br>Dorsalis pedis—3 left, 4 right<br>Posterior tibialis—4 bilaterally | **Peripheral Pulse Scale**<br><br>0—Absent<br>1—Markedly diminished<br>2—Moderately diminished<br>3—Slightly diminished<br>4—Normal |

**Abdomen**

Abdomen swollen, very tender to touch, unable to palpate due to patient's guarding of abdomen. Active bowel sounds present in all four quadrants.

**Musculoskeletal**

Muscular development appears normal for age. Some extremity joint tenderness bilaterally. ROM not able to be measured due to pain. Decreased ROM in knees and ankles bilaterally. Muscle strength and gait not tested.

**Neurological**

*Mental Status.* Alert, oriented × 3
*Cranial Nerves.* I–XII intact
*Sensory.* Increased sensation to pain, light touch in chest, abdomen, legs.

*Deep Tendon Reflexes*

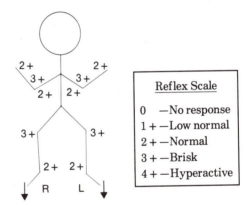

Reflex Scale

0   —No response
1 + —Low normal
2 + —Normal
3 + —Brisk
4 + —Hyperactive

**Rectal**

Deferred.

**Genitalia**

Normal appearing male. Denies urethral discharge, pain.

## Laboratory Data/Diagnostic Studies

**Laboratory Data**

*CBC.* Normocytic, normochromic anemia

*RBC.* Count 4.2

*Hgb.* 7.2 gm/100 ml

*Hct.* 38.4%

*Reticulocyte count.* 4.2% of erythrocytes

*Sickle Cell Test.* Positive (Sickledex)

*Erythrocyte Sedimentation Rate.* 12 mm in 1 h (Westergren)

*Indirect Serum Bilirubin.* 5.6/100 ml

*Blood Smear.* Variable RBCs, abnormal shapes, nucleated RBCs, target cells, spherical cells

*Diagnostic Studies*

*KUB.* normal
*Culture and Sensitivity of ankle ulcer.* *Staphlococcus aureus*

## COLLABORATIVE PLAN OF CARE

*Diet*

Regular diet as tolerated

*Medications*

Acetominophen tabs: q3–4 prn
Morphine sulfate: 10 mg s.c. STAT
Morphine sulfate (after initial s.c. dose) in 15-mg increments orally. Starting with 15 mg, increase q20min until adequate analgesia obtained. Thereafter, give adequate dose (not to exceed 60 mg) q2–3h.
Trimethobenzamide suppository: 25 mg q6h prn for nausea
Folic acid tab: 1 po qd

*Intravenous Therapy*

Dextrose 5% and ½ saline:
6000ml/24 — 100 – 125/kg/day

*Therapeutic Measures*

Bedrest; up on commode for BM only
Routine VS
Egg-crate foam mattress
Wound care, NS wet to dry dressing to left ankle TID
Force oral fluids 2000 cc/day
Warm soaks to knees TID and prn

*Consults*

Social service

## NURSING DIAGNOSES DEVELOPED IN CARE PLAN

Alteration in Tissue Perfusion, p. 350
Noncompliance, p. 348
Pain, p. 349

## ADDITIONAL NURSING DIAGNOSES TO BE CONSIDERED

Activity Intolerance
Alteration in Sensory Perception, visual
Alteration in Skin Integrity
Coping, Ineffective Family
Disturbance in Self Concept, Potential
Fluid Volume Deficit, Potential
Infection, Potential For
Intermittent Constipation Pattern
Knowledge Deficit
Powerlessness

## NURSING CARE PLAN BASED ON IDENTIFIED NURSING DIAGNOSES

*Noncompliance*

*Related to:* Perceived nonsusceptibility and adolescent developmental need.

***Evidenced by:*** Stated by significant other describing non-compliance and lack of adherence to sleep/rest and nutritional needs.

*Desired Patient Outcomes*

***By Discharge, the Patient Will:***
• Verbalize intent to adhere to dietary and sleep activities that conform to health/illness needs.

*Evaluation Criteria*

***By Discharge, the Patient Will:***
• Verbalize a more positive intent for self-care activities.
• Choose self-care activities based on appropriate information.

## Interventions

Assess contributing factors about management of this disease that the patient sees as negative.

Assess for recent changes in lifestyle or developmental stressors.

Reduce or eliminate causative or contributing factors if possible.

Assist person to manage stressors by sharing information with family and trusted friends.

Formulate a contract with the client to achieve a series of steps toward health-related behavior changes.

## Rationale

The diagnosis must *not* be used as a reflection of the nurse's value judgment, but rather that of a clear assessment of the client's perception of the problem (Carpenito, 1987, p. 410).

When confronted with crises or stressors, patients and family members may respond with panic, anger, or apathy (Foster, Hunsberger, and Anderson, 1989, p. 434).

Patients and families need to be better educated about the disease; improved knowledge results in a realistic approach and better comprehension of contributing factors. Prevention or reduction of these factors can result in a decrease of disabilities (Pack, 1983, p. 229).

Functional family characteristics include positive, open communication without fear, on any topic (Foster, Hunsberger, and Anderson, 1989, p. 432).

A contract can establish new behaviors by providing positive consequences (Steckel, 1980, p. 1596).

*Pain*

***Related to.*** Viscous blood and tissue hypoxia 2° to sickle cell anemia (Carpenito, 1987, p. 240).
***Evidenced by:*** Patient report of discomfort, Guarded position, and facial mask of pain.

*Desired Patient Outcomes*

• Patient will relate relief of pain after use of consistent plan of both invasive and noninvasive methods.

*Evaluation Criteria*

***By Discharge, the Patient Will:***
• verbalize relief and/or reduction of pain.
• acknowledge understanding of noninvasive pain relief techniques.

## Interventions

Assess pain tolerance

## Rationale

Pain tolerance differs in individuals and may vary in one individual from time to time (Carpenito, 1987, p. 163).

| Interventions | Rationale |
|---|---|
| Monitor slow administration of packed red cells, if procedure is ordered. | The use of slow administration of blood products can relieve symptoms of crisis (Luckmann & Sorenson, 1987, p. 1051). |
| Limit energy expenditure, but encourage passive ROM exercises. | Limiting exercise may decrease pain of crisis by decreasing oxygen need (Doenges, Jeffries, and Moorhouse, 1984, p. 367; Whaley and Wong, p. 1531). |
| Keep affected joints supported and in proper position for pain relief, immobilize and evaluate. | Keeping joints positioned will minimize stress on joints, and pain (Doenges, Jeffries, and Moorhouse, 1984, p. 367). |
| Provide prescribed analgesia on a consistent schedule. | "The preventative approach to pain is a regular schedule for medication administration to treat the pain before it becomes severe, rather than the prn approach" (Carpenito, 1987, p. 163). |
| Medicate as much as possible with oral pain medication. | The oral route of administration is preferable; oral narcotics alleviate pain as effectively as parenteral with none of the serious complications (Down the Hatch in Sickle Cell Crisis, 1987, p. 109). |
| Teach use of noninvasive pain management techniques (guided imagery and progressive relaxation). | Studies show that the human brain secretes endorphins, which have opiate-like properties that relieve pain. This release of endorphins may be responsible for the positive effect of noninvasive pain relief measures (Carpenito, 1987, p. 163; Gagan, 1984, p. 24). |

| | |
|---|---|
| **Alteration in Tissue Perfusion** | **Related to:** Viscous blood and occlusion of microcirculation 2° to sickle cell anemia (Carpenito, 1987, p. 240) <br> **Evidenced by:** Aching pain in knee joints, left leg ulcer |
| **Desired Patient outcome** | **The Patient Will:** <br> • Identify factors that increase peripheral circulation. <br> • Report a decrease in pain. <br> • Acceptable perfusion is maintained. |
| **Evaluation Criteria** | **By Discharge, the Patient Will:** <br> • Identify factors such as the medical regimen, diet, exercise, and sleep that will encourage oxygenation and perfusion. <br> • Report fewer sickle cell crises. |

| Interventions | Rationale |
|---|---|
| Teach factors that promote avoidance of recurrences: avoid infection, strenuous physical activity, emotional stress, dehydration, high altitude. | These factors may precipitate sickling crisis by increasing the sickling tendency (Luckmann and Sorenson, 1987, p. 1051). |
| Reduce Activity | Reduced activity, helps to reduce oxygen need, thereby compensating for hemoglobin decrease (Doenges, Jeffries, and Moorhouse, 1984, p. 365). |
| Administer oxygen as ordered. | Increased oxygen serves to decrease cardiac workload (Luckmann and Sorenson, 1987, p. 1052). |

| *Interventions* | *Rationale* |
|---|---|
| Administer anti-pyretics. | To reduce fever and to decrease evaporative fluid loss that might precipitate dehydration and sickling (Doenges, Jeffries, and Moorhouse, 1984, p. 365). |
| Administer fluids. | Fluids cause hemodilution and help decrease thrombosis; electrolyte replacement to correct metabolic acidosis. |

## QUESTIONS FOR DISCUSSION

1. Relate the concept of noncompliance to the case situation with Lonnie Campbell considering his age and developmental stage.
2. Identify any precipitating physiological or psychological factors that may have contributed to this hospital admission.
3. Identify any abnormal laboratory values that were seen in this case.
4. If you were to choose between "activity intolerance" and "self-care deficit" for a care plan in this case, which would you choose and why? Use defining characteristics and cues to defend your choice.
5. Identify five nursing interventions that would promote compliance after Lonnie's discharge.

## REFERENCES

Carpenito, LJ: Nursing Diagnosis: Application to Clinical Practice. JB Lippincott, Philadelphia, 1987.

Doenges, M, Jeffries, M, and Moorhouse, M: Nursing Care Plans: Nursing Diagnosis in Planning Patient Care. FA Davis, Philadelphia, 1984.

Down the hatch in sickle cell crisis. Emerg Med 3(15):109–110, 1987.

Foster, R, Hunsberger, M, and Anderson, J: Family-Centered Nursing Care of Children. WB Saunders, Philadelphia, 1989.

France-Dawson, MF: Sickle cell disease: Implications for nursing care. J Advanced Nurs 11:729–737, 1986.

Gagan, JM: Imagery: An overview with suggested application for nursing. Perspec Psychiatr Care 22(1):20–24, 1984.

Gordon, M: Manual of Nursing Diagnosis. McGraw-Hill, New York, 1987.

Gradolf B: Sickle cell anemia in children. Issues Comprehensive Pediatr Nurs Sept–Dec 6(5–6):295–307, 1983.

Korn, E: The user of altered states of consciousness and imagery in physical and pain rehabilitation. J Ment Imagery 7(1):25–34, 1983.

Luckmann, J and Sorenson, K: Medical-Surgical Nursing, A Psychophysiologic Approach. WB Saunders, Philadelphia, 1987.

Pack, B, et al: Symposia on sickle cell disease. Nurs Clin North Am 18(1):129–229, 1983.

Phipps, WJ, Long, BC, and Woods, NF. Medical Surgical Nursing, Concepts and Clinical Practice, CV Mosby, St. Louis, 1987.

Steckel, SB: Contracting with patient-selected reinforcers. AJN pp 1596–1599, September, 1980.

Vichinsky and Lubin, BH: Suggested guidelines for the treatment of children with sickle cell anemia. Hematol/Oncol Clin North Am 1(3):483–501, 1987.

Waechter, E, Phillips, J, and Holaday, B: Nursing Care of Children. Philadelphia, JB Lippincott, 1985.

Whaley, L and Wong, D: Nursing Care of Infants and Children. CV Mosby, St. Louis, 1987.

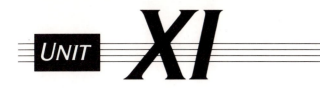

# THE PATIENT WITH ALTERATIONS IN THE IMMUNE RESPONSE SYSTEM

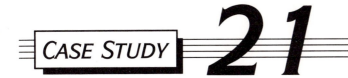
# A PATIENT WITH SYSTEMIC LUPUS ERYTHEMATOSUS

Alice L. Rose, M.S.N., R.N.

## PATHOPHYSIOLOGY OF SYSTEMIC LUPUS ERYTHEMATOSUS

Systemic lupus erythematosus (SLE) is defined as a chronic remitting, inflammatory, autoimmune disease of connective tissues, which may affect skin, joints, pleural, and pericardial membranes, kidneys, and the hematologic and central nervous systems (CNS). (Ziegler, 1984, p. 673). The disease process involves an abnormal reaction of the body to its own connective tissue and is accompanied by certain characteristic immunological phenomena. SLE is often referred to as a collagen disease. The relationship to collagen is important. Collagen is 1 of 3 main fibers in connective tissue, a protein synthesized by fibroblasts whose main function is to support and protect tissues and cells. Collagen constitutes one third of body protein. If one third of the body's protein is attacked by the body's immune system, the implications for the degree of involvement of all organ systems should be clear.

### Risk Factors, Predisposition

There are an estimated 500,000 cases of SLE in the United States. Women develop the disease 8 times more often than men. The ratio of black women to white women is 3:1. Often the disease is thought to typically affect young women who present with a characteristic butterfly rash on the face over the nose and forehead; however, not all patients develop the rash, and the disease is diagnosed in both sexes and in persons of any age (Neuberger and Neuberger, 1984, p. 722; Ziegler, 1984, p. 674).

Discoid lupus erythematosus (DLE) should be differentiated from SLE. DLE is a more benign disease in most cases; only 5%–10% of patients progress to SLE (Blau, 1986, p. 96). Patients with DLE have a rash with erythema, raised patches, and scaling with possible scarring, which may occur anywhere on the body. Some laboratory findings may mimic SLE, but unless symptoms are present, patients are usually not treated for DLE.

### Etiology

A single, specific etiology for SLE has not been identified. One theory indicates a genetic predisposition. Serologic abnormalities and positive antinuclear antibodies (ANA) have been found in the relatives of patients with SLE. SLE has also been associated with certain inherited deficiencies of complement (Blau, 1986, p. 104). There is also speculation about a genetic link with certain immunologic abnormalities. In patients with SLE, T-cell hypoactivity and hyperactivity of B cells result in a variety of autoantibodies found during diagnosis.

An SLE-like syndrome may be induced by certain medications, including hydralazine. Withdrawal of the medication may result in eventual relief from all symptoms. Certain other medications are felt to trigger or reactivate SLE, including sulfa, penicillin, oral contraceptives, and others.

An infection may cause exacerbations of SLE or impede existing therapy, but bacterial infections have not been implicated as the cause of the disease. At this time, no virus has been isolated either. Regardless of the possible etiologies, the disease is characterized by the development of autoantibodies against a wide variety of self-antigens.

## Immunologic Occurrences

SLE is a disease of disordered immunologic regulation. Individuals who are disease-free may make autoantibodies. Autoimmunity under certain circumstances is rather common, such as in aging. The B-lymphocytes apparently are capable of making autoantibodies, just as normal antibodies are made by B-lymphocytes. Normally, the T-cell population (suppressor and helper cells) regulate and control immune responses, so people do not all develop autoantibodies leading to disease. It is possible that immune-response genes may act by influencing immunologic regulation (the normal T-cell and B-cell functions), thus creating the tie of genetic and immunologic occurrences causing SLE (Koffler, 1987, p. 5). In sum, there is a primary derangement in equilibrium of regulatory forces, especially in the balance between helper and suppressor T-cells.

It is felt that antibodies (protein) combine with cell constituents to form immune complexes. These immune complexes are deposited in organs such as the kidney. Then, white blood cells invade to destroy the immune complexes (the inflammatory process occurs). Increasing complexes mean increased inflammation. The neutrophil or white blood cells contain enzymes (lysozomes). As the white blood cells engulf the immune complexes, enzymes spill out and kill immune complexes as well as causing extensive tissue damage that lead to all the complicating multisystem involvement of SLE.

## Relationship of Complement

Complement consists of a group of serum proteins. The complement system is one of the effectors of the inflammatory response. When an antibody attaches to a cell membrane, complement combines with the antigen. When immune complexes are formed, as in SLE, complement is used up or fixed by the role it plays in the inflammatory process (activated by the deposition of the immune complexes), thus serum complement levels fall (Massicot, 1985, p. 11).

There are many immunologic occurrences in patients with SLE. These account for the many abnormal laboratory findings in SLE, but these may or may not have an impact on the exact course of the disease and the treatment modalities. Some of these include anti-DNA antibody, positive LE cell, elevated ESR, positive Coombs' test, positive (false) VDRL, positive rheumatoid factor.

# COMMON CLINICAL FINDINGS

The American Rheumatism Association has proposed that 4 of the following criteria must occur at any given time for a patient to be diagnosed with SLE for the purposes of clinical trials: Malar rash, discoid rash, photosensitivity, oral ulcers, arthritis, serositis, renal disorder, neurologic disorder, hematologic disorder, immunologic disorder, or antinuclear antibody. (Blau, 1986, p. 97).

A brief review of system involvement clarifies the complex nature of the disease (Nass, 1987, p. 69; Steinberg, 1987, p. 131).

The muco-cutaneous system may involve a butterfly rash, lesions on exposed body parts, alopecia, edema, or oral or nasopharyngeal erosions. The musculoskeletal system may show joint involvement with pain, arthritis, or mysositis as the presenting symptoms. Anemia, decreased platelets, elevated ESR, decreased complement, positive rheumatoid factor, positive LE cell, or anti-DNA antibodies are evidence of hematological-serological involvement. In renal involvement, hematuria, mild proteinuria, abacterial pyuria progressing to casts, or increased proteinuria may occur. Cardiovascular signs include pericarditis, myocarditis, endocarditis, or vasculitis.

Central nervous system involvement may include seizures, organic brain disease, peripheral neuropathy, psychoses, depression, anxiety, or stroke. Pleurisy, pneumonitis, dyspnea, or cyanosis indicate respiratory involvement. Gastrointestinal symptoms include decreased appetite, nausea and vomiting, abdominal pain, decreased peristalsis, or peritonitis. Ocular symptoms included retinal exudates, papilledema, or corneal involvement with photophobia.

Another finding may be infection. This is the second, most frequent cause of death for patients with SLE. With an increased susceptibility to infection and decreased resistance as a result of medications taken, symptoms of infection require early intervention.

# TREATMENT MODALITIES

The treatment for patients with SLE consists of medications, emotional support, and extensive education for the patient and significant others to promote avoidance of those factors that trigger the exacerbations, and to manage the signs and symptoms that are present.

Initial medications for minor organ involvement are based on the symptoms that the patient displays (Steinberg, 1987, p. 145). Hydroxychloroquine is often used for skin involvement. Nonsteroidal anti-inflammatory agents are used in arthritis, and for fever. If these agents do not produce effective results, low doses of steroids are tried. Moderate doses of steroids, 40 mg/d, are used for major organ involvement. If the renal biopsy results indicate increased disease, then high doses of steroids and possibly immunosuppressants such as Azothioprine are used.

For emotional support, referral for counselling or to the Lupus Foundation or to a local support group may be advised.

Coordination of the educational program is important to avoid confusion and promote trust. Physicians, social workers, nurses, dietitians, and other health-team members all play a significant role.

# PATIENT ASSESSMENT DATA BASE

## Health History

*Client:*
Mrs. Beth Crown

*Address:* 1009 Bellaire Ave, Dayton, Ohio 45420
*Telephone:* 216-555-1625
*Contact:* James W. Crown (husband)
*Address of contact:* Same
*Telephone of contact:* Same
*Age:* 32    *Sex:* Female    *Race:* White
*Educational background:* Liberal Arts Degree
*Religion:* Protestant    *Marital status:* Married
*Usual occupation:* Formerly Airline Stewardess; Currently Child-Care Worker
*Present occupation:* On leave from position in Child Care Center
*Source of income:* Husband's salary
*Insurance:* Blue Cross Master Health Plus
*Source of referral:* Self
*Source of history:* Self
*Reliability of historian:* Reliable
*Date of interview:* January 12, 1990
*Reason for visit/Chief complaint:* "I am totally exhausted and want to know for sure what is going on; if this is as serious as it sounds, I have to decide how to care for the children."

### HEALTH PERCEPTION/HEALTH MANAGEMENT PATTERN

*Present Health Status*

Mrs. Crown was in generally good health until 1 year ago when she noticed she was feeling unusually tired and, in the morning, felt aching and joint tenderness. After several months of the aching, joint tenderness, and tiredness, Mrs. Crown was seen by her physician for a routine annual examination. The physician

**Present Health Status — Continued**

detected an elevated BP and abnormal urinalysis. He recommended she return for further evaluation, but she did not do so until she noticed a rash on her forehead and cheeks. She was seen by her physician who performed tests, including laboratory studies. He recommended a brief hospital admission for diagnostic studies, including kidney biopsy. She was told she had lupus. Due to the non-emergent nature of the illness, Mrs. Crown will be maintained at home with admission scheduled in 1 month.

**Past Health Status**

*General Health.* Mrs. Crown had 1 major illness, in her early twenties, necessitating hospitalization for an acute pulmonary inflammatory condition of undetermined origin. She has been seen annually by her physician for routine examinations, including birth control for the past 18 months.
*Prophylactic Medical/Dental Care.* Visits dentist annually; physician annually
*Childhood Illnesses.* Usual childhood illnesses excluding mumps, but including rheumatic fever
*Immunizations.* Usual childhood, tetanus 4 years ago

*Major illnesses/Hospitalizations*
Hospitalized 12 years earlier for acute pulmonary inflammation
No history of major infections

*Current Medications*
*Prescriptions:* Ovulen-21 for birth control for 18 months since marriage
*Nonprescription:* None.
*Allergies.* None.

*Habits*
*Alcohol:* On rare occasions
*Caffeine:* One cup/d
*Tobacco:* Nonsmoker

***Family Health History***

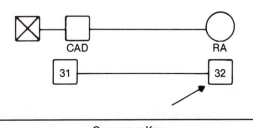

| Genogram Key | |
|---|---|
| ○—Female | CAD—Coronary Artery Disease |
| □—Male | RA—Rheumatoid Arthritis |
| A&W—Alive and Well | X —Deceased |

## Nutritional/Metabolic Pattern

**Nutritional**

*Usual Daily Menu*
*Breakfast:* Cereal, toast, juice, 1 cup of coffee
*Lunch:* Sandwich, fruit
*Dinner:* Meat, rice, vegetable, drinks water with meals
*Note:* Does not like milk.

**Metabolic**

*Height:* 5 ft. 6 in. (168 cm); *Weight:* 118 lb (54 kg)

## ELIMINATION PATTERN

### Bowel

Has a bowel movement each day with regularity.

### Bladder

Noticed slight decrease in urine output over the past month; hands and feet are slightly swollen.

## ACTIVITY/EXERCISE PATTERN

### Activity/Exercise

As an assistant at a local day-care center, Mrs. Crown was required to walk and stand for each of the 5 8-hour workdays she worked per week. Four months ago, she changed from working 5 shifts to working two 8-hour shifts. She made this change because of her extreme tiredness when working full-time. She attributed this exhaustion to her changed lifestyle with additional responsibilities since marrying. Mrs. Crown indicated the reason she really sought medical care at this time was the exhaustion and inability to work and care for her 2 stepchildren. She has not been able to work at all for the past month and has been considering other arrangements for care of the children, at least during the day. Has not been out of her house for the past 2 weeks since her appointment with the physician.

**Self-Care Ability**

| | |
|---|---|
| Feeding—0 | Grooming—0 |
| Bathing—0 | General mobility—0 |
| Toileting—0 | Cooking—II |
| Bed mobility—0 | Home maintenance—II |
| Dressing—0 | Shopping—IV |

> ### Functional Levels Code
> 0—Full self-care
> I—Requires use of equipment or device
> II—Requires assistance or support from another person
> III—Requires assistance or supervision from another person and equipment or device
> IV—Is dependent and does not participate

## SLEEP/REST PATTERN

### Sleep/Rest

Used to sleep 7 h/night but has more recently required more sleep as well as a nap in the late afternoon or early evening. Her sleep is described as fitful and she awakens not feeling rested. She describes herself as feeling restless, but without energy to do anything. Increased sleep and rest do not seem to help her feel more rested. No sleep aids used.

## COGNITIVE/PERCEPTUAL PATTERN

### Hearing

No reported difficulty hearing; no aids used.

### Vision

Wears glasses for reading; prescription new 1 year ago.

### Sensory Perception

No change noticed

### Learning Style

Enjoys learning by use of visual aids such as television. No alteration in memory or ability to concentrate.

*Pain/Discomfort*

Feels aching and joint tenderness. Feels malaise much of time.

## Self-Perception/Self-Concept Pattern

*Self-concept*

Has always been thought of as pretty; worked as an airline attendant until a lay-off occurred. Decided to work with children to see how she liked children and because others told her she was bubbly and could make children happy. Describes self as usually energetic, always on-the-go until this illness. Is now feeling confused about her disease and what it means for her. She waited to marry because she felt marriage did not fit her busy life. She is now unsure what she thinks of herself.

*Interpersonal Style*

Usually confident and relates readily to others; puts others at ease. Since the physical changes of facial rash and puffiness, has been embarrassed to go out and be seen by others.

## Role/Relationship Pattern

*Role/Relationship*

Mrs. Crown lives in home owned by husband before marriage. She has been married 18 months to a widowed airline pilot, who has two children aged 2½ and 4 years. Their home is in the country, about 40 miles outside of a major urban area. Mrs. Crown feels isolated by being outside the city but was starting to adjust. At this time is feeling very concerned about her responsibilities and what her husband will think about her illness. Her 2 children are staying with their closest neighbor, 1 mile from her home. Although her parents live 50 miles away, her mother cannot care for the children because she is partially disabled by arthritis. Her husband is trying to take time off from work; his parents live in another state, as does Mrs. Crown's sister. Family relationships are positive, but family members are limited by health or distance from providing much assistance. Although finances are not a problem at this time, other resources in terms of friends are limited. Mrs. Crown has many friends but most of them were from her work as an airline attendant, so are not local.

## Sexuality/Reproductive Pattern

*Sexuality/Reproductive*

Currently taking birth control pills. Had hoped to have children in the future. Normal menstruation since age 12. No pregnancies. No perceived problems with taking birth control pills. Feels especially close to husband even though his work requires that he travel.

## Coping/Stress Tolerance Pattern

*Coping/Stress Tolerance*

Stressors in life have increased markedly since marriage, especially in the month previous to interview due to illness and the manifestations, in particular the rash and fatigue. Assuming the role change from full-time career with the airlines to stepmother and work in day-care center was a major transition that involved changes in support systems. Until marriage would have relied on friends at work for support, now relies on husband who is frequently away. Feels a need for more adult company to verbalize her concerns.

## VALUE/BELIEF PATTERN

*Value/Belief*

She and family are Protestant. Finds religion helpful in times of crisis. Highly values her family life and relationships.

# Physical Examination

*General Survey*

Thirty-two-year-old white female, attractive, well-dressed, oriented.

*Vital Signs*

**Temperature.** 99°F (oral)
**Pulse.** 96 and regular
**Respirations.** 22
**BP.** 124/88 (right arm, seated)

*Integument*

**Skin.** Warm, supple, moist. Red, flat, dry rash on cheeks and forehead.
**Mucous Membranes.** Pink
**Nails.** Pink, smooth

*HEENT*

**Head.** Symmetrical, short brown hair. Scalp is clean with no lesions. Face is symmetrical, no tenderness, rash as above.
**Eyes.** Pupils equal, round, reactive to light and accommodation (PERRLA). No nystagmus, normal vision with glasses
**Ears.** Normal hearing, symmetrical
**Nose.** No septal deviation
**Mouth/Throat.** Teeth in good repair, mucous membranes pink and moist, without tonsils

*Neck*

No nodes, trachea midline

*Pulmonary*

Lungs clear to auscultation, respirations regular, unlabored

*Breast*

No masses or tenderness, does self-breast examination

*Cardiovascular*

Apical pulse 96, no murmurs

*Peripheral Vascular*

**Peripheral Pulses**
Temporal—4+ bilaterally
Carotid—4+ bilaterally
Brachial—4+ bilaterally
Radial—4+ bilaterally
Femoral—4+ bilaterally
Popliteal—4+ bilaterally
Posterior tibial—4+ bilaterally
Dorsalis pedis—4+ bilaterally

**Peripheral Pulse Scale**

| |
|---|
| 0—Absent |
| 1—Markedly impaired |
| 2—Moderately impaired |
| 3—Slightly impaired |
| 4—Normal |

*Abdomen*

Flat, bowel sounds present, no masses palpable, no liver palpable

*Musculoskeletal*

Full ROM both arms. Knees and ankles stiff and painful with diminished ROM.

*Neurological*

**Mental Status.** Alert, oriented × 3; stated anxiety; reliable.
**Sensory.** Light touch, pain and vibration to the face, trunk and extremities within normal limits with joints at knees and ankles painful

*Neurological—Continued*                    ***Deep Tendon Reflexes***

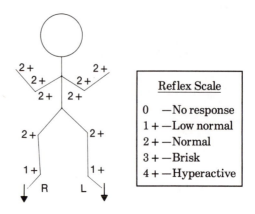

| Reflex Scale | |
| --- | --- |
| 0 | —No response |
| 1 + | —Low normal |
| 2 + | —Normal |
| 3 + | —Brisk |
| 4 + | —Hyperactive |

*Genitalia*               Deferred

*Rectal*                  Normal, no palpable masses

## Laboratory Data/Diagnostic Studies

*Laboratory Data*
***Anti-DNA Antibody.*** Positive
***Serum complement.*** C3 and C4 diminished
***Rheumatoid Factor.*** Present
Positive LE cell test
***Hemoglobin.*** 13.2 g/dl
***Hematocrit.*** 39%
***Na.*** 140 meq/L
***K.*** 3.5 meq/L
***Cl.*** 98 meq/L
Mild Proteinuria
***Leukopenia.*** less than 4000/$\mu$l

*Diagnostic Studies*
***Chest x-ray.*** Normal
***Electrocardiogram.*** Normal
***Kidney biopsy.*** To be done

## COLLABORATIVE PLAN OF CARE

*Diet*                    Low sodium regular

*Medications*             Prednisone: 15 mg qid. with milk or food

*Intravenous Therapy*     Does not apply

*Therapeutic Measures*
Take temperature bid
Activity ad lib with at least 30/min rest periods bid
Weigh self each day
Return for visit in 1 week

*Consults*
Occupational therapy, physical therapy, consider recommending
  a counselor

# NURSING DIAGNOSES DEVELOPED IN CARE PLAN

# ADDITIONAL NURSING DIAGNOSES TO BE CONSIDERED

Altered Role Performance
Anxiety
Comfort, Altered: Pain, Chronic
Fatigue
Fear
Fluid Volume, Altered: Excess
Impaired Home Maintenance Management
Knowledge Deficit, Disease Process, Therapeutic Measures, Diagnostic Procedures
Potential for Infection
Potential Impaired Skin Integrity

# NURSING CARE PLAN BASED ON IDENTIFIED NURSING DIAGNOSES

| *Disturbance in Self-Concept: Body Image* | ***Related to:*** Obvious changes in appearance caused by facial rash.<br>***Evidenced by:*** Expressed concerns over ability to face friends and family with this appearance. |
|---|---|
| *Desired Patient Outcomes* | ***The Patient Will:***<br>• Verbalize a positive self-concept.<br>• Discuss plans to socialize.<br>• Identify positive feelings about appearance.<br>• Use cosmetics to enhance appearance.<br>• Return to previous activities without undue stress related to appearance. |
| *Evaluation Criteria* | ***The Patient:***<br>• Verbalizes a positive self-image.<br>• Discusses social activities in which she is involved.<br>• Demonstrates comfort about appearance by interacting openly with others.<br>• Wears appropriate cosmetics.<br>• Identifies a return to previous activities. |

## Interventions

Offer support to patient, including time to discuss feelings about appearance and identification of positive aspects of self

Teach patient methods to minimize the

## Rationale

The opportunity to freely discuss concerns about body image may occur only in the safe environment of the office where the nurse is nonjudgmental and open. Initiating the discussion in a gentle manner may provide an opportunity for dealing with this very sensitive issue (Phillips, 1984, p. 192).

Offering the patient strategies to positively affect the cause of

## Interventions

cause of the body image disturbance including:
• Avoiding exposure to ultraviolet light
• Refer to cosmetologist for appropriate make-up to use over rash

Consider referral for counseling if preceding interventions are unsuccessful.

## Rationale

the disturbance should contribute to a feeling of regaining some control over the problem (Nass, 1987, p. 74).

The potential long-term nature of the symptoms may be overwhelming and not relieved by infrequent interventions such as those provided by routine followup. The symptoms such as a facial rash are only 1 component of a disease that may have life-threatening complications. The need for support to handle this situation on an ongoing basis is often indicated (Lockshin and Rothfield, 1988, p. 92).

---

### Activity Intolerance

*Related to:* Severe fatigue, weakness and aching
*Evidenced by:* Inability to carry out usual activities, including working, care of stepchildren, and home maintenance

### Desired Patient Outcomes

*The Patient Will:*
• Prioritize activities based on her own value for each activity.
• State that she feels less fatigue.
• State that she feels she has control of her schedule to allow for adequate rest.

### Evaluation Criteria

*The Patient Will:*
• Look and state that she feels less fatigued.
• Arrange or is investigating child-care arrangements and assistance with home management.

---

## Interventions

Discuss sleep/rest patterns prescribing 8–10 h of sleep per night and 2 short rest periods during the day.

Discuss measures to promote conservation of energy including use of proper body mechanics; use of outside resources such as a housekeeper and child-care.

Refer to occupational therapy and/or physical therapy for program to structure activities, increase strength, and conserve energy.

## Rationale

Additional sleep and rest periods have been shown to decrease fatigue associated with SLE (Kinash, 1984, p. 33).

Support for use of outside help to manage the home situation may make this intervention acceptable to the patient who is used to working, managing the home, and caring for children. Pacing activities to allow for rest has been beneficial to patients (Kinash, 1984, p. 34).

Offering concrete assistance in learning energy conservation may contribute to the patient feeling support (Nass, 1987, p. 74).

---

### Alteration in Tissue Perfusion

*Related to:* Lupus nephritis.
*Evidenced by:* Moderate edema hands and feet, mild proteinuria, and slight decrease in urine output.

### Desired Patient Outcomes

*The Patient Will:*
• Demonstrate controlled renal symptoms including de-

creased edema of hands and feet, decreased proteinuria, and normal amount of urine output.
- Identify the parameters that should be monitored to detect increase in symptoms.

*Evaluation Criteria*

*The Patient:*
- Over several weeks of treatment with steroids as an outpatient, states she has decreased edema of hands and feet.
- Identifies measures she will use to monitor and treat renal symptoms: assess and record edema; monitor urine output; collect urine specimen as needed; take prescribed medication safely.
- Takes prescribed prednisone without evidence of gastro-intestinal irritation.
- Identifies side effects of long-term use of steroids as well as verbalizes when to report these.

## *Interventions*

## *Rationale*

Assess and record edema

Early renal involvement may or may not be manifested with common signs. Early detection and treatment may delay serious disease (Blau, 1986, p. 98).

Collect appropriate urine specimens

Although an early sign of renal involvement is mild proteinuria, some patients have normal urine with evidence by biopsy of renal damage. Urine should be assessed at regular intervals (Clinical Highlights, 1985, p. 241).

Instruct the patient about renal involvement in SLE to include her own role in monitoring the disease process: Assess and record edema, provide urine specimens, safely take prescribed medications.

There is some evidence that earlier detection of the disease and effective management are contributing to an increase in life expectancy for patients with SLE (Kinash, 1984, p. 32). A key component in this process is the ability of the patient and family to learn about the disease and seek treatment as needed.

# QUESTIONS FOR DISCUSSION

1. What additional signs, symptoms, and complications should this patient monitor, report, and seek medical attention for before the life-threatening stage is reached?
2. What ideas and strategies would you use with this patient to allow her to participate as much as possible in monitoring the disease process without overwhelming her completely?
3. What teaching would you provide when asked about a kidney biopsy?
4. What suggestions would you offer to this patient to allow her more-effective rest when she tries to rest, but feels restless and fatigued instead? How important is this ability to gain adequate rest?
5. What strategy would you use to promote involvement of her husband at this time in managing the home situation, including child-care?
6. Because of the serious side-effects and the potential long-term use of anti-inflammatory agents/immuno-suppressants, what teaching would you offer? What strategies would you recommend to promote as normal a lifestyle as possible while fostering adherence to prescribed medical therapies?
7. What would you discuss with this patient about childbearing abilities and birth-control?
8. Are there any resources and written materials you would suggest for this patient that present information about others' ability to cope with this condition?

# REFERENCES

Blau, SP: In Management, less is often more. Consultant 26:96, 104, 1986. Clinical highlights: Useful laboratory findings in systemic lupus erythematosus. Hosp Med 21:241, 1985.

Kinash, RG: Physiologic responses of patients with systemic lupus and implications for rehabilitation. Rehabilitation Nurs 9:33, 1984.

Koffler, D: Immunology of systemic lupus erythematosus and related rheumatic diseases. Clin Symp 39:5, 1987.

Lockshin, MD and Rothfield, NF: A better prognosis in lupus. Patient Care. p. 92, 1988.

Massicot, JG: Current immunologic research on systemic lupus erythematosus. Health Values: Achieving High Level Wellness 9:11, 1985.

Nass, T: Helping the patient who has lupus. RN 50:69, 1987.

Neuberger, JS and Neuberger, GB: Epidemiology of the rheumatic diseases. Nurs Clin North Am 4:722, 1984.

Phillips, RH: Coping with Lupus. Avery Publishing Group, Wayne, NJ, 1984.

Sonnett, R: Serodiagnosis of systemic lupus erythematosus. J Med Tech 5:280, 1986.

Steinberg, AD: Systemic lupus erythematosus, part II. Hosp Med 23:145, 1987.

Ziegler, GC: Systemic lupus erythematosus and systemic sclerosis. Nurs Clin North Am 19:673, 1984.

# BIBLIOGRAPHY

Benson, MD: Effective use of highly regarded and often disregarded tests. Consultants. 1985.

Birmingham, JJ: Home Care Planning Based on DRGs: Functional Health Pattern Model. JB Lippincott, Philadelphia, 1986.

Bullock, BL and Rosendahl, PP: Physiology: Adaptations and Alterations in Functions. Little, Brown & Co, Boston, 1984.

Burgess, S and Joyce, K: Case study: Systemic lupus erythematosus and renal insufficiency. ANNA 13:168, 1986.

Carpenito, LJ: Nursing Diagnosis: Applications to Clinical Practice. JB Lippincott, Philadelphia, 1983.

Doenges, ME, Jeffries, MP, and Moorhouse, MF: Nursing Care Plans: Nursing Diagnoses in Planning Patient Care. FA Davis, Philadelphia, 1984.

Fauci, AS: Corticosteroids in autoimmune disease. Hosp Pract 18:103, 1983.

Gordon, M: Manual of Nursing Diagnosis. McGraw-Hill, New York, 1987.

Gordon, M: Nursing Diagnosis: Process and Application. McGraw Hill, New York, 1982.

Hamilton, HK: Nursing Drug Handbook. Springhouse Corporation, Springhouse, Pa, 1987

Hooker, RS: Systemic lupus erythematosus. Physician Assistant. 12:71, 1988.

Hurley, ME: Classification of Nursing Diagnosis: Proceedings of the Sixth Conference. CV Mosby, St. Louis, 1986.

Hurst, JW: The Heart, Arteries, and Veins. McGraw-Hill, New York, 1982.

Joyce, KM, Austin, HA, and Balow, JO: The patient with lupus nephritis: A nursing perspective. Heart Lung 14:75, 1985.

Long, B and Phipps, WJ: Essentials of Medical-Surgical Nursing: A Nursing Process Approach. CV Mosby, St. Louis, 1985.

Maehara, KT: Laboratory Diagnosis of Systemic Rheumatic Disease. Am J Med Tech. 49:477, 1983.

Malasanos, L, et al: Health Assessment. CV Mosby, St. Louis, 1986.

Martens, JM, et al: Respiratory muscle dysfunction in systemic lupus erythematosus. Chest 84:170, 1983.

McClelland, F, et al: Continuity of Care: Advancing the Concept of Discharge Planning. Grune and Stratton, Orlando, FL, 1985.

Nursing '86 Books. Diagnostics. Nurses Reference Library. Springhouse Corporation, Springhouse, Pa, 1986

Nursing '86 Books. Diagnostics. Nurses Reference Library. Springhouse Corp, Springhouse, Pa, 1986

Sala, DJ and Lentz, JR: Pregnant women with systemic erythematosus. MCN 11:382, 1986.

Scherer, JC: Lippincott's Nurses Drug Manual. JB Lippincott, Philadelphia, 1985.

Searle, L: Honoring the personal side of chronic illness. Nursing '85 11:53, 1985.

Steinberg, AD: Systemic lupus erythematosus, part I. Hosp Med 23:131, 1987.

Sudbury, F: Rheumatology nursing assessment. CONA 9:4, 1987.

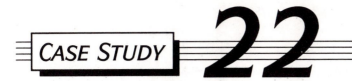

# A PATIENT WITH ACQUIRED IMMUNE DEFICIENCY SYNDROME

Susan Caloggero, M.S.M., R.N. and
Julia Hodsdon Basque, M.S., R.N.

When the original Communicable Disease Center (CDC) surveillance definition for acquired immune deficiency syndrome (AIDS) was developed in 1981, those indicator diseases that were included represented an array of unusual infections and malignancies thought to be specific for the newly recognized syndrome. Since that time, HIV serology and specific viral culture techniques have been developed and, in 1985, the definition was expanded.

As of September, 1987, a third version of the case definition of AIDS was released by the CDC. The new case definition now includes human immunodeficiency virus, (HIV) encephalopathy (dementia complex), wasting syndrome, and a broader range of indicator diseases (such as disseminated or miliary tuberculosis [TB] and recurrent nontyphoid salmonella septicemia) in patients with laboratory evidence of HIV antibody.

## ANATOMY AND PHYSIOLOGY

The immune system protects the body against infections and certain cancers. It is made up of several types of white blood cells, lymph nodes and lymphatic ducts.

- Lymph nodes: Lymph nodes are centers for lymphocyte production and removal of foreign bodies; these become larger and/or tender in the presence of infection.
- Lymphocytes: Two important types of lymphocytes are the B cell and T cell. B cells are involved in humeral immunity of the body; T cells are involved in the cell-mediated immunity of the body

### TYPES OF T CELLS

$T_S$ = *T-suppressor cells*           T-suppressor cells suppress or inhibit immune response.

$T_H$ = *T-helper cells*              T-helper cells signal other immune system cells and stimulate immune response to fight off infection.

*T-killer cells*                T-killer cells destroy invading infection directly.

## TYPES OF IMMUNITY

*Humoral immunity*

Humoral immunity produces antibodies in response to infection; these antibodies are specific, and circulate in the bloodstream. Most humoral response in AIDS remains intact.

*Cell-mediated immunity*

Cell-mediated immunity confers protection against bacteria that live and grow inside host cells (i.e., mycobacteria) and against certain viruses. AIDS damages this aspect of the immune system (in particular, T-helper cells).

# PATHOPHYSIOLOGY

HIV belongs to the family of viruses known as *retroviruses*. Retroviruses carry their genetic information on RNA chromosomes rather than DNA chromosomes. They utilize an enzyme, *reverse transcriptase*, to replicate. HIV has been shown to specifically target monocytes, macrophages, T-helper cells and other cells bearing the $T_4$ receptor sites (Gee and Moran, 1988). HIV enters the host cell after attaching to these receptor sites. Once inside the host cell, HIV uses reverse transcriptase to create viral DNA. Eventually, the viral DNA will become integrated into the ($T_4$ cell) host cell's DNA structure; the result is a "genetic hybrid called a provirus" (Gee and Moran, 1988, p. 97). "HIV can remain dormant in the provirus form without replicating as long as the $T_4$ host cell remains immunologically inactive" (Gee and Moran, p. 97, 1988). However, if the $T_4$ host cell becomes activated by another infectious process, the provirus becomes activated, begins to replicate, and "expresses" HIV virus. The host cell, therefore, becomes a "virus-producing factory," resulting in the eventual cell death of the infected $T_4$ cell. Because the $T_4$ helper cells are affected chiefly, the immune response becomes increasingly ineffective. The ratio of $T_4$ cells to $T_8$ cells becomes unbalanced. The $T_8$ (suppressor) cell count increases, and the immune system cannot provide feedback to signal the system appropriately. Both the cell-mediated and humoral systems are affected. B cells become less-effective in producing antibodies to combat infections. Antibodies to HIV are produced, but they are also ineffective in fighting off the virus.

The clinical course of infection with HIV seems to begin with an acute viral illness lasting up to 14 days. This acute illness has been described by various research groups as appearing before the development of antibodies against HIV (Stage I HIV infection). Researchers believe that patients might be highly infectious during this acute phase. The body's humoral response (antibody production) takes up to 8–12 weeks after exposure before anti-HIV antibodies can be detected in the serum by standard testing (seroconversion). Following the acute illness, there is a dormant period in which the virus is basically inactive. This incubation period may last anywhere from 2 months to 5 years, with the average time being 2–3 years (Gee and Moran, 1988). Generally, individuals do not experience any signs of illness during this time; however, they are presumed infectious (Stage II HIV infection). Within 5–7 years of infection, clinical manifestations of HIV infection usually become apparent and will then be labeled AIDS or AIDS-related complex (ARC) (Stages III and IV HIV infections).

Research has focused on the potential role of "co-factors" in the development of AIDS from asymptomatic to symptomatic. Some co-factors that could activate the immune response and potentially trigger rapid replication of HIV are the Epstein–Barr virus, cytomegalovirus, sexually transmitted diseases, intravenous (IV) drug use, allergies, and poor nutrition. These represent only a few potential co-factors that could activate the virus. Scientists are attempting to test the validity of the co-factor theory.

## Risk Factors

HIV is found in any bodily fluid or substance that contains lymphocytes. Such substances include blood, semen, saliva, tears, breast milk, vaginal secretions, urine, and feces. Thus far, the bodily fluids that have been implicated in the *transmission* of HIV are blood, semen, vaginal/cervical secretions, and breast milk. HIV is transmitted through the following activities:

- Sexual contact (anal and vaginal intercourse)
- Blood-to-blood exposure via
  - Needlesticks or mucous membranes
  - Blood transfusion
  - Sharing needles as in IV drug use
  - Artificial insemination

*High-risk activities* are identified as unprotected anal and/or vaginal intercourse (without condom use), unprotected oral sexual contact, and sharing needles in IV drug use. Engaging in high-risk activities with multiple sexual partners also places an individual at a greater risk.

Recommendations regarding prevention of HIV transmission basically involve avoidance of unprotected sexual activity, and use of a latex barrier so as to prevent exchange of blood and bodily fluids; avoidance of sharing needles, as in the use of IV drugs; implementation of universal precautions in the health-care setting; and screening of all women of child-bearing age who are within the high-risk categories.

# COMMON CLINICAL FINDINGS AND TREATMENT MODALITIES

Due to the syndrome's profound immunologic disturbances, the person with AIDS is susceptible to multiple opportunistic infections and unusual malignancies. Opportunistic infections are caused by agents that usually exist in the human body or external environment without being a threat to health, but become active and health-threatening when given the opportunity presented by the depressed immune system of the person with AIDS. Persons with AIDS usually develop protozoan infections (*Pneumocystis carinii* pneumonia, toxoplasmosis), fungal infections (cryptococcal meningitis, candidiasis), bacterial infections (*Mycobacterium avium-intracellular*, pulmonary TB), viral infections (cytomegalovirus, herpes simplex II) and cancers (Kaposi's sarcoma, lymphoma).

*Pneumocystis carinii pneumonia* (PCP) is characterized by a nonproductive cough, fever, progressive dyspnea on exertion or at rest, and increasing malaise and fatigue. Usually there is a gradual onset of symptomatology; however, a small percentage of patients have an acute onset accompanied by severe hypoxemia and progressive respiratory failure. Diagnosis is made by chest x-ray and sputum induction or bronchoscopy. The initial treatment regimen usually consists of IV administration of trimethoprim and sulfamethoxazole (Bactrim) for a total of 14–21 days. If a patient develops drug toxicity at any point during the 21-day regimen, Pentamidine isethionate (Pentam 300) may be substituted to complete the course. Bactrim is initially given intravenously and may be switched to the oral route on an outpatient basis. Side-effects commonly appear 7–14 days into treatment and include rash, nausea and vomiting, fever, neutropenia, thrombocytopenia, nephrotoxicity, hepatotoxicity, and hyponatremia. Pentamidine is given intravenously. Side-effects are anemia, neutropenia, renal and heptatotoxicity, hypoglycemia, and orthostatic hypotension. Aerosolized pentamidine is utilized as an alternative to parenteral therapy for both treatment and prophylaxis of PCP. Systemic side-effects are avoided because the drug is not systematically absorbed and does not achieve significant blood levels.

*Kaposi's sarcoma* (KS) is a rare cancer of the skin's blood vessels that first appears as small, blue violet-to-brownish lesions on the trunk, arms, head and neck, and invades the lungs and other organs. Diagnosis is usually made by biopsy of a single lesion. Treatment of KS depends largely on the clinical status of the patient. Radiation therapy can help control localized disease. Chemotherapeutic agents are used to treat KS when a systemic effect is desired. Potential side-effects must be considered when evaluating patients for chemotherapy.

*Lymphomas* are neoplasms involving the cells of the lymphoid system, which are composed of either lymphocytes or reticular cells. In persons with AIDS, non-Hodgkin's lymphoma is more virulent and response to treatment differs dramatically from non-AIDS non-Hodgkin's lymphoma. Diagnosis is made by a lymph-node biopsy.

*Primary Central Nervous System (CNS) Lymphoma* patients may present with confusion, short-term memory loss, personality and behavior alterations, headaches, or seizures. Computer Axial Tomography (CT) scans or Magnetic Resonance Imaging (MRI) usually will detect a space-occupying lesion in the brain. Primary CNS lymphomas are generally unresponsive to therapy; however, the lesions are somewhat radiosensitive, making radiation therapy the treatment of choice.

*Toxoplasma gondii* is a protozoan infection. These parasites are found in under cooked meats, cats' feces, and contaminated water. In AIDS patients, the infection affects the brain and manifests as seizures and other neurologic deficits. Patients may present with a gradual onset of symptoms of fulminating disease. Diagnosis is complicated. MRI/CT may be useful diagnostic tools, along with the assessment of clinical symptoms. Treatment consists of drug therapy with a combination of pyrimethamine and sulfadiazine sodium. Duration of the therapy is a minimum of 6–8 weeks. However, many patients continue on a maintenance therapy program due to the increased incidence of relapse after discontinuing drug therapy.

*Candidiasis* is a fungal infection. Oral thrush is often one of the first manifestations of HIV infection and is usually treated with Nystatin mouthwash. Esophageal thrush, however, is usually treated with ketoconazole. Side effects include nausea and hepatotoxicity. Most patients will describe painful swallowing and retrosternal pain. The barium swallow procedure is used for diagnostic evaluation.

*Cryptococcal neoformans* is a fungal infection in the CNS, usually presenting as meningitis. Patients most-often present with chronic symptoms of high fevers, malaise, and headaches. Other symptoms, such as photophobia, stiff neck, nausea and vomiting, and mental status changes may not occur until several weeks after initial symptoms are noted. Diagnostic evaluation involves careful examination of cerebral spinal fluid (CSF) along with CT scan and/or MRI if CSF examination is negative. Treatment of choice is fungizone intravenous (Amphotericin B). Initial reaction to the drug is quite common. Often premedication with antihistamines and antipyretics is recommended before infusion of Amphotericin B. Gradual increase of daily doses of the IV drug is advised until a therapeutic dose is achieved. Careful monitoring of renal function is crucial. Bone marrow suppression may occur, and localized phlebitis is a common problem.

Cytomegalovirus (CMV) causes a mononucleosis-like syndrome with infection of internal organs other than the liver, spleen, or lymph nodes. It may also manifest as pneumonia or colitis. The most common manifestation is spots in the retina, which may lead to blindness. Diagnostic evaluation depends on presenting symptoms. Treatment for retinitis is ganciclovir. Patients require an initial induction period of 14–21 days, 2 doses per day, then daily maintenance therapy of 1 dose per day for 5 days per week indefinitely. The most common side effect is bone marrow suppression (neutropenia).

*Myobacterium Avium—Intracellular* (MAI) is a mycobacterial infection, sometimes referred to as *atypical tuberculosis*. "MAI disease in AIDS is believed to be a reactivation of a previous environmentally acquired infection" (Gee and Moran, 1988, p. 166). It is not considered contagious. It is quite resistant to pharmacological therapy and usually carries a poor prognosis when diagnosed in AIDS patients. Persistent fevers are frequently noted; however, they are cyclical throughout the day and usually remain low grade (<101°F). Other general AIDS-related symptoms may be present (i.e., weight-loss, fatigue, and debilitation). Because MAI usually invades the bone marrow, most patients will be pancytopenic. Some patients may present with a syndrome of gastrointestinal disease related to MAI. MAI in AIDS is typically a disseminated disease process. Diagnosis is made by positive culture of organisms from one extra-pulmonary site. Combination drug therapy is under investigation.

*Mycobacterium tuberculosis* is a frequent cause of disease in HIV-infected patients. About 50% of patients will present with a pulmonary manifestation. Diagnostic evaluation of sputum usually demonstrates the presence of acid-fast organisms. Treatment is isoniazid, rifampin, and either ethambutol (Myambutol) or pyrazinamide (Pyrazinamide).

# CURRENT TREATMENTS

Aside from the specific treatments used to combat opportunistic infections and malignancies in AIDS patients, there is no effective cure for AIDS at this time. Research currently being conducted is looking at ways of killing HIV or restoring the damaged immune system.

A number of antiviral agents are in various stages of clinical trials. These drugs are attempting to intervene in some stage of the viral life cycle and prevent further replication. One such agent recently approved by the Food and Drug Administration, is zidovudine (Azidothymidine [AZT]). AZT does not kill the virus; it stops viral replication. It does this by "fooling" the enzyme, reverse transcriptase, into thinking that AZT is the same building block used to create viral DNA. AZT prevents viral replication by preventing the completion of viral DNA strands. AZT must be taken continuously in order to maintain an effective level of drug in the system. If treatment is interrupted, it may be re-started once the underlying cause has been remedied.

Current protocols are underway to evaluate the potential effectiveness of AZT taken by HIV-asymptomatic carriers. Early trials of AZT use demonstrated longer survival times, weight gain, and fewer relapses of the opportunistic infections. Usually drug side effects are the mechanism that prevents patients from taking AZT on a long-term basis. Most-common side effects are bone marrow suppression, nausea, and headaches.

# PATIENT ASSESSMENT DATA BASE

## Health History

*Client*
Mr. George Marshall

*Address:* 33429 Hawthorne Blvd, Torrance, California
*Telephone:* (213) 555-9692
*Contact:* Marjorie Marshall (mother)
*Address of contact:* 33429 Hawthorne Blvd, Torrance, California
*Telephone of contact:* (213) 555-9692
*Age:* 36    *Sex:* Male    *Race:* White
*Educational background:* MSM (Masters of Science in Management)
*Religion:* Protestant    *Marital status:* Single
*Usual occupation:* Department Manager in Medical Equipment Company
*Present occupation:* Unemployed
*Source of income:* Social Security Disability; applying for Medicaid
*Insurance:* BC/BS: Master Health Plus
*Source of referral:* Marjorie Marshall
*Source of history:* Patient
*Reliability of historian:* Reliable
*Date of interview:* January 2, 1990
*Reason for visit/Chief complaint:* 36-year-old-male recently discharged from hospital, requiring hospice support.

### HEALTH PERCEPTION/HEALTH MANAGEMENT PATTERN

*Present Health Status*

Patient states, "I just got out of the hospital. I still feel weak. I'm concerned that my mother is all by herself and won't be able to care for me. And I'm so much sicker than I was before."

*Past Health Status*

*General Health.* Patient states, "I was healthy up until 9 months ago when I developed a serious pneumonia called PCP. The AIDS diagnosis was made at the same time. I finally recovered from the PCP and was out of the hospital on prophylactic Bactrim and an experimental medication. I did okay until a month ago. I started having thick mucus and high fevers. I went into the hospital where they discovered I had TB."
*Prophylactic Medical/Dental Care.* Before AIDS diagnosis, visited doctor "regularly" once a year. More frequent doctor visits in the last 6 months, at least monthly. Mr. Marshall rarely visits dentist unless he is experiencing a dental problem.
*Childhood Illnesses.* Mumps at age 5, chicken pox at age 7.
*Immunizations.* Patient states, "The usual ones I guess."
*Major Illnesses/Hospitalizations.* Two hospitalizations for major opportunistic infections within a 9-month period.
*History of Related Infections.* Before diagnosis, frequent colds, sinus infections that "I couldn't get rid of." History of oral candidiasis, *Pneumocystis carinii* pneumonia, and TB. "Repeated infections have become a real concern of mine; it seems I can't stay healthy."

**Past Health Status — Continued**

**Current Medications**
*Prescription:* Bactrim, rifampin, streptomycin sulfate, Myambutol, pyridoxine.
*Nonprescription:* None.
**Allergies.** None.

**Habits**
*Alcohol:* Drinks "socially"
*Caffeine:* 1–2 cups coffee/d; 3–4 Pepsi colas/d
*Drugs:* None
*Tobacco:* Non-smoker

**Family Health History**

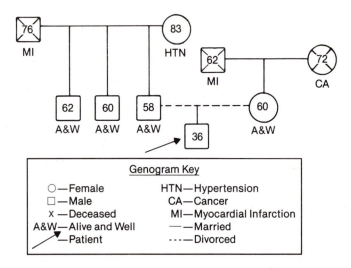

Genogram Key

○ —Female     HTN—Hypertension
□ —Male     CA—Cancer
x —Deceased     MI—Myocardial Infarction
A&W—Alive and Well     —Married
—Patient     · · · —Divorced

## NUTRITIONAL/METABOLIC PATTERN

**Nutritional**

**Usual Daily Menu**
*Breakfast:* Milk, toast, coffee
*Lunch:* Peanut butter and jelly sandwich, pudding, soup, Pepsi cola
*Dinner:* Meatloaf, potato, peas, coffee
*Snacks:* Crackers; 3 8-oz. Pepsi colas

**Metabolic**

*Height:* 5 ft. 7 in. (170 cm); *Weight:* 125 lb (57 kg). Weight six months ago: 140 lb (64 kg). Had lost weight secondary to decreased appetite, difficulty in swallowing (thrush), and dislike of "hospital food." Weight now stabilized. History of candidiasis (thrush) in mouth, now resolved. No history of lesions or skin breakdown.

## ELIMINATION PATTERN

**Bowel**

Usual pattern is once/d, soft stool; current pattern is twice/d, slightly soft/watery.

**Bladder**

Usual pattern is 4–5 times/d with "moderate amounts each time." Current pattern is same. No complaints of burning, pain, urgency, or dribbling on urination. Notes red tinge to urine ("due to one of my medications").

## ACTIVITY/EXERCISE PATTERN

**Activity/Exercise**

George states that he has barely enough energy for desired or required activities. "I get fatigued very easily. It seems all I can do is get myself out of bed to go to the bathroom. It helps if I pace myself, so I do a lot of resting."

### Self-Care Ability

| | |
|---|---|
| Feeding — 0 | Grooming — II |
| Bathing — II | General mobility — I |
| Toileting — I | Cooking — II |
| Bed mobility — 0 | Home maintenance — II |
| Dressing — II | Shopping — II |

---

### Functional Levels Code

   0 — Full self-care
    I — Requires use of equipment or device
  II — Requires assistance or support from another person
 III — Requires assistance or supervision from another person
       and equipment or device
 IV — Does not participate in self care

---

**Oxygenation/Perfusion**

History of shortness of breath associated with pulmonary infections. States no difficulties at present.

### Cardiac Risk Factors

| | Positive | Negative |
|---|---|---|
| Sedentary life-style | X | |
| Hyperlipidemia | | X |
| Cigarette smoking | | X |
| Diabetes | | X |
| Obesity | | X |
| Hypertension | | X |
| Hypervigilant personality | X | |
| Family history of heart disease | X | |

## SLEEP/REST PATTERN

**Sleep/Rest**

Sleeps 8–10 hours a night. Normally feels tired. Occasional night sweats. Naps during day (1–3 hr). Denies use of sleep aids.

## COGNITIVE/PERCEPTUAL PATTERN

**Hearing**

No expressed difficulty, able to respond to normal conversation.

**Vision**

Vision normal; wears glasses for reading.

**Sensory Perception**

Oriented × 3, memory intact, no expressed difficulties with taste, smell or sensation, left-handed, no complaints of pain.

**Learning Style**

Highly educated man who states he likes to have information about his illness and his treatment options. Learns best by "careful reading, then discussion." Requests information about AIDS support group. Feels knowledgeable about current health status.

## SELF-PERCEPTION/SELF-CONCEPT PATTERN

**Self-Perception/Self-Concept**

Describes himself as "independent" and "creative." States he used to view himself as healthy, but now realizes the severity of his illness. "I'm well aware of the stigma of AIDS. It makes you feel alone."

## ROLES/RELATIONSHIP PATTERN

*Role/Relationship*

George lived in New York City and worked as a Department Manager in a medical equipment company before most recent hospitalization (4 weeks ago). Is on a leave of absence from work and is currently living with his mother in Torrance. He is an only child. Parents divorced 15 years ago. No contact with father. It has been only 3 months since mother learned of patient's homosexuality and diagnosis of AIDS. During recent interview with mother, she states that she is having enormous difficulty accepting the fact that her son may be dying. At times, she appears angry at the medical community for not being able to cure her son. She is working full-time and is concerned about who will care for her son in the daytime hours.

## SEXUALITY/REPRODUCTIVE PATTERN

*Sexuality/Reproductive*

George is a homosexual man. He was celibate for 1 year before diagnosis to avoid AIDS and has no significant relationships at present. No history of other venereal diseases.

## COPING/STRESS TOLERANCE PATTERN

*Coping/Stress Tolerance*

"I used to handle stress by working harder at my job—I'm a bit of a workaholic." Described his initial diagnosis of AIDS as a stressful past event, "At first I couldn't talk about it . . . I was overwhelmed with fear . . . I read that I probably have only 2 years to live, if that . . . I'm beginning to see how sick I really am. [tearfully] I still can't talk about it much."

## VALUE/BELIEF PATTERN

*Value/Belief*

Patient values relationships in his life, but feels socially isolated because most of his friends are in New York City and are not accessible to him right now. States formal religion has never been helpful to him.

# Physical Examination

*General Survey*

36-year-old slight, white man who appears older than stated age, lying in bed. Does not appear to be in acute distress. Speaks directly to interviewer and maintains occasional eye contact.

*Vital Signs*

**Temperature:** 98.4°F oral
**Pulse:** 88 per minute (regular)
**Respirations:** 26/min, shallow
**BP:** 124/82 right arm, sitting position

*Integument*

**Skin.** Warm, dry, no evidence of lesions, turgor slightly decreased.
**Mucous membranes.** Pink, slightly dry, no lesions noted.
**Nails.** Beds smooth, no clubbing.

*HEENT*

**Head.** Normocephalic, without bruises or lesions. Hair is sparsely distributed; thin, straight, and brown. Face is symmetrical, with smile and eyebrow raise, jaw closure appropriate.
**Eyes.** Vision (R) 20/40, (L) 20/40; EOMs intact bilaterally, conjunctiva clear; pupils equal, round, reactive to light and accommodation (PERRLA).
**Ears.** Auricles intact bilaterally; can hear whisper up to 2 feet

**HEENT—Continued**

bilaterally. Rinne test: air conduction twice .bone conduction.
**Nose.** Nares patent, septum midline, no sinus tenderness on palpation.
**Mouth/Throat.** Swallow and gag intact; uvula midline; tongue midline, protrudes without tremor.
**Neck.** The submental and submaxillary lymph nodes palpable, size approximately 2 cm and 1½ cm, respectively. Other nodes not palpable.

**Pulmonary**

Thorax oval. Antero-posterior diameter 2:1. Diaphragmatic expansion equal bilaterally. Diffuse crackles auscultated bilaterally at base of both lungs.

**Breast**

No masses, pain, or discharge noted.

**Cardiovascular**

Patient examined in lying position. No pulsations observed or palpated. Point of maximum intensity at fifth left intercostal space. No murmurs or extra heart sounds noted.

**Peripheral Vascular**

**Peripheral Pulses**
Temporal—4 bilaterally
Carotid—4 bilaterally
Brachial—4 bilaterally
Radial—4 bilaterally
Femoral—4 bilaterally
Popliteal—4 bilaterally
Posterior tibial—4 bilaterally
Dorsalis pedis—4 bilaterally

**Peripheral Pulse Scale**

| |
|---|
| 0—Absent |
| 1—Markedly diminished |
| 2—Slightly diminished |
| 3—Slightly diminished |
| 4—Normal |

**Abdomen**

Abdomen slightly concave, smooth, without scars. Bowel sounds heard in all 4 quadrants. No masses felt on palpation. No complaints of pain or tenderness.

**Musculoskeletal**

ROM within normal limits in all joints including fingers and toes. Strength against resistance equal bilaterally. Gait steady.

**Neurological**

**Mental Status.** Alert and oriented × 3; thought processes and general behavior appropriate.
**Cranial Nerves.** Cranial nerves I–XII intact.
**Motor.** Able to move all extremities.
**Sensory.** Able to distinguish sharp vs dull sensations on all extremities.

**Deep Tendon Reflexes**

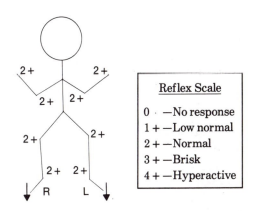

| Reflex Scale |
|---|
| 0 · —No response |
| 1 + —Low normal |
| 2 + —Normal |
| 3 + —Brisk |
| 4 + —Hyperactive |

| | |
|---|---|
| *Rectal* | Deferred. |
| *Genitalia* | Normal adult male. |

## Laboratory Data/Diagnostic Studies

*Laboratory Data*

*Na.* 133 mmol/L
*K.* 3.6 mmol/L
*CL.* 102 mmol/L
*CO$_2$.* 24 mmol/L
*BUN.* 25 mg/100 ml
*Creatinine.* 0.6 mg/100 ml
*Hemoglobin.* 9.2 g/100 ml
*Hematocrit.* 27.7%

*White blood cells.* 2000 mm$^3$
*% Lymphocytes.* 20%
*Platelets.* 93,000 mm$^3$
*Sputum culture.* Moderate mycobacterium tuberculosis
*Blood culture.* Negative

*Diagnostic Studies*

*Chest x-ray.* Diffuse interstitial infiltrates

### COLLABORATIVE PLAN OF CARE

*Diet*

Diet as tolerated; encourage eating but avoid raw fruits and vegetables (cook first)

*Medications*

Bactrim: 1 DS tablet bid
Rifampin: 600 mg po qd
Streptomycin Sulfate: 1 gm IM once weekly
Ethambutol: 1200 mg po qd
Pyridoxine: 50 mg po qd

*Intravenous Therapy*

Not applicable

*Therapeutic Measures*

Encourage ambulation
Monitor calories/weight qd
Universal precautions with respiratory precautions (mask) until sputum smears are negative.
Obtain sputum smear for culture and sensitivity and acid-fast bacillus once weekly until negative.

*Consults*

Consult Hospice home care
Home health aide
Hospice volunteers
Homemaker services
Social service

*Preoperative Plan*

Not applicable

## NURSING DIAGNOSES DEVELOPED IN CARE PLAN

Anticipatory Grieving, p. 378
Ineffective Family Coping: Compromised, p. 379
Potential for Infection, p. 377
Social Isolation, p. 379

## ADDITIONAL NURSING DIAGNOSES TO BE CONSIDERED

Activity Intolerance
Nutrition, alteration in: Less than Body Requirements
Self Care Deficit: Bathing/Hygiene
Self Care Deficit: Dressing/Grooming

# NURSING CARE PLAN BASED ON IDENTIFIED NURSING DIAGNOSES

| | |
|---|---|
| **Potential for Infection** | ***Related to:*** Immunocompromised state.<br>***Evidenced by:*** Two opportunistic infections within a 9-month period; decreased WBC count and decreased lymphocyte count. |
| **Desired Patient Outcomes** | ***The Patient Will:***<br>• Describe the usual modes of transmission of microorganisms.<br>• Describe precaution techniques that may protect him from opportunistic infections.<br>• Describe early signs/symptoms of infection. |
| **Evaluation Criteria** | ***Within 2 Days, the Patient Will:***<br>• Verbalize the usual transmission of organisms<br>• Verbalize precaution techniques that may protect him from opportunistic infections<br><br>***Within 4 Days, the Patient Will:***<br>• Demonstrate the above precaution techniques in his immediate environment.<br>• Verbalize the signs and symptoms of infection.<br><br>***Throughout Patient's Illness:***<br>• If an infection does occur, the signs and symptoms will be noted by the patient and will be reported to a health-care provider. |

## Interventions

Discuss with George the usual modes of transmission of microorganisms. Encourage mother to join in discussions.

Discuss techniques that may protect patient from opportunistic infections:

• Good handwashing techniques (by himself, family, and other health-care providers)

• Keep home environment clean (especially kitchen and bathroom)

• Avoid raw vegetables/fruit (cook first)

• Minimize stress (e.g., relaxation techniques, acupuncture, positive imagery)

## Rationale

The best defense against the spread of an infection is to break the infection chain (Potter and Perry, 1985, p. 864). Teaching the patient the usual means of transmission of organisms (air, direct contact, indirect contact, food, body fluids, etc.) can be the rationale for motivating Mr. Marshall to use precaution techniques that may protect him from further infections. (Stair and McNally, 1985).

Thorough handwashing is the most important means of preventing and controlling the transmission of organisms (Potter and Perry, 1985, p. 140).

Keeping the home environment clean will reduce the possibility of opportunistic infections (Gong and Rudnick, 1986, p. 230).

Raw fruits and vegetables may transmit microbes to the patient (Wolff and Colletti, 1986, p. 76).

Minimizing personal stress by using relaxation, positive thinking, positive imagery, or acupuncture can help provide emotional support and may, in fact, increase the body's autoimmune response (Callan, 1987, p. 38).

## Interventions

• Maintain a balanced diet

Discuss with George the early signs and symptoms of infection:

• Redness
• Swelling
• Pain, soreness, stiffness, aches
• Ulcerations, skin breakdown
• Fever
• Increased fatigue, sputum production, or cough

## Rationale

A balanced diet will improve resistance to infection (Potter and Perry, 1985, p. 878).

If infections are noted early, then treatment can begin promptly and the spread of the infection can be minimized. (Stair and McNally, 1985, p. 141).

---

| | |
|---|---|
| **Anticipatory Grieving** | **Related to:** Recent acute illness, subsequent dependent state, and anticipated early death. **Evidenced by:** Verbalization of severity of illness, tears, and sad affect during portions of interview. |
| **Desired Patient Outcomes** | The patient will identify areas of loss (both actual losses and potential losses) that have occurred or have the potential to occur as a result of his AIDS diagnosis. |
| **Evaluation Criteria** | **Within 4 Days, the Patient Will:** |
| | • Refer to himself and others with AIDS as "persons with AIDS" (PWAs). |
| | • Participate in planning his personal care, and will state that he feels informed and able to make decisions regarding his care. |
| | **Within 1 Week, the Patient Will:** |
| | • Identify areas of actual loss and areas of potential loss. |
| | • State he is aware that death is a possibility, but that he chooses to focus on positive experiences whenever possible. |

---

## Interventions

Encourage George to refer to himself as a PWA, not a *victim* of AIDS.

Maintain George's independence and control over his physical care. Involve him in all decisions regarding his care. Keep him informed of his condition. Encourage questioning.

Discuss with George those losses that he has already experienced and those that he perceives as potential losses. In these discussions help him to balance the possibility of survival with the possibility of death. Offer him bereavement counsel from a hospice volunteer, if available.

## Rationale

Referring to people as victims of AIDS makes many AIDS people feel victimized and passive. AIDS task force groups encourage use of the term "PWA" (Callan, 1987, p. 128).

The course of AIDS is unpredictable and often beyond a PWA's control. Maintaining independence and control over decisions regarding personal care will help George to feel more in control. Keeping George informed and educated about AIDS and his treatment plans will help him to make educated decisions about his care (Callan, 1987, p. 130).

Giving George opportunities to discuss his losses will help him to work through his grief. Balancing hope with the possibility of death is critical in coping with AIDS. (Callan, 1987, p. 33).

| | |
|---|---|
| ***Social Isolation*** | ***Related to:*** Loss of support network.<br>***Evidenced by:*** Patient's verbalization of feeling alone once diagnosed with AIDS; and patient no longer living or working in pre-illness location (currently unable to return to work and friends, and support network is not in immediate vicinity). |
| ***Desired Patient Outcomes*** | Increase patient's support network in immediate community from 1 to greater than 3. |
| ***Evaluation Criteria*** | ***Within 4 days, the Patient Will:***<br>• State that he has information and telephone numbers of local AIDS support group.<br><br>***Within 1 week, the Patient Will:***<br>• Name 2 people with whom he feels he can discuss his concerns or fears. |

## Interventions

Discuss with George those community supports available to him, such as:

• Hospice volunteers
• AIDS Action "Buddy System"
• AIDS support groups; discuss all potential benefits
• Assist in making contact with an AIDS support network.
• Provide sample reading material/pamphlets from local or regional AIDS Action or Task Force publications.
• Provide telephone number and contact person of local or regional AIDS Action or Task Forces.

## Rationale

"Specialized AIDS services can augment health care, not only enhancing support but also counteracting the sense of isolation that PWAs often experience" (Schietinger, 1986).

There are many support groups and individuals willing to assist the PWA. Often all that is needed to gain information/assistance is a phone call by the PWA to the local or regional AIDS task force (Turner and Williamson, 1986).

| | |
|---|---|
| ***Ineffective Family Coping: Compromised*** | ***Related to:*** Mother feels overwhelmed with son's condition and care.<br>***Evidenced by:*** Mother's verbalization of frustration with medical community being unable to cure her son; son's verbalization of concern that mother is his only support person and she may not be able to care for him alone; and mother working full-time and caring for her son at home. |
| ***Desired Patient/Family Outcomes*** | ***Within 1 Week, the Mother Will:***<br>• Name 2 people whom she feels she can openly talk to about her son's care.<br><br>***Within 1 Week, the Mother and Son Will:***<br>• Describe a realistic home-care plan that<br>  ○ Maintains son's maximum level of independence.<br>  ○ Involves community supports. |
| ***Evaluation Criteria*** | ***Throughout Patient's Illness, the Mother Will:***<br>• State a realistic picture of her son's condition, prognosis, and care needs. |

| *Interventions* | *Rationale* |
|---|---|
| Provide time (approximately 20 min/visit) for RN to spend with mother to review patient's care and condition. Keep mother updated and with a realistic view of son's progress. | The mother should benefit from updated, realistic information from a consistent caregiver such as the RN (Robinson, 1984, p. 82). |
| Offer mother opportunity (i.e., name and number) of various people or organizations to gain personal support. Suggest:<br><br>• Social worker in home-care agency<br>• Spiritual advisor, if appropriate<br>• Family support groups, such as "Mothers with AIDS" | Often the greatest support comes from those who have experienced a similar experience ("Mothers with AIDS") or from professionals trained to help people in crisis such as a social worker, or minister (Durham and Cohen, 1987, p. 174). |

## QUESTIONS FOR DISCUSSION

1. How would you prioritize George's nursing diagnoses?
2. Can you generalize about what the common nursing diagnoses are for a given AIDS patient? Why or why not?
3. Distinguish among HIV+, ARC, and AIDS.
4. What precautions should a nurse take while caring for a PWA?
5. What is considered to be "safe sex"?
6. If you were educating the public on the transmission of AIDS, what would you emphasize?

## REFERENCES

Callan, M (ed): Surviving and Thriving with AIDS. People with AIDS Coalition, Inc, New York, 1987.

Durham, JD and Cohen, FL: The Person with AIDS: Nursing Perspectives. Springer Publishing, New York, 1987.

Gee, G and Moran, TA: AIDS: Concepts in Nursing Practice. Williams & Wilkins, Baltimore, 1988.

Gong, V and Rudnick, N: AIDS: Facts and Issues. Rutgers University Press, New Brunswick, 1986.

Potter, P and Perry, A: Fundamentals of Nursing: Concepts, Progress and Practice. CV Mosby, St. Louis, 1985.

Robinson, L: Acquired immunodeficiency syndrome: An update. Crit Care Nurse 4(5):75–83, 1984.

Schietinger, H: A home care plan for AIDS. Am J Nurs 86(9):1021–1028, 1986.

Stair, TC and McNally, JD: Injury, Potential for, Related to Infection. In McNally, JC, Stair, TC and Somerville, E (eds): Guidelines for Cancer Nursing Practice. Harcourt Brace Javanovich, Orlando, 1985.

Turner, J and Williamson, K: AIDS: A challenge for contemporary nursing, part II: Clinical AIDS. Focus on Critical Care 13(4):41–50, 1986.

Wolff, PH and Colletti, MA: AIDS: Getting past the diagnosis and onto discharge planning. Crit Care Nurse 6(4):76–81, 1986.

## BIBLIOGRAPHY

Bakerman, S: Understanding AIDS. Interpretive Laboratory Data, Inc, North Carolina, 1988.

Ho, DD, Pomerantz, RJ and Kaplan, J: Pathogenesis of infection with human immunodeficiency virus. N Engl J Med 317(5): 278–286, 1987.

Jennings, C: Understanding and Preventing AIDS. Harvard University Press, Cambridge, MA, 1988.

Massachusetts Hospital Associates and Massachusetts Department of Public Health: AIDS: An Education Reference Manual. MHA, Inc, Burlington, MA, 1988.

Nichols, EK: Mobilizing Against AIDS. Harvard University Press, Cambridge, MA, 1986.

Wormser, GP, Stahl, RE and Buttone, EJ: AIDS and Other manifestations of HIV Infection. Noyes Publications, Park Ridge, NJ, 1987.

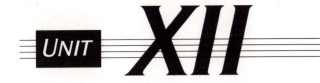

# UNIT XII

# THE PATIENT WITH MULTISYSTEM ALTERATIONS

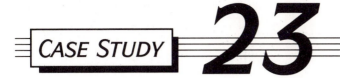

# A PATIENT WITH A MAJOR BURN INJURY

Anne Keiran Manton, M.S., R.N., C.E.N.

The number of people who suffer burn injuries each year in the United States is believed to exceed 2 million. Of these, it is estimated that more than 100,000 require hospitalization. Deaths resulting from burn injuries may be as many as 12,000 per year. (Achauer, 1987; Johnson, O'Shaughnessy, and Ostergren, 1981; Wagner, 1981). Although heart disease, cancer, and stroke are responsible for more deaths per year than burn injuries, burn injuries result in a greater number of productive years lost because of the slow recovery and rehabilitation processes necessitated by burn injuries, the frequent functional impairment, and also the relatively young mean age of burn victims (Wagner, 1981). Major burns should be viewed as a catastrophic event that may be the beginning of prolonged hospitalization, painful treatments, frequent surgeries, possible multiple complications, financial difficulties, and physical and emotional scarring.

Most significant burns occur in the home, with industry as the next most-common site. In addition, it is estimated that about 75% of deaths from burn injury are sustained in fires occurring in the home (Achauer, 1987). The literature is inconclusive with regard to the population at highest risk for burns; however, it is clear that children younger than 6 years of age and those between 17 and 35 years of age are in high-risk categories.

## ANATOMY AND PHYSIOLOGY OF THE SKIN

A review of the anatomy and physiology of the skin is needed to fully appreciate the many possible sequellae of thermal injury. Damage to the skin contributes, either directly or indirectly, to all other complications that occur in the patient who has sustained major burns.

The skin is composed of three layers: the *epidermis*, the *dermis*, and the *hypodermis* (Figure 23-1). The outermost layer is the epidermis, which is about 0.07 mm to 0.12 mm in depth. The epidermis contains 5 layers (or *strata*), which are, in descending order from the outermost to the innermost: the *stratum corneum*, the *stratum lucidum*, the *stratum granulosum*, the *stratum spinosum*, and the *stratum germinativum*. The stratum corneum and the stratum germinativum are most important to the present discussion because the stratum corneum functions to restrict fluids from entering or leaving the body and to protect against micro-organisms and most chemicals; the stratum germinativum is where new epithelial cells are produced and so is responsible for the regenerative capability of the skin.

The layer of skin next to the epidermis is the *dermis*, which is about 1 mm to 2 mm thick. It is composed of fibrous connective tissue, collagen, elastic fibers, nerves, and blood and lymph vessels. The dermis contains epidermal appendages, including hair follicles, sebaceous glands, sweat glands, the entire vascular supply for the skin, and also both sensory (*afferent*) and motor (*efferent*) nerves.

The innermost layer of the skin, called the *hypodermis*, is not well differentiated from the dermis. The hypodermis contains fat (*panniculus*), smooth muscle (*arrectoris pilorum*), and the areolar bed (*tela subcutanea*). The hypodermis is also referred to as *subcutaneous tissue*.

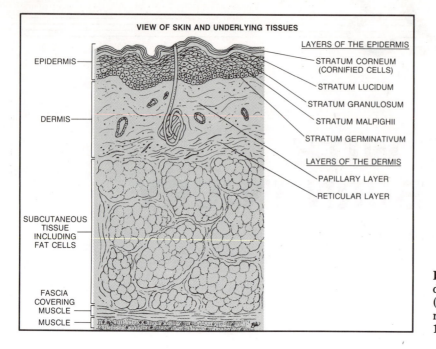

**FIGURE 23–1.** View of skin and underlying tissues. (From Thomas, CL (ed): Taber's Cyclopedic Medical Dictionary, ed 16. FA Davis, Philadelphia, 1989, p. 1687.)

The structure of the skin is well suited to its function. The cutaneous surface of the epidermis is coated with a layer of lipids and organic salts, which is known as the *acid mantle*. It is believed that the acid mantle, with its pH of 4.5 to 6, has antibacterial and antifungal properties. The epidermis contains keratin, which limits fluid loss. Between the stratum corneum and the stratum granulosum is a barrier layer, which is an electronegatively charged field with the smallest interstices in the skin, and which forms both a physiological and structural barricade to entrance by external substances. When damaged, the epidermis, which is a reproductively self-sufficient system, is capable of regenerating entirely from the remaining cells, provided the basal layer is intact and the appendages are still present. The diffuse distribution of afferent nerve endings throughout the epidermis allows the skin to be considered the principle sensory end organ.

In addition to providing mechanical strength and an anchor for the epidermis, the dermis supplies support and nourishment for the epidermis and its appendages. The dermis also assists in preventing infection and repairing wounds. The vascular system of the dermis is important in thermoregulation, given the ability of the vessels to dilate or constrict. The hypodermis is a thermal insulator, a shock absorber and an energy storer.

"To summarize, five general functions of skin include: (1) protection from potentially injurious external influences, (2) a barrier to invasion by microorganisms, (3) reception of sensory impulses, (4) regulation of heat exchange with the environment, (5) excretion as well as limited absorption of various substances" (Freeman, 1984, p. 54).

# PATHOPHYSIOLOGY OF BURNS

Burns are classified according to their etiology as *thermal, electrical,* or *chemical* in origin. The category of thermal burns can be subdivided with regard to more-specific etiology as *scald burns, flame burns, flash burns,* and *contact burns.* It has been demonstrated that the degree of tissue injury is a result of the intensity of heat and the duration of exposure. There is an inverse relationship between these 2 factors (i.e., the more intense the heat, the shorter time needed to produce cellular destruction). The other factor that determines the extent of injury is the conductance of the tissue involved. Conduction, or the state of dissipation or absorption of heat, is related to several factors. These factors include peripheral circulation, thickness of the skin, water content of the tissue (hydration), and the presence or absence of insulating substances such as hair and skin oils.

The traditional classification of burn injury into *first, second,* and *third degree burns* is used infrequently at present. The more-descriptive and more-functional classifications of *superficial burn, partial-thickness burn,* and *full-thickness burn* are more often the categories used in practice and in the literature (Figure 23-2).

**CLASSIFICATION OF BURNS**

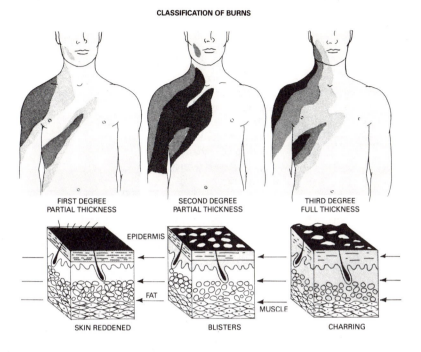

FIGURE 23–2. Classification of burns. (From Thomas, CL (ed): Taber's Cyclopedic Medical Dictionary, ed 15. FA Davis, Philadelphia, 1985, p. 243.)

The partial-thickness classification is frequently subdivided into the categories, *superficial partial-thickness burn*, and *deep partial-thickness burn*.

Superficial burns involve only the epidermis. This type of burn most often results from long exposure to low-intensity heat (e.g., sunburn), but may also result from a brief exposure to high-intensity heat. Such exposure results in erythematous, edematous skin that is painful to touch. The burn heals rapidly and does not scar. Such burns are considered to be minor and do not usually require hospitalization.

A deep partial-thickness burn involves all of the epidermis and varying depths of the dermis. Blistering is typical of this burn category. Nerve endings are irritated, and these injuries are quite painful. When intact, the blister membrane forms a sterile environment and prevents excessive fluid loss from the wound. These wounds heal without scarring in 10–14 days, although some discoloration may result if a large number of melanocytes have been destroyed.

Burns that result in complete destruction of the epidermis and significant disruption of the dermal layer, but with appendages such as sweat glands and hair follicles left intact, are termed deep partial-thickness burns. The sparing of the appendages, which are lined with epidermis, allows the potential for regeneration. The burn wound is red, painful, and weeps fluid. Blistering may or may not occur. Fluid loss may be extensive if a large body surface area is burned. A significant feature of the deep partial-thickness burn is the loss of the cellular barrier that protects against bacterial invasion and wound sepsis. In addition, wound healing takes longer because of the damage to deeper skin layers.

In a full-thickness injury, the epidermis, dermis, and dermal appendages are destroyed. Coagulation necrosis of cells characterize the wound. A thick, leathery eschar forms, which allows large fluid losses and is unable to prevent bacterial invasion and wound sepsis.

In addition to estimates of the burn depth, it is important to determine the size of the burn. The burn size is expressed as a percentage of total body surface area (TBSA). There are several techniques for estimating the burn size. Perhaps the most simple and widely used is the "rule of nines" (Table 1 and Figure 23-3). The rule of nines divides the body into areas, each of which represents 9% of the total body surface. This method is inexact, and should be used only for gross estimates of the burned area. It is sufficient, however, to allow some guidance in fluid resuscitation needs in the immediate post-burn period.

An early effect of burn injury is edema formation. This is due mostly to marked vasodilatation and microvascular permeability. If the area of burn injury is large enough (>25%–30%), the edema is not localized to the area of damage, but rather, the response becomes generalized. It is estimated that twice the normal plasma pool of albumin is lost from the vascular space in the first few days following a moderately sized burn injury. Approximately half remains within the interstitial space while the rest is lost through the wound surface. Bonaldi and Frank (1987, p. 30, 31) discuss the role of inflammatory mediators in edema formation, "Histamine is thought to be the first vasoactive substance released following burn injury . . . the early transient stage of vasodilation and increased venular permeability is probably due to this substance . . . fol-

### TABLE 1. RULE OF NINES

| BODY AREA | PERCENT-AGE |
|---|---|
| Head and neck | 9% |
| Right upper extremity | 9% |
| Left upper extremity | 9% |
| Anterior trunk | 18% |
| Posterior trunk | 18% |
| Right lower extremity | 18% |
| Left lower extremity | 18% |
| Perineum | 1% |

lowing thermal injury, coagulated protein located outside of blood vessels is thought to activate the complement cascade which then acts as a trigger stimulus for the acute inflammatory process. Once the complement system is activated, a host of permeability factors are liberated at the site of injury . . . The formation of edema following thermal injury is a complex balance between many systems which regulate microvascular permeability."

Loss of fluid occurs through the surface of the burn wound itself. Water vaporization has been found to be at least 4 times as rapid through burned skin as through normal skin. This fluid loss, when combined with the fluid lost from the vascular space due to edema, places the burn victim at high risk for hypovolemia.

At 2–3 days post-burn, capillaries begin to regain their integrity and fluid begins to move from the interstitial space back into the vasculature. This causes diuresis, and at this time, fluid and electrolyte balance must be monitored closely. Although a variety of electrolyte imbalances may occur, the patient is most at risk for hyponatremia and hypokalemia. Hemoglobin and hematocrit levels should be closely monitored, because anemia secondary to red-cell breakdown may also occur at this time.

Thermal injury affects virtually every organ system. The loss of skin as a barrier to invading pathogenic organisms places an additional burden on the system of specific immune responses. It has been noted, however, that immunosuppression follows burn injury. Many factors are believed to contribute to this phenomenon, such as burn-generated toxins, hormonal changes that occur as a result of the injury, increased prostaglandins, and host deficiency.

Numerous hematologic changes occur after major thermal trauma. These changes include increased platelet adhesiveness, decreased platelet survival, elevated fibrinogen levels, increased fibrin split levels, increased levels of factors V and VIII, thrombocytopenia, secondary thrombocytosis, and increased destruction of erythrocytes. Post-burn anemia is a frequent occurrence and should be anticipated.

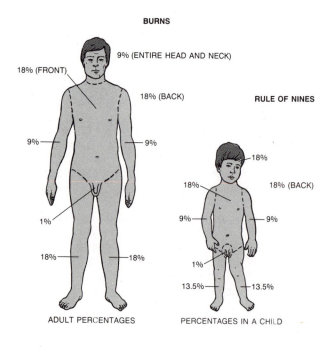

**FIGURE 23–3.** Estimation of body surface area for determining percentage of burns. (From Thomas, CL (ed): Taber's Cyclopedic Medical Dictionary, ed 16, FA Davis, Philadelphia, 1989, p 260).

A significant increase in metabolic rate and heat production follows burn injury. Studies have shown that although patients with substantial burn injury may feel subjectively cold, their core body temperature may be elevated above normal due to the increase in metabolism. The physical energy demands that result from the increase in metabolic rate and heat production may double or triple, so that the caloric requirements of a patient with major burns may be 4000 to 5000 calories per day. This need is met initially by the use of liver and muscle glycogen, but these stores are quickly depleted and fat and protein are then used.

## Risk Factors

While anyone is a potential burn victim, there are demographic and other variables that may place some people in a higher risk category than others. Survey data demonstrate that the southeastern states, especially South Carolina and Mississippi, have a higher incidence of thermal injury than do other geographic areas. Incidence of burn injury is higher among lower socioeconomic groups and among nonwhite populations. Because many burn injuries and nearly one half of burn deaths result from cigarettes or other smoking materials (Choctaw, Eisner, and Wachtel, 1987), smoking or living with someone who smokes also increases the risk of burns. "Burns remain primarily accidents of the home caused by carelessness and ignorance and would not occur if caution and normal safety measures were enforced" (Crawford, 1981, p. 2).

# COMMON CLINICAL FINDINGS AND COMPLICATIONS OF BURNS

Loss of skin, and therefore loss of its protective and homeostatic function, as a result of thermal injury can lead to important complications. Such complications can involve the respiratory system, the musculoskeletal system, the gastrointestinal system, the cardiovascular system, the immune system, and the genitourinary system. An awareness of possible complications may help in their prevention.

Increased metabolic demand may lead to muscle wasting. In addition, the burn injury itself may involve muscle, or infection may lead to involvement and destruction of muscle tissue. Infection of major extremity burns may lead to amputation as a life-saving measure. Contractures, both of the burn wound scar and muscles, are complications that can be minimized by aggressive preventive measures.

It is estimated that pulmonary complications occur in 15%–18% of patients admitted to burn centers. When respiratory failure occurs in the burn patient, the mortality is 70%–90% (Achauer, 1987). In view of these estimates, aggressive preventive measures must be undertaken with all victims of major burn injury.

Respiratory problems following burns can be classified as to etiology: inhalation injuries, restrictive complications, or adult respiratory distress syndrome (ARDS). Carbon monoxide is inhaled as a gaseous component of smoke, however, the danger is not as a result of physical damage to the lung, but rather as a result of carbon monoxide's affinity for the oxygen-binding site of hemoglobin, with the resulting displacement of oxygen. This leads to low circulating volumes of oxygen, tissue hypoxia, inadequate cellular and organ function, and eventually death.

Both the heat of inhaled smoke and toxic chemicals can cause inhalation injuries. Damage to the respiratory epithelium as a result of the heat of inhaled smoke is usually limited to the upper airway. Usually, the damage consists of cellular necrosis and surrounding inflammatory reaction. Upper-airway obstruction or compromise due to edema may result. Injury that results from the inhalation of toxic chemicals produced by the combustion of materials is not restricted to the upper airway but, rather, occurs throughout the respiratory tract, including the small airways and alveoli. Injuries caused by inhaling heat or toxic substances may result in a loss of cilial activity and therefore poor clearance of bronchiotracheal secretions, a predisposition to alveolar fluid accumulation, generalized interstitial edema of the lung parenchyma, decreased lung compliance, and pulmonary infection.

Circumferential burns of the neck may result in edema that compresses the trachea or occludes the airway. Circumferential burns of the thorax may produce edema that constricts chest excursion and thus decreases tidal volume.

Gastrointestinal complications are not unusual following a major thermal injury. Gastric and duodenal erosions have been reported in 66% of severely burned patients, with significant ulceration in nearly 20% (Meyer and Trunkey, 1987). Ileus, which accompanies the early systemic response to burn injury, can also cause complications. The increased metabolic needs of the burn patient must be addressed; however, in the presence of ileus, tube feedings to meet metabolic requirements may lead to gastric distention and possible aspiration. Parenteral hyperalimentation as a substitute also carries the risk of complications such as pneumothorax, hemothorax, catheter sepsis, or embolization. Other gastrointestinal complications of burns include acalculous cholecystitis, hepatic dysfunction, and pancreatitis.

Elderly patients may be at greater risk for complications of the cardiovascular system. The stress imposed on the heart during fluid resuscitation and subsequent diuresis may not be tolerated by the elderly or those with previous cardiac disease. Myocardial infarction, as a result of increased cardiac workload and increased metabolic activity, is not uncommon in elderly burn patients. Vascular complications may result from the burn injury or as a consequence of therapy. Thrombophlebitis may occur in superficial venous channels adjacent to burn wounds or may result from intravenous therapy. The latter may pose a more-serious threat to the patient because of the potential for infection. Septic phlebitis can be a serious complication because it may result in septic emboli to the heart or lungs.

Because of current practice in the management of burns, which involves close attention to fluid resuscitation and management of hypovolemia, renal complications are relatively uncommon, however the potential exists. When renal failure does follow, it is often secondary to sepsis, septic shock, or nephrotoxic substances.

Sepsis, as a result of immunological compromise, is a major complication of major thermal injury. "Infection is directly or indirectly responsible for nearly 95 percent of deaths from burns that occur more than two days after the injury" (Meyer and Trunkey, 1987, p. 172). The combination of loss of the protective skin barrier and the immune-system depression that follows a burn injury results in a seriously elevated risk of post-burn sepsis.

# TREATMENT MODALITIES

Because of the potentially devastating effects of burn injury, prompt and appropriate implementation of treatment modalities is of utmost importance. Whether the burn is minor or major, 1 of the priorities of treatment is to stop the burning process. This can be accomplished by removing the source of the burning and by the application of cold water. Ice and ice water are to be avoided because the extreme cold may serve to extend the injury.

Another priority of treatment is attention to the airway. Many burn victims also incur injury as the result of inhalation of heated air or noxious fumes. Treatment should include careful assessment and frequent reassessment of respiratory status. Contingent upon the extent of injury, treatment may include humidified oxygen administration by nasal cannula or mask, administration of bronchodilators and mucolytic agents, bronchial suctioning, or may require endotracheal intubation and mechanical ventilation.

In major burn injuries, fluid loss is of great concern. Intravenous fluids must be administered promptly and in large quantities. There are several formulas for fluid resuscitation of patients with major burn injuries. An example of a fluid resuscitation formula is the "Consensus Formula," which recommends, "Lactated Ringer's solution (or other balanced salt solution): 2–4 ml × kg body weight × % body surface area (BSA) burned. Half to be given in first 8 hours; second half to be given over next 16 hours" (Bruner and Suddarth, 1988, p. 1301). Some formulae also include administration of colloids. Regardless of the specific formula used, it is important to remember that major burns require massive fluid resuscitation. After the first 48 hours, fluid resuscitation is administered at a rate needed to maintain a urine output of at least 0.5–1 ml/kg of body weight.

Such massive fluid resuscitation, combined with the physiological effects of the injury, necessitates careful monitoring of the patient with major burns. Frequent checks of vital signs, including central venous pressure or pulmonary artery pressure, are imperative for this patient. A bladder catheter must be in place to enable the frequent measurement of urinary output and observation/analysis of the urine.

Care of the burn wound must include strict adherence to principles of aseptic technique. In addition, persons who have contact with the patient must wear gowns, masks, and hair covering. Use of specific topical agents and other details of wound care will vary with institutions and particular burn injuries.

Because of the evaporative heat loss resulting from major thermal injury, attention should be given to maintaining a warm environment. The patient's temperature should be monitored closely. The patient's temperature should be maintained between 97°–101°F, to minimize metabolic stress.

Pain management is of great importance of treatment of the burn-injured patient. Because of the likelihood of altered absorption, analgesics should be administered intravenously. Specifics of pain management will vary with institutions and the extent and location of injury.

Care of the burn-injured patient is complex. Of necessity, the treatment modalities described above are general guidelines. They do, however, represent areas of concern in the treatment of all patients with major burn injuries.

# PATIENT ASSESSMENT DATA BASE

## Health History

*Client:*
Mr. Brian Byrnes

*Address:* 99 Ocean Drive, Ft. Lauderdale, Florida 33314
*Telephone:* (305) 555-4567
*Contact:* Mr. and Mrs. Edward Byrnes (parents)
*Address of contact:* 18 Shore Road, Miami, Florida 33136
*Telephone of contact:* (305) 555-4321
*Age:* 20    *Sex:* Male    *Race:* White
*Educational background:* College (2 years completed)
*Religion:* Christian    *Marital status:* Single
*Usual occupation:* Student
*Present occupation:* Gasoline station attendant
*Source of income:* Part-time work and parents
*Insurance:* Blue Cross/Blue Shield (subscriber Edward Byrnes)
*Source of referral:* Fire Department ambulance crew
*Source of history:* Client and his mother
*Reliability of historian:* Good
*Date of interview:* 6-11-89
*Reason for visit/Chief complaint:* Major thermal injury

## HEALTH PERCEPTION/HEALTH MANAGEMENT PATTERN

### Present Health Status

Brian was well until approximately 44 hours before the interview, when his clothing ignited at the gasoline station where he is employed. Trouser legs, on which a moderate amount of gasoline had been spilled, ignited from sparks of a torch in use in the auto repair area of the garage. Patient sustained partial and full thickness burns on 30% TBSA. Distribution of burns is: right leg = 14%, left leg = 8%, right buttock = 3%, right hand and forearm = 5%.

### Past Health Status

*General Health.* Brian describes his health as excellent before the accident; no chronic illnesses, no somatic complaints, able to participate fully in all desired or required activities.

*Prophylactic Medical/Dental Care.* Has yearly routine physical examination by primary-care physician as required by the athletic department of college (plays football). Has dental prophylaxis appointment once or twice a year, hasn't had cavities "for years."

*Childhood Illnesses.* Had chicken pox and several episodes of otitis media.

*Immunizations.* Up-to-date on all immunizations. Received tetanus immune globulin and tetanus toxoid in the Emergency Ward this admission.

*Major Illnesses/Hospitalizations.* None

*Current Medications.*
*Prescription:* None

**Past Health**
**Status — Continued**

*Nonprescription:* Occasional aspirin for headache or muscle ache, frequent multivitamins.
**Allergies.** Lactose intolerance as young child, no other allergies known.

**Habits**
*Alcohol:* Beer on weekends and occasionally during the week; average amount about 1–2 six-packs per week.
*Caffeine:* Rarely drinks coffee (less than once per week) cola 2 or 3 times per day.
*Drugs:* Denies use of recreational drugs at present time; admits to past occasional experimentation.
*Tobacco:* None

### Family Health History

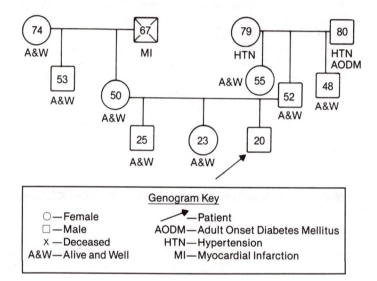

### NUTRITIONAL/METABOLIC PATTERN

**Nutritional**

Brian and his mother agree he has a good appetite except when feeling stressed. Enjoys most foods, few dislikes. Favorite foods: ice cream, pizza, steak, hamburgers, french fries, and desserts of all kinds. Dislikes: fish, except shellfish.
Present status: NPO at this time.

**Usual Daily Menu**
Deferred due to patient's condition.

**Metabolic**

Denies recent weight loss or gain, cannot recall any problems with healing or heat/cold intolerance. *Weight:* 205 lb (93.2 kg); *Height:* 6 ft. 2 in. (187.9 cm)

### ELIMINATION PATTERN

**Bowel**

Denies difficulty with bowel elimination. Moves bowels "almost every day" without straining or discomfort. Denies laxative use.

**Bladder**

Denies pain or burning on urination or history of urinary tract infections. No discharge or difficulty with beginning stream. No history of incontinence.

## Activity/Exercise Pattern

*Activity/Exercise*

Before accident, exercised frequently. Daily exercise routine included swimming laps in college pool and lifting weights each morning and running about 5 miles each afternoon. Is on the college football team and participates informally in other sports activities with friends. Mother states it was important for him to stay in shape for football. Full self-care abilities before accident.

*Self-Care Ability*

| | |
|---|---|
| Feeding — II | General mobility — III |
| Bathing — II | Cooking — Not applicable |
| Toileting — III | Home maintenance — Not applicable |
| Dressing — II | |
| Grooming — II | Shopping — Not applicable |

> ### *Functional Levels Code*
> 0 — Full self-care
> I — Requires use of equipment or device
> II — Requires assistance or supervision from another person
> III — Requires assistance or supervision from another person and equipment or device
> IV — Is dependent and does not participate

*Oxygenation/Perfusion*

Denies any chest pain, dyspnea, chronic cough, or shortness of breath in past. Is able to participate in all desired activities without limitation. No recollection of ever having chest xray or electrocardiogram until this admission.

*Cardiac Risk Factors*

| | Positive | Negative |
|---|---|---|
| Sedentary life-style | | X |
| Hyperlipidemia | | X |
| Cigarette smoking | | X |
| Diabetes | | X |
| Obesity | | X |
| Hypertension | | X |
| Hypervigilant personality | | X |
| Family history of heart disease | X | |

## Sleep/Rest Pattern

*Sleep/Rest*

Usually sleeps about 7 hours per night. Is likely to sleep more on weekends if time permits. Occasionally naps in daytime, between classes. Believes amount of sleep/rest is adequate, feels rested on awakening, falls asleep easily and does not require sleep aids. At present, states has not slept well since the accident. Pain, fear, and the frequent monitoring activities have allowed only brief naps. States he feels exhausted.

## Cognitive/Perceptual Pattern

*Hearing*

Denies uncompensated sensory deficits. States hearing is fine.

*Vision*

Uses glasses for reading, states vision is otherwise "OK." Last visit to ophthalmologist was before beginning college 2 years ago.

*Sensory Perception*

Right hand is dominant, and Brian is concerned about implications of the burn injury to that hand. Until now, he says, his only pain experience has been minor football injuries (i.e., "bumps and bruises"). Believes he usually tolerates pain well, but describes present situation as "excruciating" and "unbelievable." (Because of this, health history was collected over course of a day, with aspects abbreviated, deferred, or supplemented with information from mother when possible.)

*Learning Style*

Mother states Brian has always been a "quick learner" and a good student, particularly in math and sciences. Brian is studying engineering at college.

## SELF-PERCEPTION/SELF-CONCEPT PATTERN

*Self-Perception/Self-Concept*

Brian states he used to feel pretty good about himself. "I had everything going for me. I was doing well in school, with football, and in my social life. All that's changed now. I don't know how I feel about myself now. I'm certainly not going to look the same." Mrs. Byrnes says that Brian was very proud of his football accomplishments, including a football scholarship to college, which now may be discontinued. Maintaining his physical attractiveness was also important to Brian. He enjoyed the role of "jock" and all the attention it brought him. Mother quotes Brian as saying, "I guess I'm going to be pretty useless now, a burden. These legs aren't going to take me far now. Guess my beach days are over too, I'll look like a freak." Mrs. Byrnes states that this attitude is most unlike Brian, and she is concerned.

## ROLE/RELATIONSHIP PATTERN

*Role/Relationship*

Brian recently completed his second year of college. Last month he leased an apartment with some friends, after living in the dormitory for the past 2 years. He began working at the gasoline station several months ago, after football season, to supplement money given to him by his parents. Brian's relationships with his parents and siblings are positive and loving. He especially admires his older brother. Brian has many friends, both male and female, and has enjoyed an active social life both in his hometown and at college.

## SEXUALITY/REPRODUCTIVE PATTERN

*Sexuality/Reproductive*

Brian is heterosexual and comfortable with his sexuality. Does not have a steady girlfriend at this time, but had a serious relationship with a girlfriend during high school and his first year of college. This relationship was terminated by mutual agreement. They remain friends.

## COPING/STRESS TOLERANCE PATTERN

*Coping/Stress Tolerance*

Mother describes Brian as even tempered. She feels that he seems to handle stress well. Uses exercise as an outlet for stress and frustration, especially swimming and running. Accepts challenges willingly. Mother states at times he seems to thrive on challenge. Only loss mother can remember Brian experiencing was the death of his grandfather when he was much younger. Although understandably sad for a while, he seemed to cope with this loss without difficulty.

## VALUE/BELIEF PATTERN

*Value/Belief*

Mother is Protestant; father is Catholic. Brian has been raised with an awareness of both religions but has not declared a preference for either, according to mother. Mother believes he has a strong sense of right and wrong and his actions are true to those beliefs. There are no ethnic traditions or customs practiced in the parental home.

# Physical Examination

*General Survey*

Twenty-year-old male lying in bed in obvious physical discomfort, with frequent facial grimacing. Right hand, forearm, and both legs wrapped in bulky dressing. Somewhat pale, moist skin on face and neck. Lying on left side. Generalized edema is apparent. Breathing is without difficulty.

*Vital Signs*

*Temperature:* 99.8°F
*Pulse:* 88/min, regular (apical)
*Respirations:* 24/min, regular
*BP:* 100/60 (left arm, semi-Fowler's)

*Integument*

*Skin.* Pale, moist, and edematous; areas of second and third degree burns as depicted below.

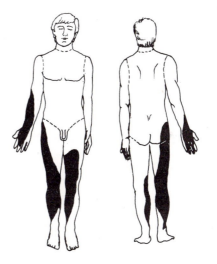

*Nails.* On left hand and both feet intact, no clubbing, good capillary refill on left side, slightly slower refill on right foot. Right hand not examined due to dressing.
*Mucous membranes.* Pale and moist.

*HEENT*

*Head.* Symmetrical, normal adult size and shape. Hair is reddish-blonde, thick, and straight; scalp is clean, no lesions noted. Face is edematous, no evidence of thermal injury.
*Temporomandibular joint:* Not evaluated.
*Eyes.* Pupils equal, round, reactive to light and accommodation (PERRLA); peripheral vision equal to examiner's, ocular movements intact. Eyelids edematous, but able to open and close.
*Ears.* Auricles symmetrical, no drainage or lesions; hearing level is such that the client is able to repeat whispered phrases.
*Nose.* Nares edematous but patent, nasal hairs not singed, nasogastric tube in place.

| | |
|---|---|
| *HEENT — Continued* | *Mouth/Throat.* Able to swallow without difficulty, gag reflex intact, no hoarseness noted. |
| *Neck* | Full range of motion (ROM), some edema, no burn lesions, trachea midline, carotids and trachea palpable without difficulty. |
| *Pulmonary* | Chest wall is without injuries, expansion symmetrical, excursion of diaphragm about 4 cm, lungs clear to percussion, slight rales at bases bilaterally, no wheezing noted on inspiration or expiration. |
| *Breast* | Minimal breast tissue, no masses or tenderness. |
| *Cardiovascular* | No murmurs, rubs, or extra sounds noted. Point of maximal impulse (PMI) palpable at the fifth intercostal space. Apical pulse rate 88 and regular. Central line in place in right subclavian vein. |

*Peripheral Vascular*

*Peripheral Pulses*
Temporal — 4 bilaterally
Carotid — 4 bilaterally
Brachial — 4 on left, right not evaluated
Radial — 4 on left, right not evaluated
Femoral — 4 bilaterally
Popliteal — not evaluated bilaterally
Posterior tibial — 4 on left, right not evaluated
Dorsalis pedis — 4 bilaterally

*Peripheral Pulse Scale*

| |
|---|
| 0 — Absent |
| 1 — Markedly diminished |
| 2 — Moderately diminished |
| 3 — Slightly diminished |
| 4 — Normal |

| | |
|---|---|
| *Abdomen* | Symmetrical, slight distention, bowel sounds absent. No pain or tenderness on palpation, liver and spleen not palpated. |
| *Musculoskeletal* | Full ROM without difficulty of all joints not affected by the burn injury. ROM for right elbow, wrist, knee, and ankle limited due to pain from burns. Similar restriction for left knee. Large muscles developed symmetrically, strength good despite injury. Right lower extremity has recent escharotomy incisions. |
| *Neurological* | *Mental Status.* Oriented to person, place, and time; aware of circumstances preceding hospitalization.<br>*Cranial Nerves.* Cranial nerve I not tested, cranial nerves II–XII intact.<br>*Motor.* Able to perform coordinated movements as directed, remainder of motor examination deferred.<br>*Sensory.* Sensation intact on face, trunk and all 4 extremities.<br>*Deep Tendon Reflexes.* Deferred. |
| *Rectal* | Examination deferred. |
| *Genitalia* | Circumcised adult male, no burns noted, indwelling bladder catheter in place, scrotum edematous. |

## Laboratory Data/Diagnostic Studies

| | |
|---|---|
| *Laboratory Data* | *Hemoglobin.* 14.3 gm/100 ml<br>*Hematocrit.* 42.5/100 ml (42.5%)<br>*Na.* 140 mEq/l |

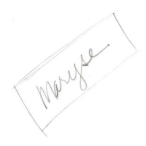
*Maryse*

**K.** 3.6 mEq/l
**Cl.** 101 mEq/l
**Co2.** 24 mEq/l
**BUN.** 13.4 mg/100 ml — *5-25 mg/dL*
**Carboxyhemoglobin level.**
  1.5% of total hgb — *<2% saturation of Hb*
**Arterial Blood Gases**
**pH.** 7.39  *7.35 - 7.45*
**pO$_2$.** 94 torr  *75-100*
**pCO$_2$.** 40 torr  *35-45*
**Oxygen saturation.** 97%

**Urinalysis**
**Color.** Yellow
**Specific gravity.** 1.02
**pH.** 5.5
**Hemoglobin.** Trace
**Protein (albumin).** 8 mg/dl
**Glucose.** Trace
**Ketones.** Trace

**Diagnostic Studies**

**Central Venous Pressure.** 5 cm H$_2$O
**Chest X-ray.** Normal, no infiltrates noted
**Electrocardiogram.** Normal sinus rhythm, no abnormalities

# COLLABORATIVE PLAN OF CARE

**Diet**

Nothing by mouth (npo)

**Medications**

Morphine 2–3 mg/h via continuous IV drip

**Intravenous Therapy**

IV 5% D/W with 20 mEq Kcl per 1000 ml to run at 100 ml/h.
  Increase to 150 ml/h if urine output < 50 ml and notify MD.

**Therapeutic Measures**

Vital signs q1h. Include temperature and peripheral pulses CVP
  q1h—notify house officer if <2 cm.
Hourly urine output—notify house officer if >50 ml/h
Continuous cardiac monitor
Daily weights
Nasogastric tube to intermittent suction irrigate q4h and prn.
Test gastric aspirate for guiac q12h
Test all stools for occult blood
Daily electrolytes, Hgb, Hct, and ABGs. If Hct <35 or Hgb
  <12, give 1 unit of packed cells and notify MD.
Keep head of bed elevated 30°
Wound care: daily washing using shower cart apparatus and
  bid application of silver sulfadiazine–cerium nitrate, and
  dressings
Active and passive ROM of involved joints q2–3h when patient
  is awake
Splint to right hand continually except during exercise and to
  other involved joints at night
Protective isolation precautions

**Consults**

Nutrition consult
Exercises per physical therapist
Position of involved joints as per physical therapist

**Preoperative Plan**

Prepare patient for excision and grafting this afternoon—pre-op
  medication orders per anesthesia department.

# NURSING DIAGNOSES DEVELOPED IN CARE PLAN

Body Image Disturbance, p. 398
Pain, p. 396
Potential for Infection, p. 397

# ADDITIONAL NURSING DIAGNOSES TO BE CONSIDERED

Altered Nutrition: Less than Body Requirements
Altered Patterns of Urinary Elimination
Altered Tissue Perfusion
Fear
Fluid Volume Deficit
Fluid Volume Excess
Impaired Gas Exchange
Impaired Physical Mobility
Post-trauma Response
Potential Altered Body Temperature
Sleep Pattern Disturbance

# NURSING CARE PLAN BASED ON IDENTIFIED NURSING DIAGNOSES

| | |
|---|---|
| **Pain** | ***Related to:*** Thermal injury.<br>***Evidenced by:*** Verbal report of pain, grimacing, facial expressions, pallor and sweating. |
| **Desired Patient Outcomes** | ***The Patient:***<br>• Describes pain as tolerable and is able to cooperate with treatment methods.<br>• Is able to employ nonpharmacologic methods to assist in pain management. |
| **Evaluation Criteria** | ***The Patient Will:***<br>• Use both pharmacologic and nonpharmacologic methods of pain reduction after instruction.<br>• Be able to manage pain sufficiently, to participate in care, and to tolerate procedures throughout hospital stay. |

| Interventions | Rationale |
|---|---|
| Administer narcotic intravenously as prescribed in dosage needed for patient to tolerate pain. | Pain medication should not be administered on a prn basis for patients in severe pain. If prn method is used, the patient is probably under medicated (Friedmann, Shapiro and Plon, 1987, p. 249).<br>Intravenous administration is necessary because of altered absorption and circulation resulting from the burn injury (Brunner and Suddarth, 1988, p. 1307). |
| Teach patient pain-reduction techniques such as relaxation, meditation, imagery, or self-hypnosis. | These techniques enhance the effect of analgesics and can provide the patient with a sense of control (Brunner and Suddarth, 1988, p. 1307), and can decrease perception of pain or increase pain tolerance (Kibbee, 1984, p. 61). |

## Interventions

Provide emotional support and reassurance. Spend time (not associated with treatments) with patient to give him the opportunity to express his feelings, help him deal with his feelings, and to provide feedback on his progress.

Give information about the patient's treatment plans, and the expected outcomes.

Assist patient with appropriate means of expressing pain, such as verbalization to nurse when pain is not relieved by usual methods.

Teach patient about the usual pain trajectory in burn recovery.

Provide for uninterrupted sleep to the extent possible.

## Rationale

Helps to reduce fear and anxiety and, thus, helps to reduce pain (Brunner and Suddarth, 1988, p. 1307); pain is increased by anxiety (Robertson, Cross, and Terry, 1985 p. 43).

Promotes trust and helps patient to accept painful treatments (Brunner and Suddarth, 1988, p. 1307).

Allows/encourages patient to express pain and discomfort (Brunner and Suddarth, 1988, p. 1320).

Reduces fear of the unknown and may provide patient with a sense of control (Brunner and Suddarth, 1988, p. 1320).

Sleep deprivation can exacerbate pain (Freeman, 1984, p. 65).

---

| *Potential for Infection* | *Related to:* Pathophysiology of major thermal injury. *Evidenced by:* Damage to the epidermis and dermis, (loss of defense against microbial invasion due to 30% burn wound). |
|---|---|
| *Desired Patient Outcomes* | *The Patient Will:* • Be free of infection and sepsis. |
| *Evaluation Criteria* | *Throughout the Hospital Stay:* • The risk of infection will be minimized as evidenced by adherence to technique in all interactions with the patient. • Episodes of infection (should they occur) will be recognized and treated promptly and effectively. *Upon Discharge:* • The patient will not exhibit any signs of infection. |

---

## Interventions

Wash hands thoroughly before and after any patient contact.

Use barrier gowns, gloves, masks, and hair cover when wounds are exposed or when in direct contact with patient or bed.

Assure adequate nutrition once gastrointestinal motility resumes by careful attention to dietary intake. Serve desired food. Implement other strategies if necessary in consultation with dietitian, patient, and family.

## Rationale

Minimizes risk of cross contamination (Brunner and Suddarth, 1988, p. 1319).

Decreases contamination of wound with normal or pathogenic flora by health-care providers (Brunner and Suddarth, 1988, p. 1319).

Nutritional deficiencies contribute to immune defects after burn injury (Hansbrough, Zapata-Sirvent, and Peterson, 1987, p. 70). Adequate nutrition is essential for improving immunologic response and healing (Brunner and Suddarth, 1988, p. 1306).

| *Interventions* | *Rationale* |
|---|---|
| Prevent pressure on wounds; position patient carefully and change position frequently. | Minimizes trauma and allows for adequate perfusion to burn wounds (Brunner and Suddarth, 1988, p. 1319). |
| Cleanse and dress insertion site of central and peripheral IV lines using sterile technique at least q/d. | IV sites are often an additional source of infection in the burned patient (Grube, Marvin, and Heimbach 1988, p. 194). |
| Indwelling catheter care bid and after bowel movements. Anchor catheter securely to minimize excessive movement. | Frequent cleansing decreases chance of infection (Doenges, Moorhouse, and Geissler, 1989, p. 553). |
| Assist with and promote meticulous personal hygiene of nonburned areas, teeth and mouth, perineum, and hair. | Reduces bacterial contamination from patient's normal flora and pathogenic organisms (Brunner and Suddarth, 1988, p. 1306). |
| Assess wound with each dressing change for signs of healing or infection. | Enables early detection and therefore early treatment of infection (Brunner and Suddarth, 1988, p. 1319). |
| Be alert for and report changes in mental status, respiratory rate, increased pulse, and fever. | May be signs of septicemia. (Brunner and Suddarth, 1988, p. 1306). |
| Instruct patient and visitors: concerning the necessity of near-sterile technique and protective precautions. | Can aid in the prevention of contamination (Doenges, Moorhouse, and Geissler, 1989, p. 718). |
| In addition to performing chest physiotherapy, encourage deep-breathing exercises and incentive spirometry. | Pneumonia represents a serious complication for burn patients and is a hazard of immobility. (Bayley and Smith, 1987, p. 40). |

---

| | |
|---|---|
| ***Body Image Disturbance*** | ***Related to:*** Thermal injury and anticipated subsequent disfigurement.<br>***Evidenced by:*** Patient's statements, such as "I don't know how I feel about myself now. I'm certainly not going to look the same," and "I'll look like a freak." |
| ***Desired Patient Outcome*** | ***The Patient Will:***<br>• Verbalize acceptance of alterations in appearance as a result of burn injury. |
| ***Evaluation Criteria*** | ***Following Excision and Grafting, the Patient Will:***<br>• Begin to verbalize acceptance of his altered body image.<br>***By Time of Discharge, the Patient Will:***<br>• Be able to discuss his healing and scarring in a positive manner<br>• Verbalize strategies to respond to questions or stares regarding his injury<br>• Be more focused on function than on appearance, demonstrated by active participation in the work to attain full function of involved extremities<br>• Verbalize acceptance of present body image |

## Interventions

Allow patient to use coping mechanisms such as denial, regression, withdrawal, or anger, but attempt to discover reasons for these behaviors.

Support use of effective pre-burn coping mechanisms to the extent possible. Because physical activity seems to have been a past coping mechanism for the patient, exercises such as ROM may be helpful in this regard, once his physical condition permits. Also, explore use of new coping mechanisms.

Allow patient to mourn the loss of previous body image and function.

Provide opportunity for expression of thoughts, feelings, fears, and anxieties.

Anticipate behaviors and coping mechanisms such as crying, sobbing, anger, or frustration, and avoid negative staff reactions. If patient's behavior must be modified, be clear as to reasons why.

Maintain an honest but positive approach in giving information and responding to questions.

Foster independence to the extent possible.

Enlist family and friends in support/acceptance of the patient.

Encourage and assist significant others to verbalize their personal needs, fears, feelings, and concerns.

Demonstrate acceptance of the patient by maintaining a positive attitude toward the patient as a whole person.

## Rationale

Although the patient's coping mechanisms may seen abnormal, they may be defense mechanisms maintaining an intact psyche for the patient (Freeman, 1984, p. 65).

Encourages patient to use familiar coping mechanisms that have been successful in the past (Brunner and Suddarth, 1988, p. 1321).

Mourning is necessary before acceptance can occur (Heffley, 1981, p. 239, 240).

Awareness of the patient's concerns and understanding the basis for them enables the nurse to provide support and to cooperate with other members of the health-care team in developing a plan to help the patient handle these feelings (Brunner and Suddarth, 1988, p. 1323).

Patient may view negative reactions as rejection because of disfigurement (Heffley, 1981, p. 240).

"Delaying truth delays rehabilitation . . . mature individuals are capable and desirous of knowing facts" (Friedmann, Shapiro, and Plon, 1987, p. 254). Encourages patient to ask questions and voice concerns in a trusting atmosphere (Brunner and Suddarth, 1988, p. 1321).

Independence helps patient view self as a productive human being (Heffley, 1981, p. 239).

Single most important determinant in rehabilitation of a patient is the social support available to the patient (Friedmann, Shapiro, and Plon, 1987, p. 254).

Can facilitate significant others' acceptance of the patient (Ulrich, Canale, and Wendell, 1986, p. 765).

Acceptance by others increases self-esteem and aids in acceptance of altered body image (Doenges, Moorhouse, and Geissler, 1989, p. 294).

## QUESTIONS FOR DISCUSSION

1. Discuss the three depths of burn injury. How can they be differentiated from each other? What are the implications for management of each?
2. If Brian had sustained an inhalation injury, what signs and symptoms would he exhibit?
3. How is the burn size determined? Why is this information important?

4. How are fluid replacement needs determined in the first 24 hours post burn injury? Discuss the advantages and disadvantages of different types of fluid used in resuscitation of the burn patient.

5. In the list of possible nursing diagnoses, both fluid volume deficit and fluid volume excess are listed. Explain how Brian could be at risk for both these diagnoses at the time the assessment data were collected.

6. Brian will soon be receiving nutrition by mouth. How will his nutritional needs be determined? What strategies can the nurse employ to assure his nutritional requirements are met?

7. Brian is scheduled for early excision and grafting of his burn sites. What are the advantages and disadvantages of this treatment modality? Why might this method of treatment have been selected for Brian?

8. Discuss issues of contracture prevention, positioning, and splinting as general principles and those you would use for Brian.

9. When should rehabilitation begin?

# REFERENCES

Achauer, BM: Management of the Burned Patient. Appleton & Lange, Norwalk, Conn, 1987.

Bayley, EW and Smith, GA: The three degrees of burn care. Nursing 87 17(3):34–41, 1987.

Bonaldi, LA and Frank, DH: Pathophysiology of the burn wound. In Achauer, BM (ed): Management of the Burned Patient. Appleton & Lange, Norwalk, Conn, 1987.

Brunner, LS and Suddarth, DS: Textbook of Medical–Surgical Nursing, ed 6. JB Lippincott, Philadelphia, 1988.

Choctaw, WT, Eisner, ME, and Wachtel, TL: Causes, preventions, prehospital care, evaluation, emergency treatment, and prognosis. In Achauer, BM (ed): Management of the Burned Patient. Appleton & Lange, Norwalk, Conn, 1987.

Crawford, JL: Incidence and prevention of burn injuries. In Wagner, MM (ed): Care of the Burn-Injured Patient: A Multidisciplinary Involvement. PSG Publishing, Littleton, Mass, 1981.

Doenges, ME, Moorhouse, MF, and Geissler, AC: Nursing Care Plans: Guidelines for Planning Patient Care, ed 2. FA Davis, Philadelphia, 1989.

Freeman, JW: Nursing care of the patient with a burn injury. Crit Care Nurse 4(6):52–68, 1984.

Friedmann, JK, Shapiro, J, and Plon, L: Psychosocial treatment and pain control. In Achauer, BM (ed) Management of the Burned Patient. Appleton & Lange, Norwalk, Conn, 1987.

Grube, BJ, Marvin, JA, and Heimbach, DM: Candida: A decreasing problem for the burned patient? Arch Surg 123:194–196, 1988.

Hansbrough, JF, Zapata-Sirvent, RL, and Peterson, VM: Immunomodulation following burn injury. Surg Clin N Am 67(1):69–88, 1987.

Heffley, DL: Burn care—a nursing perspective. In Wagner, MM (ed): Care of the Burn-Injured Patient: A Multidisciplinary Involvement. PSG Publishing, Littleton, Mass, 1981.

Johnson, CL, O'Shaughnessy, EJ, and Ostergren, G: Burn Management. Raven Press, New York, 1981.

Kibbee, E: Burn pain management. Crit Care Q 7(4):54–62, 1984.

Meyer, AA and Trunkey, DD: Preventing and treating complications. In Achauer, BM (ed): Management of the Burned Patient. Appleton & Lange, Norwalk, Conn, 1987.

Robertson, K, Cross, PJ, and Terry, JC: Burn care: The first crucial days. Am J Nurs 85(1):29–50, 1985.

Ulrich, SP, Canale, SW, and Wendell, SA: Nursing Care Planning Guides. WB Saunders, Philadelphia, 1986.

Wagner, MM: Care of the Burn-Injured Patient. PSG Publishing, Littleton, Mass, 1981.

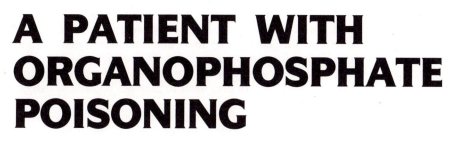

# CASE STUDY 24

# A PATIENT WITH ORGANOPHOSPHATE POISONING

Anne Keiran Manton, M.S., R.N., C.E.N.

Since the early 1970s, the use of the pesticide DDT has been severely restricted. Since the virtual banning of DDT, organophosphates, which are more rapidly hydrolized than DDT and therefore have less-harmful cumulative environmental effects, have increased in general usage. Despite the fact that organophosphates have a toxicity that is high for insects but relatively low for human beings, they are the pesticides most-frequently involved in serious human poisoning (Bryson, 1986). The many varieties of organophosphates are widely used as pesticides and all are cholinesterase inhibitors. A brief review of the autonomic nervous system will aid in understanding the action of organophosphates and their danger.

## PHYSIOLOGY OF THE AUTONOMIC NERVOUS SYSTEM

The *autonomic nervous system* is the division of the nervous system that controls the visceral functions of the body, including gastrointestinal motility and secretion, body temperature, sweating, arterial pressure, pupillary reaction and other activities to greater or lesser extent. The autonomic nervous system has 2 major subdivisions, the *sympathetic* and the *parasympathetic*, by which impulses are transmitted.

Acetylcholine is a transmitter substance (i.e., it plays an important role in the transmission of nerve impulses at synapses and myoneural junctions). The preganglionic neurons of both the sympathetic and parasympathetic systems secrete acetylcholine at their nerve endings. The postganglionic neurons of the parasympathetic system also secrete acetylcholine. Because they secrete acetylcholine at their nerve endings, these fibers are called *cholinergic*. Most of the postganglionic endings of the sympathetic nervous system secrete the transmitter substance norepinephrine and are referred to as *adrenergic*. The sympathetic or parasympathetic effects on the different organs are caused by the acetylcholine and norepinephrine secreted by the postganglionic neurons (Guyton, 1986).

The terminal endings of the cholinergic nerve fibers secrete acetylcholine continually. Once secreted, most of the acetylcholine is split off within seconds, or fractions of seconds, into choline and acetate ion by the enzyme cholinesterase, which is present in the terminal nerve ending and also on the surface of the receptor organ. The choline that is formed is used again in the synthesis of new acetylcholine.

Stimulation of the particular organ is a result of the reaction of the transmitter substance (acetylcholine or norepinephrine) with receptor substances in the cells of the organ. It is believed that the receptor is most likely a protein or lipoprotein in the cell membrane. Two different types of receptors are activated by acetylcholine. These receptors are referred to as *muscarinic receptors* and *nicotinic receptors*.

Most organs are controlled dominantly by either the sympathetic or the parasympathetic nervous system. Both systems cause excitatory effects in some organs and inhibitory effects in others. Sometimes the systems work reciprocally to each other (i.e., when sympathetic stimulation excites an organ and parasympathetic stimulation inhibits it). There is, however, no generalization that can be made with regard to whether sympathetic or parasympathetic stimulation will result in the excitation or the inhibition of function in a particular organ.

## Organophosphates

During World War II, as part of research to develop an effective insecticide and an effective nerve gas, it was found that refinements of the alkyl esters of phosphoric acid (organophosphates) were effective for both purposes. Their popularity as insecticides has grown not only because of their effectiveness in controlling insects, but also because they are rapidly hydrolized and therefore do not accumulate in the environment or in the bodies of animals. When used in agricultural settings, the presence of residue on the food grown has not been a problem. In addition to agricultural use, organophosphates are also used to manage household insect problems such as fleas and flies.

Organophosphates are powerful inhibitors of acetylcholinesterase. This inhibition is a result of the "firm binding of phosphate radicals of the organophosphates to the active enzyme sites, forming phosphorylated enzymes. The pharmacologic and toxicologic effects of organophosphates are probably entirely due to inhibition of acetylcholinesterase, resulting in excess accumulation of acetylcholine at cholinergic synapses. This overabundance initially stimulates and subsequently paralyzes cholinergic synaptic transmission in the central nervous system (CNS), somatic nerves, autonomic ganglia, parasympathetic nerve endings, and some sympathetic nerve endings (e.g. sweat glands)" (Goldfrank, Bresnitz, and Kirstein, 1982, p. 283).

## Risk Factors

Those most at risk for organophosphate poisoning are persons who come in contact with the insecticide as part of their daily work environment. Agricultural workers, pilots of crop-dusting planes, and workers in chemical plants where organophosphates are produced are at greatest risk. Also at risk are smaller-amount users of the insecticides, who use these compounds for household or small-garden application. As is the case with other poisons, children who may have access to these insecticides or be exposed to them during their utilization are at particular risk.

## COMMON CLINICAL FINDINGS

Because of its anticholinesterase effects, the signs and symptoms of organophosphate poisoning are predictable and can be classified as follows: *muscarinic effects, nicotinic effects*, and CNS manifestations. Muscarinic (parasympathetic) manifestations of organophosphate poisoning are those affecting the bronchial tree, the gastrointestinal system, the heart, the lacrimal and sweat glands, pupil and ciliary body, and the bladder. The muscarinic effects can be remembered by the acronym "SLUDGE" (i.e., the muscarinic effects may include *s*alivation, *l*acrimation, *u*rination, *d*efecation, *g*astrointestinal cramps, and *e*mesis). Nicotinic effects (sympathetic and somatic motor) are those that act on striated muscle and sympathetic ganglia and result in weakness, muscle fasciculations, areflexia, tachycardia, hypertension, and pallor. CNS manifestations may include headache, restlessness, drowsiness, confusion, emotional lability, ataxia, convulsions, and coma (See Table 1 for a summary of the most-common signs and symptoms of organophosphate poisoning).

## TREATMENT MODALITIES

Initial treatment of organophosphate poisoning includes attention to airway maintenance, decontamination if necessary, and administration of atropine and pralidoxime (PAM). Atropine is used to block the action of acetylcholine on parasympathetic receptors while the organophosphate is being metabolized. Atropine does not, however, affect the rate of restoration of the inhibited acetylcholinesterase, nor does it have an effect on skeletal muscle and autonomic ganglia. Pralidoxime is useful in the treatment of organophosphate poisoning because it does reactivate acetylcholinesterase. It also acts to detoxify the organophosphorus molecules and has an anticholinergic effect. It is suggested that both atropine and pralidoxime be administered in nearly all cases of organophosphate poisoning (Milby, 1971; Namba et al, 1971; Bayer and Rumack, 1983; Haddad and Winchester, 1983; Bryson, 1986).

**TABLE 1. SIGNS AND SYMPTOMS OF ORGANOPHOSPHATE POISONING\***

| | |
|---|---|
| CNS Manifestations | Restlessness, emotional lability, headache tremor, drowsiness, confusion, slurred speech, ataxia, generalized weakness, coma, convulsions, depression of respiratory and cardiovascular centers |
| Muscarinic Manifestations | |
| Salivary Glands | *S*alivation increased |
| Lacrimal Glands | *L*acrimation increased |
| Bladder | *U*rinary frequency, incontinence |
| Gastrointestinal | *G*astrointestinal, diarrhea, incontinence |
| | *G*astrointestinal cramps, tenesmus |
| | *E*mesis, nausea, anorexia |
| Bronchial tree | *B*ronchoconstriction, dyspnea, cyanosis, increased bronchial secretions, pulmonary edema |
| Sweat Glands | Increased sweating |
| Cardiovascular | Bradycardia, hypotension |
| Pupils | Miosis, occasionally unequal |
| Ciliary body | Blurred vision |
| Nicotinic Manifestations | |
| Sympathetic ganglia | Hypertension, tachycardia, pallor |
| Striated muscle | Muscular fasciculations, cramps, weakness, areflexia |

\*Adapted from Goldfrank, 1982, p. 283.

# PATIENT ASSESSMENT DATA BASE

## Health History

***Client:***
Mrs. Rose Gardner

*Address:* Farm Lane, Kansas City, Kansas
*Telephone:* (913) 555-2468
*Contact:* P. Gardner (husband)
*Address of contact:* Same as client
*Telephone of contact:* Same as client
*Age:* 53    *Sex:* Female    *Race:* Black
*Educational background:* Secretarial school
*Religion:* Protestant    *Marital status:* Married
*Usual occupation:* Homemaker
*Present occupation:* Same
*Source of income:* Husband and family vegetable stand
*Insurance:* Blue Cross/Blue Shield (husband is subscriber)
*Source of referral:* Self
*Source of history:* Client and husband
*Reliability of historian(s):* Good
*Date of interview:* 6/28/88 (in emergency department)
*Reason for visit/Chief complaint:* Sudden onset of weakness, headache, and nausea.

## HEALTH PERCEPTION/HEALTH MANAGEMENT PATTERN

**Present Health Status**

Mrs. Gardner states that she was working in her garden this morning using an insecticide for some particularly resistant insects. After about an hour, she began to feel quite ill. Her specific symptoms at that time were nausea, headache, weakness, and sweating. As she returned to the house, her symptoms increased to include abdominal cramps, diarrhea, and vomiting. She and her husband agreed she should come to the emergency department. In response to questions regarding the specific insecticide and her possible exposure Mrs. Gardner relates that as she lifted the makeshift container (in which the insecticide had been given her by a neighbor) from the shelf, the cover fell off, and a good deal of the insecticide spilled on her. She brushed the insecticide from her skin and clothing and thought no more about the incident until she started feeling ill. Neither Mrs. nor Mr. Gardner knew the name of the insecticide, and the container was unlabeled. Attempts are being made to contact the neighbor to ascertain the nature of the insecticide.

**Past Health Status**

*General Health.* Mrs. Gardner considers herself to be in good health usually. She denies any chronic illnesses or past health problems.

*Prophylactic Medical/Dental Care.* Has a routine physical examination every "couple of years." Last physical exam was about a year ago. Given a "clean bill of health" at that time. Routine dental exam about every 6–8 months. Last visit about 4 months ago. Sees periodontist about once a year. Past history of periodontal disease. No current problems.

*Childhood Illnesses.* Mumps, chicken pox, measles, and german measles.

*Immunizations.* Diphtheria and tetanus shot 2–3 years ago for small laceration on hand from work in garden. Does not know of other immunizations.

*Major Illnesses/Hospitalizations*
Only hospitalizations were for birth of children. Two vaginal deliveries and twins by caesarian section.
No major illnesses.

*Current Medications*
*Prescription:* None.
*Nonprescription:* Occasional Tylenol
*Allergies.* None.

*Habits*
*Alcohol:* Rare social drink, less than 1 per month
*Caffeine:* 1–2 cups of coffee in the morning, rare tea or cola.
*Drugs:* Denies use of recreational drugs.
*Tobacco:* Smokes about a half pack per day at present. Used to smoke more than 1 pack per day. (Total equals approximately 36 pack years).

## Family Health History

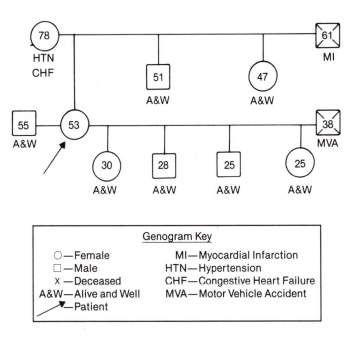

Genogram Key
○ —Female          MI—Myocardial Infarction
□ —Male            HTN—Hypertension
X —Deceased        CHF—Congestive Heart Failure
A&W—Alive and Well  MVA—Motor Vehicle Accident
➤ —Patient

## NUTRITIONAL/METABOLIC PATTERN

**Nutritional**

Mrs. Gardner has a good appetite; no recent changes. No dietary limitations. States she eats a well-balanced diet. 24-hour diet recall deferred until after admission and patient condition more stable.

**Metabolic**

Denies recent weight loss or gain. *Weight:* 137 lb (62.3 kg); *Height:* 5 ft. 5 in. (165.1 cm). No problems with skin, with healing, or with temperature intolerance.

## ELIMINATION PATTERN

**Bowel**

Bowels regular (every day or every other day), stool formed, brown. Denies use of laxatives or any recent changes in bowel habits.

**Bladder**

No history of urinary tract infections, burning on urination, or incontinence.

## ACTIVITY/EXERCISE PATTERN

**Activity/Exercise**

Mrs. Gardner states she has a high energy level. "That's why I knew right away when I was feeling so weak that something was very wrong." She is usually able to perform all desired and required activities without limitations and has full self-care abilities. Maintains a large vegetable garden and sells the produce at a small vegetable stand, which she runs herself. Occasionally hires neighborhood youngsters to help with the stand in the summer.

**Activity/Exercise — Continued**

**Self-Care Ability**

Feeding — 0                                    Grooming — 0
Bathing — 0                                    General mobility — 0
Toileting — 0                                  Cooking — 0
Bed mobility — 0                               Home maintenance — 0
Dressing — 0                                   Shopping — 0

---

**Functional Levels Code**
  0 — Full self-care
  I — Requires use of equipment or device
 II — Requires assistance or supervision from another person
III — Requires assistance or supervision from another person
      and equipment or device
 IV — Is dependent and does not participate

---

**Oxygenation/Perfusion**

States that she usually has no dyspnea at rest or on exertion. Can climb 2 flights of stairs without discomfort. At present, admits to feeling of "chest tightness" and although she feels the need to cough, is having some difficulty raising secretions. No complaints of chest pain, palpitations, or feeling of irregular heart beat.

**Cardiac Risk Factors**

|                                  | Positive | Negative |
|----------------------------------|----------|----------|
| Sedentary life-style             |          | X        |
| Hyperlipidemia                   |          | X        |
| Cigarette smoking                | X        |          |
| Diabetes                         |          | X        |
| Obesity                          |          | X        |
| Hypertension                     |          | X        |
| Hypervigilant personality        |          | X        |
| Family history of heart disease  | X        |          |

## SLEEP/REST PATTERN

**Sleep/Rest**

Mrs. Gardner states she sleeps soundly 7–8 hr/night. Claims she has no difficulty falling asleep, uses no sleep aids, has no difficulty staying asleep. She denies waking during the night, and says she feels rested upon awakening.

## COGNITIVE/PERCEPTUAL PATTERN

**Hearing**

States no difficulty with hearing

**Vision**

Wears glasses for reading, otherwise no problems with vision. Last ophthalmology visit about 2 years ago.

**Sensory Perception**

Mrs. Gardner is alert, oriented to person, place, and time. Memory is intact. Right hand is dominant. No usual difficulty with pain, feels she has a "high pain threshold," says she "can tolerate a lot."

**Learning Style**

States she learns best by verbal instruction followed by demonstration, "Tell me, then show me and I'm okay."

## SELF-PERCEPTION/SELF-CONCEPT PATTERN

*Self-Perception/Self-Concept*

Considers herself a "good, down-to-earth person." Says she is usually very strong and self-sufficient, but admits to being very afraid in the present situation. She asks, "Will I be all right? Do you think I might die? I've never felt anything like this before. I hope they'll do the right thing to make me better, I'm so afraid. I can't believe this is happening."

## ROLE/RELATIONSHIP PATTERN

*Role/Relationship*

Was widowed 15 years ago. Has been married to present husband for 9 years. States they have a good marriage. Lives in a rural area. House has "plenty of land" around it, and she takes pleasure in gardening. All of her children live away from home, but nearby.

Relationships with children are good. Two oldest children are married, and Mrs. Gardner smiles as she mentions that she has 3 grandchildren.

## SEXUALITY/REPRODUCTIVE PATTERN

*Sexuality/Reproductive*

Content with sexuality and sexual expression. Gravida 3; Para 4. States she's in the "midst of menopause"; has had 2 periods in the past year. Has not been "particularly bothered" by symptoms. Does not take estrogen. Negative pap smear at last physical exam.

## COPING/STRESS TOLERANCE PATTERN

*Coping/Stress Tolerance*

States she copes well with most stresses. "I'm not coping well now though. I'm really scared on top of feeling so sick." Says gardening is the way she best copes with stress. She also says "You do what you have to do," when talking about being widowed when her children were younger.

## VALUE/BELIEF PATTERN

*Value/Belief*

Attends church services "often," but is not very involved in church activities. She defines "often" as more than once a month. Believes in the value of hard work. Does not adhere to any specific religious or ethnic customs.

# Physical Examination

*General Survey*

Fifty-three-year-old woman, who is pale, diaphoretic, has generalized muscular twitching, and appears anxious.

*Vital Signs*

**Temperature:** 98°F (oral).
**Pulse:** 72 regular (apical).
**Respirations:** 24 regular, somewhat shallow.
**BP.** 106/60 (right arm in semi-Fowler's position).

*Integument*

**Skin.** Pale, very diaphoretic, no lesions, bruises, or rash noted
**Mucous Membranes.** Intact, moist, pale, no lesions noted
**Nails.** Beds are smooth, no clubbing noted

*HEENT*

**Head.** Head symmetrical, normocephalic. Scalp and hair have no lesions or tenderness. Face is symmetrical, no tenderness noted. Temporomandibular joint is deferred.

**HEENT — Continued**

*Eyes.* Full range of extraocular movements, no nystagmus, pupils equal, round, *only slightly* reactive to light.
*Ears.* Able to hear whispered voice, no tenderness noted
*Nose.* Deferred
*Throat.* Teeth in good repair, mucous membranes intact and very moist (excess salivation). Throat — deferred.

**Neck**

Full range of motion (ROM) no enlarged nodes

**Pulmonary**

Thorax oval, AP diameter 2:1, muscle fasciculations evident, coarse rales bilaterally, diffuse wheezes

**Breasts**

Symmetrical, no tenderness, no masses felt

**Cardiovascular**

Regular rhythm, no extra sounds, no murmurs

**Peripheral Vascular**

*Peripheral Pulses*
Temporal — 4 bilaterally
Carotid — 4 bilaterally
Brachial — 4 bilaterally
Radial — 4 bilaterally
Femoral — 4 bilaterally
Popliteal — 4 bilaterally
Posterior tibial — 4 bilaterally
Dorsalis pedis — 4 bilaterally

*Peripheral Pulse Scale*

0 — Absent
1 — Markedly diminished
2 — Moderately diminished
3 — Slightly diminished
4 — Normal

**Abdomen**

Slightly rounded, muscle fasciculations evident, hyperactive bowel sounds in all 4 quadrants, percussion and palpation deferred due to patient's discomfort

**Musculoskeletal**

No deformities noted, muscle development symmetrical, muscle strength decreased, no limitations in ROM noted, however, full ROM of all joints not tested; gait not tested. No tenderness or crepitation.

**Neurological**

*Mental status.*   Alert, oriented × 3, memory intact for recent and past events
*Cranial nerves.* Cranial nerves II–XII intact
*Motor.* Generalized muscle fasciculations noted
*Sensory.* Deferred.

*Deep Tendon Reflexes*

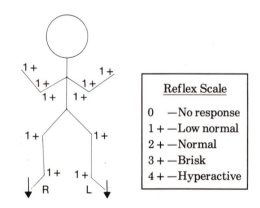

Reflex Scale

0   — No response
1 + — Low normal
2 + — Normal
3 + — Brisk
4 + — Hyperactive

| Genitalia | Deferred |
|---|---|
| Rectal | Deferred |

## Laboratory Data/Diagnostic Studies

**Laboratory Data**

*Hemoglobin.* 12.4 g/100 ml
*Hematocrit.* 38/100 ml (38%)
*WBC.* 10,000/mm³; Serum acetylcholinesterase level 20% of normal
*Na.* 140 mEq/l
*K.* 3.9 mEq/l
*Cl.* 99 mEq/l
*BUN.* 33 mg/100 ml
*Blood sugar.* 144 mg/dl (nonfasting)

*Arterial blood gases*
*pH.* 7.37
*Po₂.* 88 torr
*Pco₂.* 40 torr
*Routine urinalysis.* normal
*Analysis for metabolites.* not yet available

**Diagnostic Studies**

Chest x-ray done, no report available yet. Electrocardiogram normal, no ischemic changes, no dysrhythmias.

## COLLABORATIVE PLAN OF CARE

**Diet**

Does not apply (patient is in the emergency department).

**Medications**

Atropine 2 mg IV stat, repeat in 15 min if no observed adverse effect. Thereafter, repeat every 30 min until sweating and excess salivation disappears or adverse effect noted. May be repeated prn for reappearance of symptoms and notify MD.
Pralidoxime chloride 1 gm/100 ml 5% D/W IV stat. Administer over 15 min, repeat in 1 h if muscle weakness and fasciculations persist.

**Intravenous Therapy**

1000 ml normal saline IV at rate to keep vein open.

**Therapeutic Measures**

Oxygen 2L/min via nasal prongs.
Vital signs, including neuro v/s, q30 min for 4 h, then q1h × 10, if stable.
Admit to telemetry unit for observation.
Continuous cardiac monitor.
Seizure precautions; padded bedsides.
Send repeat urine for urinalysis in 12 h.
Repeat arterial blood gases q4h × 4.

**Consults**

Does not apply.

**Preoperative Plan**

Does not apply.

# NURSING DIAGNOSES DEVELOPED IN CARE PLAN

# ADDITIONAL NURSING DIAGNOSES TO BE CONSIDERED

Decreased Cardiac Output
Knowledge Deficit
Impaired Gas Exchange
Ineffective Breathing Pattern
Potential for Injury: Seizures

# NURSING CARE PLAN BASED ON IDENTIFIED NURSING DIAGNOSES

| | |
|---|---|
| *Ineffective Airway Clearance* | *Related to:* Systemic response to organophosphates. *Evidenced by:* Increased secretions, muscle weakness. |
| *Desired Patient Outcomes* | *The Patient Will:*<br>• Maintain an adequate airway and respiratory effort. |
| *Evaluation Criteria* | *Throughout the Patient's Hospital Stay:*<br>• Her airway will be sufficiently free from secretions to allow adequate gas exchange as measured by arterial blood gases. |

## Interventions

Encourage patient to cough.

Place patient in Fowler's or semi-Fowler's position if able to tolerate.

Place hand on patient's upper abdomen and exert upward pressure during exhalation.

Ensure presence of catheters and other suctioning equipment.

Keep endotracheal intubation nearby and available for immediate use if needed.

Suction prn

## Rationale

The most serious manifestation of organophosphate poisoning is respiratory failure from weakness of the respiratory muscles and excessive bronchial secretions (Namba et al, 1971, p. 481).

Allows most effective use of accessory muscles (Ulrich, Canale, and Wendell, 1986, p. 306).

Augments cough efforts (Ulrich, Canale, and Wendell, 1986, p. 306)

Copious bronchial secretions may require suctioning (Kline and Bayer, 1983, p. 79).

Respiratory arrest may occur early or even after initial therapy appears to have been successful (Kline and Bayer, 1983, p. 79). Necessary equipment must be at hand for the first 48 h after poisoning (Dreisbach, 1980, p. 113).

To mechanically clear airway when patient's efforts are ineffective or inadequate, and to stimulate cough (Taylor, Lillis, and LeMone, 1989, p. 925).

## Interventions

Continuously evaluate level of consciousness, restlessness, and respiratory status. Report changes immediately.

Administer atropine as needed to diminish secretions (see Collaborative Plan of Care).

Teach patient the importance of raising secretions and of expectoration. Provide suitable means of disposal such as tissues and paper bag or basin.

## Rationale

These are early signs of hypoxia and may represent decreasing respiratory muscle strength and ability to manage secretions (Haddad and Winchester, 1983, p. 710).

Atropine is given as needed to achieve and maintain control of excess salivary and bronchial secretions. Adequacy of dose is judged by the absence of excessive secretions and the presence of a tachycardia of more than 100 beats/min (Kipling and Cruickshank, 1985, p. 282).

Patient may find expectoration offensive and attempt to limit or avoid it (Doenges, Jeffries, and Moorhouse, 1984, p. 111).

---

| **Potential For Poisoning** | ***Related to:*** Present exposure to toxic substance and lack of awareness/disregard for environmental hazards. |
| --- | --- |
| | ***Evidenced by:*** Present signs and symptoms that indicate exposure to toxic substance and, patient's description of her behavior with regard to toxic substances. |
| **Desired Patient Outcomes** | ***During Hospitalization:*** |
| | • The potential for further poisoning related to the present exposure will be eliminated. |
| | ***By Discharge:*** |
| | • The patient will be able to identify situations that place her at risk for poisoning and take appropriate measures to eliminate or minimize future hazards. |
| **Evaluation Criteria** | ***By the Time of Discharge, the Patient Will:*** |
| | • Identify toxic risks in her home environment. |
| | • Relate strategies to eliminate or minimize those risks. |

---

## Interventions

To prevent further poisoning from the contamination present, continued absorption must be prevented. Remove all clothing and wash skin and hair thoroughly with copious amounts of soap and water. A second washing of skin with ethyl alcohol is also recommended. In addition, staff should wear protective gear during this procedure to prevent becoming contaminated themselves. (This task was performed on admission to emergency department, but may need to be repeated.)

To decrease the possibility of future poisoning, discuss in a nonjudgmental manner the importance of proper storage, labeling, use, and disposal of pesticides and their containers.

## Rationale

Organophosphate on the skin can continue to be absorbed into the system. Many of these substances are more soluble in alcohol than water (Bayer, Rumack, and Wanke, 1984, p. 244).

Proper use, storage, and disposal are important in the prevention of poisoning (Miller, 1982, p. 294).

| *Interventions* | *Rationale* |
|---|---|
| Inform the patient about the toxic potential of most pesticides and suggest strategies for their safe use. | Knowledge about the danger associated with the use of pesticides may aid in poisoning prevention (Newton et al, 1987, p. 13). |
| Teach the patient techniques for decontamination of skin and clothing | Should the patient find herself or another person in a similar situation, tragedy may be averted if proper decontamination is performed. (Miller, 1982, p. 294). |
| Instruct the patient to have the telephone number of the Poison Control Center near her phone and to call immediately for advice if other poisoning exposures should occur. | Poison Control Centers can provide accurate treatment instructions for prompt treatment of poisoning emergencies (Taylor, Lillis, and LeMone, 1989, p. 489). |

---

| *Fear* | *Related to:* Sudden onset of symptoms associated with a life-threatening emergency.<br>*Evidenced by:* Patient's verbalization of fear. |
|---|---|
| *Desired Patient Outcomes* | *The Patient Will:*<br>• Experience a reduction in fear and increased security with her treatment and caregivers. |
| *Evaluation Criteria* | *By the Time the Patient is Transferred from the Emergency Department to the Telemetry Unit, She Will:*<br>• Verbalize a reduction in fear.<br>• Verbalize comfort with the staff's ability to manage her current situation to result in a positive outcome. |

---

| *Interventions* | *Rationale* |
|---|---|
| Acknowledge the patient's fear. Give her the opportunity to explore her concerns further. | Feelings are real and it is helpful to bring them out into the open so they can be discussed and dealt with (Doenges, Moorhouse, and Geissler, 1989, p. 775). |
| Provide, at a level the patient can understand, information about the patient's problem and its treatment. | Allows the patient to anticipate symptoms and actions of the caregivers, and to participate in the decision process (Doenges, Moorhouse, and Geissler, 1989, p. 750). |
| Emphasize that symptoms can be controlled or eliminated, and describe and explain how. | Allows patient to anticipate actions of caregivers in response to symptoms, thus allows a sense of control (Doenges, Moorhouse, and Geissler, 1989, p. 776). |
| Explain tests, procedures, and treatments. | Knowledge can help decrease fear (Doenges, Moorhouse, and Geissler, 1989, p. 750). |
| Direct all caregivers to address Mrs. Gardner by her name and to introduce self to patient. | Personalization decreases anxiety and established rapport (Doenges, Jeffries, and Moorhouse, 1984, p. 81). |
| Include Mr. Gardner in explanations. | Provides an opportunity to enhance support systems (Doenges, Moorhouse, and Geissler, 1989, 310). |
| Be available for and encourage verbalizations and questions. | Demonstrates concern and willingness to help (Doenges, Moorhouse, and Geissler, 1989, p. 776) Can help decrease stress. |

| *Interventions* | *Rationale* |
|---|---|
| Do not leave patient alone during times of respiratory distress; if this is not possible assure her that staff are nearby. | Presence of a caregiver reduces fear and anxiety (Ulrich, Canale, and Wendell, 1986, p. 305). |

## QUESTIONS FOR DISCUSSION

1. What were the dangers in Mrs. Gardner's environment that led to the poisoning? In what ways could this situation have been avoided?
2. What populations are at high risk for poisoning? Why is this so? Discuss contributing factors.
3. Discuss nursing concerns/precautions when decontaminating a patient such as Mrs. Gardner.
4. Why is Mrs. Gardner on a cardiac monitor? What should the nurse be observing for?
5. If the pesticide had been swallowed by Mrs. Gardner instead of its dermal and possibly inhalation route of entry, what additional measures would need to be taken?
6. Can you describe how in your area you would get help for a poisoning emergency?

## REFERENCES

Bayer, MJ and Rumack, BH: Poisoning & Overdose. Aspen Systems Corp, Rockville, Md, 1983.

Bayer, MJ, Rumack, BH, and Wanke, LA: Toxicologic Emergencies. Robert J. Brady, Bowie, Md, 1984.

Bryson, PD: Comprehensive Review in Toxicology. Aspen Systems Corp, Rockville, Md, 1986.

Doenges, ME, Jeffries, MF, and Moorhouse, MF: Nursing Care Plans: Nursing Diagnosis in Planning Care. FA Davis, Philadelphia, 1984.

Doenges, ME, Moorhouse, MF, and Geissler, AC: Nursing Care Plans: Guidelines for Planning Patient Care, ed 2. FA Davis, Philadelphia, 1989.

Dreisbach, RH: Handbook of Poisoning. Lange Medical Publications, Los Altos, Calif, 1980.

Goldfrank, LR: Toxicologic Emergencies: A Comprehensive Handbook in Problem Solving. Appleton-Century-Crofts, New York, 1982.

Goldfrank, LR, Bresnitz, EA, and Kirstein, R: Organophosphates. In Goldfrank, LR (ed): Toxicologic Emergencies: A Comprehensive Handbook in Problem Solving. Appleton-Century Crofts, New York, 1982.

Guyton, AC: Textbook of Medical Physiology. WB Saunders, Philadelphia, 1986.

Haddad, LM and Winchester, JF: Clinical Management of Poisoning and Drug Overdose. WB Saunders, Philadelphia, 1983.

Kipling, RM and Cruickshank, AN: Organophosphate insecticide poisoning. Anaesthesia 40:281–284, 1985.

Kline, S and Bayer, MJ: Insecticide poisoning. In Bayer, MJ and Rumack, BH (eds): Poisoning and Overdose. Aspen Systems Corp, Rockville, Md, 1983.

Milby, TH: Prevention and management of organophosphate poisoning. JAMA 216(13):2131–2133, 1971.

Miller, M: Pesticide poisoning. J Emerg Nurs 8(6):288–294, 1982.

Namba, T, et al: Poisoning due to organophosphate insecticides. Am J Med 50:475–492, 1971.

Newton, M, et al: General treatments of household poisonings. J Emerg Nurs 13(1):12–15, 1987.

Taylor, C, Lillis, C, and LeMone, P: Fundamentals of Nursing: The Art and Science of Nursing Care. JB Lippincott, Philadelphia, 1989.

Ulrich, SP, Canale, SW, and Wendell, SA: Nursing Care Planning Guides: A Nursing Diagnosis Approach. WB Saunders, Philadelphia, 1986.

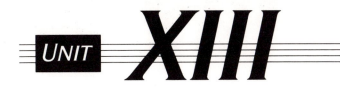

# THE PATIENT WITH
# A PSYCHIATRIC DISORDER

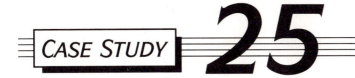

# A PATIENT WITH DRUG ABUSE: COCAINE

Marie C. Femino Esposito, R.N., M.S., CPNP

Cocaine use originated at least several thousand years ago. As early as the 1500s, the Inca Indians in the Andes chewed the leaves of the coca plant with an alkaline substance such as ash; the ash helped to extract the alkaloid and increase dosage. The leaves were chewed to increase endurance — hunger, thirst, and fatigue were auspiciously tolerated under the euphoric phenomenon created by coca chewing. The Incas recognized the coca leaf as a stimulant and anorexiant. Runners were rewarded with the coca leaf and also used the leaf to endure their run. After the Spanish conquest, the coca leaf became the emotionally sustaining substance of the conquered people.

Writings on the wonders of the coca leaf made their way to Spain around the mid-1500s. The coca leaf came under scientific inspection, and around 1859 Neimann isolated the alkaloid cocaine. Freud, after experiencing the effects of cocaine on himself around April 1884, recommended it for asthma, alcohol and morphine addiction, digestive disorders, cachexia, and diminished sexual desire. Later he and his colleague Koller administered cocaine as an anesthetic to the eye of Freud's father during an operation to relieve glaucoma. Simultaneously, in another part of the world, Halsted performed the first nerve block using cocaine. Both Freud and Halsted became addicted to cocaine.

The new wonder drug began to increase in popularity. A Bordeaux wine created by Angelo Francois Mariani's use of coca leaves in the wine container was endorsed by 3 popes, 16 heads of states, and 8000 physicians who sampled the "vin Mariani." Another popular use of coca was that of the Coca-Cola Company. The company advertised their soft drink as "delicious and refreshing" and that it "relieves fatigue." The soft drink became very popular and continues to be well liked today although its recipe has been decocainized. Cocaine was also once thought to cure tuberculosis. Under this assumption, Robert Louis Stevenson was treated with cocaine and, under its influence, wrote *The Strange Case of Dr. Jekyll and Mr. Hyde* in 6 days and 6 nights.

Cocaine abuse in the early 1900s was sensationalized in the media, in songs, and in the movies. With the onset of World War II the rate of cocaine abuse declined; however, cocaine use began a comeback around 1969. Historically, cocaine has been reported as a safe nonaddictive drug until as recently as 7–10 years ago. Despite the recent warnings about the dangers of cocaine use, the sale of cocaine now amounts to approximately $30 billion a year in the United States alone. Cocaine mortality and emergency department visits have increased 200%, and admissions to government treatment programs have increased 500% over the past 10 years. The total number of Americans who have tried the drug is rising yearly. In 1986, approximately 20–25 million people had used cocaine at least once. Of the above total, as many as 5–6 million use cocaine on a regular, monthly basis, and 1–2 million people are dependent abusers. Every day, some 5000 people try cocaine for the first time. These estimates were made before the use of crack became popular and therefore are conservative.

Early research allowed for the development of many medicinal uses of cocaine, but the legalized use of cocaine for medical purposes has declined over the years. The 2 forms of cocaine currently used are alkaloid cocaine and cocaine hydrochloride, Schedule II drugs under the provisions of the Comprehensive Drug Abuse

Prevention and Control Act of 1970. Medicinal cocaine is used for ears, nose, and throat procedures as an anesthetic and vasoconstrictor.

## PATHOPHYSIOLOGY OF COCAINE USE

Coca is the dried leaf of *Erythroxylon coca*, and the commercial drug is derived from 3 plant varieties indigenous to the mountainous eastern Andes regions of South America such as Peru, Bolivia, Java, and Colombia.

The schematic representation of the commercial and street chemistry of coca derivatives is presented in Figure 25-1 (Kunkel, 1986, p. 133).

Benzoylmethylecgonine is an ester of benzoic acid and the nitrogen-containing base ecgonine, found in the leaves of Erythroxylon coca and other species of Erythroxylon. Ecgonine is an amino alcohol closely related to tropine, the amino alcohol in atropine. Cocaine is a potent sympathomimetic-like amphetamine and a local anesthetic of the procaine family. The main difference between amphetamines and cocaine that

**COMMERCIAL AND STREET CHEMISTRY OF COCA DERIVATIVES**

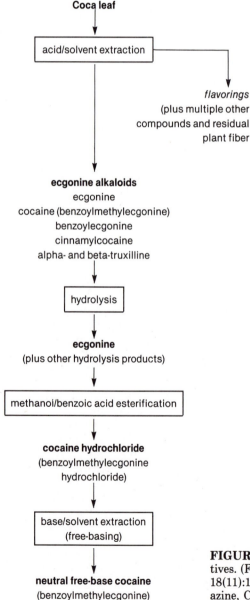

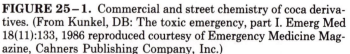

**FIGURE 25–1.** Commercial and street chemistry of coca derivatives. (From Kunkel, DB: The toxic emergency, part I. Emerg Med 18(11):133, 1986 reproduced courtesy of Emergency Medicine Magazine, Cahners Publishing Company, Inc.)

pertains to abuse is duration of action. The half-life of cocaine in plasma is 90 minutes, whereas amphetamine half-life is 4–8 times longer. Both produce a pharmacodynamic tachyphylaxis, resulting in rapidly declining effects despite the continued presence of the stimulant in plasma. Amphetamine availability in the United States is now quite limited.

The action of cocaine is only partially understood. Cocaine blocks nerve conduction by increasing the threshold for electrical excitability. Cocaine decreases or blocks permeability of the nerve membrane to sodium, probably by binding to a receptor in the sodium channel of the membrane and physically obstructing the movement of ions through the channels.

Cocaine stimulates nerves by blocking the active reuptake of norepinephrine, and perhaps dopamine and serotonin, into the presynaptic nerve terminal. This seems to create excess norepinephrine in the nerve synapse, thereby resulting in a stimulatory effect on the adrenergic nerves of the central nervous system (CNS), creating a euphoric effect and on the peripheral sympathetic nervous system with stimulation similar to the "fight/flight/fright" phenomenon. Another theory hypothesizes that the blockage of the dopaminergic pathways in the brain is responsible for the euphoric effects of cocaine. Neurobiologically, cocaine *initially* increases the mental well-being and thus creates a feeling of euphoria. Repeated cocaine use is further hypothesized to lead rapidly to presynaptic dopamine depletion and postsynaptic dopamine receptor super-sensitivity, which results in tolerance, craving, dysphoria, paranoia, hallucinations, and depression. The vicious cycle of addiction relates to obtaining the relief from the depression or striving for the initial great "rush" or euphoric pleasure by repeating or increasing the dose.

Cocaine produces a rapid immunization to a toxic dose by previous usage of small doses of the same substance (*pharmacodynamic tachyphylaxis*), resulting in rapidly declining effects. Cocaine abuse is characterized by "binges" in which the drug is readministered up to every 10 minutes, lasting from a few hours to 7 days, with the average binge being approximately 12 hours. Cocaine is rapidly distributed and metabolized. Its half-life ranges from 30 minutes to 2 hours. Cocaine is quickly distributed to fatty tissue (lipophilic). The brain has a large blood supply and a high lipid content and thus tends to concentrate the drug. Plasma concentrations of 50 $\mu$g/L–500 $\mu$g/L have been associated with a "high" after a single dose. Cocaine can be administered nasally (*insufflated*), intravenously, orally, or in the free-base form can be inhaled as a vapor (*free-basing*). Peak plasma concentrations are obtained within 15–30 minutes of ingestion, the brain cocaine concentration at this time is over 4 times the plasma cocaine concentration.

The major urinary metabolite of cocaine is benzoylecgonine. This compound is produced in the body by hydrolysis. Urine testing is best accomplished by screening for the presence of cocaine with the Syva EMIT enzymeimmunoassay, radioimmunoassays, or the chromatographic test, which are intended for use with urine samples and recognize primarily the major urinary product, benzoylecgonine. The radioimmunoassays, a type of urine test, can detect cocaine metabolites for up to a week after a single, large dose. Two other types of urine tests that can detect cocaine metabolites are: (1) the enzymeimmunoassay for 2–5 days after use of the cocaine; and (2) chromatographic confirmation techniques for less than 24 hours after use of cocaine. Test results come back either positive or negative and detect a threshold level of the metabolite in body fluids. False positive results can occur, particularly when the assay is applied to samples other than urine. The inactive metabolite benzoylecgonine remains in the body longer than cocaine, a positive immunoassay result may not correspond to the presence of the active drug or clinical symptoms. Because the Syva EMIT immunoassay is based on an enzymatic reaction, it is advisable to check and buffer the pH to normal physiologic levels before testing. Extremely low or high pH will inhibit the EMIT reaction, leading to false-negative results. Interference of urine pH by substance abusers is common in their attempt to avoid detection. Therefore a pH check should be done on any urine sample submitted for analysis by an EMIT immunoassay.

## Risk Factors

There is no systematic way of evaluating the potential for an individual to become a heavy cocaine abuser or a noncompulsive user. Is vulnerability a component of individual personality, or motivated by specific features of personality or psychopathology? There are many variables that must be taken into consideration, such as demographic characteristics, personality traits, and the ability to distinguish cocaine-induced organic mental disorders from coexisting mood disorders. To what degree does drug usage correct ego deficits and support adaptive needs? Apart from coexisting psychiatric disorders, no predispositions to stimulant abuse have been identified.

More compulsive use of cocaine, as a transition from recreational use, may result with either increased access to the drug and a resulting escalation in dosages, or when a more-rapid route of administration is chosen (e.g., intravenous or smoking). Clinicians suggest that an understanding of the route of administration of cocaine and of the pattern of cocaine use can define critical components of cocaine abuse. Approximately 90% of cocaine abusers report intensive bingeing as one of the characteristics of compulsive abuse.

# COMMON CLINICAL FINDINGS

The clinical effects of cocaine vary from individual to individual, and within the different timeframes in a person's life. Many drug abusers experience a precipitating crisis that usual adaptive capacities are not able to handle, and therefore are vulnerable to an adaptive benefit such as the feeling of euphoric pleasure or the "rush" felt with cocaine use. Determination of the social milieu is therefore helpful. The personality and state of mind of the cocaine abuser should be considered within the context of the maturational factors and developmental inadequacies as a continuum incorporated with the psychological and physiological responses of the individual. The dosage, chronicity of use, and route of administration are additional considerations when trying to predict common human clinical findings. The *Boston Globe* recently reported "It's not a rich person's drug, it's not a black person's drug, it's not a poor person's drug . . . It's an equal opportunity drug, and unfortunately people have not realized how dangerous it really is." (Ribadeneira, 1988, p. 1).

Signs and symptoms of cocaine use or toxicity are increased heart rate (tachycardia and/or severe arrhythmias), vasoconstriction, rise in blood pressure, intracranial hemorrhage, high-output congestive heart failure, pupillary dilation, relaxation of bronchial airways, increased mental alertness and concentration, and increased motor activity that becomes less and less coordinated as the dose increases. Some people may experience restlessness, tremors, clonic-tonic seizures, emesis, an elevation in temperature, and death.

The scenario might develop as follows. An individual takes small doses of cocaine once in a while and for a short time feels "an intoxicating wave of the highest rapture," (Brenner and Kostant, 1986, p. 8) a very strong, intense, euphoric feeling that leaves the person breathless. There is a strong sense of well being, contentment, and invulnerability associated many times with a burst of energy. The individual goes on to experience a suppression of appetite, a sense of timelessness, and has heightened perceptions.

The euphoric episode may be replaced with negative sequelae, especially as the dosage and duration of intake increase and if the drug use occurs under adverse conditions. Some of the negative sequelae noted are nausea, vertigo, and headache, which precede later more-profound effects. More-profound adverse effects of advanced cocaine toxicity are dysphoria or emotional lability and paranoia. Hallucinations in the form of tactile ("cocaine bugs"), visual ("snow lights"), and other sensory hallucinatory effects may also be experienced. A full-cocaine psychosis may develop, with disorientation, fearfulness, delusions, and feelings of hopelessness and worthlessness. Chronic cocaine abusers "crashing" after a prolonged "high" may experience insomnia, anorexia and weight loss, and an accelerated heart rate and increased blood pressure. The worst-case scenario might terminate with convulsions, severe cardiac problems, and death.

The major complications of cocaine with placental vasoconstriction and abruptio placentae associated with acute hypertension. Third-trimester use of cocaine has been reported to induce a sudden onset of uterine contractions, fetal tachycardia, and excessive fetal activity.

The effects of cocaine on the newborn due to exposure of the fetus in utero are ambiguous at this time. Infants tend to be smaller, lower in birth weight, and have a small head circumference. Neurological signs exhibited are irritability, tremulousness, muscle rigidity, and increased startle response. Chasnoff, et al (1985, p. 669) report differences in neurobehavior detected by the Brazelton scale, (a) depressed interactive behavior, and (b) state control, impairment in organizational abilities of the infant. Other signs in the newborn associated with cocaine use by the mother during pregnancy are increased heart rate and respiratory rate, diarrhea, disturbed sleep patterns, and poor tolerance for oral feedings. Some correlations have also linked perinatal cerebral infarction and sudden infant death syndrome (SIDS). Further research and longitudinal studies need to be done to ascertain the short-term and long-term sequelae of cocaine ingestion on the fetus and newborn.

# TREATMENT MODALITIES

In devising an individualized treatment program for the cocaine drug abuser, the clinician must first assess the psychological, physical, social, and pharmacological factors that have contributed to the cocaine-abusing behavior.

The psychological assessment should include a complete history of self and family illnesses, including a psychiatric predisposition to bi-polar illness, attention-deficit disorder, personality disorders, and depression. Several researchers have observed an increased prevalence of psychopathology with cocaine abuse and have suggested that patients may be "self-medicating" (Gawin and Kleber, 1986, p. 573–583; Millman, 1988, p. 27–32; Pollack, Brotman, and Rosenbaum, 1989, p. 31–44). It is sometimes difficult for the clinician to discern substance-abuse symptomatology or withdrawal from a substance from psychopathology. Therefore it is clinically important to recognize concomitant psychopathology. Pharmacological interventions are assessed according to individual needs.

Pharmacological interventions in the cocaine-abusive client are presently being studied. There is some evidence that disipramine, a tricyclic antidepressant, when combined with individual therapy can help to decrease craving for cocaine (Millman, 1988, p. 32; O'Brien, et al, 1988, p. 22). Weiss (1988) found that disipramine may cause relapse to cocaine abuse since symptoms similar to cocaine usage were caused by the use of disipramine (jitteriness syndrome/early tricyclic syndrome) in 3 clients. Pharmacological treatment should be structured around a full psychiatric assessment and consideration of the exact efficacy of medicinal interventions such as in the treatment of severe symptoms of the acute sequelae of cocaine intoxication; treatment of underlying psychopathology; treatment of combined drug use (alcohol and cocaine; heroin and cocaine); or reduction of craving. Much caution should be taken in giving a substance abuser medications that are addictive in nature.

A complete physical examination will determine present medical problems or medical sequelae from frequent drug abuse (i.e., underweight, vitamin deficiency, various body excoriations or ulcers, and liver disease). Liver disease can result from alcohol abuse. Many patients are polydrug users (Pollack, Brotman, and Rosenbaum, 1989, p. 36; Zuckerman, et al, 1989, p. 764). Essential laboratory testing should be done to substantiate or determine adverse sequelae of existing or suspected medical problems, including screening urine for toxic substances.

The initial assessment process should also include the evaluation of the client's social milieu. Positive family support and peer support will help the client with the recovery process. Conversely, negative family or peer support can obstruct the rehabilitative process. It is important to understand how the client functions within his or her complex environmental system. How does the client integrate and utilize support from family and friends? The family with a substance-abuse problem is at risk. In such cases, the family system, itself including the extended-family-system members who may also have substance-abuse problems, places the client at extreme risk. Relapse prevention strategies are sabotaged when the individual is re-exposed to stimuli that condones substance abuse.

Another component of the assessment should include a complete drug history, including types of drugs used in the present and past; route of administration; frequency; amount of the drug used; the desired effects of the drug obtained; and the environmental climate at the time of consumption of the drug.

In establishing a rehabilitative program, the clinician and the client may initiate a written contract, which serves to establish the intrinsic guidelines of an individualized program. The essential components of a cocaine-abuse rehabilitative program are (1) commitment to all drug abstinence, which component is supported by random urine testing; (2) frequent attendance of a support group and individualized counseling sessions; (3) regular attendance of a 12-step program or similar self-help group (12-step programs include the belief of the "powerlessness" over cocaine use, an examination of lifestyle and moral choices, an acceptance of the need for help, and admitting drug addiction and personal needs); (4) a comprehensive drug-education program that includes relapse-prevention strategies, including extinction of conditional cues, recognition of the early warning signs of the resumption of substance abuse, development of coping strategies, and incorporation of stress reduction strategies; and (5) the development of family (including extended family) and social-support systems.

In order for a cocaine drug-abuse-treatment program to succeed, there must be complete abstinence from drug use. Many professionals think that the development of a "trusting" relationship, combined with educating the client on the perils of drug abuse, can increase self-awareness and self-esteem, and thus promote positive decision-making skills (i.e., decreased drug usage). But in essence these professionals may be permitting continued use of cocaine. The problem in assessment by professionals of continued cocaine abuse is in underestimating the highly addictive qualities of the drug, which encode in the brain a powerful, euphoric, conditioned response to continue use of the drug. Therefore initial treatment should include random urine testing 2–3 times per week for at least a 4-week period to ensure abstinence. Spot urine testing should be continued for the length of the drug rehabilitative program, approximately 6–12 months. Urine testing helps to promote self-control efforts and is an objective monitor of a patient's progress (Millman, 1988, p. 28).

Relapse prevention strategies may consist of development of coping strategies to decrease susceptibility to drug cravings and urges. Some programs have tried to expose the patient repeatedly, in a controlled environment, to conditioned cues that might precipitate drug usage in order to decrease the power of the cues, give practice in use of coping skills to resist resumption of drug use, or to promote extinction of drug responses (O'Brien, et al, 1988 p. 18). O'Brien, et al (1988, pp. 18–20) found that with cocaine abuse the programs should be geared to the route of administration that is familiar to the cocaine abuser (i.e., intranasal, smoking, or intravenous). The programs may use audiotapes, videotapes, slides, and paraphernalia, that is, drug administering equipment specific to their method of using cocaine (intranasal, intravenous, or freebase) (O'Brien, et al, 1988, p. 20).

Discerning appropriate stimuli for the individual is difficult because there are many factors that may serve as a reminder or cause a craving response. There are some individuals who do not respond at all to the types of stimuli used in stimuli/craving extinction programs. The client's mood at the time of the extinction program may be 1 factor that contributes to a negative response to the stimuli presented. Drug cravings were elicited in a client who was in an angry mood when previously no response was noted to the same stimuli (O'Brien, et al, 1988, p. 19).

It is important to recognize that early warning signals of resumption of cocaine use happen before actual drug use is resumed. The client may be over-confident in his or her abstinence of drug use and place his or her self in high-risk situations. The therapist must continually challenge distorted views of "safe situations" and help the client to formulate realistic views.

As with all addictions, there may be times when it is impossible for the client to resist usage of the drug. Relapses produce "feelings profound failure and expectation of continued failure" (Washton, 1986, p. 569). Washton (1986, p. 569) suggests that clients should be prepared for these "slips" so that abstinence may be resumed, and refers to the effect of the isolated usage of the drug on the client as "abstinence violation effect (AVE)." The client should be taught that an isolated use of a drug does not mean defeat, but can be viewed as a learning experience to prevent other isolated events.

Coping strategies and stress-reduction strategies also must be incorporated into a treatment program in order to help the individual make appropriate lifestyle changes.

A treatment program should support a drug-free environment, relapse-prevention strategies, psychotherapy via group and individual counseling, regular attendance of a 12-step program or similar self-help program and individual therapy, development of lifestyle changes, and emotional support. A holistic view of a rehabilitation program sees the client within his or her environment, and thus focuses on increasing self-esteem through the development of parenting skills, healthy relationships, alternative lifestyle changes (exercise programs, coping strategies, stress-reduction strategies, meditation, and religion), educational support, professional support, occupational and vocational support.

# PATIENT ASSESSMENT DATA BASE

## Health History

*Client:*
Ms. Susan Clark

*Address:* 2 Prospect Street, Louisville, Kentucky
*Telephone:* (555) 584-8967
*Contact:* Ms. Anne Walker (mother)
*Address of contact:* Same as client
*Telephone of contact:* Same as client
*Age:* 21   *Sex:* Female   *Race:* White
*Educational background:* High School
*Religion:* Protestant   *Marital status:* Single
*Usual occupation:* Receptionist
*Present occupation:* Mother
*Source of income:* General Welfare
*Insurance:* Medicaid
*Source of referral:* Greg Halsted, MD
*Source of history:* Self
*Reliability of historian:* In Process of evaluating
*Date of interview:* 9/10/89
*Reason for visit/Chief complaint:* "I'm here because I have been using cocaine."

## HEALTH PERCEPTION/HEALTH MANAGEMENT

*Present Health Status*

*Status of Patient.* Present health evaluation occurred 7 days after her daughter's birth. Susan was well known to a small community hospital. She is a 21-year-old woman who is an unemployed receptionist with a 6-year history of drug and alcohol abuse. At age 15 years, she began daily use of marijuana and admits to experimenting with speed, caffeine, and mescaline on different occasions. She describes heavy alcohol intake (5–10 drinks/night) on the weekends. At 18 years of age, Susan reports being introduced to cocaine at a party, "Someone brought it out at a party and we all did a few lines."

She has been seeing the same boyfriend for the last few years. He is the putative (alleged) father of her baby. Susan reports that she and her boyfriend started to do cocaine mainly on the weekends, a few lines now and then with occasional bingeing (lasting only a few hours). Gradually over the next 2 years, her use of cocaine increased from occasional use on the weekends to use every day, "Prior to my knowledge that I was pregnant, I found myself doing lines of cocaine throughout the entire day." She states that binges could last up to 2 days (usually on the weekends), but no longer, "I needed to get up for work the next day." She denies smoking cocaine or intravenous use of the drug. Susan stated that at the same time as her boyfriend began to smoke cocaine (approximately 1 year ago) she noticed that they had begun to fight more often.

Susan was in her twentieth gestational week before she knew that she was pregnant, "I kept spotting with my period for a few months and didn't even think that I was pregnant." During the pregnancy, she denied drug and alcohol abuse but was inconsistent with keeping prenatal appointments and unable on 2 occasions to give urine for drug screening. On the 1 occasion when urine was obtained, no toxic substances were detected. She had been using cocaine regularly until she found out that she was pregnant. She tried to stop usage of cocaine, but found that she would revert back to cocaine use at least once a month while pregnant. It was difficult for her to stop "because everyone else was using cocaine." Just after she found out that she was pregnant, her boyfriend hit her once during a time when they were both "high" on cocaine. She states that she became enraged and unable to control her anger, had picked up a baseball bat and hit him on the head. He was in the hospital for a couple of days. This act frightened her because she knew that she could have killed him. At this time, she asked him to get out of her life and she moved in with a girlfriend.

***Status of Patient's Infant.*** The baby is described as having intrauterine growth retardation (IUGR)—less than expected rate of intrauterine growth. The nurses in the nursery noted 8 h postpartum that the baby was jittery with increased irritability, and was difficult to feed. Due to the mother's past drug history, inconsistency with prenatal appointments, and the baby's IUGR (4.5 lb at 40 weeks gestation), and unexplained increased irritability and jitteriness (all other lab values for the infant were within normal limits), a urine specimen was taken from the neonate for a toxic screen. (A toxic screen on the urine of the neonate can be obtained when the physician feels that the observed signs and symptoms in the neonate are inconsistent with reported data and suspects toxic substance abuse. If the mother refuses the test, a court order can be obtained to perform the test for diagnostic purposes in the best interest of the neonate. Rules may differ depending on the state.) The urine came back positive for cocaine.

***Treatment Plans.*** A family conference was held with Susan, her doctor, social worker, Department of Social Service's (DSS) intake worker, and primary nurse. The team recommended that

**Present Health Status — Continued**

she enter an outpatient drug-rehabilitation program. As a part of their recommendations, a visiting nurse would monitor the nutrition of the infant and provide a home-health aide for the infant, due to the increased needs of an infant with a feeding problem (potential failure to thrive) and the inability of the mother to focus on such needs. Early intervention would monitor the growth and development of the infant, and the DSS worker would coordinate, monitor, and support the mother's compliance to the drug-rehabilitation program and day care while attending a drug rehabilitation program and the transition to a drug-free family life-style. Susan thought cocaine to be relatively harmless to her and her baby, "I never wanted to hurt my baby," but has seen a downhill trend in her lifestyle. This has recently frightened her, along with her thoughts about losing her baby. Seven days postpartum, Susan agreed to enter the drug-rehabilitation program.

*Situational factors.* Susan's boyfriend has left the state because "the law was after him and he also wanted to get away from his friends and their use of cocaine." Her boyfriend has been calling her every day and would like her to come and live with him. He has told her that he does not use cocaine anymore. Susan states that she never had to pay for cocaine because her friends always had the drug available. Her boyfriend had started to sell the drug in order to pay for his increased usage. For the last few months, she notes, she has felt increased depression and fatigue. She attributes these feelings to an increased number of arguments between her boyfriend and herself, and the eventual demise of the relationship; increased arguments with her mother; instability in a home ("flipflopping" from mother's home to boyfriend's home, to a girlfriend's home, and occasionally being without a home); the birth of her baby; confusion about her and her baby's future; and her inability to completely quit cocaine use. Susan states that for the last year she has not felt like having sex. Many times she would have sex just because her boyfriend wanted it. She doesn't ever remember feeling good about having sex. Her mood when she first started to use cocaine was "happy," but that didn't last long—all she remembers now is being sad and unsettled. She describes situations (within the last year) involving "problems with breathing" that have left her feeling very scared. Susan states that during these situations she would feel uneasy and unsettled, her rate of breathing would increase, she would feel a "little spacey," and then could feel herself panicking because she could not catch her breath. Some friends suggested that she breathe into a bag, and that seemed to help.

**Past Health Status**

*General Health.* General health status has been good up until now, "I have always been in good physical condition."

*Prophylactic Medical/Dental Care.* Receives annual dental examinations, but does not have routine medical checkups. Susan has had pap smears done in the past, but has been inconsistent with the examinations and cannot remember the date of her last pap smear. Her past pregnancy has made it necessary for her to be more consistent with her health care.

*Childhood Illness.* Had chickenpox in the second grade, remembers no other childhood illnesses.

*Immunizations.* Received all childhood vaccinations; received last tetanus booster when she was 13 years old.

***Major Illness/Hospitalizations.*** At age 13, Susan sprained and partially tore the medial lateral ligament in her right leg while skiing. Since the accident, she has felt it necessary to regularly work out with weights to maintain muscle strength in her right leg; if she does not, the leg begins to bother her. About April, 1984, she was admitted to Louisville General Hospital after being hit on her left eye. She was vague as to how the accident occurred. She stated that she stayed in the hospital for 1 week "because they were watching for increased pressure in her left eye." She states that there were no serious consequences after this injury and has had no problems with her eye since the incident.

### Current Medications
Ferrous sulfate 325 mg qd
(decreased hemoglobin [Hgb] secondary to recent delivery and stated poor nutritional habits).
***Allergies.*** No known allergies to food or medications.

### Habits
*Alcohol:* "I don't abuse alcohol, but I have a maximum of 5 drinks a night on the weekend when I'm out with my friends, and an occasional drink during the week."
*Caffeine:* 3–6 cups of coffee/d with occasional use of caffeine pills to "give me more energy."
*Drugs:* Daily abuse of cocaine with bingeing for 3h–2d up until a few months ago; infrequent use lately.
*Tobacco:* Does not smoke

### Family Health History

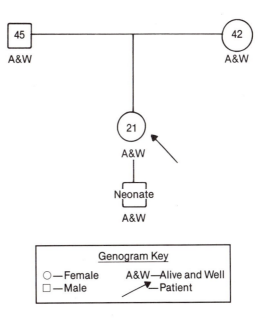

Family history includes: father with high cholesterol, "many heart problems," and status post angioplasty (2 years ago); mother has no known illnesses.

## NUTRITIONAL/METABOLIC PATTERN

### Nutritional

The patient states that she does not usually eat well-balanced meals, especially when using cocaine. "I don't like fruits and I

**Nutritional—Continued**

don't like vegetables." While Susan was using cocaine, she exhibited anorexic tendencies and lost 22 lb. She states that she now is trying to eat more, but just is not hungry.

*Usual Daily Menu*
*Breakfast:* 1½ cups of rice pilaf, 1 can of Diet cola, 16 oz water, 2 cups of coffee.
*Lunch:* Boneless Chicken breast, 1 baked potato, 16 oz orange juice.
*Dinner:* 1 bowl of spaghetti, 1 porkchop, 16 oz of water, 2 cups of coffee.

**Metabolic**

*Height:* 5 ft. 4 in. (162.6 cm); *Weight:* 110 lb (50 kg) presently; weight 2 years ago—120 lb; weight before pregnancy—98 lb; weight gain during pregnancy—22 lb.
**Dentition:** "I may have a few cavities . . . I don't remember when I was last at the dentist."

## ELIMINATION PATTERN

**Bowel**

Patient reports constipation, bowel movement approximately every third to fourth day. Has used laxative once a month approximately if constipation is severe.

**Bladder**

Susan reports no difficulty with urination, no burning or frequency.

## ACTIVITY/EXERCISE PATTERN

**Activity/Exercise**

The patient describes herself as a person who likes to be very active. "I love to ski, run, walk long distances, and work out with weights at the gym." Since her pregnancy, she has not been very active. The most activity recently has been taking long walks.

*Self-Care Ability*

| | |
|---|---|
| Feeding—0 | Grooming—0 |
| Bathing—0 | General mobility—0 |
| Toileting—0 | Cooking—0 |
| Bed mobility—0 | Home maintenance—0 |
| Dressing—0 | Shopping—0 |

> *Functional Levels Code*
> 0—Full self-care
> I—Requires use of equipment or device
> II—Requires assistance or support from another person
> III—Requires assistance or support from another person and equipment or device
> IV—Is dependent and does not participate

**Oxygenation/Perfusion**

*Last chest X-ray.* Can't remember having a chest x-ray
*Last EKG.* Has never had one done
*Normal Sinus Rhythm.* Unable to assess

### Cardiac Risk Factors

|  | Positive | Negative |
|---|:---:|:---:|
| Sedentary life-style |  | X |
| Hyperlipidemia |  | X |
| Cigarette smoking |  | X |
| Diabetes |  | X |
| Obesity |  | X |
| Hypertension |  | X |
| Hypervigilant personality | X |  |
| Family history of heart disease | X |  |

## SLEEP/REST PATTERN

### Sleep/Rest

Susan states that sleep was limited while she was on cocaine. At present, she has been having nightmares for no apparent reason. She cannot remember her dreams. Her mother is helping her watch the baby so that she can try to get more sleep, but her sleep is not restful because she is concerned about the baby's needs. Sleep may remain an issue while the baby is young.

## COGNITIVE/PERCEPTUAL PATTERNS

### Hearing

Patient denies problems with hearing.

### Vision

Patient denies problems with vision.

### Sensory Perception

Patient denies problems with taste, touch, or smell.

### Learning Style

Susan quit school in the eleventh grade and would like to go back to school to get her GED. She relates that she did well while in school, but was bored. Susan states, "I am a quick learner." She spends free time during the day reading books related to care of the newborn and watching soap operas. She is left-hand dominant.

## SELF-PERCEPTION/SELF-CONCEPT PATTERN

### Self-Perception/Self-Concept

"Now that I look back on things, I see that I've made some pretty silly decisions. I like myself off drugs, I did not like what was happening to me on cocaine. I would like to believe that I will be a good mother, have a nice relationship with someone, and be independent and support myself, but I'm scared. I don't know if I can do it, and I'm not sure I know how to make the change." The anger and depression that she felt while on cocaine was very scary. "I have never had a relationship that I have really felt good about. I need to feel confident in what I'm doing and believe in myself and I'm not sure that I do yet."

## ROLE/RELATIONSHIP PATTERN

### Role/Relationship

Susan would like to be a good mother first. She also would like to finish school and go on to be a lawyer. "Can a single mother go back to school and become independent of the system? Will I be able to get some help with what I want to do?" She states that her mother and she are getting along better since she has moved back home. She further states that her mother is supportive and does not tell her what to do, but helps her reason through situations. Susan wonders if she is having trouble with men because her father left when she was only 2 years old and her mother has

*Role/Relationship — Continued*

not had many other relationships. Her father does come and visit and she enjoys this time with him. "I miss not having a father around."

## SEXUALITY/REPRODUCTIVE PATTERN

*Reproductive*

"I have not ever experienced a good sexual relationship. I'm not sure I know what to expect." She states that she has been interested in boys since age 11. Susan began to menstruate irregularly at around 12 years of age. She does not routinely obtain gynecological exams. Susan reports being sexually active since age 15. "I'm aware of AIDS, but I'm not sure I can get a guy to wear a condom." At present she is considering using the Pill when her postpartum time is over, but "I'm afraid of the side-effects and therefore would like some contraceptive teaching."

## COPING/STRESS-TOLERANCE PATTERN

*Coping/Stress Tolerance*

At this time, Susan reports that her main support system is her mother. She has never considered counseling before, but sees the experience as positive. "At times I feel alone, especially when all my friends do coke. I have been with them during the last few months of my pregnancy and only doing cocaine maybe once a month. I had to sit with them while they were doing it to know that I could resist. Just before the baby was born, I was very down and there was a party and I just felt that 2 lines wouldn't hurt and then I went into labor." Susan feels that she is strong within herself and that she wants things to be better for her baby's future. Her resistance "most of the time" to using cocaine with her friends has given her the confidence that she can stop.

## VALUE/BELIEF PATTERN

*Value/Belief*

Susan describes herself as an agnostic. "I don't find religion or talking to God helpful at all." She is unsure about her values in relation to being a single mother and the ability to make the right choices, but she feels that she is learning to develop good reasoning skills.

# Physical Examination

*General Survey*

*Interview:* Drug Rehabilitation Clinic, Louisville, Kentucky. Attractive, slim (especially for a woman only 1-wk postpartum), 21-year-old female. Susan delivered a baby boy on 9/3/89. She presents herself as a personable, concerned young woman. Oriented to person, time, and place.

*Vital Signs*

*Temperature.* 98.8°F or 37.1°C (oral)
*Apical Pulse.* 88 regular
*BP.* 120/88, LA
*Respirations.* 22, regular

*Integument*

*Skin.* The appearance of the skin is slightly dry, warm, and pale. No lesions or bruising were noted.
*Mucous Membranes.* Pink, moist, and intact.
*Nails.* "I tend to bite my nails." Nails were short and not well groomed.

| | |
|---|---|
| **HEENT** | **Head.** Symmetrical, hair thick with nice luster, no palpable masses.<br>**Eyes.** Pupils equal, round, reactive to light and accommodation (PERRLA). Extra-ocular movements intact (EOM). Normal fundi, without edema, hemorrhage or exudate. Gross visual acuity intact.<br>**Ears.** Bilaterally symmetrical, similar in size and shape, right and left tympanic membranes clear with no abnormalities. Weber and Rinne within normal limits, air conduction greater than bone conduction.<br>**Nose.** Nostrils pink, patent, no septal deviation, no scarring.<br>**Mouth/Throat.** Mucosa is pink and moist, no deviation of uvula, gums slightly pale, tonsils not swollen.<br>**Neck.** Supple, no palpable nodes, normal-size thyroid, trachea midline, no visible vasculature. |
| **Pulmonary** | Bilateral clear, equal, breath sounds throughout. Symmetrical, bilaterally, equal chest expansion. |
| **Breasts** | Well developed, warm, firm, slightly nodular, slightly tender with a small amount of milk leaking occasionally from nipples. Nipples with no cracks or fissures. |
| **Cardiovascular** | Apical pulse 82, regular, no murmurs; no rub; point of maximal impulse at fifth intercostal space, midclavicular line, S1 and S2 of good quality. |
| **Peripheral Vascular** | Bilateral pulses symmetrical and of normal strength. No edema noted. |

*Peripheral Pulse*
Temporal — 4 bilaterally
Carotid — 4 bilaterally
Brachial — 4 bilaterally
Radial — 4 bilaterally
Femoral — 4 bilaterally
Popliteal — 4 bilaterally
Posterior tibial — 4 bilaterally
Dorsalis pedis — 4 bilaterally

*Peripheral Pulse Scale*

| |
|---|
| 0 — Absent |
| 1 — Markedly diminished |
| 2 — Moderately diminished |
| 3 — Slightly diminished |
| 4 — Normal |

| | |
|---|---|
| **Abdomen** | Lax and weak in midline, slightly tender; fundus 4 finger breaths below umbilicus; bowel sounds present and active in all quadrants; nonpalpable liver, spleen, and kidneys; no bruits. |
| **Musculoskeletal** | Normal, symmetrical-appearing, bilateral upper and lower extremities with full range of motion (ROM); equal strength; no redness or signs of joint inflammation. |
| **Neurological** | **Mental Status.** Alert and oriented to time, person, and place.<br>**Cranial Nerves.** Intact, I–XII<br>**Motor.** Symmetrical, equal tone, strength, and muscle mass with full ROM in both upper and lower extremities.<br>**Sensory.** Normal sensation to touch. |

*Deep Tendon Reflexes*

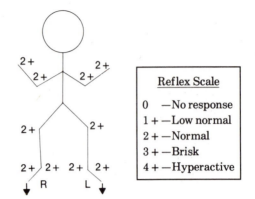

| Reflex Scale | |
|---|---|
| 0 | —No response |
| 1+ | —Low normal |
| 2+ | —Normal |
| 3+ | —Brisk |
| 4+ | —Hyperactive |

**Rectal/Perineum**

No loss of sphincter control, WNL, guaiac negative. Well healing 4+ episiotomy incision (to the rectum) noted.

**Genitalia**

Genitalia still somewhat swollen, but normal in appearance. Pelvic exam deferred; status postpartum; lochia: color—maroon, amount—scant

## Laboratory Data/Diagnostic Studies

**Laboratory Data**

*Status as of 9/10/89*
*Hct.* 30
*WBC.* 9.5/mm$^3$
*Hgb.* 10.3g/dl

*Toxic Screen*
*9/3/89.* Urine—cocaine = positive
*9/10/89.* Urine—cocaine = negative

## COLLABORATIVE PLAN OF CARE

**Therapeutic Measures**

Initial intake meeting, written contract established.
*Random Urines.* Taken for toxic screen. The urine must remain negative per contract or program could be extended. If unable to remain drug-free, inpatient hospitalization for detoxification mandated in order to break cycle of recurrent stimulant binges or of daily use.
*Group/Individual Counseling.* Regular attendance of support group and counseling sessions (initially recommended daily).
*Regular Self-Help Group Attendance.* Attendance of a 12-step program or similar self-help group recommended.

**Consults**

*Home Visits.* Visiting nurse to evaluate and assess home environment; assess and teach nutrition of mother and infant; postpartum course, including involution of the uterus, growth and development of the infant and signs and symptoms of the effects of cocaine use on the fetus during pregnancy. Teach parenting skills, including recognition of infant cues. Provide support and make referrals to community agencies when indicated.
*Social Worker.* Either a social worker or DSS worker to coordinate and monitor care of infant and mother. Collaborative

plan developed between outpatient facility and community resources to formulate a comprehensive drug rehabilitation program.

**Medications**                    Ferrous sulfate 1 tab (325 mg/tab) qd

# NURSING DIAGNOSES DEVELOPED IN CARE PLAN

Coping, Ineffective: Individual, p. 438
Parenting, Alteration in: Actual, p. 434
Self-Concept, Disturbance in: Self-Esteem, p. 431

# ADDITIONAL NURSING DIAGNOSES TO BE CONSIDERED

Altered Nutrition: Less than Body Requirements
Altered Thought Processes
Anxiety (Self Care; Parenting)
Bathing/Hygiene Self-Care Deficit
Bowel Elimination, Alteration in: Diarrhea
Breathing Pattern, Ineffective
Comfort, Alteration in
Family Coping: Potential for Growth
Fluid Volume Deficit, Potential
Grieving, Anticipatory
Health Maintenance, Alteration in
Home Maintenance Management, Impaired
Ineffective Family Coping: Compromised
Injury, Potential for
Knowledge Deficit (Self-Care; Parenting)
Mobility, Impaired, Physical
Noncompliance, Nonadherence to Therapeutic Regimen
Parenting, Alteration in: Actual or Potential
Self Concept, Disturbance in: Body Image
Sensory Perceptual, Alteration in
Sexual Dysfunction
Sleep Pattern Disturbance
Skin Integrity, Impairment of: Actual or Potential
Social Isolation
Violence, Potential for

# NURSING CARE PLAN BASED ON
# IDENTIFIED NURSING DIAGNOSES

| *Self-Concept, Disturbance in: Self-Esteem* | *Related to:* Pathophysiological — six-year history of drug abuse; situational — new single-parent status; maturational — adolescent and parent |
| --- | --- |
| | *Evidenced by:* Inconsistency in keeping prenatal appointments; destructive behavior to self and fetus by use of cocaine and alcohol while pregnant; and changing usual pattern of responsibility: new infant, single parenthood, changing relationships with peers and family. |

*Desired Patient Outcomes*

*The Patient Will:*
- Verbalize increased sense of self-esteem in ability to accomplish desired personal goals.
- Begin to assume role-related responsibilities, (i.e., health management for self and infant).
- Actively participate in the decision-making process in relation to statement of personal goals and development of treatment regimen.
- Maintain abstinence from all mood-altering chemicals.
- Identify feelings, strategies, and methods in development and reconstruction of positive perception of self.

*Evaluation Criteria*

*Upon Discharge, the Patient Will Be Able to Independently:*
- Maintain abstinence from all mood-altering chemicals and be "drug free"
- Regularly attend a 12-step program or similar self-help program
- Attend ongoing individual therapy sessions that are structured around a chemical-dependency program.
- Identify coping strategies that help to promote a "good feeling" about oneself and decrease dependence on mood-altering chemicals.
- Initiate participation in activities to attain personal goals, and make fundamental lifestyle changes needed to abstain from the use of mood-altering chemicals (e.g., exercise program, vocational program, educational program, a parenting program, pursuit of professional endeavors, and development of a support system).

## Interventions

Assess causative and contributing factors

Assess environmental system

Assess Behavioral system

Assess value/belief system

## Rationale

Rehabilitation is dependent upon the understanding and prediction of behavior (Thompson, 1986, p. 1814).

In determining peer use of drugs, peer approval drug use, and model for drug use, the nurse will be able to identify cues and make inferences necessary to understand past environmental influences, and help in the development of a treatment regimen (Semlitz and Gold, 1986, p. 468). Peer influences promote initial use of all drugs (Semlitz and Gold, 1986, p. 469).

Assessment of previous problem behaviors, such as use of cigarettes, other illicit drugs, alcohol, and engagement in minor delinquent acts, will help the nurse identify cues and make inferences necessary to understand past patterns of behavior, and help in development of a treatment regimen (Semlitz and Gold, 1986, p. 468).

Assessment of the patient's attitude, values, beliefs, and expectations will help in identification of cues and in making inferences necessary to understand past values and belief systems, and help in development of a treatment regimen (Semlitz and Gold, 1986, p. 468). A predisposition toward nonconformity, rebellion, and independence are intrapersonal characteristics with high correlation as precursors of drug use (Semlitz and Gold, 1986, p. 468).

| *Interventions* | *Rationale* |
|---|---|
| Assess family system | Assessment of the members of the family system, individually and collectively, including parental use of drugs, parent–child relationships (especially with respect to lack of closeness to parents), extended family, cultural factors, and parental value/belief system will help to establish cues and make inferences necessary to understand past influences within the family unit, and help in the development of a treatment regimen (Semlitz and Gold, 1986, p. 468). |
| Assess cognitive development | Low academic performance and motivation are important antecedents in drug abuse (Semlitz and Gold, 1986, p. 469). Understanding past influences will help in the development of a treatment regimen (Semlitz and Gold, 1986, p. 469). |
| Promote a positive sense of self through:<br>• Communication techniques<br>• Acceptance of the patient as a worthwhile, trusted human being who has intrinsic value<br>• Avoidance of a judgmental attitude<br>• Establishment of clear and consistent limits<br>• Flexibility in allowing for individual growth<br>• Listening | The nurse's attitude can hinder or facilitate the patient's adaptation to an alteration in self-concept (Carpenito, 1983, p. 392). Positive reinforcement is based on the principle of human behavior that any positive stimulus that follows a behavior or response strengthens that response (Travers, 1982, p. 30). The development of negative self-esteem is learned through repeated negative personal experiences. High self-esteem is correlated with parenting skills, management techniques, and consistent discipline, coupled with high parental interest in the child (Coon, 1980, p. 371). |
| Assist the patient in recognition, acceptance, and development of internal sense of self-esteem by promoting positive use of "I" statements. | "Self" can only be identified through subjective feelings. By designating the self with "I" pronouns, and identifying self rather than nonself ("he," "she," "we," "they") stronger emotions are produced and thus the sense of responsibility for one's own behaviors increases rather than diffusing onto other persons' actions (Thompson, et al, 1986, p. 1814). |
| Encourage recognition of strengths and positive experiences. | Nursing strategies involving repeated identification, development, and recognition of positive experiences over time (positive feedback) help the client to reconstruct an increased acceptance of self (Thompson, McFarland, Hirsch, Tucker, and Bower, 1986, p. 1817). |
| Facilitate the development of problem-solving strategies. | The nurse promotes expression of feelings, and helps the patient maintain a reality orientation. Once a problem is identified, the nurse facilitates the evaluation of possible outcomes and alternative solutions. Problem-solving reduces ambiguity and feelings of loss of control; the way back to health is a learning process (Wykle, 1983, p. 184). |
| Promote wellness/relapse-prevention strategies | Relapse-prevention techniques gradually reduce the external controls that are initially placed on the patient during abstinence, with the goal of facilitating the development of the abuser's internal control system (Gawin and Ellinwood, 1988, p. 1177). |
| Encourage the development of new interpersonal and social skills. | Rehabilitation of cocaine is difficult. The "rush" from the "high" is thought to be encoded into the cocaine abuser's memory, easily remembered through association with other environmental stimuli, (e.g., increased socialization and approximation with cocaine user friends, dealers, drug paraphernalia, and drug supplies) and |

| *Interventions* | *Rationale* |
|---|---|
| | places the patient in a high-risk situation with less probability to remain drug free) (Washton, 1986, p. 569). One common precipitant of relapse is unrealistic justification of occasional use of cocaine (Washton, 1986, p. 565). |
| Encourage development of behavior strategies as a response to conditioning factors in habitual drug cravings, extinguishing conditioned cues. | Urges to use cocaine can be sublimated with substitute behaviors such as vigorous exercising or talking with a support person (Washton, 1986, p. 568). |
| Teach recognition of early warning signals of relapse. | Teach the patient that use of rationalization and denial sets up the potential for a relapse (i.e., placing self in high-risk situations and developing overconfidence) (Washton, 1986, p. 569). |
| Encourage the demystification of the cocaine "high." | Increased susceptibility to relapse is perpetuated by remembering the pleasurable and good effects of cocaine rather than the adverse effects. The nurse facilitates strengthening memories of the negative consequences of abuse in order to counteract memories of drug euphoria (Washton, 1986, p. 569; Garwin and Ellinwood, 1988, p. 1177). |
| Prepare patient to cope with "abstinence violation effect" (AVE). | The patient experiences intense negative reactions (feelings concerned with guilt, personal weakness, profound failure, and helplessness) on using the drug after a stretch of abstinence. Negative reactions could increase chances of a second "slip", and progression to a complete relapse (Washton, 1986, p. 569). There is a potential for a patient to "slip" into a full relapse from a single use of cocaine if she or he does not view the "slip" as an isolated event, and a learning experience to be used to prevent future relapses. Patients are taught about AVE, the feelings that might be experienced, and how to cope with these feelings so that a "slip" does not become total destruction of the program (Washton, 1986, p. 569). |
| Teach stress reduction. | Stress-reduction teaching consists of developing a behavior modification program that helps the patient develop strategies for managing stimulant-associated temptation (i.e., vigorous exercise) (Washton, 1986, p. 570; Garwin and Ellinwood, 1988, p. 1177). The nurse must also recognize and share with the patient that a lifestyle without drugs is a major "loss," and that utilization of stress-management strategies helps the patient to develop adaptive coping skills. |
| Encourage the patient to participate in various treatment modalities in order to maintain successful abstinence (group or family therapy). | Group sessions provide positive role models and the peer support needed to counteract episodic re-emergence of stimulant cravings (Washton, 1986, p. 566; Garwin and Ellinwood, 1988, p. 1178). |
| Teach patient self-care, problem-solving strategies, and communication skills. | All responses are learned. Teaching appropriate responses and interactions help to strengthen, develop, and maintain a positive sense of self (Miles, 1986, p. 350). |

| *Parenting, Alteration in: Actual* | *Related to:* Intrauterine growth retardation of the fetus; use of cocaine; lack of support from putative father of the infant; lack of knowledge in parenting skills and behaviors; mother's unmet social and emotional needs. |
|---|---|

*Evidenced by:* Denial, rationalization, and lack of knowledge of the effects of cocaine on fetal development; inconsistencies in keeping appointments with primary health care providers; father left state prior to birth of the infant; verbalization of role inadequacy; lack of a father figure; increased stress, financial burdens, and lack of support during parent's childhood; plus low academic accomplishment (has not finished high school).

**Desired Patient Outcomes**

*The Patient Will:*
- Identify and resolve parenting problems resulting from cocaine abuse.
- Verbalize fears and needs related to own unmet social and emotional nurturing.
- Express realistic expectations regarding infant growth and development.
- Exhibit positive attachment behaviors to the infant (use positive statements in reference to the infant, assumes *enface* [face-to-face] *position*, initiate an active role in infant's care, express appropriate concerns, maintain consistency in health care of the infant with a primary caretaker, verbalizes problem-solving strategies as inconsistencies develop, and utilizes a support system).

**Evaluation Criteria**

*Upon Discharge, the Patient Will Be Able to:*
- Maintain continuity of health care for self and infant by keeping clinic appointments and by following prescribed treatment regimen including use of preventive health maintenance strategies (drug abstinence and "safe" sexual practices).
- Initiate positive parenting behaviors: offer age-appropriate amounts and types of food; provide appropriate verbal and tactile stimulation; provide age-appropriate toys; provide for scheduled rest periods for the infant; verbalize realistic expectations regarding infant's growth and development; demonstrate realistic perception of infant's growth and development; provide positive outlets for own recreation or relaxation; show initiative in attempts to manage infant's problems*; verbalize positive statements regarding mother-infant relationship.
- State strategies to cope with stress.
- Identify support system.
- Utilize existing support system appropriately.
- Continue to attend ongoing individual and group therapy sessions.
- Identify strengths and positive parenting experiences providing a foundation for the development and expansion of parenting skills.

(*Very important for plan to succeed)

**Interventions**

Assess causative and contributing factors.

**Rationale**

Planning, implementing, and evaluating health care involves assessment of every individual in the patient's family system (mother, father, grandmother, and infant) and how they interact as a family unit. The assumption is that family members are dependent upon each other for their physical, emotional, cognitive, and social needs (Sciarillo, 1980, p. 242). The family oper-

| *Interventions* | *Rationale* |
|---|---|
| | ates as a system, any problems with one member will affect all members (Johnson, 1986, p. 1). How well the family system functions individually and as a unit directly affects a child's well-being; each member's health status; the family as a unit; and, ultimately, their school and community environment (Pasternack, 1982, p. 16). |
| | Assessment provides a framework for objective appraisal and for the identification of mothers who need further assessment, either requiring medical or nursing care and supportive interventions (Pasternack, 1982, p. 16). |
| Assess attachment behaviors (maternal behavioral cues, verbal, visual, and tactile). | Attachment is an observable, active, sensual, specific, affective, reciprocal process between mother and infant. Attachment behaviors form the foundation of the dynamic relationship between parent and child that will ultimately nurture and develop the infant and the family system (Neeson and May, 1986, p. 1196). |
| Assess previous pregnancies and responses to the birthing process. | The mother's attitude about her pregnancy may influence her feelings about her infant; (factors that may be negative experiences can include an unplanned pregnancy; increased stress associated with the emotional, physical, or financial burden of the pregnancy; the presence or lack of substance abuse; and the presence or lack of a supportive person) (Cropley, 1986, p. 16). |
| Assess supportive system. | Assessment of the support system (nuclear family, extended family, friends, peers, and use of community resources, support groups, social agencies, institutions such as church or school) helps the nurse to ascertain who could help problem-solve and could support the mother in times of trouble (Miller, 1982, p. 19; Neeson and May, 1986, p. 1202). The assessment of the support system also provides information on unhealthy relationships that may contribute to high-risk situations. The patient will need support on how to recognize, avoid, and cope with high-risk situations that could contribute to poor parenting and eventual drug relapse (Washton, 1988, p. 34–38). The clinician must also keep in mind that parenting is a learned behavior. In general, people parent as they were parented (Carpenito, 1983, p. 319). |
| Assess cocaine use and its effect on the mother and infant. | The nurse should know that further research in this area is needed, therefore accurate assessment is essential (see Coping, Ineffective: Individual, p. 438; and Self-Concept, Disturbance in: Self-Esteem, p. 431). A parent who uses cocaine introduces a toxic substance into the system of the fetus or nursing infant, resulting in drug addiction of their child with possible physical and neurobehavioral sequelae (Rosecan, Spitz, and Gross, 1987, p. 307). |
| Assess preparation for childbearing and childrearing. | Assessment helps to predict patterns that assist the nurse recognizing in actual or potential adaptation problems to the birth of a new baby (i.e., lack of experience with infants, and positive and negative learned maternal behaviors) (Cropley, 1986, p. 19). |
| Assess growth and development of the infant. | Infants born to mothers who use cocaine may exhibit short stature, low birth weight, small head circumference, mild-to-moderate tremulousness, increased irritability, increased muscular rigidity (*hypertonic*), increased startle response, increased respiratory rate, increased heart rate, poor tolerance of oral feedings, diarrhea, and disturbed sleep patterns (Smith, 1988, p. 177). If the mother is a polydrug user, it can be difficult to discern |

| Interventions | Rationale |
|---|---|
| | which signs and symptoms are attributable to which drug. Some mothers use IV cocaine and heroin ("speedball"). Other mothers drink alcohol, smoke cigarettes, smoke marijuana, take "downers" (Librium, Valium), and take cocaine (IV, intranasal, or inhale). Recently, it has been noted that cocaine-addicted infants may have problems with "state control" or impairment in the organizational abilities of the infant, aversion of gaze from the caretaker's voice, difficulty engaging enface contact, difficulty consoling self, and lability of skin color (Chasnoff, et al, 1985, p. 668). |
| Assess parental learning needs in relation to self-care and infant care. | Many learning needs (i.e., nutrition, mother-and-infant hygiene, involution of the uterus, hormonal changes and emotions, recognition of infant cues, sleep/rest patterns, neonatal stimulation, infant safety, exercise, and contraception) must be met so that the new parent can effectively take care of herself, her infant, and the family unit (Neeson and May, 1986, pp. 925–926). |
| Provide a therapeutic environment (i.e., listen attentively, sit and talk with the patient, validate, offer feedback, promote trust, set limits, assist in goal setting, and evaluate). | The nurse needs to convey to the patient a nonjudgmental, sensitive, caring, attitude when asking questions. Questions need to be asked matter-of-factly to elicit information about needs and concerns regarding self-care and infant care, and the use of cocaine. In establishing such an atmosphere the nurse will be more likely to facilitate communication, and to obtain the needed information to make appropriate nursing interventions (Smith, 1988, p. 177; Neeson and May, 1986, p. 1187). |
| Observe parent–infant interactions. | Frequent assessment of parent–infant relationships is essential in identifying patterns of behaviors that place the parent–infant relationship at risk (Cropley, 1986, p. 32). Situations that contribute to potential or actual alteration in parenting are often related to ineffective individual or family coping (see Coping Ineffective: Individual p. 438) (Carpenito, 1983, p. 320). |
| Identify existing support system. | The nurse should encourage family members to use supports and resources already available to them. The critical aspect of self-care is the use of appropriate supportive resources during times of stress (Neeson and May, 1986, p. 1205). |
| Encourage the patient to identify current strengths and positive experiences in the parenting role. | The nurse needs to use all opportunities to help the parent discover and use her or his strengths. By facilitating the discovery of strengths in the patient, the nurse can help to foster a positive climate that increases the parent's functioning and self-esteem (Miles, 1986, p. 353). |
| Provide health and parent education in response to observed and established needs through mutual goal setting. | Mastering the basics of infant care requires information, reinforcement, practice, and feedback that is reciprocal between the parent and infant; and nursing activity that supports parental feelings and needs (Neeson and May, 1986, p. 1194). |
| Facilitate and coordinate access to and utilization of health and community resources as needed—the drug rehabilitation program and needed support systems should be the priority. | The nurse can help expand the knowledge base and support system of the parent (Neeson and May, 1986, p. 1203). |
| Evaluate the effects of nursing interventions and the need to revise plans or validate achievements. | Nursing efforts are needed to identify attainment of established patient goals, and the effectiveness of the nursing interventions in goal achievement or lack of goal achievement, and, if necessary, to revise the plan. |

| | |
|---|---|
| **Coping, Ineffective: Individual** | ***Related to:*** maturational crisis—young adult and parent-hood; personal vulnerability; knowledge deficit; problem-solving skills deficit; inadequate support system.<br>***Evidenced by:*** Verbalization of inability to cope; confusion of roles; destructive behavior toward self and infant; difficulty using problem-solving skills and decision-making skills. |
| **Desired Patient Outcomes** | ***The Patient Will:***<br>• Develop an awareness of own emotional and coping responses.<br>• Discuss coping mechanisms other than drugs to deal with stress of daily living and negative mood changes.<br>• Demonstrate ability to use healthful coping mechanisms (e.g., skills in problem-solving, decision-making, goal-setting, and relaxation) other than drugs to deal with stress of daily living and negative mood changes.<br>• Develop an awareness of own emotional reactions and coping responses.<br>• Maintain adequate health care for self and infant including use of preventive health strategies.<br>• Participate in clear realistic plans for long-term care.<br>• Evaluate coping responses in respect to goals, emotional responses, plans, and actions. |
| **Evaluation Criteria** | ***Upon Discharge, the Patient Will Be Able to:***<br>• Verbalize an awareness that avoidance of all mood-altering substances is a lifelong process and can only be maintained by a positive attitude and life-style changes.<br>• Verbalize an awareness of the warning signs of relapse.<br>• Verbalize feelings and thoughts regarding self in response to stressful situations.<br>• Demonstrate an ability to learn from occasional "slips" by formulating improved coping strategies and continuing with abstinence program (development of problem-solving skills).<br>• Actively participate in formulating realistic plans for self and infant (i.e., education, child care, health management for self and infant, financial management, home management, and professional or occupational advancement).<br>• Demonstrate an ability to use healthful responses when in actual stressful situations (development of decision-making skills).<br>• Regularly attend a 12-step program or similar self-help program and/or individual therapy.<br>• Participate in a parenting program.<br>• State increased positive statements about self and infant.<br>• Actively seek support at appropriate times. |

| Interventions | Rationale |
|---|---|
| Assess the degree of impairment. | In assessing the patient's functional health patterns, the nurse is able to move toward understanding the overall role-relationship pattern and the client's perceptions; use Gordan's (1982, pp. 82–110) functional health pattern assessment tool. |
| Develop a written treatment plan of care. | A written plan of care, or contract, provides a framework for evaluating interactions that occur between client and others, |

| *Interventions* | *Rationale* |
|---|---|
| | consistency amongst caretakers and family, individualization of patient needs, and maximizes individual strengths and resources (Washton, 1986, p. 566). |
| Set firm and consistent limits. | Establishment of boundaries provides predictability, clarification, reinforcement of roles and purposes, and facilitates coordinated efforts toward common goals (Phipps, Long, and Woods, 1983, pp. 117–118). |
| Reinforce positive social behaviors. | *Positive reinforcement* is when a reward or pleasant event follows an action, increasing the probability of the action happening again (Coon, 1980, p. 187 and p. 203). Examples of social behaviors to reinforce: discussing problems related to drug use, initiating a friendly conversation, keeping appointments, caring for self and infant, recognizing the reality of own behaviors, participating in group, and actively participating in problem-solving strategies. |
| Provide positive feedback on observed acceptable behaviors. | Positive feedback includes the social, verbal, and nonverbal responses (either real or perceived) that indicate acceptance of one person by another (Jensen and Bobak, 1985, p. 777). Positive feedback is a learning experience used to improve performance of the individual (Coon, 1980, p. 203). |
| Use cognitive restructuring to help the client become cognizant of unacceptable behaviors. | Constructively point out unacceptable behaviors (e.g., manipulation and "acting-out") and assist in development of an awareness between emotional response patterns and resulting behaviors. Awareness of unacceptable behaviors is the first step in the development of acceptable coping responses (Thompson, et al, 1986, p. 1896). |
| Promote positive sense of self. | See Nursing Diagnosis, Self-Concept, Disturbance in: Self-esteem, p. 431. |
| Allow the patient to express feelings. | Use of open-ended questions helps in eliciting the patient's thoughts and feelings. Spending time exploring the meaning of feelings with the patient helps the nurse ascertain the meaning of both verbal and nonverbal communications and allows for the development of adaptive coping strategies by utilizing strengths, interests, and abilities of the patient (Miles, 1986, p. 349). |
| Assist the patient with stress/anxiety reduction by use of concrete strategies (e.g., recreation, relaxation, and diversional activities). | See Nursing Diagnosis, Self-Concept, Disturbance in: Self-esteem, p. 431. |
| Promote wellness/relapse prevention strategies. | See Nursing Diagnosis, Self-Concept, Disturbance in: Self-esteem, p. 431. |

## QUESTIONS FOR DISCUSSION

1. What are the legal, ethical and moral issues that must be confronted during delivery of care to maternal substance abusers? a) Women's rights with respect to the rights of the unborn b) Should substance abusing mothers be prosecuted for child abuse? c) If substance abuse during pregnancy is a prosecutable offense, are other behaviors which may have adverse effects on the fetus also prosecutable?
2. What nursing observations might help detect a pregnant mother who is using cocaine?

3. What strategies will assist the mother in making her own decision to stop using cocaine?
4. What educational interventions motivate the pregnant substance abuser to quit the use of the drug?
5. Does physical dependence or psychological dependence cause the greater harm in perpetuating cocaine abuse?

# REFERENCES

Carpenito, LJ: Nursing Diagnosis: Application to Clinical Practice. JB Lippincott, Philadelphia, 1983.

Chasnoff, IJ, et al: Cocaine use in pregnancy. N Engl J Med 313(11):666–669, 1985.

Coon, D: Introduction to Psychology. West Publishing, New York, 1980.

Cropley, C: Assessment of Mothering Behaviors. In Johnson, SH: Nursing Assessment and Strategies for the Family at Risk—High-Risk Parenting. JB Lippincott, Philadelphia, 1986, pp. 15–40.

Garwin, FH and Ellinwood, EH: Cocaine and other stimulants: Actions, abuse, and treatment. N Engl J Med 318(18):1173–1182, 1988.

Garwin, FH and Kleber, H: Pharmacologic treatment of cocaine abuse. Psychiatr Clin North Am 9(3):573–574, 1986.

Gordan, M: Nursing Diagnosis. McGraw-Hill, New York, 1982, pp. 81–91.

Jensen, MD and Bobak, IM: Maternity and Gynecological Care. CV Mosby, Toronto, 1985.

Johnson, SH: Nursing Assessment and Strategies for the Family at Risk—High-Risk Parenting. JB Lippincott, Philadelphia, 1986.

Kunkel, DB: The toxic emergency, part I. Emerg Med 18(11):125–138, 1986.

Miles, MS: Counseling strategies. In Johnson, SH (ed): Nursing Assessment and Strategies for the Family at Risk—High-Risk Parenting. JB Lippincott, Philadelphia, 1986, pp. 343–360.

Miller, JR: Family structure and development. In Smith, MJ, et al (eds): Child and Family. McGraw-Hill, New York, 1982, pp. 17–37.

Millman, R: Evaluation and clinical management of cocaine abusers. J Clin Psychiatry 49(2):27–33, 1988.

Neeson, J and May, K: Comprehensive Maternity Nursing: Nursing Process and the Child Bearing Family. JB Lippincott, Philadelphia, 1986.

O'Brien, C, et al: Pharmacological and behavioral treatments of cocaine dependence: Controlled studies. J Clin Psychiatry 49(2):17–22, 1988.

Pasternack, SB: Conceptual Framework. In Smith, MJ, et al (eds): Child and Family. McGraw-Hill, New York, 1982, pp. 3–16.

Phipps, WJ, Long, BC, and Woods, NF: Medical Surgical Nursing. CV Mosby, Toronto, 1983.

Pollack, M, Brotman, A, and Rosenbaum, J: Cocaine abuse and treatment. Compr Psychiatry 30(1):31–44, 1989.

Ribadeneira, D: Cocaine—Boston's 'equal opportunity' drug. Boston Globe 233(135):1, 18, 1988.

Rosecan, JS, Spitz, HI, and Gross, B: Contemporary issues in the treatment of cocaine abuse. In Rosecan, JS and Spitz, HI (eds): Cocaine Abuse. Brunner/Mazel, New York, 1987, pp. 299–322.

Semlitz, L, and Gold, MS: Adolescent drug abuse: Diagnosis, treatment, and prevention. Psychiatr Clin North Am 9(3):455–474, 1986.

Sciarillo, WG: Using Hymovich's framework in the family-oriented approach. Maternal Child Nursing 5:242–248, 1980.

Smith, J: The dangers of prenatal cocaine use. Maternal Child Nursing 13:174–179, 1988.

Thompson, J, et al: Clinical Nursing. CV Mosby, Toronto, 1986.

Travers, JF: The Growing Child, ed 2. Scott, Foresman and Co, London, 1982.

Washton, AM: Nonpharmacologic treatment of cocaine abuse. Psychiatr Clin North Am 9(3):563–571, 1986.

Washton, AM: Preventing relapse to cocaine. J Clin Psychiatry 49(2):34–38, 1988.

Weiss, R: Relapse to cocaine abuse after initiating desipramine treatment. JAMA 260(17):2545–2546, 1988.

Wykle, M: Adaptive behavior. In Phipps, WJ, Long, BC, and Woods, NF (eds): Medical Surgical Nursing, ed 2. CV Mosby, London, 1983.

Zucherman, B, et al: Effects of maternal marijuana and cocaine use on fetal growth. N Engl J Med 320(12):762–768, 1989.

# BIBLIOGRAPHY

## Articles

Abramowicz, M (ed): Crack. The Medical Letter 28(718):69–72, 1986.

Bass, A: As cocaine use shifts, so does clientele. Boston Globe 233(139):8, 1988.

Baxter, J, et al: Localization of neurochemical effects of cocaine and other stimulants in the human brain. J Clin Psychiatry 49(2):23–26, 1988.

Cregler, L and Mark, H: Special report: Medical complications of cocaine abuse. N Engl J Med 315(23):1495–1500, 1986.

Fischman, M: Behavioral pharmacology of cocaine. J Clin Psychiatry 49(2):7–10, 1988.

Garwin, FH: Chronic neuropharmacology of cocaine: Progress in pharmacotherapy. J Clin Psychiatry 49(2):11–16, 1988.

Gomez, L: The history of cocaine: 1884–1984 from Freud to Delorean. Life pp. 56–67, 1984.

Kleber, H: Introduction to cocaine abuse: Historical, epidemiological, and psychological perspectives. J Clin Psychiatr 49(2):3–6, 1988.

Kunkel, DB: The toxic emergency, part II. Emerg Med 18(13):168, 170–173, 1986.

Madden, J, Payne, T, and Miller, S: Maternal cocaine abuse and effect on the newborn. Pediatr 77(2):209–211, 1988.

Pearsall, HR and Altesman, RI: Cocaine abuse. Hosp Med 126–139, 1987.

Spiehler, V: Cocaine and metabolites. Clin Chem News 24–26, 1986.

Ventura, WP: Cocaine use: Your choice now—no choice later. NSNA/Imprint 34–38, 1988.

Washton, AM: Preventing relapse to cocaine. J Clin Psychiatr 49(2):34–38, 1988.

## Books

Brenner, JH and Kostant, AR: Cocaine—The Drug That Fell From Social Grace. ARK Publications, Inc, Newton, Mass, 1986.

Gold, MS: 800-Cocaine. Bantam Books, New York, 1984.

Wilde, JL: The school-aged child. In Smith, MJ, et al (eds): Child and Family. McGraw-Hill, New York, 1982, pp. 267–290.

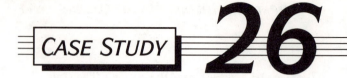
# AN ELDERLY PATIENT WITH DEPRESSION

J. Elaine Souder, Ph.D., R.N.,
Dorothy Bagnell Kelliher, M.S., R.N.

The term *depression* is commonly used to convey a wide range of mood states, from temporary unhappiness to life-threatening psychotic depression with suicidal intent. When used in the clinical sense, depression indicates a sustained lowering of mood, which is accompanied by alterations in cognitive, emotional, social, and physiological functioning. Depression is the most common mental disorder in the elderly.

There are a number of theories about the etiology of depression, including psychodynamic, behavioral, sociological, existential, and biological models. Conceptualization of depression from a particular perspective informs treatment decisions, and guides development of relevant research questions. There is a growing emphasis on neurobiological approaches to understanding and treating major mood disorders.

## ANATOMY AND PHYSIOLOGY OF DEPRESSION

The basic anatomic and functional unit of the central nervous system (CNS) is the neuron. The neuron contains a cell body, dendrites, and an axon. The cell body contains the nucleus and cytoplasm. The axon carries electric impulses from the cell body to other neurons. Dendrites permit electric messages to be conducted to the cell body. The basis of behavior is thought to lie with interneuronal and intraneuronal communication. This communication occurs by means of electric impulses along the neurons and between neurons by firing at the synapse. Transfer of information is dependent on neuronal integrity. The integrity of neurons may be altered due to the aging process (Blazer, 1982, p. 50).

Neurotransmitters are chemicals that permit electric impulses to be transmitted from an axon to the dendrite of an adjacent neuron at a structure known as the synapse. Neurotransmitters, particularly norepinephrine and serotonin, are believed to be involved in mood-regulating pathways of the brain (Brown and Mann, 1985, p. 142).

## PATHOPHYSIOLOGY OF DEPRESSION

Clinical depression is thought to be associated with altered biochemical processes at the synaptic sites in the neural pathways. It is unclear if the hypothesized biochemical alteration is the cause or consequence of altered mood. It is believed that neurotransmitter substances, specifically serotonin and norepinephrine, are decreased in clinical depression, leading to a decrease in neurotransmission. Norepinephrine is a catecholamine, found in the hypothalamus and brainstem, which is involved in CNS response to emergencies.

442

Serotonin, found in the pineal gland, the hypothalamus, and the raphe nuclei of the CNS as well as in other parts of the body, is synthesized from tryptophan and is implicated in sleep–wake cycles. Although the mechanisms of action differ with type of drug, all antidepressants produce an increase in one or more neurotransmitter substances (Brown and Mann, 1985, p. 144).

Depressive states may also be associated with hypersecretion of cortisol, and alterations in circadian rhythms.

## Classification System

Psychiatric clinicians use the well-known *Diagnostic Statistical Manual III-R* (DSM3-R) to classify depression and other psychiatric disorders. Specific criteria have been identified to describe bipolar affective disorder, major depression, dysthymia, and cyclothymia. *Bipolar disorder*, also know as *manic depressive illness*, is diagnosed by a history of at least 1 episode of manic behavior and usually distinct episodes of depression as well. In contrast, *cyclothymia* is a mood disorder characterized by clearly defined mood swings that are not as severe as manic depressive illness. *Dysthymia* is a persistent lowered mood state characterized by symptoms of depression that are not severe enough to meet the criteria for major depression.

A DSM3-R diagnosis of major depression requires that, in addition to either loss of interest or pleasure, or dysphoric mood, the individual has experienced 4 of the following criteria over the previous 2 weeks (American Psychiatric Association, 1987, p. 222):

• Poor appetite or significant weight loss
• Insomnia or hypersomnia
• Psychomotor agitation or retardation
• Fatigue, or loss of energy
• Feelings of worthlessness, or excessive guilt
• Recurrent thoughts of death, or suicidal ideation
• Complaints or impairment of cognitive abilities

Earlier classification systems utilized descriptive terminology (e.g., endogenous and exogenous, retarded or agitated, neurotic vs psychotic, reactive and involutional) to categorize depression. These terms have not provided a systematic organization for understanding depressive disorders, and are no longer in common use.

## Risk Factors

Across age groups, women have a higher incidence of reported depression than men. There has been some controversy as to whether this represents a true difference in incidence of depression or a difference associated with reporting. It has also been suggested that men may not seek treatment for depression as readily as women, or that men may self-medicate depression with alcohol.

Family history of affective disorders is a major risk factor for depression (Zarit, 1980, p. 197). Because older adults are not as likely to acknowledge psychiatric disorders as younger adults in today's society, assessment should be used to learn if parents, aunts, uncles, grandparents, or other family members have had a "breakdown," received "shock treatments," attempted suicide, or have had definite periods of dysfunction.

A third factor associated with depression in the elderly is losses (Zarit, 1980, p. 198). Losses may involve spouses, siblings, parents, children, or significant others. In addition, old age commonly brings loss of status, health, economic security, useful employment, and independence. The necessity to grieve fully for losses is essential to mental health. If grieving is denied, delayed, distorted, or dysfunctional, depression may result (Zarit, 1980, p. 241).

Polypharmacy is another risk factor implicated in depression in the elderly. A number of drugs commonly prescribed for conditions in the elderly are known to cause depression (e.g., antihypertensives, anti-inflammatory agents, and CNS depressants) (Salzman and Shader, 1978, p. 304).

It is important to search for physiological and organic etiologies of depression in the elderly because many overt and occult illnesses can cause mental depression. A thorough medical work-up is indicated before psychiatric intervention, particularly if there is no prior history of affective disturbance (Lazar and Karasu, 1980, p. 48).

Negative thought patterns and irrational beliefs about self, the world, and others may cause depression. Specific therapies to address this risk factor are well known and have proven effective in certain types of depression (Gallagher and Thompson, 1983, p. 168). Researchers and authors have also described a link between depression, stress, and alcoholism.

## COMMON CLINICAL FINDINGS

There is no definitive diagnostic test for depression, although the dexamethasone suppression test (DST) may be employed by some clinicians. Weight loss greater than 10 lb is common. Performance on psychological and cognitive testing may be impaired due to psychomotor retardation, difficulty in concentration, and motivational deficits.

Symptoms of depression may be grouped into several categories (Blazer, 1982, p. 23). Common emotional symptoms are sadness, loss of interest in the social environment, inability to experience pleasure (*anhedonia*), irritability, worry, emptiness, hopelessness, and helplessness. In addition to the cited symptoms, it is important when assessing a patient's emotional state to consider any deviations from the patient's *usual* emotional state. Cognitive symptoms in the depressed elderly person include "unwarranted pessimism" about the future, rumination about problems, delusions of uselessness, and suicidal thoughts or preoccupation with death. Delusions and hallucinations may be present in psychotic depression. Complaints about impaired memory and concentration are also common. Physical symptoms are very common among depressed elderly persons. Problems with the gastrointestinal tract are cited most frequently, although sleep difficulties are also common. Vegetative symptoms of depression include decreased appetite, weight loss, constipation, decreased libido, and fatigue. Diurnal variation and hypochondriasis are also common. Volitional symptoms include apathy, regression, withdrawal, decreased initiative and motivation, and suicidal impulses.

### COMPLICATIONS

The major concern in depression is that the patient may attempt or commit suicide. In addition, untreated depression may lead to physical deterioration due to self-neglect or a chronic depressive state. Depression in the elderly may be misdiagnosed as dementia (Archibald and Ullman, 1983, p. 49).

## TREATMENT MODALITIES

Treatment of depression consists of psychological and somatic therapies. Psychosocial interventions include supportive relationships, encouragement to grieve for losses, and structured meaningful activities. Psychotherapy can assist depressed individuals in verbalizing painful and negative feelings, working through losses, and learning more-effective ways to meet personal needs (Stuer, 1982, p. 195).

Somatic therapies are indicated in the presence of vegetative signs, anhedonia, history of depressive episodes, and positive family history of affective disorders. Somatic therapy includes antidepressants and electroconvulsive treatment (ECT). Antidepressants are categorized according to chemical structure, and fall into several broad categories (e.g., tricyclics, monamine oxidase inhibitors). Elderly individuals should be started on very low doses of antidepressant medication. ECT is particularly useful for agitated depression in the elderly patient with somatization, in suicidal depression, or in individuals who have had previous successful treatment with ECT (Lazar and Karasu, 1980, p. 53).

# PATIENT ASSESSMENT DATA BASE

## Health History

**Client:**
Mrs. Blue

**Address:** 229 Buckingham Place, Phoenix, Arizona
**Telephone:** (602) 331-0179
**Contact:** Robert Blue (son)
**Address of contact:** 165 South Erwin Drive, Austin, Texas
**Telephone of contact:** (512) 337-4088
**Age:** 71    **Sex:** Female    **Race:** White
**Educational background:** High school graduate
**Religion:** Presbyterian    **Marital status:** Widowed
**Usual occupation:** Retired secretary
**Present occupation:** Same
**Source of income:** Social security, modest retirement pension
**Insurance:** Medicare
**Source of referral:** Internist—Dr. Jacobs (who has followed Mrs. Blue's condition during her admission to Medical IV and who has arranged for her transfer to the Neuropsychiatric Unit)
**Source of history:** Patient
**Reliability of source:** Reliable
**Date of interview:** 2/2/89
**Reason for visit/Chief complaint:** "My bowels are turning to concrete, and they can't find anything wrong with me."

## HEALTH PERCEPTION/HEALTH MANAGEMENT PATTERN

**Present Health Status**

Mrs. Blue has been transferred from Medical IV to the Neuropsychiatric Unit following a negative workup for severe constipation and nausea of 3 months duration. When asked to describe her current health, she responds, "Something is wrong with my bowels—they're turning to concrete. But the tests didn't find the problem." Denies other health problems, though admits to fatigue and lethargy.

**Past Health Status**

**General Health.** Good.
**Prophylactic Medical/Dental Care** "If it ain't broke, don't fix it." Does not engage in routine preventive health care; states that she has dentures because she didn't take care of her teeth. Before current difficulty, last saw her physician 2 years ago when she had pneumonia.
**Childhood Illnesses** Measles, mumps.
Immunizations. Smallpox vaccination at age 6.
**Major illnesses** Denies any major illnesses, although was hospitalized for pneumonia 2 years ago following the flu; reports a hospitalization 12 years ago for phlebitis in her left leg.

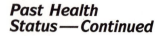

*Past Health
Status—Continued*

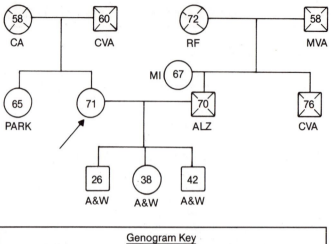

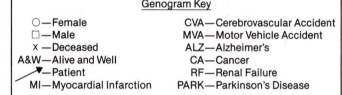

Genogram Key
○—Female
□—Male
X —Deceased
A&W—Alive and Well
—Patient
MI—Myocardial Infarction

CVA—Cerebrovascular Accident
MVA—Motor Vehicle Accident
ALZ—Alzheimer's
CA—Cancer
RF—Renal Failure
PARK—Parkinson's Disease

## NUTRITIONAL/METABOLIC PATTERN

*Nutritional*

Reports loss of interest in eating and anorexia secondary to gastrointestinal complaints. When asked about weight loss, admits that her weight has dropped from 130–115 lb (59–52.2 kg) over the past several months.

**Usual Daily Menu**
*Breakfast:*   orange or half grapefruit; tea with lemon.
*Lunch:*   ½ chicken sandwich on white bread.
*Snack:*   2 vanilla wafers and 4 oz whole milk.
*Dinner:*   2 oz sherry, 3 fish sticks, ½ c peas.
*Night Snack:*   4 oz warm prune juice.

*Metabolic*

Mrs. Blue has lost approximately 15 lb (6.8 kg) over the past 4 months.

## ELIMINATION PATTERN

*Bowel*

Normally has a daily bowel movement mid-morning following tea and a walk. However, for several months before admission has experienced severe constipation (bowel movement weekly) that has been responsive only to Ex-Lax.

*Bladder*

Voids without difficulty at 3–4 hour intervals while awake.

## ACTIVITY/EXERCISE PATTERN

*Activity/Exercise*

Usually takes a leisurely 20-minute walk in morning. Has discontinued this practice recently, citing fatigue and lack of interest. Mrs. Blue cares for her 6-room ranch house, and since her retirement 3 years ago, naps and watches television in the afternoon and evening hours.
*Self-Care Ability.* Mrs. Blue is usually able to care for her self and home activities, though recently acknowledges difficulty in doing usual household chores. Personal hygiene appears to be neglected.

*Self-Care Ability*

Feeding — 0

Bathing — II

Toileting — II

Bed mobility — 0

Dressing — 0

Grooming — II

General mobility — 0

Cooking — II

Home maintenance — II

Shopping — II

---

*Functional Levels Code*

  0 — Full self-care

  I — Requires use of equipment or device

  II — Requires assistance or supervision from another person

  III — Requires assistance or supervision from another person

      and equipment or device

  IV — Dependent and does not participate

---

**Oxygenation/Perfusion**

Chest x-ray on admission; experiences dyspnea on exertion — feels this is due to increasing fatigue; no paroxysmal dyspnea. No history of rheumatic fever or lung disease. EKG on this admission — no changes noted — medical doctor told her it was normal.

*Cardiac Risk Factors*

|  | Positive | Negative |
|---|---|---|
| Sedentary life-style |  | X |
| Hyperlipidemia |  | X |
| Cigarette smoking |  | X |
| Diabetes |  | X |
| Obesity |  | X |
| Hypertension | X |  |
| Hypervigilant personality |  | X |
| Family history of heart disease |  | X |

## SLEEP/REST PATTERN

**Sleep/Rest**

Normally has 6 hours of uninterrupted sleep, awakening at 5 AM. However, in the past several months reports frequent interruption in sleep and early morning awakening (EMA). Believes that she currently sleeps 2–3 hours each night. Wakens feeling sad and despairing.

## COGNITIVE/PERCEPTUAL PATTERN

**Hearing**

Experienced some difficulty hearing questions during nursing assessment and appeared reluctant to request that questions be repeated. Denies any hearing problems.

**Visual**

Vision corrected with bifocal lenses; eyes last checked 3 years ago.

**Sensory Perception**

Often feels cold. No other changes noted.

**Learning Style**

Alert and oriented to time, place, and person. Thought it was a different day of the week, explaining that she has not felt like reading a newspaper recently. States that she learns best by watching someone do something and finds it too tiring to read. Is right handed. Appears not to understand the implications of the negative work-up and her transfer to the psychiatric unit, stating "What tests do they have here for my bowel problems?" Recall of remote and past memory appears adequate. Can accurately identify information about hospitalization. Immediate recall of named objects is poor. Abstract thinking is impaired. When asked to explain the meaning of "Don't cry over spilled milk," responded, "The cows don't care."

## SELF-PERCEPTION/SELF-CONCEPT PATTERN

### Self-Perception/Self-Concept

Mrs. Blue describes herself as a quiet, hard-working woman who was devoted to her children and husband. Although employed as a secretary for a small plumbing firm for many years, she describes her work as "merely a job." As her children left home, her life focused increasingly on her husband. She reports that life feels very empty since her husband's death 1 year ago. Identifies successes in life as being a good wife. Currently feels a failure as a mother because her youngest son is "in trouble with the law." Declines to expand further on this disappointment.

## ROLE/RELATIONSHIP PATTERN

### Role/Relationship

Mrs. Blue describes receiving much satisfaction from her role as mother and wife. Her 3 children, now aged 42, 38, and 26, no longer live in the area, and her contact with them consists of occasional telephone calls, and visits at major holidays. Does not feel close to neighbors or friends. Her closest friend died several years ago. One has the sense that the death of her husband a year ago was a crucial loss.

## SEXUALITY/REPRODUCTIVE PATTERN

### Sexuality/Reproduction

Has 3 children from planned pregnancies; her children are of adult age. Reports regular sexual relations with her husband of many years. Since his death has no interest in "sexual matters."

## COPING/STRESS-TOLERANCE PATTERN

### Coping/Stress Tolerance

Describes her life as being relatively easy. However, admits difficulty in coping since husband's death last year. When asked to elaborate, states that she is very lonely and thinks of him continually. Expresses many pessimistic, hopeless, and helpless feelings about the future. Admits to frequent thoughts of dying, though denies any suicidal plan. States that she copes by watching television and by sleeping, but she is now having a lot of difficulty sleeping through the night.

## VALUE/BELIEF PATTERN

### Value/Belief

Mrs. Blue values traditional family structure, individual responsibility, and honesty. She is troubled particularly by frequent reports of crime and violence in the city and believes that she may leave for a safer area. Active involvement with her religion has provided much guidance and structure for her life, though she describes more recently receiving less comfort from her religious faith. Regarding medical care, she responded that she trusts her doctor because he is the expert and wants him to make decisions about her care.

## Physical Examination

A complete physical examination was done on admission to the medical unit. All findings were negative, including blood studies, thyroid function tests, and bowel work-up.

Mrs. Blue is to be transferred to the Neuropsychiatric Unit to rule out the diagnosis of a major depressive episode from one of uncomplicated bereavement.

## Mental Status Examination

**General Survey**

Mrs. Blue presented as a 69-year-old female, dressed in a food-stained hospital gown and her own ripped robe. She was transferred by wheelchair from a medical unit. She exhibited poor eye contact, flat-affect, hunched posture, a generally low activity level, and apathetic behavior.

**Speech**

Speech pattern was notable for slowness, hesitancy, low volume, and brief responses. Thought progression appeared logical though some blocking was evident.

**Emotional State**

Mood was depressed with constricted range of affect; was tearful at one point when discussing her relationship with her son.

**Thought Processes**

Pessimistic, hopeless, and helpless; admits to frequent thoughts of dying, denies any suicidal plan; interpretation of proverbs indicates disturbance in abstract thinking; seems preoccupied with the state of her bowels.

## Laboratory Data/Diagnostic Studies

**Laboratory Data**

*Red Blood Cell (RBC).* 3 million/mm$^3$
*Hematocrit (HCT).* 31%
*Free thyroxine (T$_4$).* 2.1 ng/dl
*Free Triiodthyromine (T$_3$).* 275 pg/100 ml
*Thyroid Stimulating Hormone (TSH).* 25. μIU/ml
*Thyroxine (Total T$_4$).* 10 μg/dl
*Blood Sugar.* 105 mg/100 ml

**Diagnostic Studies**

*Mini-mental State Exam.* 27/30
*Computed Axial Tomography (CAT) Scan (Head).* No evidence of tumor or pathologic activity.
*Magnetic Resonance Imaging (MRI).* No evidence of a cerebral mass or infarction.
*Abdominal Ultrasound.* No abdominal mass evident.
*Barium Enema.* Normal contour, filling, and rate of passage in the colon.
*Stool Guiaic.* Negative.

## COLLABORATIVE PLAN OF CARE

**Diet**

- Encourage fluids, fruits, bran, and vegetables.
- Offer 2 oz sherry before dinner daily.

**Medications**

- Nortriptyline 25 mg po, tid
- Halcion 0.125 mg po HS, prn × 14 days
- Metamucil 1 packet in juice q AM
- Milk of Magnesia 30 cc po HS prn
- Tylenol 650 mg po q 4–6 h prn

**Therapeutic Measures**

- Patient observation every 15 min
- Pulse, postural blood pressure readings tid
- Weigh every Monday in AM

- Maintain sleep record—discourage daytime sleeping
- Encourage patient to assume responsibility for grooming and hygiene

**Consults**
- Psychiatric social worker
- Occupational and recreational therapy consults
- Nutrition consult

# NURSING DIAGNOSES DEVELOPED IN CARE PLAN

Potential for Violence, Self-Directed, p. 451
Self-Esteem Disturbance p. 452
Social Isolation, p. 450

# ADDITIONAL NURSING DIAGNOSES TO BE CONSIDERED

Altered Thought Processes
Altered Nutrition: Less than Body Requirements
Bathing-Hygiene: Self-Care Deficit
Constipation
Diversional Activity Deficit
Dysfunctional Grieving
Hopelessness
Ineffective Individual Coping
Sleep Pattern Disturbance

# NURSING CARE PLAN BASED ON IDENTIFIED NURSING DIAGNOSES

| | |
|---|---|
| **Social Isolation** | **Related to:** Depressed mood, impaired hearing, life patterns. **Evidenced by:** Withdrawn behavior, absence of significant others, decreased number of social visits and phone calls. |
| **Desired Patient Outcomes** | **The Patient Will:** • Engage in meaningful social interactions. |
| **Evaluation Criteria** | **By Date of Discharge, the Patient Will:** • Express positive feelings about her interpersonal relationships on the unit. • Initiate social contact with a friend. • Identify a community group that she will contact upon discharge. |

## Interventions

Develop nurse–patient relationship and spend time with patient even if she does not talk.

Use touch deliberately when speaking with patient.

## Rationale

Spending time with a person demonstrates interest and is therapeutic when self-esteem is low (Townsend, 1988, p. 128).

Touch is an effective means of making contact with the elderly depressed individual (Blazer, 1982, p. 124).

## Interventions

Assess adequacy of social skills.

Teach social skills as needed by providing feedback, role plays, and discussion.

Provide acknowledgement and positive feedback for efforts.

Encourage participation in group work.

Consult social worker for appropriate community resources.

Explore possibility of getting a pet after discharge.

## Rationale

Lack of appropriate social skills may play a role in social isolation and depression (Zarit, 1980, p. 204).

Social skills are behaviors that can be learned (Zarit, 1980, p. 237).

Reinforcement encourages repetition of desired behavior (Townsend, 1988, p. 120).

Group work provides opportunities for socialization and the instilling of hope (Love, 1988, p. 1022).

Following discharge, involvement with community groups/agencies offers opportunities for social support and interaction (Mann and Graham, 1986, p. 158).

Pet therapy, if acceptable to the older adult, has been found to be helpful in alleviating feelings of loneliness (Haggard, 1985, p. 1375).

---

| | |
|---|---|
| **Potential for Violence, Self-Directed** | **Related to:** Dysfunctional grieving, depression, inadequate social network.<br>**Evidenced by:** Verbalization of hopelessness, references indicating wish to die. |
| **Desired Patient Outcome** | **The Patient Will:**<br>• Not harm self during hospitalization. |
| **Evaluation Criteria** | **By Date of Discharge, the Patient Will:**<br>• No longer acknowledge suicidal ideation.<br>• Be able to identify someone to contact should she feel hopeless.<br>• Make plans indicating a desire to live.<br>• Express feelings more appropriately.<br>• Demonstrate normal mood. |

---

## Interventions

Avoid extreme cheerfulness and "pep talks."

Assess suicide risk daily.

Check patient every 15 minutes.

## Rationale

Such attempts to cheer a depressed person may communicate that sad feelings are unacceptable (Janosik and Davies, 1986, p. 127).

Regular assessment of suicidal ideation is warranted during depression to determine changes in level of ideation (Rawlins and Heacock, 1988, p. 406).

Communicates caring, concern, and provides opportunity for ongoing assessment of mood and activity; minimizes opportunities for self-harm. This is particularly important in initial work with newly admitted depressed patient (Rawlins and Heacock, 1988, p. 406).

## Interventions

Develop a contract with patient that stipulates she will remain safe for the negotiated period of time and will contact staff if she feels like harming herself.

Renegotiate contract at regular intervals.

Remove potentially dangerous items from patient's belongings and environment.

Encourage verbalization and ventilation of feelings.

## Rationale

Communicates concern and shared responsibility for her safety and helps decrease chance of impulsive self-destructive acts (Rawlins and Heacock, 1988, p. 406).

Current feelings of depression and hopelessness may preclude long-term contract (Rawlins and Heacock, 1988, p. 406).

The responsibility for a safe environment is a major nursing priority in caring for depressed individuals (Rawlins and Heacock, 1988, p. 406).

Feelings of anger and frustration are thought to play a role in depression (Archibald and Ullman, 1983, p. 49).

---

**Self-Esteem Disturbance**

*Related to:* Lack of meaningful roles; feelings of abandonment by children and spouse.
*Evidenced by:* Lack of eye contact; not taking responsibility for self-care; inability to recognize own accomplishments.

**Desired Patient Outcome**

*The Patient Will:*
• Demonstrate feelings of self-worth.

**Evaluation Criteria**

*By Date of Discharge, the Patient Will:*
• Maintain good eye contact.
• Acknowledge positive aspects of self.
• Care for self independently.
• Communicate her needs in clear and assertive manner.

---

## Interventions

Spend time with patient.

Assist with activities of daily living (ADL)

Plan activities that utilize patient's skills and strengths.

Give "permission" to express negative feelings.

Encourage discussion of past events and accomplishments.

Recognize efforts to assume responsibility for personal hygiene and care.

## Rationale

This action communicates caring and demonstrates that the individual is worth your time (Townsend, 1988, p. 123).

Appearance affects sense of self-worth. Nursing assistance conveys sense of caring (Archibald and Ullman, 1983, p. 50).

Successful activities will increase self-esteem (Townsend, 1988, p. 123).

Verbalization of anger, sadness, and frustration will facilitate grieving and resolution of losses (Archibald and Ullman, 1983, p. 51).

Reminiscence allows life review and acknowledgement of important roles (Ebersole, 1976, p. 1304).

Consistent encouragement and reinforcement increases the likelihood that patient will continue to care for self (Archibald and Ullman, 1983, p. 51).

# QUESTIONS FOR DISCUSSION

1. What factors contribute to the high incidence of depression in the elderly population?
2. Identify the signs and symptoms of depression. How does depression in elderly persons differ from depression in younger individuals?
3. What verbal and nonverbal clues may suggest suicidal intent?
4. What is the nurse's role when an individual is receiving a tricyclic antidepressant?
5. What are the nursing responsibilities in caring for a depressed individual receiving ECT?
6. What changes in the care plan would be made for an acutely suicidal patient?

# REFERENCES

American Psychiatric Association: Diagnostic and Statistical Manual of Mental Disorders. American Psychiatric Association, Washington, DC, 1987.

Archibald, JW and Ullman, MA: Is it really senility or just depression. RN November:46, 49–51, 1983.

Brown, RP and Mann, JJ: A clinical on the role of neurotransmitters in mental disorders. Hospital Community Psychiatry 36(2):141–149, 1985.

Ebersole, P: Reminiscing. Am J Nurs 76(8):1304–1305, 1976.

Gallagher, D and Thompson, LW: Cognitive therapy for depression in the elderly: A promising model for treatment and research. In Breslau, DC and Haug, MR (eds): Depression and Aging. Springer, New York, 1983, p. 168.

Haggard, A: A patient's best friend. Am J Nurs 85(12):1375–1376, 1985.

Janosik, EH and Davies, JL: Psychiatric Mental Health Nursing. Jones and Bartlett, Boston, 1986.

Lazar, I and Karasu, TB: Evaluation and management of depression in the elderly. Geriatrics 35(12):47–53, 1980.

Love, C: Applying the nursing process with the elderly. In Wilson, HS and Kneisl, CR: Psychiatric Nursing, ed 3. Addison-Wesley, Reading, Mass, 1988, p. 1022.

Mann, AH and Graham, N: Management of depression of the elderly at home. Churchill Livingston, New York, 1986.

Rawlins, RP and Heacock, PE: Clinical Manual of Psychiatric Nursing. CV Mosby, St. Louis, 1988.

Salzman, C and Shader, RI: Depression in the elderly, Part II. Possible drug etiologies: Differential diagnostic criteria. J Am Geriatr Soc 26(7), 1978.

Stever, J: Psychotherapy for depressed elders. In Blazer, D (ed): Depression in Late Life. CV Mosby, St. Louis, 1982, p. 195.

Townsend, MC: Nursing diagnosis in psychiatric nursing. Philadelphia, FA Davis, 1988.

Zarit, SH: Aging and mental disorders. New York, Free Press, 1980.

# BIBLIOGRAPHY

Akisal, H and McKinney, WT: Overview on recent research on depression: Integration of ten conceptual models into a comprehensive clinical frame. Arch Gen Psychiatry 32:285–304, 1975.

Beck, CK, Rawlins, RP, and Williams, SR: Mental Health—Psychiatric Nursing. CV Mosby, St. Louis, 1988.

Chaisson, GM, et al: Treating the depressed elderly client. J Psychosoc Ment Health 22(5):25–30, 1984.

Murphy, E: Affective disorders in the elderly. London, Churchill Livingston, 1986.

Pierre, J, Craven, RF, and Bruno, P: Late life depression: Guide for assessment. J Gerontol Nurs 12(7):5–10, 1986.

# BIBLIOGRAPHY

*Anatomy, Physiology, and Pathophysiology*

Carrieri, VK, et al: Pathophysiological Phenomena in Nursing: Human Response to Illness. WB Saunders, Philadelphia, 1986.

Guyton, AC: Textbook of Medical Physiology, ed 7. WB Saunders, Philadelphia, 1987.

Hole, JW, Jr.: Human Anatomy and Physiology, ed 4. WC Brown, Dubuque, IA, 1987.

Porth, C: Pathophysiology: Concepts of Altered Health States, ed 2. JB Lippincott, Philadelphia, 1986.

Price, SA and Wilson, LM: Pathophysiology: Clinical Concepts of Disease Processes, ed 3. McGraw-Hill, New York, 1986.

Thibodeau, GA: Anatomy and Physiology. CV Mosby, St. Louis, 1987.

Tortora, GJ and Anagnostakos, NP: Principles of Anatomy and Physiology, ed 5. Harper & Row, New York, 1986.

*Community Health Nursing*

Clemen-Stone, S, et al: Comprehensive Family and Community Health Nursing, ed 2. McGraw-Hill, New York, 1987.

Jarvis, LL: Community Health Nursing: Keeping the Public Healthy, ed 2. FA Davis, Philadelphia, 1985.

Logan, BB and Dawkins, CE: Family-Centered Nursing in the Community. Addison-Wesley, Menlo Park, CA, 1986.

Pender, NJ: Health Promotion in Nursing Practice, ed 2. Appleton & Lange, Norwalk, CT, 1987.

Stanhope, M and Lancaster, J: Community Health Nursing: Process and Practice for Promoting Health, ed 2. CV Mosby, St. Louis, 1988.

*Critical Care Nursing*

Alspach, JG and Williams, SM: Core Curriculum for Critical Care Nursing, ed 3. WB Saunders, Philadelphia, 1985.

Dolan, JT: Critical Care Nursing: Clinical Management through the Nursing Process. FA Davis, Philadelphia, in preparation.

Holloway, NM: Nursing the Critically Ill Adult, ed 3. Addison-Wesley, Menlo Park, CA, 1988.

Hudak, CM, et al: Critical Care Nursing: A Holistic Approach, ed 4. JB Lippincott, Philadelphia, 1986.

Kenner, CV, et al: Critical Care Nursing: Body, Mind, Spirit, ed 2. Little, Brown, Boston, 1985.

Moorhouse, MF, et al: Critical Care Plans: Guidelines for Patient Care. FA Davis, Philadelphia, 1987.

*Fundamentals of Nursing*

Kozier, B and Erb, G: Fundamentals of Nursing: Concepts and Procedures, ed 3. Addison-Wesley, Menlo Park, CA, 1987.

Kozier, B and Erb, G: Techniques in Clinical Nursing: A Nursing Process Approach. Addison-Wesley, Menlo Park, CA, 1987.

Perry, AG and Potter, PA: Clinical Nursing Skills and Techniques: Basic, Intermediate, and Advanced. CV Mosby, St. Louis, 1986.

Potter, PA and Perry, AG: Basic Nursing: Theory and Practice. CV Mosby, St. Louis, 1987.

Potter, PA and Perry, AG: Fundamentals of Nursing: Concepts, Process, and Practice, ed 2. CV Mosby, St. Louis, 1989.

Sorensen, KC and Luckmann, J: Basic Nursing: A Psycho-physiologic Approach, ed 2. WB Saunders, Philadelphia, 1986.

*Health Assessment*

Bates, B: A Guide to Physical Examination and History Taking, ed 4. JB Lippincott, Philadelphia, 1987.

Bowers, AC and Thompson, JM: Clinical Manual of Health Assessment, ed 3. CV Mosby, St. Louis, 1988.

Malasanos, L, et al: Health Assessment, ed 3. CV Mosby, St. Louis, 1986.

Seidel, HM, et al: Mosby's Guide to Physical Examination. CV Mosby, St. Louis, 1987.

*Maternity Nursing*

Bobak, IM and Jensen, MD: Essentials of Maternity Nursing: The Nurse and the Childbearing Family, ed 2. CV Mosby, St. Louis, 1987.

Doenges, ME, et al: Maternal/Newborn Care Plans: Guidelines for Client Care. FA Davis, Philadelphia, 1988.

Malinowski, JS: Nursing Care during the Labor Process, ed 3. FA Davis, Philadelphia, 1989.

Neeson, JD: Clinical Manual of Maternity Nursing. JB Lippincott, Philadelphia, 1987.

Neeson, JD and May, KA: Comprehensive Maternity Nursing. JB Lippincott, Philadelphia, 1986.

Olds, SB, et al: Maternal-Newborn Nursing: A Family-Centered Approach, ed 3. Addison-Wesley, Menlo Park, CA, 1988.

Reeder, SJ, et al: Maternity Nursing, ed 16. JB Lippincott, Philadelphia, 1987.

*Medical-Surgical Nursing*

Brunner, LS and Suddarth, DS: Textbook of Medical-Surgical Nursing, ed 6. JB Lippincott, Philadelphia, 1988.

Cella, JH and Watson, J: Nurse's Manual of Laboratory Tests. FA Davis, Philadelphia, 1989.

Fischbach, FT: A Manual of Laboratory Diagnostic Tests, ed 3. JB Lippincott, 1988.

Kneisl, CR and Ames, SW: Adult Health Nursing: A Biopsychosocial Approach. Addison-Wesley, Menlo Park, CA, 1986.

Lewis, S: Medical-Surgical Nursing: Assessment and Management of Clinical Problems, ed 2. McGraw-Hill, New York, 1987.

Luckmann, J and Sorensen, KC: Medical-Surgical Nursing: A Psychophysiologic Approach, ed 3. WB Saunders, Philadelphia, 1987.

Patrick, ML, et al: Medical-Surgical Nursing: Pathophysiological Concepts. JB Lippincott, Philadelphia, 1986.

Phipps, WJ, et al: Medical-Surgical Nursing: Concepts and Clinical Practice, ed 3. CV Mosby, St. Louis, 1986.

*Nursing Process/Nursing Diagnoses*

Alfaro, RA: Application of Nursing Process: A Step-by-Step Guide to Care Planning. JB Lippincott, Philadelphia, 1986.

Bulechek, GM and McCloskey, JC: Nursing Interventions: Treatments for Nursing Diagnoses. WB Saunders, Philadelphia, 1985.

Carpenito, LJ: Handbook of Nursing Diagnosis 1989–90. JB Lippincott, Philadelphia, 1989.

Carpenito, LJ: Nursing Diagnosis: Application to Clinical Practice, ed 2. JB Lippincott, Philadelphia, 1987.

Doenges, ME and Moorhouse, MF: Nurse's Pocket Guide:

Nursing Diagnoses with Interventions, ed 2. FA Davis, Philadelphia, 1988.

Doenges, ME, et al: Nursing Care Plans: Guidelines for Planning Patient Care, ed 2. FA Davis, Philadelphia, 1989.

Gettrust, KV: Applied Nursing Diagnosis: Guides for Comprehensive Care Planning. John Wiley, New York, 1985.

Gordon, M: Manual of Nursing Diagnosis 1988–1989. CV Mosby, St. Louis, 1989.

Gordon, M: Nursing Diagnosis: Process and Application, ed 2. McGraw-Hill, New York, 1987.

Iyer, PW, et al: Nursing Process and Nursing Diagnosis. WB Saunders, Philadelphia, 1986.

Kim, MJ, et al: Pocket Guide to Nursing Diagnoses, ed 3. CV Mosby, St. Louis, 1989.

Ulrich, S, et al: Nursing Care Planning Guides: A Nursing Diagnosis Approach. WB Saunders, Philadelphia, 1986.

*Nutrition*

Dudek, SG: Nutrition Handbook for Nursing Practice. JB Lippincott, Philadelphia, 1987.

Lewis, CM: Nutrition and Nutritional Therapy in Nursing. Appleton & Lange, Norwalk, CT, 1985.

Robinson, CH: Normal and Therapeutic Nutrition, ed 17. MacMillan, New York, 1986.

Stanfield, P and Hui, YH: Nutrition and Diet Therapy: Self-Instruction Modules. Jones & Bartlett, Boston, 1986.

*Pediatric Nursing*

Foster, RLR, et al: Family-Centered Nursing Care of Children. WB Saunders, Philadelphia, 1989.

James, SR: Child Health Nursing: Essential Care of Children and Families. Addison-Wesley, Menlo Park, CA, 1988.

Marlow, DR and Redding, BA: Textbook of Pediatric Nursing, ed 6. WB Saunders, Philadelphia, 1988.

Mott, SR, et al: Nursing Care of Children and Families: A Holistic Approach. Addison-Wesley, Menlo Park, CA, 1985.

Whaley, LF and Wong, DL: Essentials of Pediatric Nursing, ed 3. CV Mosby, St. Louis, 1988.

Whaley, LF and Wong, DL: Nursing Care of Infants and Children, ed 3. CV Mosby, St. Louis, 1986.

*Pharmacology*

Baer, C and Williams, B: Clinical Pharmacology and Nursing. Springhouse Corp, Springhouse, PA, 1988.

Clark, JB, et al: Pharmacological Basis of Nursing Practice, ed 2. CV Mosby, St. Louis, 1986.

Deglin, JH and Vallerand, AH: Davis's Drug Guide for Nurses. FA Davis, Philadelphia, 1988.

Govoni, L and Hayes, J: Drugs and Nursing Implications, ed 6. Appleton & Lange, Norwalk, CT, 1988.

Malseed, RT and Harrigan, GS: Textbook of Pharmacology and Nursing Care: Using the Nursing Process. JB Lippincott, Philadelphia, 1989.

Mathewson, MK: Pharmacotherapeutics: A Nursing Process Approach. FA Davis, Philadelphia, 1986.

McHenry, LM and Salerno, E: Mosby's Pharmacology in Nursing, ed 17. CV Mosby, St. Louis, 1989.

Shlafer, M and Marieb, EN: The Nurse, Pharmacology, and Drug Therapy. Addison-Wesley, Menlo Park, CA, 1989.

Spencer, RT, et al: Clinical Pharmacology and Nursing Management, ed 2. JB Lippincott, Philadelphia, 1986.

*Psychiatric/Mental Health Nursing*

Beck, CK, et al: Mental Health-Psychiatric Nursing: A Holistic Life-Cycle Approach, ed 2. CV Mosby, St. Louis, 1988.

Diagnostic and Statistical Manual of Mental Disorders, ed 3, revised. American Psychiatric Association, Washington, DC, 1987.

Doenges, ME, et al: Psychiatric Care Plans: Guidelines for Client Care. FA Davis, Philadelphia, 1989.

Johnson, BS: Psychiatric-Mental Health Nursing: Adaptation and Growth, ed 2. JB Lippincott, Philadelphia, 1989.

Stuart, GW and Sundeen, SJ: Principles and Practice of Psychiatric Nursing, ed 3. CV Mosby, St. Louis, 1987.

Townsend, MC: Nursing Diagnoses in Psychiatric Nursing: A Pocket Guide for Care Plan Construction. FA Davis, Philadelphia, 1988.

Wilson, HS and Kneisl, CR: Psychiatric Nursing, ed 3. Addison-Wesley, Menlo Park, CA, 1988.

# Appendix A:
# Classification of NANDA Nursing Diagnoses by Gordon's Functional Health Patterns *

Health Perception-Health Management Pattern
   Health maintenance, altered
   Noncompliance (specify)
   Infection, potential for
   Injury, potential for
   Injury, potential for: trauma
   Injury, potential for: poisoning
   Injury, potential for: suffocating
Nutritional-Metabolic Pattern
   Nutrition, altered: potential for more than body requirements
   Nutrition, altered: more than body requirements
   Nutrition, altered: less than body requirements
   Swallowing, impaired
   Tissue integrity, impaired: oral mucous membrane
   Fluid volume deficit: potential
   Fluid volume deficit: actual (1)
   Fluid volume deficit: actual (2)
   Fluid volume excess
   Skin integrity, impaired: potential
   Skin integrity, impaired: actual
   Tissue integrity, impaired
   Body temperature, altered: potential
   Thermoregulation, ineffective
   Hyperthermia
   Hypothermia
Elimination Pattern
   Bowel elimination, altered: constipation
   Bowel elimination, altered: diarrhea
   Bowel elimination, altered: incontinence
   Urinary elimination, altered patterns
   Incontinence, functional
   Incontinence, reflex
   Incontinence, stress
   Incontinence, urge
   Incontinence, total
   Urinary retention
Activity-Exercise Pattern
   Activity intolerance: potential
   Activity intolerance
   Mobility, impaired physical
   Self-care deficit: bathing/hygiene
   Self-care deficit: dressing/grooming
   Self-care deficit: feeding
   Self-care deficit: toileting
   Diversional activity, deficit
   Home maintenance management, impaired
   Airway clearance, ineffective
   Breathing pattern, ineffective

   Gas exchange, impaired
   Cardiac output, altered: decreased
   Tissue perfusion, altered: renal, cerebral, cardiopulmonary, gastrointestinal, peripheral
   Growth and development, altered
Sleep-Rest Pattern
   Sleep pattern disturbance
Cognitive-Perceptual Pattern
   Comfort, altered: pain
   Comfort, altered: chronic pain
   Sensory/perceptual alterations: visual, auditory, kinesthetic, gustatory, tactile, olfactory
   Unilateral neglect
   Knowledge deficit (specify)
   Thought processes, altered
Self-Perception-Self-Concept Pattern
   Fear
   Anxiety
   Hopelessness
   Powerlessness
   Self-concept, disturbance in: body image
   Self-concept, disturbance in: personal identity
   Self-concept, disturbance in: self-esteem
Role-Relationship Pattern
   Grieving, anticipatory
   Grieving, dysfunctional .
   Role performance, altered
   Social isolation
   Social interaction, impaired
   Family processes, altered
   Parenting, altered: potential
   Parenting, altered: actual
   Communication, impaired verbal
   Violence, potential for: self-directed or directed at others
Sexuality-Reproductive Pattern
   Sexual dysfunction
   Sexuality, altered patterns
   Rape trauma syndrome
   Rape trauma syndrome: compound reaction
   Rape trauma syndrome: silent reaction
Coping-Stress Tolerance Pattern
   Coping, ineffective individual
   Adjustment, impaired
   Post-trauma response
   Coping, family: potential for growth
   Coping, ineffective family: compromised
   Coping, ineffective family: disabled
Value-Belief Pattern
   Spiritual distress (distress of the human spirit)

*Based on Gordon, M.: Nursing Diagnosis: Process and Applications. McGraw-Hill, New York, ed 2, 1987, with permission.

# Appendix B:
## DOENGES' DIAGNOSTIC DIVISIONS

**ACTIVITY/REST**
Activity intolerance
Activity intolerance, potential
Disuse syndrome, potential for
Diversional activity deficit
Fatigue
Sleep pattern disturbance

**CIRCULATION**
Cardiac output, altered: decreased
Dysreflexia
Tissue perfusion, altered: (specify)

**EGO INTEGRITY**
Adjustment, impaired
Anxiety [specify]
Coping, defensive
Coping, ineffective individual
Decisional conflict (specify)
Denial, ineffective
Fear
Grieving, anticipatory
Grieving, dysfunctional
Hopelessness
Post-trauma response
Powerlessness
Rape trauma syndrome
Self-concept, disturbance in: body image; personal identity; role performance; self-esteem
Self-esteem, chronic low
*Self-esteem, disturbance in
Self-esteem, situational low
Spiritual distress (distress of the human spirit)

**ELIMINATION**
Bowel elimination, altered: constipation
Constipation, colonic
Constipation, perceived
Bowel elimination, altered: diarrhea
Bowel elimination, altered: incontinence
Incontinence, functional
Incontinence, reflex
Incontinence, stress
Incontinence, total
Incontinence, urge
Urinary elimination: altered patterns
Urinary retention [acute/chronic]

**FOOD/FLUID**
Breastfeeding, ineffective
Fluid volume, altered: excess
Fluid volume deficit, actual 1 [regulatory failure]
Fluid volume deficit, actual 2 [active loss]
Fluid volume deficit, potential
Nutrition, altered: less than body requirements
Nutrition, altered: more than body requirements
Nutrition, altered: potential for more than body requirements

*Revised.

Oral mucous membranes, altered
Swallowing, impaired

**HYGIENE**
Self-care deficit: feeding; bathing/hygiene; dressing/grooming; toileting

**NEUROSENSORY**
Neglect, unilateral
Sensory-perceptual alteration: visual; auditory; kinesthetic; gustatory; tactile; olfactory
Thought processes, altered

**PAIN/COMFORT**
Comfort, altered: pain, acute
Comfort, altered: pain, chronic

**RESPIRATION**
Airway clearance, ineffective
Aspiration, potential for
Breathing pattern, ineffective
Gas exchange, impaired

**SAFETY**
Body temperature, potential altered
Health maintenance, altered
Home maintenance management, impaired
Hyperthermia
*Hypothermia
Infection, potential for
Injury, potential for: poisoning; suffocation; trauma
Mobility, impaired physical
Skin integrity, impaired: actual
Skin integrity, impaired: potential
Thermoregulation, ineffective
Tissue integrity, impaired
Violence, potential for: directed at self/others

**SEXUALITY (Component of Social Interaction)**
Sexual dysfunction
Sexuality patterns, altered

**SOCIAL INTERACTION**
Communication, impaired: verbal
Coping, family: potential for growth
Coping, ineffective family: compromised
Coping, ineffective family: disabling
Family process, altered
Parental role conflict
Parenting, altered: actual or potential
Self-concept, disturbance in: role performance
Social interaction, impaired
Social isolation

**TEACHING/LEARNING**
Growth and development, altered
Health seeking behaviors (specify)
Knowledge deficit [learning need] (specify)
Noncompliance [compliance, altered] (specify)

# Appendix C:
# MEDICAL/SURGICAL ASSESSMENT TOOL

EXCERPTED FROM **DOENGES, MOORHOUSE, AND GEISSLER**
NURSING CARE PLANS, EDITION 2, © 1989 F. A. DAVIS COMPANY

This Medical/Surgical Assessment Tool can be used to create a patient data base organized by Diagnostic Divisions with related Nursing Diagnoses. Using this tool will allow the nurse to *individualize* the Patient Assessment Data Base included with each of the 92 prototype care plans in *Nursing Care Plans: Guidelines for Planning Patient Care.** As necessary, Diagnostic Divisions, with their associated nursing diagnoses, may be added to or deleted from the Patient Assessment Data Base presented for each care plan, thus permitting the nurse to *tailor* the care plan to meet the particular needs of each patient.

*This Assessment Tool is also included on page 14.

Name: _____

Age: _____ DOB: _____ Sex: _____ Race: _____

Admission date: _____ Time: _____ From: _____

Source of information: _____ Reliability (1–4): _____

Family member/Significant other: _____

## ACTIVITY/REST

### Reports (Subjective)

Occupation: _____ Usual activities/Hobbies: _____

Leisure time activities: _____

Complaints of boredom: _____

Limitations imposed by condition: _____

Sleep: Hours: _____ Naps: _____ Aids: _____

    Insomnia: _____ Related to: _____

    Rested upon awakening: _____

### Exhibits (Objective)

Observed response to activity: Cardiovascular: _____

                           Respiratory: _____

Mental status (i.e., withdrawn/lethargic): _____

Neuromuscular assessment:

    Muscle mass/tone: _____

    Posture: _____ Tremors: _____

    ROM: _____ Strength: _____

    Deformity: _____ Other: _____

## CIRCULATION

### Reports (Subjective)

History of: Hypertension: _____ Heart trouble: _____

         Rheumatic fever: _____ Ankle/leg edema: _____

         Phlebitis: _____ Slow healing: _____

         Claudication: _____ Other: _____

Extremities: Numbness: _____Tingling: _____

Cough/hemoptysis: _____

Change in frequency/amount of urine: _____

### Exhibits (Objective)

BP: R: Lying: _____ Sitting: _____ Standing: _____

    L: Lying: _____ Sitting: _____ Standing: _____

    Pulse pressure: _____ Ausculatory gap: _____

Pulse (palpation): Carotid: _____ Temporal: _____

                Jugular: _____ Radial: _____

                Femoral: _____ Popliteal: _____

                Post Tibial: _____ Dorsalis pedis: _____

*459*

Cardiac (palpation): PMI: _____
    Thrill: _____ Heaves: _____
Heart sounds:  Rate: _____ Rhythm: _____ Quality: _____
    Friction rub: _____ Murmur: _____
Breath sounds: _____
Vascular bruit: (specify): _____
Jugular vein distention: _____
Extremities:  Temperature: _____ Color: _____
    Capillary refill: _____
    Homan's sign: _____ Varicosities: _____
    Nails (describe abnormalities): _____
    Distribution/quality of hair: _____
Color/cyanosis: Overall: _____ Mucous membranes: _____ Lips: _____
    Nail beds: _____ Conjunctiva: _____ Sclera: _____

## EGO INTEGRITY

### Reports (Subjective)

Report of stress factors: _____ ____
Ways of handling stress: _____
Financial concerns: _____
Relationship status: _____
Cultural factors: _____
Religion: _____ Practicing: _____
Lifestyle: _____ Recent changes: _____
Feelings of:  Helplessness: _____ Hopelessness: _____
    Powerlessness: _____

### Exhibits (Objective)

Emotional status (check those that apply):
    Calm: _____ Anxious: _____ Angry: _____
    Withdrawn: _____ Fearful: _____ Irritable: _____
    Restive: _____ Euphoric: _____ Other (specify): _____
Observed physiologic response(s): _____

## ELIMINATION

### Reports (Subjective)

Usual bowel pattern: _____ Laxative use: _____
Character of stool: _____ Last BM: _____
History of bleeding: _____ Hemorrhoids: _____
Constipation: _____ Diarrhea: _____
Usual voiding pattern: _____ Incontinence: _____ When: _____
    Urgency: _____ Frequency: _____ Retention: _____
Character of urine: _____
Pain/burning/difficulty voiding: _____
History of kidney/bladder disease: _____

### Exhibits (Objective)

Abdomen: Tender: _____ Soft/Firm: _____
    Palpable mass: _____ Size/girth: _____
    Bowel sounds: _____
Hemorrhoids (per rectal exam):  Internal: _____ External: _____
Bladder palpable: _____ Overflow voiding: _____

## FOOD/FLUID

### Reports (Subjective)

Usual diet (type): _____ No. meals daily: _____

Last meal/intake: _____ Dietary pattern: _____

Loss of appetite: _____ Nausea/vomiting: _____

Heartburn/indigestion: _____ Related to: _____ Relieved by: _____

Allergy/Food intolerance: _____

Mastication/swallowing problems: _____

    Dentures: Upper: _____ Lower: _____

Usual weight: _____ Changes in weight: _____

Use of diuretics: _____

### Exhibits (Objective)

Current weight: _____ Height: _____ Body build: _____

Skin turgor: _____ Mucous membranes moist/dry: _____

Hernia/masses: _____

Edema: General: _____ Dependent: _____

    Periorbital: _____ Ascites: _____

Jugular vein distention: _____

Thyroid enlarged: _____ Halitosis: _____

Condition of teeth/gums: _____

Appearance of tongue: _____

  Mucous membranes: _____

Bowel sounds (previously assessed): _____

Breath sounds (previously assessed): _____

Urine S/A or Chemstix: _____

## HYGIENE

### Reports (Subjective)

Activities of daily living: Independent: _____

    Dependent (specify): Mobility: _____ Feeding: _____

                Hygiene: _____ Dressing: _____

                 Toileting: _____ Other: _____

    Equipment/prosthetic devices required: _____

    Assistance provided by: _____

    Preferred time of bath: _____ AM _____ PM

### Exhibits (Objective)

General appearance: _____

Manner of dress: _____ Personal habits: _____

Body odor: _____ Condition of scalp: _____

Presence of vermin: _____

## NEUROSENSORY

### Reports (Subjective)

Fainting spells/dizziness: _____

Headaches: Location: _____ Frequency: _____

Tingling/Numbness/Weakness (location): _____

Stroke (residual effects): _____

Seizures: _____ Aura: _____ How controlled: _____

Eyes: Vision loss: R: _____ L: _____

    Glaucoma: _____ Cataract: _____

Ears: Hearing loss:  R: _____  L: _____

Nose:  Epistaxis: _____  Sense of smell: _____

## Exhibits (Objective)

Mental status:

    Oriented/disoriented:  Time: _____

                        Place: _____

                        Person: _____

    Alert: _____  Drowsy: _____  Lethargic: _____

    Stuporous: _____  Comatose: _____  Other: _____

    Cooperative: _____  Combative: _____  Delusions: _____

    Hallucinations: _____  Affect (describe): _____

Memory:  Recent: _____  Remote: _____

Speech pattern: _____  Content: _____

    Word choice: _____  Congruence: _____

Glasses: _____  Contacts: _____  Hearing Aids: _____

Pupil size/reaction:  R: _____  L: _____

Facial droop: _____  Swallowing: _____

Handgrip/release:  R: _____  L: _____  Posturing: _____

Deep tendon reflexes: _____  Paralysis: _____

## PAIN/COMFORT

### Reports (Subjective)

Location: _____  Intensity (1–10): _____  Frequency: _____

Quality: _____  Duration: _____  Radiation: _____

Precipitating factors: _____

How relieved: _____

### Exhibits (Objective)

Facial grimacing: _____  Guarding affected area: _____

Emotional response: _____  Narrowed focus: _____

## RESPIRATION

### Reports (Subjective)

Dyspnea (related to): _____

Cough/sputum: _____

History of Bronchitis: _____  Asthma: _____

    Tuberculosis: _____  Emphysema: _____

    Recurrent pneumonia: _____  Other: _____

    Exposure to noxious fumes: _____

Smoker: _____  Packs/day: _____  Number of years: _____

Use of respiratory aids: _____  Oxygen: _____

### Exhibits (Objective)

Respiratory:  Rate: _____  Depth: _____  Symmetry: _____

Use of accessory muscles: _____  Nasal flaring: _____

Fremitis: _____

Breath sounds: _____

Egophony: _____

Cyanosis: _____  Clubbing of fingers: _____

Sputum characteristics: _____

Mentation/restlessness: _____

Other: _____

## SAFETY

### Reports (Subjective)

Allergies/Sensitivity: _____ Reaction: _____

Previous alteration of immune system: _____ Cause: _____

History of sexually transmitted disease (date/type): _____

Blood transfusion: _____ When: _____

    Reaction (describe): _____

History of accidental injuries: _____

Fractures/dislocations: _____

Arthritis/Unstable joints: _____

Back problems: _____

Changes in moles: _____ Enlarged nodes: _____

Impaired: Vision: _____ Hearing: _____

Prosthesis: _____ Ambulatory devices: _____

Expressions of ideation of violence (self/others): _____

### Exhibits (Objective)

Temperature: _____ Diaphoresis: _____

Skin integrity: _____

    Scars: _____ Rashes: _____

    Lacerations: _____ Ulcerations: _____

    Ecchymosis: _____ Blisters: _____

    Burns (degree/percent): _____

Mark location of above on diagram:

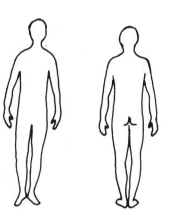

General strength: _____ Muscle tone: _____

    Gait: _____ ROM: _____

    Paresthesia/Paralysis: _____

## SEXUALITY

Sexual concerns: _____

### Female

### Reports (Subjective)

Age at menarche: _____ Length of cycle: _____ Duration: _____ _____

Last menstrual period: _____ Menopause: _____

Vaginal discharge: _____ Bleeding between periods: _____

Practices breast self-exam: _____ Last PAP smear: _____

Method of birth control: _____

**Exhibits (Objective)**

Breast exam: _____

Vaginal warts/lesions: _____

### *Male*

**Reports (Subjective)**

Penile discharge: _____ Prostate disorder: _____

Vasectomy: _____ Use of condoms: _____

Practices self-exam:  Breast: _____ Testicles: _____

Last proctoscopic exam: _____ Last prostate exam: _____

**Exhibits (Objective)**

Exam:  Breast: _____ Testicles: _____

## SOCIAL INTERACTION

**Reports (Subjective)**

Marital status: _____ Years in relationship: _____

    Living with: _____

    Concerns/Stresses: _____

Extended family: _____

Other support person(s): _____

Role within family structure: _____

Report of problems related to illness/condition: _____

Coping behaviors: _____

Do others depend on you for assistance? _____

    How are they managing? _____

Frequency of social contacts (other than work): _____

**Exhibits (Objective)**

Speech:  Clear: _____ Slurred: _____

    Unintelligible: _____ Aphasic: _____

    Unusual speech pattern/impairment: _____

    Laryngectomy: _____ Speech aids: _____

Verbal/nonverbal communication with family/SO(s): _____

_____

Family interaction (behavioral) pattern: _____

## TEACHING/LEARNING

**Reports (Subjective)**

Dominant language (specify): _____

Education level: _____

Learning disabilities (specify): _____

Cognitive limitations (specify): _____

Health beliefs/practices: _____

Special health care practices: _____

Familial risk factors (indicate relationship):

    Diabetes: _____ Tuberculosis: _____

    Heart disease: _____ Strokes: _____

    High BP: _____ Epilepsy: _____

    Kidney disease: _____ Cancer: _____

    Mental illness: _____ Other (specify): _____

Prescribed medications (circle last dose):

| Drug | Dose | Times | Takes regularly | Purpose |
|------|------|-------|-----------------|---------|
| _____ | _____ | _____ | _____ | _____ |
| _____ | _____ | _____ | _____ | _____ |
| _____ | _____ | _____ | _____ | _____ |

Nonprescription drugs: OTC: _____

    Street drugs: _____ Smokeless tobacco: _____

Use of alcohol (amount/frequency): _____

Admitting diagnosis (physician): _____

Reason for hospitalization (patient): _____

History of current complaint: _____

Patient expectations of this hospitalization: _____

Previous illnesses and/or hospitalizations/surgeries: _____

_____

Evidence of failure to improve: _____

Last complete physical exam: _____ By: _____

## Discharge Plan Considerations

Date data obtained: _____

1. Anticipated date of discharge: _____

2. Resources available: Persons: _____

    Financial: _____

3. Do you anticipate changes in your living situation after discharge? _____

4. If Yes: Areas that may require alteration/assistance:

    Food preparation: _____ Shopping: _____

    Transportation: _____ Ambulation: _____

    Medication/IV therapy: _____ Treatments: _____

    Wound care: _____ Supplies: _____

    Self-care assistance (specify): _____

    Physical layout of home (specify): _____

    Homemaker assistance (specify): _____

    Living facility other than home (specify): _____

## Additional Notes:

# INDEX

An *italic* page number indicates a figures. A "T" following a page number indicates a table.

Umbilical artery, 305
Urease, 114
Uremia, 128–129
Uremic frost, 129
Ureter, 305
Urethral orifice, 304
Urex. *See* Methenamine hippurate
Uric acid, blood. *See* Laboratory data
Uric acid stone, 113
Urinalysis, 128. *See also* Laboratory data
  in renal calculi, 121
Urinary tract
  infection of, 114, 117, 124–125
  obstruction of, 128
Urine, 111–112
  concentration of, 113, 129
  pH of, 114, 126
Urine culture. *See* Laboratory data
Urine testing, for drugs, 419, 421
Urolithiasis. *See* Renal calculi
Uterine artery, 304–305
Uterine vein, 305
Uterus, 304

Vagina, 304
Vaginal examination, 314
Valium. *See* Diazepam
Value/belief pattern
  in AIDS, 374
  in Alzheimer's disease, 10
  in breast cancer, 294
  in burn injury, 393
  in cerebrovascular accident, 78
  in chronic obstructive pulmonary disease, 154
  in chronic otitis media, 25
  in chronic renal failure, 135
  in cirrhosis of liver, 206
  in cocaine abuse, 428
  in Crohn's disease, 188
  in depression, 448
  in diabetes mellitus, 221
  in hip fracture, 272
  in hyperthyroidism, 235
  in leukemia, 331
  in lung cancer, 169
  in myocardial infarction, 57
  in organophosphate poisoning, 407
  in peripheral vascular disease, 42
  in pregnancy-induced hypertension, 312
  in renal calculi, 119
  in rheumatoid arthritis, 253–254
  in sickle cell anemia, 346
  in spinal cord injury, 96
  in systemic lupus erythematosus, 361
Valvular disease, 72
Varices, 197
Vascular lab, 223
Vasculitis, 356
Vasoconstriction, 52, 420
Vasodilation, 52
Vasospasm, 306
VDRL test, 315
  false positive, 356
Vein, 35
Ventilation, 147

  in spinal cord injury, 90
Ventilation-perfusion mismatch, 157–158
Ventilatory assistance, 158
Ventral root, 88
Ventricle, 51
Verbal communication. *See* Impaired verbal
  communication
Vertebral artery, 69, 72
Vertebral column, 86
Vertebral-basilar system, cerebrovascular accident
  involving, 73
Visceral pleura, 145
Violence. *See* Potential for violence
Vision. *See also* Cognitive/perceptual pattern
  in cirrhosis of liver, 204
  in Crohn's disease, 186
  falls and, 267
  in hyperthyroidism, 234
Visiting nurse, 424, 430
Vital signs
  in AIDS, 374
  in Alzheimer's disease, 10
  in breast cancer, 294
  in burn injury, 388, 393
  in cerebrovascular accident, 78
  in chronic obstructive pulmonary disease, 154
  in chronic otitis media, 25
  in chronic renal failure, 135
  in cirrhosis of liver, 206
  in cocaine abuse, 428
  in Crohn's disease, 188
  in diabetes mellitus, 221
  in hip fracture, 272
  in hyperthyroidism, 235
  in leukemia, 331
  in lung cancer, 170
  in myocardial infarction, 58–59
  in organophosphate poisoning, 407
  in peripheral vascular disease, 42
  in pregnancy-induced hypertension, 313
  in renal calculi, 119
  in rheumatoid arthritis, 254
  in sickle cell anemia, 346
  in spinal cord injury, 97
  in systemic lupus erythematosus, 361
Vitamin
  deficiency of, 200
  prenatal, 315–316
Vitamin A deficiency, 163
Volume overload, 129
Vulva, 304

Walker, 279
Wasting syndrome, 367
Weight control, 48–49, 64
Weight gain, 306
Weight loss, 229, 231, 233, 426, 444, 446
Wernicke's area, 71
Wheelchair, 101–102
Wheezing, 164
White blood cells, 356, 367. *See also* Laboratory data
  differential count, 324
  formation of, 324, *325*
  function of, 325–326
White matter, 86, 89